B. Martin Middleton, M.D.

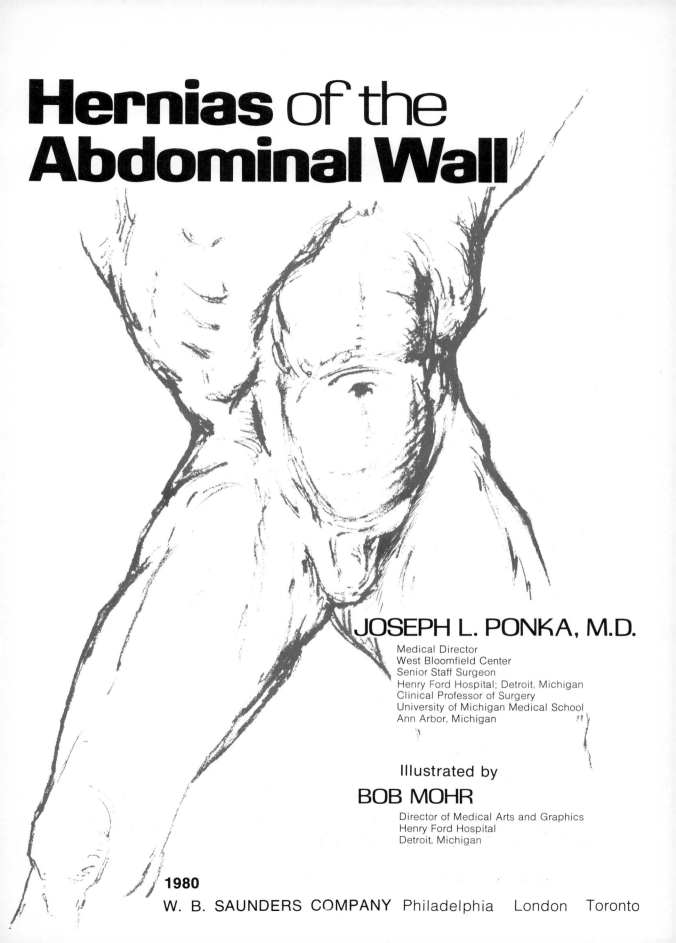

# Hernias of the Abdominal Wall

## JOSEPH L. PONKA, M.D.

Medical Director
West Bloomfield Center
Senior Staff Surgeon
Henry Ford Hospital; Detroit, Michigan
Clinical Professor of Surgery
University of Michigan Medical School
Ann Arbor, Michigan

Illustrated by

## BOB MOHR

Director of Medical Arts and Graphics
Henry Ford Hospital
Detroit, Michigan

1980

W. B. SAUNDERS COMPANY    Philadelphia    London    Toronto

W. B. Saunders Company:  West Washington Square
Philadelphia, PA  19105

1 St. Anne's Road
Eastbourne, East Sussex BN21 3UN, England

1 Goldthorne Avenue
Toronto, Ontario M8Z 5T9, Canada

**Library of Congress Cataloging in Publication Data**

Ponka, Joseph L

Hernias of the abdominal wall.

Includes index.

1. Hernia—Surgery.     2. Abdomen—Surgery.     I. Title.
   [DNLM: 1. Hernia, Ventral. WI955 P797h]

RD621.P66        617′.559′059        77–16965

ISBN 0–7216–7274–4

Hernias of the Abdominal Wall                    ISBN  0-7216-7274-4

Last digit is the print number:     9    8    7    6    5    4    3    2    1

DEDICATED TO

Claire Margaret Straub Ponka
Claire Suzette, Katherine Ann and John Ditsky
Carol Jo and David Sarkozy
Joseph L. Ponka, Jr.
Missy, Rebecca Marie, Stephen George and George Jan Ponka

Each contributed to this volume through
encouragement, patience, understanding,
and unselfishness.

And to the memory of my parents
who gave so much but received so little.

# foreword

The operative correction of hernias remains basic surgery and epitomizes all that is surgery as a profession. Uniform success—always the determined goal of surgeons—demands personal discipline, exquisite technical skill, precise and experienced judgment, extensive knowledge of recorded information, thorough appreciation of anatomy, basic comprehension of applied pathophysiology, careful preoperative management, conscientious postoperative care, and meticulous evaluation of results. Near-perfection is expected in the operative correction of hernias—a worthy standard for the evaluation of the results of all surgery.

Dr. Ponka has documented, in an atmosphere of all that is the best in our profession, the wherewithal for treating hernias. He demands the ultimate, and a lifetime at this level of conduct is obvious for each item considered in the book. Dr. Ponka repeatedly emphasizes that there is no "simple" hernia, and that each hernia must be approached as an individual problem. The unusual as well as the usual is considered. Literally hundreds of surgical residents have developed into mature surgeons as a result, in part, of the transfer of Dr. Ponka's interest in the correction of hernias to the teaching of fundamental surgery. These surgeons and this book will live as an eternally viable monument.

Although principles in the correction of the anatomic defect of an abdominal wall hernia remain constant, each patient presents a unique set of circumstances. Thus the repair of an abdominal wall hernia for each patient remains a challenge. The necessity of knowing each patient, from the newborn to the aged, as a medical whole, is evident in the material presented in Chapter Four. Unique features of groin hernias in the female—including the relatively high incidence of femoral hernias in the elderly female—are included in Chapter Seven. The famous seven steps to local anesthesia developed by Dr. Ponka are particularly important at this time of emphasis on improving operative safety and increasing the practice of ambulatory surgery. In Chapter Eighteen, the difficult and challenging sliding and recurrent hernias receive the depth of discussion that only experience can provide. A new classification of sliding hernias, based on the relationship of the viscus to the peritoneum and mesentery facilitates appropriate repair for each variety.

The use of synthetic mesh to reinforce hernia repair, particularly with the large incisional hernias, has been a landmark in surgery. Unless properly executed as described, relaxing incisions and the Hoguet maneuver can result in aggravation of the inguinal hernial defect rather than correction.

Abdominal wall hernias will always remain an important surgical problem. It may be thought that surgery has reached a level, during its past golden decade, that will not permit great advances. Yet, as this text reveals, refinements for the treatment of hernias are still to come. The "perfect" suture remains under review. Safer operations by reduction of complications must be a major goal. In sum, Dr. Ponka clearly displays the epitome of surgery for hernias of the abdominal wall as it is known today. But he indicates also the avenues for even greater achievement.

DR. MELVIN A. BLOCK
Chairman, Department of Surgery
Scripps Clinic Medical Group, Inc.
La Jolla, California
Formerly Chairman, Department of Surgery
Henry Ford Hospital; Detroit, Michigan

# preface

Progress in surgery results from the contributions of many observers. I would like to acknowledge my good fortune in having benefited from the teaching of Dr. L. S. Fallis and Dr. Henry N. Harkins. And, since circumstances dictated that I spend a great deal of time wrestling with the problem of hernia, I felt I should record my views—based on extensive experience of over 30 years—in the hope that they may prove helpful to other individuals.

In order to identify important observations and current trends, I made an extensive study of the existing literature on the subject of hernia. What emerged from my effort as being of paramount importance was the need for individualized consideration of each type of abdominal wall hernia in terms of its appearance as well as its subsequent treatment. Although this text does focus on the common varieties of hernia, various other aspects of the total problem are also discussed.

Two topics covered in depth in this text are anesthesia and recurrent hernias. The improvement, both pharmacologically and technically, of local anesthesia is a significant advance and is especially advantageous where ambulatory surgery is practiced. Recurrent hernias provide the opportunity to observe errors of diagnosis, choice of method for repair and errors of technical execution.

Wound disruption, of fundamental importance to all surgeons, is thoroughly discussed in the text, with emphasis on wound dehiscence as a factor in the genesis of incisional hernia.

A 25 year interest in prosthetics prompted my including a practical discussion of the nature and fate of prosthetic implants, in which I weigh the advantages and disadvantages and illustrate and describe the technical methods for implantation. Unusual hernias are described briefly but adequately, with appropriate illustrations, in this text. Intraoperative complications are listed in detail, and emphasis is placed on the rare encounter of intraoperative complications by the surgeon who is expert in anatomy. Postoperative complications are listed and discussed at length—the incidence of these complications is far greater in variety and degree than most surgeons realize.

The fact that enormous progress has been made in surgical treatment of hernias does not preclude the necessity of further progress. Recurrence rates can and should be reduced, as should the incidence of postoperative wound infection, and complications can be generally reduced both in number and severity.

The possibility of increased ambulatory surgical procedures will, undoubtedly, initiate in the future from improvement in postoperative management. And the causative factors associated with the aging process, in regard to connective and elastic tissues, will contribute to a better understanding of acquired hernias.

Finally, paralleling the recognition of the complexity and importance of the total hernia problem, there will be the recognition of the importance of specialization in herniology during a surgical career; this, of course, is practical in centers treating large numbers of patients.

Although this book is directed primarily at the herniologist, I believe it will also provide important surgical insights for other surgical disciplines dealing with wound disruption, use of prosthetic materials, and intraoperative and postoperative complications.

JOSEPH L. PONKA, M.D.

# acknowledgments

The elegantly drawn illustrations appearing in this book are largely the result of the dedicated work of the Director of the Department of Medical Arts and Graphics of the Henry Ford Hospital, Mr. Robert Mohr, who captured expertly the principles I wished to display.

Special recognition and gratitude is given to Ms. D. A. Newman, without whose help this volume would not have been possible. Her assistance in securing medical records and scientific articles, typing, and proofreading was invaluable. She also made worthwhile suggestions, which improved the presentation of material in several chapters; and her many hours of extra work contributed to the timely completion of this effort.

I wish to thank Mr. William Loeschel, Medical Artist, for his contributions. My appreciation is also given to those other authors and publishers who so kindly lent me their illustrations.

I would like to express my gratitude to Marie Low, former Medical Editor of the W. B. Saunders Company, for her support, confidence, and encouragement in my endeavor. Appreciation is also given to other Saunders staff members — particularly Suzanne Boyd, Associate Editor; Joanne Shore, Manuscript Editor; Peggy Klina, Illustrations Coordinator; Frank Polizzano, Production Coordinator; and Joan DeLucia, Designer — for their meticulous care in the preparation and production of the finished book.

My thanks to the Medical Records Department of the Henry Ford Hospital for providing records for my research. I especially wish to thank Walter Venditelli, Manager; Yvonne Tackett, Assistant Director, OPD Section; Lily Patchak, Supervisor, and Julie Quandah, Medical Records Clerk. In addition, I would like to thank the Medical Librarians and Assistants at the Henry Ford Hospital for their help — and, particularly, Joyce Malin, Former Director; Susan Allen, Assistant Librarian; and Henrietta Koly and Annette Donar, Library Assistants. Also, my thanks to Helen Kaisels of the Henry Ford Hospital mailroom for her careful handling of the numerous items that required delivery to Philadelphia.

The support and encouragement of the West Bloomfield Center staff were refreshing. The help of Mr. Alan Case, Mr. Robert Scavone, and Ms. Linda Messina was invaluable.

# contents

Chapter 1

SIGNIFICANT CONTRIBUTIONS TOWARD UNDER-
STANDING AND SOUND TREATMENT OF HERNIAS................. 1

Introduction .................................................................. 1
Contributions Toward Understanding the Pathology
of Hernia .................................................................... 2
Contributions Toward Understanding the Anatomy
of Hernia .................................................................... 4
Adjuncts to Hernia Repair........................................... 7
Important Technical Contributions in the
Resolution of the Hernia Problem.............................. 10


Chapter 2

ANATOMY ...................................................................... 18

General Considerations ............................................... 18
Muscles of the Anterolateral Abdominal Wall........... 20
Hesselbach's Triangle .................................................. 27
Inguinal Canal and Spermatic Cord .......................... 27
Inguinofemoral Region................................................ 30
Inguinal Region........................................................... 35
Pelvic Peritoneal Fossae.............................................. 37


Chapter 3

DIAGNOSIS OF HERNIA ............................................... 40

Principal Etiologic Factors.......................................... 41
The History.................................................................. 43
Physical Examination ................................................. 44
Hernias in Infants....................................................... 47
Diagnosis of Sliding Hernias...................................... 48
Differential Diagnosis of Hernia................................ 49


Chapter 4

PREOPERATIVE EVALUATION...................................... 53

Introductory Comments............................................... 53
Clinical Appraisal of the Patient................................ 54
History ......................................................................... 55

Physical Examination ......................................................... 56
Clinical Studies for Further Assessment ................................... 58

Chapter 5

X-RAY STUDIES IN PATIENTS WITH HERNIA .......................... 64

Flat Films of the Abdomen ................................................. 65
Barium Enema Examination of the Colon ............................... 68
Upper Gastrointestinal and Small Bowel Series........................ 70
Intravenous Pyelograms..................................................... 70
Cystograms .................................................................... 70
Herniography and Peritoneography........................................ 71

Chapter 6

PREMEDICATION, PREOPERATIVE ORDERS, AND
PREOPERATIVE PREPARATION FOR ANESTHESIA .................... 76

Considerations Before Surgery and Anesthesia........................ 76
Ambulatory Surgery ......................................................... 79

Chapter 7

THE HERNIA PROBLEM IN THE FEMALE .............................. 82

Introduction ................................................................... 82
Anatomic Considerations ................................................... 82
Incidence....................................................................... 83
Statistical Analysis .......................................................... 84
Direct Inguinal Hernias in Females....................................... 86
Combinations of Direct, Indirect, and Femoral Hernias ............. 87
Incisional Hernias............................................................ 88
Umbilical Hernias............................................................ 88
Epigastric Hernias ........................................................... 89
Esophageal Hiatal Hernia................................................... 89
Summary ....................................................................... 89

Chapter 8

LOCAL ANESTHESIA FOR ABDOMINAL WALL HERNIAS.......... 91

Introduction ................................................................... 91
Historical Background ....................................................... 91
Practical Anatomy for Local Anesthesia ................................. 93
Armamentarium............................................................... 97
Pharmacologic Considerations............................................. 100
Reactions Attributed to Local Anesthesia................................ 104
Management of Reactions .................................................. 104
Advantages and Disadvantages of Local Anesthesia ................... 105

Chapter 9

SEVEN STEPS TO LOCAL ANESTHESIA FOR INGUINAL
AND FEMORAL HERNIA REPAIR ....................................... 108

Introduction ................................................................... 108
Step One ....................................................................... 108

Step Two ................................................................ 108
Step Three .............................................................. 111
Step Four ............................................................... 111
Step Five ............................................................... 111
Step Six ................................................................ 111
Step Seven ............................................................. 111


Chapter 10
CONGENITAL INDIRECT INGUINAL HERNIA AND
RELATED ABNORMALITIES ........................................ 118
   Introduction ........................................................ 118
   Related Abnormalities ............................................. 119
   Embryology ......................................................... 122
   Direct Inguinal Hernia in Infants and Children ................ 128
   Femoral Hernias in·Infants and Children ....................... 128
   Historical Notes on Repair of Congenital Indirect
   Inguinal Hernias .................................................. 129
   Summary ............................................................ 131
   Principles of Management ......................................... 132
   The Question of Contralateral Repair ........................... 135
   Fundamental Principles in Orchidopexy ......................... 142
   Clinical Study ..................................................... 146
   Complications ...................................................... 151
   Summary ............................................................ 152


Chapter 11
INDIRECT INGUINAL HERNIA ..................................... 155
   Introduction ........................................................ 155
   History ............................................................. 155
   Obsolete, Obsolescent, and Current Techniques in
   Hernia Repair ..................................................... 158
   Technique for Repair of Indirect Inguinal Hernias
   in Adults ........................................................... 159
   Technique of Closure of Subcutaneous Tissue and Skin ......... 165
   Comment on the Technique of Repair of Indirect Inguinal
   Hernias ............................................................. 168
   Clinical Study ..................................................... 168
   Summary ............................................................ 175


Chapter 12
RECURRENT INDIRECT INGUINAL HERNIA ....................... 176
   Introduction ........................................................ 176
   Statistics and Recurrent Hernias ................................ 176
   The Enigma of the Recurrent Inguinal Hernia .................. 179
   Clinical Study ..................................................... 187
   Recommended Principles for Repair of Recurrent
   Indirect Inguinal Hernias ......................................... 189
   Summary ............................................................ 193

Chapter 13
DIRECT INGUINAL HERNIA..................................................... 196
   Introduction ..................................................................... 196
   Historical Background ..................................................... 196
   Clinical Pathologic Correlation and Considerations ............ 196
   Anatomic Considerations ................................................. 197
   Sites of Protrusion........................................................... 198
   Techniques Available for Repair....................................... 198
   Technical Details of Repair of Direct Inguinal Hernias......... 204
   Clinical Study ................................................................. 209
   Summary ....................................................................... 213


Chapter 14
RECURRENT DIRECT INGUINAL HERNIAS............................. 216
   Introduction ..................................................................... 216
   Historical Background ..................................................... 216
   Incidence of Recurrent Direct Inguinal Hernias.................. 218
   The Impact of Experience on Surgical Treatment
   of Hernias........................................................................ 221
   Causes for Failure—92 Patients with Recurrent
   Direct Inguinal Hernias..................................................... 225
   Technical Errors and Poor Choice of Technique—
   Case in Point................................................................... 226
   Recurrent Direct Inguinal Hernia—Complicated Clinical
   Course; Need for Synthetic Mesh: Case in Point................. 227
   Repair of Recurrent Direct Inguinal Hernia........................ 228
   Clinical Study ................................................................. 232
   Summary ....................................................................... 235


Chapter 15
FEMORAL HERNIA............................................................... 238
   Definition ....................................................................... 238
   Anatomy ........................................................................ 238
   Etiologic Factors.............................................................. 240
   Historical Considerations.................................................. 241
   Operative Treatment—Techniques of Repair ..................... 243
   Technique of the Lotheissen-McVay Repair........................ 244
   Upper Approach—Moschcowitz Repair ............................. 245
   Lower Approach—The Bassini Repair................................ 247
   Technique of Bassini-Kirschner Repair of Femoral Hernia .......... 247
   Abdominal or Posterior Approach ..................................... 249
   Technique of Repair of Femoral Hernia Through the
   Posterior Approach........................................................... 249
   Clinical Study of Femoral Hernias..................................... 252
   Summary ....................................................................... 262


Chapter 16
RECURRENT FEMORAL HERNIAS........................................... 264
   Femoral Hernia After Repair of Inguinal Hernia ................. 264
   Etiology of Recurrent Femoral Hernias: General Discussion ....... 265

Etiology of Recurrent Femoral Hernia (The Overlooked
Femoral Hernia) ............................................................. 266
Etiologic Factors in Recurrent Femoral Hernias ............... 267
Recurrent Femoral Hernia—Clinical Study ...................... 269
Summary ........................................................................ 273


Chapter 17

COMBINED DIRECT-INDIRECT AND FEMORAL HERNIAS;
RECURRENT MULTILOCULAR INGUINAL HERNIAS ................. 275
Introduction ................................................................... 275
Incidence of Combined Direct-Indirect and Femoral Hernias ...... 276
Technique for Repair of Combination Recurrent
Direct-Indirect Inguinal Hernias ..................................... 278
Direct-Indirect-Femoral Hernias—Clinical Study .............. 279
Recurrent Direct-Indirect and Femoral Hernias ............... 284
Summary ........................................................................ 288


Chapter 18

SLIDING INGUINAL AND FEMORAL HERNIAS ......................... 289
Definition ....................................................................... 289
Historical Considerations ................................................. 289
A New Classification of Sliding Hernias ........................... 294
Developmental and Anatomic Considerations ................... 297
The Inguinal Approach for the Repair of Sliding Hernias ...... 301
Repair of Sigmoid Sliding Hernias ................................... 307
Report on 350 Sliding Inguinal Hernias: A Summary .......... 312


Chapter 19

RECURRENT INGUINOFEMORAL HERNIA ............................... 319
Description ..................................................................... 319
Historical Background ..................................................... 320
Clinical Features of Recurrent Inguinofemoral Hernia ....... 321
General Principles of Repair ............................................ 322
Case Histories of Recurrent Inguinofemoral Hernia .......... 326
Results .......................................................................... 328
Summary ........................................................................ 329


Chapter 20

WOUND DISRUPTION ......................................................... 330
Definition and Description .............................................. 330
Incidence of Wound Disruption ....................................... 331
Clinical Conditions Seen in Patients with Postoperative
Wound Disruptions ......................................................... 332
Wound Healing and Wound Disruption ............................. 338
Nutritional and Chemical Factors in Wound Healing ......... 340
Suture Materials and Suture Technique ............................ 343
Fundamental Principles of Operative Technique ................ 349
Abdominal Incisions ....................................................... 352
Closure of Abdominal Wounds ........................................ 355

Clinical Study ........................................................ 358
Summary ............................................................. 365


Chapter 21
INCISIONAL HERNIAS ........................................... 369
Introduction ........................................................ 369
Historical Summary................................................ 369
Incidence of Incisional Hernias.................................. 371
Definition ........................................................... 372
Clinical Study ...................................................... 372
Factors in Preventing Recurrence of Incisional Hernias .............. 394


Chapter 22
UMBILICAL HERNIA IN INFANTS AND ADULTS
AND OMPHALOCELES ........................................... 397
Introduction ........................................................ 397
History .............................................................. 398
Natural History..................................................... 399
Clinical Study of Umbilical Hernia in Infants and
Children ............................................................ 402
Umbilical Hernia in Adults........................................ 408
OMPHALOCELE........................................................ 417
Historical Background ............................................. 417
Embryologic Considerations of Umbilical Defects ...................... 418
Management of Omphaloceles...................................... 423
Summary ............................................................. 432


Chapter 23
EPIGASTRIC HERNIA............................................. 435
Definition ........................................................... 435
Historical Background ............................................. 435
Anatomic Considerations .......................................... 438
The Pathologic Anatomy and the Clinical Picture....................... 439
Clinical Characteristics of Epigastric Hernias........................... 441
An Approach to Repair of Epigastric Hernias ........................... 447
Summary ............................................................. 453


Chapter 24
UNUSUAL HERNIAS ............................................. 455
RICHTER'S HERNIA .................................................. 456
Incidence............................................................ 457
Anatomic Sites of Richter's Hernias .................................... 457
Definition ........................................................... 459
Historical Background ............................................. 459
Pathogenesis ....................................................... 460
Clinical and Pathologic Correlation................................ 461
Case Reports ....................................................... 462
Operative Treatment ............................................... 463
Mortality............................................................ 464
Summary ............................................................. 464

LUMBAR HERNIAS........................................................................... 465
    Definition ................................................................................ 465
    Historical Background ............................................................. 465
    Anatomic Considerations ........................................................ 466
    Classification of Lumbar Hernias ........................................... 469
    Symptoms and Signs ............................................................... 470
    Differential Diagnosis of Lumbar Hernia................................ 470
    Treatment ................................................................................ 471
    Clinical Case............................................................................ 475
    Summary .................................................................................. 477
SPIGELIAN HERNIAS...................................................................... 478
    Definition ................................................................................ 478
    Historical Background ............................................................. 479
    Incidence.................................................................................. 479
    Anatomic Considerations ........................................................ 479
    Etiologic Factors...................................................................... 481
    Clinical Features ..................................................................... 481
    Differential Diagnosis ............................................................. 482
    Treatment ................................................................................ 483
    Clinical Experience ................................................................. 483
    Summary .................................................................................. 485
SUPRAVESICAL HERNIAS............................................................... 486
    Definition of Terms................................................................. 487
    Historical Background ............................................................. 487
    Anatomy ................................................................................... 488
    Pathology.................................................................................. 489
    Clinical Features ..................................................................... 489
    Treatment ................................................................................ 490
    Summary .................................................................................. 491
INTERPARIETAL HERNIAS ............................................................. 491
    Introduction ............................................................................ 491
    Definition ................................................................................ 492
    Historical Background ............................................................. 492
    Various Types of Interparietal Hernias.................................. 492
    Preperitoneal Hernia............................................................... 492
    Interstitial Hernia ................................................................... 494
    Extra-Aponeurotic Hernia ...................................................... 494
    Clinical Features ..................................................................... 494
    Treatment ................................................................................ 495
    Summary .................................................................................. 495
REDUCTION OF HERNIA "EN MASSE" ........................................... 496
    Definition ................................................................................ 496
    Historical Background ............................................................. 496
    Incidence.................................................................................. 497
    Pathology.................................................................................. 497
    Clinical Features ..................................................................... 497
    X-Ray Examination ................................................................. 498
    Treatment ................................................................................ 499
    Mortality................................................................................... 499
    Summary .................................................................................. 499
LITTRE'S HERNIA .......................................................................... 500
    Definition ................................................................................ 500
    Historical Background ............................................................. 500

Incidence.............................................................. 501
Anatomic and Pathologic Features ......................... 502
Treatment........................................................... 503
Summary ............................................................ 503
GASTROSCHISIS ......................................................... 504
Definition ........................................................... 505
Historical Background .......................................... 505
Embryology ........................................................ 507
Clinical Features ................................................. 509
Associated Anomalies in Gastroschisis.................... 509
Treatment........................................................... 510
Immediate Nonoperative Treatment....................... 510
Surgical Repair ................................................... 510
Mortality............................................................ 512
Summary ............................................................ 512
HERNIORRHAPHY AND APPENDECTOMY......................... 514
Historical Background .......................................... 515
Hernias Containing the Appendix – Clinical Features ... 516
Clinical Study ..................................................... 518
Summary ............................................................ 520
INGUINAL HERNIA AND CARCINOMA ........................... 522
Introduction ........................................................ 522
Historical Background .......................................... 522
Discussion .......................................................... 523
Conclusion.......................................................... 524


Chapter 25

THE RELAXING INCISION........................................... 525
Historical Background .......................................... 525
Anatomy of the Relaxing Incision .......................... 530
Technique of Performing the Relaxing Incision......... 532
Advantages of the Relaxing Incision....................... 532
Summary ............................................................ 533


Chapter 26

PROSTHETICS IN HERNIA REPAIR............................... 534
Introduction ........................................................ 534
Classification of Reinforcing Materials for Use in
Hernia Repair...................................................... 537
Autografts .......................................................... 538
Homografts ......................................................... 541
Heterografts ........................................................ 541
Metallic Prostheses .............................................. 542
Synthetic Plastic Materials.................................... 544
Summary ............................................................ 547
Clinical Study ..................................................... 547
Repair of Incisional Hernias in 266 Patients in Whom
Prosthetic Implants were Used............................... 553
Repair of Inguinal and Femoral Hernias with Implants –
Clinical Experience ............................................. 563

Prosthetic Material Used for Groin Hernias ............................ 566
Indications for Implantation of Prosthetic Materials in
Repair of Recurrent Inguinal and Femoral Hernias.................... 567
Aphorisms Applicable to Prosthetic Implants ........................... 568
Summary ................................................................. 569


Chapter 27
INTRAOPERATIVE COMPLICATIONS DURING HERNIA
REPAIR........................................................................ 573
Introduction ........................................................... 573
Intraoperative Deaths................................................. 575
Hemorrhage ............................................................ 575
Bleeding from the Pampiniform Plexus ................................ 576
Vascular Injuries..................................................... 576
Injury to the Femoral Vein .......................................... 578
Accessory Obturator Artery .......................................... 578
Injury to the Testicular Blood Supply ............................... 579
Injury to the Bladder................................................ 580
Injury to the Bowel.................................................. 581
Injury to the Ilioinguinal, Iliohypogastric, and
Lateral Femoral Cutaneous Nerves.................................... 583
Injuries to the Vas Deferens......................................... 583
Injury to Fallopian Tubes and Ovaries ............................... 584
Summary ............................................................... 585


Chapter 28
EARLY AND LATE POSTOPERATIVE COMPLICATIONS
AND THEIR MANAGEMENT ....................................................... 587
Postoperative Fatalities ............................................. 587
Early Wound Complications............................................ 592
Late Wound Complications ............................................ 600
Evaluation ........................................................... 614
Summary ............................................................... 617


Chapter 29
CONCLUDING REMARKS ........................................................ 619
Anatomy ............................................................... 619
Pathology............................................................. 620
Anesthesiology ....................................................... 620
Bacteriology.......................................................... 621
Technology............................................................ 621
On the Teaching of Surgery of Hernia................................. 623
Biochemistry of Hernia............................................... 624
Comment .............................................................. 625


INDEX......................................................................... 629

# 1

# Significant Contributions Toward Understanding and Sound Treatment of Hernias

## INTRODUCTION

In retrospect, it is obvious that success in the treatment of hernias was not to be expected until certain fundamental requirements were met. First of all, the pathologic anatomy had to be clearly understood; second, the normal anatomy of the abdominal wall needed definition; third, the proposed operative procedures had to be carried out safely without pain; fourth, the hazard of infection had to be eliminated; and fifth, the sound technical methods for correction of those defects had to be developed. Early anatomists and surgeons were obviously hampered by incorrect ideas regarding the anatomy and pathology of hernia. Superstitions, inaccurate observations, and erroneous opinions took precedence over scientific facts. Objective evaluation of method and its immediate and long-term results was wanting. It is not difficult to understand why progress toward solving the hernia problem was slow. It is true, however, that significant advances in knowledge were added from time to time. Periodically, observations and discoveries of monumental importance were made in the understanding and sound treatment of hernias.

In order to visualize the interrelationship of the various factors that bear upon the hernia problem, I arrived at the politically inopportune symbol of the pentagon (Fig. 1–1); as you can see, the five components blend almost imperceptibly, one into the other, and it is only when each component is considered in relation to the other that we are able to comprehend the problem facing our surgical ancestors.

I would like to add two other factors that contributed indirectly to progress in this field: the invention of firearms in the fourteenth century and the printing press in the fifteenth century. The explosive effects of gunpowder on the human body forced military surgeons to view and study the results of such explosions. The printing press, disseminating accurate and inaccurate information, made possible the evaluation and re-evaluation of information, and truth emerged, if slowly.

Early treatment of hernia was inevitably poor at best and frequently barbaric. Iason has recorded these early surgical efforts and misadventures in an informative and entertaining manner. His summary of the treatment of hernia up to the mid-nineteenth century is quoted directly:

Surgeons carried out surgical methods, orthodox and heterodox; they hacked, hewed and slashed; they incised, cauterized, and scarified; they castrated young and old; they destroyed or saved the spermatic vessels; they dilated or cut the inguinal rings; they stood their victims on their heads; they bled and re-bled them unmercifully; they applied hot and cold poultices;

1

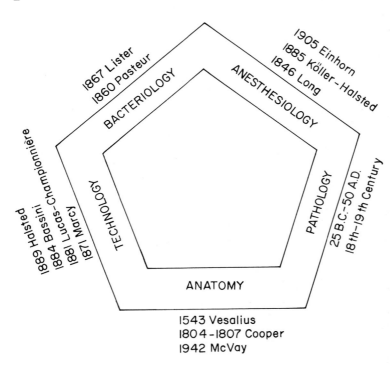

**Figure 1–1.** The pentagon offers a practical and visual relationship of the five important disciplines that have contributed toward resolution of the hernia problem.

they tortured with tobacco enemas and drastic purges; they drugged well nigh unto death; they resorted to tricks of surgical legerdemain; they tried manual manipulations; they placed iron filings on hernial tumors, hoping by magnetic action to replace them and passed patients through cleft trees with the same object in view. They used screws, pins, needles, wires — of gold, tin, lead, bronze, copper, iron — wooden spikes, ivory, testicles, animal skins, dilators, acupuncture, organic and inorganic substances (usually sutures), scalpels, scissors, salt, iodine, air, water, alcohol and acids — caustic and otherwise. Prehistoric methods solely? Roman, Greek or Byzantine? Dark or Middle Ages? Renaissance? No. Methods in vogue down to the mid-nineteenth century!

We will consider progress made toward the solution of the hernia problem from the following five aspects: *(1) Pathology, (2) Anatomy, (3) Anesthesia, (4) Asepsis and Antisepsis, and (5) Technology.* It has been through the combined progress in these interrelated areas that the hernia problem is approaching resolution. Until substantial advances were made in each of the five areas, progress could not be expected in the operative treatment of hernia. While it is not possible to include all the contributions made by different individuals, a real

effort has been made to recognize those advances that have gradually aided in understanding the hernia problem.

This chapter presents, in an unconventional manner, important contributions and observations toward the solution of the hernia problem. The important fact or observation will be recorded first, then the contributors will be identified, and a brief comment will follow. The references listed in the bibliography have been drawn upon selectively to provide many of the ideas presented in this chapter. It is most difficult to assign credit to certain individuals for new ideas without causing justifiable debate. Nevertheless, the ideas expressed here can be reasonably supported by history.

## CONTRIBUTIONS TOWARD UNDERSTANDING THE PATHOLOGY OF HERNIA

For many centuries in various countries, a hernia was directly and erroneously related to the presence of the testicle. The wanton sacrifice of the testicle, although greatly diminished, still creeps into surgical literature even today. It should be recalled that, for centuries, dissections of the human body were forbidden. Surgeons could only gain information from individuals with hernias; hence, it was logical for them to conclude that the tunica vaginalis was normally patent.

## A Description of the Hernial Sac and Its Contents

Celsus (25 B.C.–A.D. 50), in the first century B.C., was said to have described the contents of the hernial sac and to have recognized hydroceles. A description of the sac and its contents was recorded by him. He preserved the cord and testicles in his operations. However, at this stage of development in anatomic knowledge, the exact relationship between the scrotum and the peritoneal cavity was still not clearly established.

In the seventh century, Paul of Aegina (A.D. 625–690) described hernias and their contents in some detail. He called a complete, or scrotal, hernia an enterocele if it contained intestine, an epiplocele if it contained omentum, an enteroepiplocele if it contained bowel and omentum, and a hydroenteroepiplocele if bowel, omentum, and fluid were all present. He erroneously believed that the testicle was a cause of herniation.

In the first century B.C. in his *Description of Umbilical Hernia,* Celsus called it "an indecent prominence of the navel." *Exomphalos* was described by Paul of Aegina in the seventh century A.D.

PROOF THAT IN HERNIA THERE WAS NO ACTUAL RUPTURE OF THE PERITONEUM came slowly. Paul of Aegina, whose contributions were made in the seventh century, was of the opinion that ordinary hernias were due to a gradual stretching of the peritoneum. This contrasted with the belief commonly held for many centuries that the peritoneum suddenly ruptured, resulting in hernia formation. Guy de Chauliac in 1363 also agreed with the idea that there was no actual peritoneal rupture in hernia. Nevertheless, the question of peritoneal rupture was not completely settled. In his work, *Seats and Causes of Diseases,* Morgagni reviews the differences of opinion held in 1760, and it was not until the end of the seventeenth century that Ruysch finally

proved that rupture of the peritoneum did not take place in hernia formation. *Petit,* in the seventeenth century, recognized the pathologic anatomic changes resulting from large, irreducible hernias, which he stated "had lost their right of domicile."

RECOGNITION OF FEMORAL HERNIA was made by Guy de Chauliac in his *Chirurgia magna* in 1363. Sir Astley Cooper discussed the femoral hernia in his second volume on the subject of hernia, published in 1807. The term "crural hernia" was in use at that time. Scarpa also recognized the nature of femoral hernia in 1814.

DIFFERENTIATION OF DIRECT, INDIRECT, AND FEMORAL HERNIAS is attributed to Caspar Stromayr in 1559. His *Practica Copiosa* must be one of the most interesting and entertaining volumes in surgical literature. Walter von Brunn rescued this volume from oblivion after it had lain dormant for 350 years, according to Zimmerman and Veith.

AN EARLY DESCRIPTION OF DIRECT INGUINAL HERNIA is attributed to Heister in 1724. Seventy-five years passed before this important observation was appreciated. However, many more years passed before the full importance of differentiation between direct and indirect inguinal hernias was generally understood.

SLIDING INGUINAL HERNIAS were described in some detail by Antonio Scarpa (1747–1832). In his *Treatise on Hernia* in 1814, he described this entity as hernia of the large bowel. Furthermore, he differentiated between inguinal and femoral hernias and was the first to describe *perineal hernia.* Morgagni, too, noted that some hernias contained the appendix, cecum, and colon. He observed that the left side was more commonly involved in sliding hernias.

CONGENITAL HERNIA was recognized by Percival Pott in 1856. William and John Hunter, famous brothers feuding over priorities, also described congenital hernias independently. John Hunter studied the embryology of congenital hernias in detail.

RICHTER'S HERNIA was recognized as an entity by Richter in 1799. In a classic contribution, he described a hernia in which a portion of the intestinal wall was found to be incarcerated in a femoral hernia. Levater also described a similar type of hernia. Even today, 179 years later, physicians and surgeons regularly fail to recognize this interesting and life-threatening entity.

**PRESENCE OF MECKEL'S DIVERTICULUM IN A HERNIAL SAC** was recognized by Alexis Littré in 1770 when he described two such cases. Much later, in 1809, this outpouching of the ileum was to be known as Meckel's diverticulum, after the man who described it in detail.

**DESCRIPTIONS OF DIAPHRAGMATIC HERNIA** were published by Paré in 1579 and by Morgagni in 1761. Morgagni described different types of diaphragmatic hernias, and Cooper also recognized such hernias.

**EARLY RECOGNITION OF LUMBAR HERNIA** was reported by de Garengot in 1731.

**OBTURATOR HERNIA** was first described by *Ronsil* in 1724, when he reported two cases.

From this brief historical consideration, it can be seen that, even with the restrictions imposed by superstitious and religious beliefs, the nature and types of hernias were well recognized by approximately A.D. 1750. Over 100 years would pass before surgeons could treat those defects without pain or danger of infection.

## CONTRIBUTIONS TOWARD UNDERSTANDING THE ANATOMY OF HERNIA

At the time of the Greek civilization, which some observers date to 3400 B.C., Greek physicians learned from the same anatomic material that was available to sculptors. The nude body was portrayed in athletic contests, wrestling, jumping, and running. Again, it was the external appearance that was beautifully presented. By 300 B.C., anatomy was taught by Aristotle, who used animals in dissection. Galen (A.D. 131–201) gained his anatomic knowledge from dissection of apes and swine.

Guy de Chauliac (1300–1370) was an early advocate of the study of human anatomy. Up until approximately A.D. 1240, human dissection was rigorously interdicted by law and sentiment. Dissections upon monkeys centuries before had added chaos to confusion. Centers for human dissection were developed at Bologna (A.D. 1302), Venice (A.D. 1368), Florence (A.D. 1388), Vienna (A.D. 1405), Paris (A.D. 1478), and Padua (A.D. 1445). The opportunity for human dissection resulted in rapid increments in the knowledge of human anatomy, and more progress was made in the next five centuries than in the preceding five millennia. The study of human anatomy became a science under the pioneering and lasting efforts of Andreas Vesalius, who was Flemish born, but of German extraction. His works entitled *The Composition or Fabric of the Human Body (De Humani Corporis Fabrica)* appeared in A.D. 1543. The printing press (early fifteenth century) made widescale dissemination of knowledge feasible.

Knowledge of the normal anatomy of the abdominal wall is an absolute necessity if the surgeon is to repair hernias successfully. It is my impression that anatomy is currently not taught with the same enthusiasm that it was in the past.

It is interesting to review just how anatomic knowledge was gained and who made the early important contributions. Basic anatomic knowledge had already been gained well before wound infections could be controlled. Anesthesia was not yet available. Sir Astley Cooper (1768–1841) was a genius who provided many of the pieces of the anatomic puzzle of hernia in 1804 and 1807 (Fig. 1–2). Unfortunately, use of his basic knowledge had to await the development of asepsis and anesthesia.

Cooper had studied the problem of hernia and the anatomy involved more thoroughly than any single contributor. He published his well-illustrated works in two volumes, *The Anatomy and Surgical Treatment of Abdominal Hernia,* which appeared in 1804 and 1807. Every surgeon interested in the subject of hernia should inspect and study these remarkable volumes. Cooper described the following:

1. The internal abdominal ring. He made the important observation that the external ring was not situated directly over the internal abdominal ring.
2. The inguinal canal. He noted the important fact that the spermatic cord

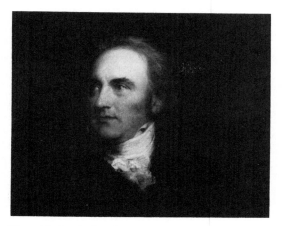

Figure 1–2.  Astley Cooper (1768–1841)

His anatomic studies of the abdominal wall and inguinal areas in 1804 and 1807 were detailed and remarkably accurate; however, lack of anesthesia and inability to control infection prevented immediate application of his knowledge of anatomy in the treatment of hernia. (By permission of the President and Council of the Royal College of Surgeons of England.)

followed an oblique course in the canal.

3. The transversalis fascia.
4. The formation of the femoral sheath from the transversalis.
5. The ligament which is appropriately known as Cooper's ligament.
6. The formation of hernias from a defect at the internal ring, rather than at the external ring.

**A Description of the Lacunar Ligament** was made in 1793 by Don Antonio de Gimbernat (1734–1816). He pointed out that the femoral ring could be enlarged medially, if necessary, without injury to the femoral vessels. Lytle has more recently provided surgeons with a detailed description and excellent illustration of the lacunar ligament in his work on femoral hernias.

**A Description of the Ligament of Cooper** was made by Sir Astley Cooper in 1804, but he never used this structure in hernia repair. Ruggi and Lotheissen recognized the usefulness of the iliopectineal ligament in repair of hernias.

**Recognition That Certain Hernias Developed from a Defect at the Internal Ring** is attributed to Sir Astley Cooper. His description of the course of an indirect inguinal hernia can hardly be improved upon. Hesselbach described the internal abdominal ring in 1814.

**The Importance of the Transversalis Fascia** was also appreciated by Cooper, who described its anatomy with remarkable thoroughness in 1807. It must be noted, however, that full recognition of the great importance of the transversalis fascia in the genesis and surgical correction of hernias is a recent development. Anson, McVay, Nyhus, and Condon have worked diligently to put the transversus abdominus lamina in proper perspective.

**The Iliopubic Tract,** a derivative of the transversalis fascia, was recognized and described by Hesselbach in 1814, but Cooper was aware of this structure as well; it was also described by Thomson, an Englishman who studied anatomy in Paris. It has been designated as Thomson's ligament and is known in the French literature as *bandelette iliopubienne.* Interest in the iliopubic tract has been stimulated through the popularity of the preperitoneal approach for hernia repair, as advocated by Nyhus and Condon.

**A Description of the Inguinal Canal** was also made by Cooper, who noted the structures of the cord as they appeared at the internal ring. He observed that the cord had an exit through the external ring and described the anterior wall as being made up of external oblique aponeurosis. He referred to the inguinal ligament as Poupart's ligament but was aware that Fallopius had described it earlier. He knew that the transversalis fascia and transversus abdominis contributed to the strength of the posterior abdominal wall, and he described the posterior wall with remarkable accuracy.

**A Description of the Femoral Sheath** was available in 1804 through the studies of Cooper. He was aware the transversalis fascia provided the anterior layer of the femoral sheath and that the pubic ramus and iliopectineal ligament formed a boundary posteriorly. He believed that the lacunar ligament formed the medial boundary, while the lateral limits were made up of connective tissue. In Cooper's publication, the femoral vessels were designated as being the crural vessels. The excellent studies of Lytle in 1957 have provided newer detailed anatomic knowledge of the femoral sheath.

**A Description of Hesselbach's Triangle** became available through the studies of Franz Kaspar Hesselbach (1759–1816). An accurate description of this triangular area in 1814 led to a better understanding of the groin area. If inguinal hernias were to be correctly repaired, the route of egress of the direct and indirect inguinal hernia through the abdominal wall required clarification; this contribution by Hesselbach was, and continues to be, of great value to students who wish to learn the anatomy of the inguinal area. The inguinal ligament, the margin of the rectus sheath, and the deep inferior epigastric artery are structures readily identifiable as important landmarks in the lower abdomen. The anatomic illustrations accompanying Hesselbach's work are remarkably clear. Furthermore, he provided illustrations depicting various types of groin hernias. He also appreciated the structure that we recognize as the internal abdominal ring.

A DESCRIPTION OF POUPART'S LIGAMENT was recorded in Paris by François Poupart in his *Historie de Academie Royal des Sciences*, in 1705. Poupart (1661–1709) was a surgeon at *l'Hotel Dieu* and a scientist of some stature. He was interested in geometry and architecture and studied the lives and habits of insects.

Poupart described the location of this ligament with reasonable accuracy at a time when other anatomists ignored it; he even suggested that this structure might be a factor in the prevention of hernias. He recognized that the three big muscles of the abdomen, *l'oblique externe, l'oblique interne*, and the *transverse*, all had a relationship to this ligament.

DETAILS OF THE ANATOMY OF THE ABDOMINAL WALL were worked out over many years. Bidloo in 1685 described the layers of the abdominal wall in general terms. His work was plagiarized by Cowper and Albinus. The printing press made this act possible. Vesling in 1677 provided an early description of the layers of the abdominal wall. Scarpa in 1809 recognized the structure we call aponeurosis, and he quite possibly recognized fascial membranes. He described the inguinal canal and the linea semicircularis. Hesselbach in 1814 described in moderate detail the external oblique aponeurosis, the transversus abdominis muscle, and

fascia. Gerrish in 1899 noted that the transversalis fascia passes posterior to the rectus muscle inferior to the linea semicircularis of Douglas.

THE SIGNIFICANCE OF THE LUMBAR TRIANGLE was recognized by Jean-Louis Petit (1674–1750), who described its boundaries as the iliac crest, the latissimus dorsi, and the external oblique muscles.

THE CONJOINED TENDON remains a controversial structure among some surgeons. Others have abandoned the concept, since it exists in reality in less than 5 per cent of anatomic specimens studied. Morton is given credit for describing this structure in 1841. The transversus abdominis and internal oblique muscles are made up of connective tissue fibers where they approach the rectus sheath and the pubis. It is difficult to describe the structure as "tendinous," since it is generally aponeurotic in nature. Condon, in the book on hernia by Nyhus and Harkins, uses the designation of transversus abdominis muscle aponeurosis to represent the same structure. He stated that in a few cases the lowermost fibers of the transversus abdominis turn downward to insert into the superior pubic ramus, lateral to the rectus abdominis. When this attachment is quite dense in its relationship to the rectus tendon, it is designated as the falx inguinalis, or conjoined tendon. Generally speaking, the structure is derived from the transversus abdominis. Infrequently, the internal oblique contributes aponeurotic fibers as well. In such instances, a conjoined tendon would be the result. It is the transversus abdominis aponeurosis that the surgeon frequently employs in the repair of groin hernias.

AN ACCURATE DESCRIPTION OF THE RELATIONSHIP OF THE TRANSVERSALIS FASCIA TO THE INGUINAL LIGAMENT was provided by McVay in 1942. He emphasized that the inguinal ligament was neither the site of the origin nor the area of insertion for the transversus abdominis and internal oblique muscles; the relationship is a matter of contiguity. McVay (Fig. 1–3) has made contributions of enduring importance to those individuals who repair groin hernias. Together with Anson, he has provided newer anatomic knowledge with sound clinical application, making hernia repair a more rational

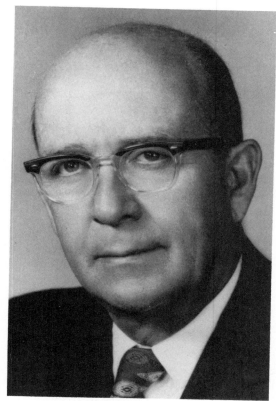

**Figure 1–3.** Chester B. McVay (1911–    )
Since 1942, he has conducted numerous research studies into important anatomic details relating to hernia. He is an anatomist-surgeon — one of a type vanishing from the current surgical scene. (Courtesy of the Yankton Clinic, S. D.)

endeavor. The following quotation from McVay is so fundamentally important that it is quoted directly.

It is pointed out that the inguinal ligament is neither the normal insertion of the inguinal strata or a suitable substitute for such attachment; on the contrary, the superior pubic ligament Cooper's ligament, which is the normal insertion is readily accessible, intrinsically strong and directly fixed to bone.

Anatomic studies by McVay, done independently and with Anson, are classics, being clearly written and well illustrated. He emphasized the importance of recognizing the various laminae of the abdominal wall and stressed the importance of the transversus abdominis layer. He has repeatedly pointed out the differences between an aponeurosis and a fascia; an aponeurosis is the fibrous continuation of

its muscle fibers, while a fascia is the thin layer of connective tissue covering both the muscle and its aponeurosis.

Currently, the anatomy appropriate to the repair of hernias is reasonably well known. It is essential that anatomic variations be appreciated when dealing with various types of groin herniations.

## ADJUNCTS TO HERNIA REPAIR

### Anesthesia

Besides the need for knowledge of normal and pathologic anatomy, advancement in the field of anesthesia was necessary if deliberate and lengthy operations were to be carried out safely and painlessly. Historically, a variety of drugs and potions were used for the relief of pain for many centuries, but in this discussion, I will touch only on those discoveries that, I feel, made the control of pain due to operative procedures a reality.

In 1842 Crawford Williamson Long, a Georgia country doctor, administered ether to James Venable for the purpose of excision of a sebaceous cyst; this report was published after 1846. In 1844 Horace Wells underwent a dental extraction under nitrous oxide anesthesia. Another dentist, William Thomas Green Morton, demonstrated that ether was an effective anesthetic in 1846. Morton served as the anesthetist for Dr. John Collins Warren in a demonstration given at Massachusetts General Hospital in Boston on October 16, 1846. Chloroform was used as an anesthetic agent in 1847.

Local anesthesia became available later than did general anesthesia. Köller in 1884 introduced cocaine as an effective anesthetic agent in ophthalmology. In 1885 Halsted demonstrated that nerve block anesthesia was possible with cocaine. Einhorn and his associates produced procaine in 1905. Other forms of anesthesia became rapidly available. Bier in 1899 administered the first spinal anesthetic to man.

Thus, it is clear that by 1885 several agents and techniques were available to produce insensibility to pain. It was now possible to ascertain with deliberation the anatomic abnormality during an operation for hernia. Correction of hernial defects was rapidly becoming more effective.

## Antisepsis and Asepsis

Prior to the antiseptic-aseptic era, nearly every operative wound was followed by infection and possibly septicemia. Mortality rates from traumatic and operative wounds were staggering. However, during this era, awareness did exist of a connection between cleanliness and infection. Oliver Wendell Holmes in 1842 and Semmelweiss in 1849 wrote of the desirability of cleansing the hands before attending patients. They suspected that the causative agent, whatever it might be, could be carried from one patient to the next. However, an a priori relationship had to be

firmly established before the ultimate conquest of infection could be realized. Two of the most influential contributors to understanding the problem of infection and the subsequent application of the antiseptic-aseptic technique were Louis Pasteur and Lord Lister.

Understanding the problem of wound infection must begin with an appreciation of the discoveries of Pasteur (Fig. 1–4), who refuted the doctrine of spontaneous generation of bacteria in 1860. This genius, although not a physician, made the initial observations that served as the foundation upon which the science of surgical bacteriology is built, and man's indebtedness to Pasteur is immeasurable. Few benefactors have contributed so much to mankind.

Lord Lister (1827–1912) was a surgeon

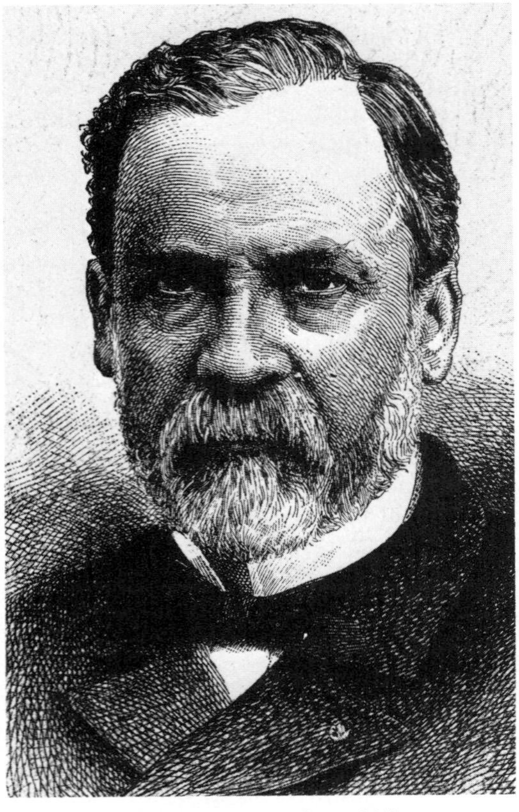

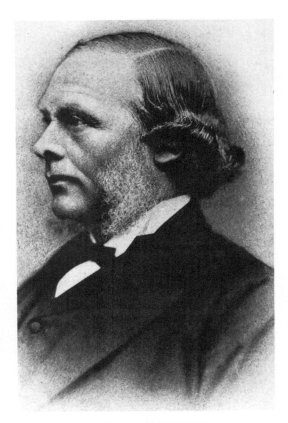

**Figure 1–4.  Louis Pasteur** (1822–1895)

His discoveries led to the eventual recognition of the relationship between wound infections and bacteria. Bacteriology became a science largely as a result of Pasteur's contributions. (Cover photograph from *The Pasteur Fermentation Centennial 1857–1957: A Scientific Symposium.* Courtesy of Bettmann Archive, Inc., New York, N.Y.)

**Figure 1–5.  Joseph Lister** (1827–1912)

Through application of knowledge provided by Pasteur, Lister advanced the antiseptic principle in the treatment of wounds. As a result, elective procedures were undertaken with a precipitous drop in morbidity and mortality. (By permission of the President and Council of the Royal College of Surgeons of England.)

who had the additional attribute of an inquiring mind (Fig. 1–5). He was prepared as a scientist to recognize the significance of Pasteur's observations. Lister was aided in his pioneering work by a colleague, a professor of chemistry, who called his attention to Pasteur's work on putrefaction and fermentation. With this preparation, Lister was able to grasp the monumental significance of Pasteur's discoveries and began applying this newly found knowledge toward the solution of the problem of infection, sepsis, and death due to microorganisms. In 1867, an important publication by Lister appeared in the British Medical Journal, entitled "On the antiseptic principles in the practice of surgery." Lister recognized that suture material could also serve as a source of wound infection. His contributions were by no means quickly accepted, for it required nearly two decades for British surgeons to fully recognize and implement Lister's ideas of antisepsis.

Although Lister receives generous and appropriate credit for his introduction of the antiseptic principle into surgery, little is said about the enormous influence he had upon other pioneers in the field of hernia surgery. Bassini, Lucas-Championnière, and Marcy all were directly exposed to his teaching and tremendously influenced thereby.

Less than 100 years ago, the great Billroth described progress made in wound care as follows:

In 1875, I first began to employ the antiseptic method regularly. In 1877, my assistant, Dr. Wölfler, journeyed to England, France and Germany and brought back with him the most recent modification of the method; whereupon we began afresh with our antiseptic treatment. The utmost precautions were taken to insure asepticity and to diminish the sources of infection. The time of making post-mortem examinations was altered; none of the servants employed about the dead-house were allowed to come near the clinic or operating theatre; all of my assistants were provided with special coats which were washed daily; special receptacles were set apart for the antiseptic dressings, and all of the sponges were most carefully and thoroughly disinfected with carbolic acid and then soaked in thymol before use. I long had an idea that some of the misfortunes met with after ovariotomy might be traced to imperfect disinfection of sponges. Professor

Frisch has shown that sponges, even after they have been soaked in 5 percent carbolic solution, are still capable of developing organic germs. In short, in every detail to the best of my power, I carried out Lister's and Volkmann's injunctions. Unfortunately, to some extent, this system is based on imperfect scientific knowledge, and thus a certain amount of faith is demanded of those who obediently carry out every detail.

Other important adjuncts were required before operative and traumatic wounds could be treated with minimal danger of infection; the simplicity of these measures in no way detracted from their efficacy.

Ernst von Bergman invented the steam sterilizer in 1891. He is also given credit for introducing the word "aseptic" into the medical vocabulary.

Halsted in 1890 contributed rubber gloves—a benefit to surgeons in particular and mankind in general. A brief quotation directly from Halsted is most interesting in regard to the motivating force that precipitated this important discovery.

In the winter of 1889 and 1890—I cannot recall the month—the nurse in charge of my operating room complained that the solutions of mercuric chloride produced a dermatitis of her arms and hands. As she was an unusually efficient woman I gave the matter my consideration and one day in New York requested the Goodyear Rubber Company to make as an experiment two pair of thin rubber gloves with gauntlets. On trial these proved to be so satisfactory that additional pairs were ordered.

The nurse, Caroline Hampton (Fig. 1–6), eventually became the wife of Dr. Halsted. The use of rubber gloves spread rapidly throughout this country and abroad. The importance of this contribution toward decreasing wound infection has not been fully appreciated. It is possible that the idea of rubber gloves was so simple that its value was de-emphasized. In my judgment, their discovery was truly one of Halsted's great contributions.

The addition of the face mask, which was devised by Mikulicz in 1896, was yet another advance toward achieving asepsis in the operating room.

Thus, by 1890 surgeons were equipped with a knowledge of bacteria and their relationship to wound infection; they were aware of methods to exclude organisms

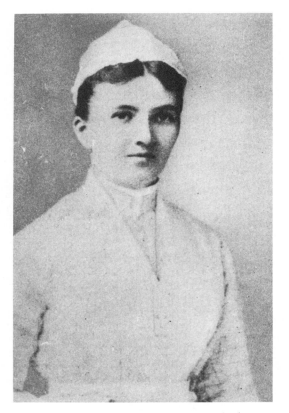

**Figure 1–6.   Caroline Hampton (1861–1922)**
While serving as nurse in W.S. Halsted's operating room, she developed a dermatitis as a result of rinsing her hands in a mercuric chloride solution. Halsted had originally intended rubber gloves to be used as protection against the irritating effects of the solution. In addition to this function, gloves were used as a means to achieve asepsis and to protect patients' wounds from possible infection arising from organisms present on the surgeon's hands. Ms. Hampton became Mrs. William S. Halsted on June 4, 1890. (Courtesy of Johns Hopkins Press, Baltimore, Md.)

from operative wounds as well as methods to destroy bacteria. Antisepsis and asepsis had become attainable realities.

## IMPORTANT TECHNICAL CONTRIBUTIONS IN THE RESOLUTION OF THE HERNIA PROBLEM

*No disease of the human body, belonging to the province of the surgeon, requires in its treatment a greater combination of accurate anatomical skill, than hernia in all its varieties.*

*Sir Astley Cooper*

Knowledge of the anatomy of hernia, despite its slow progress, made it possible for surgeons to begin using sound principles in the repair of hernias. Once the various types of hernias were differentiated, logical and effective measures could be taken to correct the particular defect.

USE OF THE GROIN OR SCROTAL INCISION FOR REPAIR. Early surgeons generally limited their incisions to the scrotum in the region of the external ring, but Celsus, who lived in the first century B.C., made use of the groin or scrotal incision in hernia repairs. Galen, in the second century A.D., utilized the groin incision and attempted to use suture techniques, as did Celsus earlier.

LIGATION OF THE HERNIAL SAC AT THE EXTERNAL ABDOMINAL RING was practiced for many centuries by a number of surgeons. Galen, a Greek surgeon, practiced ligation of the sac at the superficial ring in the second century A.D. Paul of Aegina ligated hernial sacs in the seventh century. He was known to preserve the testes in the repair of small hernias, but he excised the testicle, cord, and sac in attempting repair of larger hernias. During the Middle Ages, Lanfranc practiced ligation of the sac with gold thread. Paré, in the sixteenth century, dissected down to the sac in the inguinal canal and twisted a gold wire around the neck of the sac; this prevented the intestine from entering the sac. William of Salicet (Guglielmo Salicetti, also called Saliceto) and Roger of Palermo ligated the sac with double ligature and excised it transversely. In spite of the fact that ligation of the hernial sac at the external ring was destined to fail, it is obvious that progress was being made. Vincenz Czerny in 1877 and Banks in 1882 practiced ligation of the sac at the external ring. In addition, Czerny closed the pillars around the cord to reduce the size of the external ring. Early surgeons were constantly harassed by infection, making operative procedures dangerous for every patient; this explains the popularity of trusses into the twentieth century. Of course, the pain associated with the use of cautery or any operative procedure was unbearable.

RELEASE OF A STRANGULATED HERNIA was practiced by Pierre Franco in the sixteenth century. He inserted an instrument between the bowel and sac and then cut the constriction without injury to the intestine. The narrowed ring was enlarged and the strangulation relieved. This was the first reported (in 1561) surgical attempt at release of a strangulation obstruction.

**INCISION OR OPENING OF THE EXTERNAL OBLIQUE FASCIA** constituted one of the milestones in progress in hernia repair. This tremendously important step and frequently overlooked detail permitted high ligation of the sac and opened the way for closure of the transversalis fascia and repair of the floor of Hesselbach's triangle. Some give credit to Marcy for this contribution (1871). Lucas-Championnière (1843–1913) *incised the external oblique fascia* in 1881 (Fig. 1–7). The great importance of this step requires comment, since this significant detail permitted complete exposure of the hernial sac and eventually led to proper differentiation of

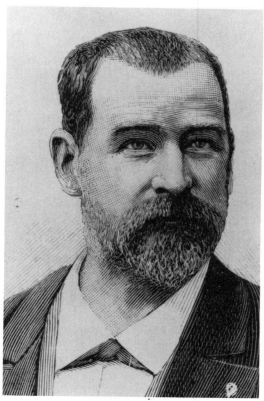

**Figure 1–7. Just Lucus-Championnière** (1843–1913)

His technique of opening the external oblique aponeurosis from the external to the internal ring permitted high ligation of the peritoneal sac and reconstruction of the transversalis fascia and internal ring. Furthermore, this indirectly resulted in a better understanding of the nature of direct hernias. (Courtesy of the New York Academy of Medicine Library, N.Y.)

direct hernias. Total excision of the peritoneal sac and visualization of the internal ring thus became possible. A rather provocative approach to the history of surgical treatment of hernia is to divide it into two eras—before and after the external oblique fascia had been opened. It took surgeons some 2000 years to progress from the external to the internal abdominal ring.

Lucas-Championnière was a follower and admirer of Joseph Lister. He practiced the antiseptic method and strongly urged its acceptance by others. An obituary of Just Lucas-Championnière appeared in the British Medical Journal in 1913 (Vol. 2, p. 1186); however, in one of the strange omissions of medical history, there was no reference to his important contribution to the surgical treatment of hernia.

**SIMPLE LIGATION OF THE PERITONEAL SAC** was advocated in 1899 by Ferguson, who recommended ligation of the sac at the internal ring without disturbing either the abdominal wall or the cord. He did, however, suture the internal oblique anterior to the spermatic cord. Czerny in 1877 and Wood in 1885 resected the peritoneal sac as high as possible; then, they closed the pillars of the external ring.

Simple ligation of the peritoneal sac is practiced today by a number of surgeons when they operate upon indirect inguinal hernias of the congenital type. The size of the internal ring is given serious consideration, and, in the presence of an enlarged ring, the transversalis fascia is approximated in order to achieve snug closure.

**HIGH LIGATION OF THE PERITONEAL SAC** was practiced by Banks in 1884. His detailed and entertaining description of dissection when there is incarcerated omentum, and its management, leaves no doubt that he practiced accurate closure of the peritoneum at the internal ring. He advocated opening the peritoneal sac for thorough inspection. Furthermore, he attempted closure of the internal ring, for he described the danger of piercing the epigastric artery when placing sutures of silver wire. Marcy in 1881, Bassini in 1887, and Halsted in 1890 also ligated the hernial sac at its neck. Herzfeld in 1912 pointed out that the causal factor in congenital hernia is the patent processus vaginalis. High ligation of the sac alone—without disturbing the abdominal wall—is adequate treatment to cure such hernias. Potts, Riker, and Lewis later affirmed the same idea.

**CLOSURE OF THE TRANSVERSALIS FASCIA** at the internal ring is an absolutely necessary detail if recurrence of an indirect inguinal hernia is to be avoided. Several surgeons have probably achieved this end using different methods.

In 1881 Marcy stated that he did not open small hernial sacs. He further stated, "In some instances it will be better to first close the peritoneum independently with a fine continuous suture; otherwise, refresh the pillars of the ring or wall of the opening and close by sutures." The importance of the transversalis fascia has been recognized slowly, but due to the contributions of Condon, McVay, and Nyhus, more surgeons are aware that this structure forms a first line of defense against groin hernias.

**USE OF THE INGUINAL INCISION OF THE UPPER APPROACH** to a femoral hernia was first made by Annandale whose report appeared in 1876. Ruggi in 1892 and Lotheissen in 1897 also used the upper, or abdominal, approach, and their descriptions are clear and understandable.

**USE OF COOPER'S LIGAMENT IN THE REPAIR OF FEMORAL HERNIA** was suggested by Cooper himself, but he never had the occasion to perform such an operation. Ruggi described his operation in 1892, advocating high ligation of the peritoneal sac, and after reading Ruggi's report, there is no doubt that he placed sutures between Cooper's ligament and the medial border of Poupart's ligament, a technique later proposed by Moschcowitz.

In 1897 Lotheissen had planned to perform a Bassini repair of a hernia upon a woman who had two earlier operations performed elsewhere, with recurrence at the operative site each time. A portion of Poupart's ligament had been sacrificed, making it impossible to complete the usual Bassini repair. It is clear that Lotheissen utilized Cooper's ligament, to which he sutured the muscular layers of the lower abdomen. Lotheissen's friend, Professor Narath of Utrecht, Holland, used a similar method of repair. Annandale is frequently and erroneously credited with having

used Cooper's ligament in his repair of an unusual hernia consisting of oblique (indirect), direct, and femoral components.

The principle by which Cooper's ligament was used for the repair of groin hernias originated with Lotheissen, but it was McVay who placed this technical advance on a firm anatomic basis and popularized its clinical use. The designation of the procedure as a McVay repair is appropriate. Socin in 1879 dissected the femoral sac, ligated it at the highest point, and returned the stump to the abdomen. No repair was attempted.

Moschcowitz reported his method of repair in 1907. He recognized that von Frey, Billroth, Czerny, Schede, Bottini, and Gaurneri had advocated suture of the inguinal ligament to pectineal fascia. Moschcowitz, however, placed sutures of chromicized catgut between Cooper's ligament with its adjacent periosteum to Poupart's ligament. He added a repair of the inguinal floor to a somewhat similar method that had been employed by Ruggi in 1892.

**USE OF THE FEMORAL OR LOWER APPROACH** was made by Bassini, who performed his operation for the repair of femoral hernia in 1884, but he did not report it until 1894. Cushing, not the world-renowned neurosurgeon, described his procedure in 1888. The modern surgeon has available all the anatomic and technical knowledge necessary to treat nearly every femoral hernia successfully, provided that he applies the available anatomic and technical knowledge effectively in each individual patient.

**CLOSURE OF THE INTERNAL ABDOMINAL RING** was not possible until surgeons had the opportunity to open or incise the external oblique fascia. There is some evidence that Marcy might have first closed the internal ring in 1871. His reports leave room for some uncertainty as to the precise nature of his repair. The techniques advocated by Bassini in 1887 and Halsted in 1890 clearly included closure of the internal ring.

**COMBINATION OF TECHNIQUES IN HERNIA REPAIR** is a relatively recent approach. This is at least a partial explanation for the success that Bassini, who first performed his operation in 1884, was able to report to the Italian Surgical

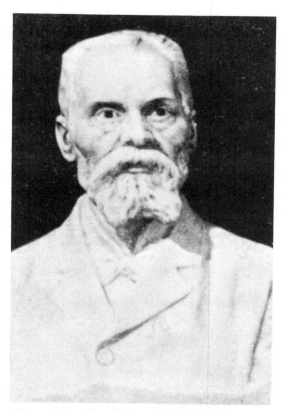

**Figure 1–8. Eduardo Bassini (1844–1924)**

A surgeon and anatomist, he was the first to employ a combination of technical details in the repair of groin hernias. His illustrations provided other surgeons with an effective method, while his statistically supported, excellent results gave them an objective worthy of attainment. (Courtesy of Consorzio Bibliografico Universitario; Padova, Italy.)

Society in 1887 regarding his results in 42 repairs. Bassini (1884–1924) was an excellent anatomist as well as surgeon (Fig. 1–8). He illustrated his method of repair with such clarity that it was possible for other surgeons to perform his operation. Furthermore, he followed his patients postoperatively with a thoroughness not previously recorded, as far as I could discover. His results were available for other surgeons to note as a point of reference. There is no doubt in my mind that his effort had an enormous impact on the surgery of hernia.

Essentially, Bassini's method included a combination of these details: (1) high ligation of the peritoneal sac; (2) repair of the floor of the inguinal canal; (3) displacement of the cord to a position in front of the reconstructed floor of the

inguinal canal resulting from repair of the floor of the inguinal canal; (4) closure performed from the internal ring to the pubic tubercle; (5) a new and important principle—closure of the abdominal wall in individual layers; and (6) use of nonabsorbable sutures of silk.

Of tremendous importance was the fact that Bassini also provided substantial statistical proof in writing that his method, practiced consistently, gave excellent results. Others presented isolated cases operated upon by a variety of techniques with no follow-up studies. Individual verbal case reports, personal opinions, and delayed publications were not uncommon sources of information. Bassini initially reported his results obtained after operating upon 64 patients. However brief, Bassini's follow-up study gave surgeons an objective worthy of attainment. His influence upon the technology of hernia repair remains indelible.

THE PREPERITONEAL APPROACH TO INGUINAL AND FEMORAL HERNIA REPAIR has been popularized by Nyhus. His chapter in the book on hernia by Nyhus and Harkins deals with the subject in depth. Although groin hernias have been repaired through abdominal incisions since 1743 (as reported by Meade), the preperitoneal or retroperitoneal approach is a relatively recent development.

The following is a brief discussion of those surgeons who used the preperitoneal approach in repairing defects in the inguinofemoral area.

According to Koontz, Tait in 1861 repaired a femoral hernia using an abdominal incision. His definition of structures used in the actual repair was not entirely clear. In 1898 Kelly repaired femoral hernias while performing laparotomies for gynecologic disorders.

Bates in 1913 reduced the indirect inguinal hernial sac after opening the peritoneum. High ligation of the sac was achieved; then the transversalis fascia was repaired around the internal ring.

Cheatle in 1920 exposed the hernial sac and internal ring using the preperitoneal approach. He practiced high ligation of the sac. Closure of the ring was an optional matter with him.

Henry in 1936 advocated this approach for repair of indirect and femoral hernias. Musgrove and McCready in 1949 and

Mikkelson and Berne in 1954 published their significant papers dealing with the repair of femoral hernias utilizing the preperitoneal approach. In 1952 Riba and Mehn, while performing a retropubic prostatectomy, repaired a direct inguinal hernia by suture of transversalis fascia to Cooper's ligament.

The credit for bringing the preperitoneal approach for repair of groin hernias to its modern popularity belongs to Nyhus and his coworkers. He has been employing this approach to repair of direct, indirect, and femoral hernias since 1955. He has utilized the transversalis fascia and its derivatives in repair of groin hernias. Such structures have been sutured to Cooper's ligament in the repair of direct and femoral hernias.

**TRANSPLANTATION OF THE CORD.** The fate of the spermatic cord in hernia repair, viewed from a historical perspective, has been traumatic and variable. Displacement of the cord has varied in degree. Bassini in 1887 described his method in which the cord remained under the external oblique muscle but rested upon the newly reconstructed floor of the inguinal canal. In 1890 Halsted described his procedure in which he reduced the size of the cord by excising the cremaster muscle and veins of the pampinoform plexus. He then placed this mini-cord in a subcutaneous position. Ferguson in 1890 advised against transplantation of the cord. In fact, he sutured the external oblique over the cord after high ligation of the peritoneal sac. At the present time, it appears that transplantation of the cord external to the external oblique is being practiced with decreasing frequency. Radical excision of the pampiniform plexus is not practiced by modern surgeons who deal with hernias.

**EXCISION OF THE CREMASTER MUSCLE** was advocated by Halsted in 1893. He preserved the vas deferens, blood vessels, and one or two veins! As a result of such extensive stripping of the cord, atrophic testicles and hydroceles were fairly common.

In spite of these results, some decrease in the size of the cord, particularly in large indirect inguinal hernias, seems desirable. This can be achieved with comparative safety by simply excising the hypertrophied cremaster muscle and sparing the veins.

**USE OF TRANSVERSE OVERLAPPING TECHNIQUE FOR REPAIR OF UMBILICAL HERNIA.** In 1898 Mayo successfully repaired, under adverse circumstances, a large umbilical hernia in an obese female. He presented the important principle of transverse closure for the first time. Farris in 1959 showed experimentally that overlapping of tissues did not improve the strength of the wound; nevertheless, as a principle, transverse closure is desirable in appropriate cases.

**CONVERSION OF THE DIRECT PERITONEAL SAC INTO AN INDIRECT SAC** is known as the *Hoguet* maneuver. This sound technique and maneuver was advocated by Hoguet in 1920. He pointed out that the peritoneum may be easily identified at the internal ring and, by means of lateral traction, withdrawn lateral to the deep inferior epigastric artery, thus converting the direct into an indirect peritoneal sac. This method minimized the possibility of bladder injury, since opening into a direct sac through the floor of Hesselbach's triangle might result in injury to the bladder. Furthermore, this simple approach decreases the possibility of overlooking a coexisting femoral hernia. Additionally, the Hoguet maneuver is useful in reducing the peritoneal component of a femoral hernia. Even today, this helpful technical procedure is overlooked by many surgeons.

**USE OF THE RELAXING INCISION.** The need for some type of procedure which permits relaxation of the lower abdominal wall and particularly the rectus sheath has gained recognition very slowly. When the interval of distance between the transversus abdominus arch and the inguinal ligament is large, as it frequently is in direct inguinal hernias, some method is necessary to permit shifting of tissues downward to strengthen the floor of Hesselbach's triangle. Some type of incision in the anterior sheath of the rectus is necessary if undue tension is to be avoided. Incision in the anterior rectus sheath had been practiced occasionally by many surgeons. Wölfler in 1892, Bloodgood in 1899, Berger in 1902, Halsted in 1903, Fallis in 1938, Rienhoff in 1940, Tanner in 1942, Mattson in 1946, and McVay in 1962 all incised the lower portion of the anterior sheath of the rectus muscle.

In my opinion, the full importance of the

relaxing incision has yet to be appreciated by many surgeons. It is essential in the repair of direct and femoral hernias in which the McVay technique is used, and it is of tremendous importance in many direct recurrent inguinal hernias where the tissue in the floor of Hesselbach's triangle has been largely destroyed. It is also useful in the repair of combination types of hernias, such as direct-indirect.

It is difficult to understand how some surgeons concerned with the problem of hernia repair state with pride that they have never resorted to the use of the relaxing incision. It is, in my opinion, one of the most useful adjuncts in modern surgery for the repair of hernias in which tissues are deficient in the floor of Hesselbach's triangle.

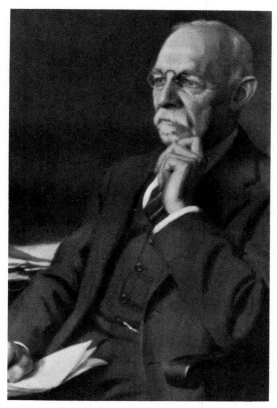

**Figure 1–9. William Stewart Halsted** (1852–1922) He is considered to have founded a "school of surgery." He insisted upon careful asepsis, meticulous dissection, accurate hemostasis, and use of fine suture material in surgical operations. He also advocated transplantation of the cord to the subcutaneous position, a technique generally recognized as the "Halsted repair." (Courtesy of Johns Hopkins University School of Medicine, Baltimore, Md.)

**DETAILS OF OPERATIVE TECHNIQUE** were carefully developed by Halsted (Fig. 1–9). Although many surgeons have emphasized the need for careful attention to detail in the repair of hernias, no one stressed their importance more than Halsted did. He insisted upon careful asepsis, meticulous and accurate dissection, thorough hemostasis, and the use of fine suture material and gentleness in the handling of tissue. He studied the hernia problem and tried a variety of techniques, abandoning those he found to be ineffective. He recognized that too great a reduction in the size of the cord resulted in atrophic testes and hydroceles. He was aware of the value of the relaxing incision. The procedure of transplantation of the spermatic cord into the subcutaneous position is popularly known as the Halsted technique of repair.

Halsted was responsible for the surgical education of Dr. Roy D. McClure, first Surgeon-in-Chief of the Henry Ford Hospital. Dr. McClure, in turn, passed much of his knowledge to Dr. Laurence S. Fallis, the second Surgeon-in-Chief, who continued his interest in the subject of hernia. Drs. McClure and Fallis shared their knowledge and experience with such well-known surgeons as W. A. Altemeier, K. W. Warren, S. F. Marshall, H. N. Harkins, C. R. Lam, B. E. Brush, D. E. Szilagyi, and James Barron. It was my unique opportunity to work with Dr. L. S. Fallis as his Chief Resident Surgeon.

The knowledge of wound healing has increased rapidly, and this information is being increasingly applied to the surgical treatment of hernias. The recognition that scar tissue is a poor substitute for normal tissue is of recent origin.

The evolution of the successful treatment of hernias could not begin to materialize until scientific fact supplanted superstition, inaccurate observation, and erroneous opinion. Incorrect ideas held by the early anatomists and surgeons regarding the pathology and anatomy of hernia delayed the establishment of any knowledgeable understanding of the nature of the hernia problem and its subsequent resolution. In order to initiate this success however, certain fundamental requirements had to be met, including the following criteria: clarification of normal and pathologic anatomy; sound surgical technology for the correction of the defects; and execution of the proposed operative procedures safely, painlessly, and with the elimination of the hazard of infection.

For more than 25 centuries, anatomists, surgeons, dentists, pharmacologists, pathologists, and bacteriologists have contributed to the total fund of medical knowledge currently available, thereby providing a cumulative effect toward the successful surgical repair of hernias. With the advent of the present century, the full importance of the transversus layer of the abdominal wall was fully recognized. In addition, the great variety of techniques that are currently available for hernia repair has created a need to define more precisely the indications for their specific use.

With their knowledge of the pathology and anatomy of hernia, the advances in technique, and the use of anesthesia, asepsis, and antisepsis, surgeons are able to achieve substantial success in the repair of abdominal wall hernias.

## REFERENCES

Annandale, T.: Case in which a reducible oblique and direct inguinal and femoral hernia existed on the same side and were successfully treated by operation. Edinb. Med. J. 21:1087, 1876.

Banks, W. M.: Notes on the radical cure of hernia. Med. Times Gaz. 2(No. 1777):72, 1884.

Bassini, E.: Nuovo metodo per la cura radicale dell' ernia. Atti Congr. Assoc. Med. Ital. 2:179, 1889.

Cheatle, C. L.: An operation for the radical cure of inguinal and femoral hernia. Br. Med. J. 2:68, 1920.

Condon, R. E.: Anatomy of the inguinal region and its relationship to groin hernias. In Nyhus, L. M. and Harkins, H. N.: Hernia. Philadelphia, J. B. Lippincott Co., 1964, p. 28.

Cooper, A. P.: The Anatomy and Surgical Treatment of Abdominal Hernia (2 vols.). London, Longman & Co., 1804 and 1807.

Czerny, V.: Studien zur Radikalbehandlung der Hernien. Wein. Med. Wochenschr. 27:497, 1877.

Farris, J. M. et al.: Umbilical hernia: An inquiry into the principle of imbrication and a note on the preservation of the umbilical dimple. Am. J. Surg. 98:236, 1959.

Ferguson, H. W.: Oblique inguinal hernia, typic operation for its radical cure. J.A.M.A. 33:6–9, 1899.

Halsted, W. S.: The radical cure of hernia. Bull. Johns Hopkins Hosp. 1:12, 1889.

Halsted, W. S.: The radical cure of inguinal hernia in the male. Bull. Johns Hopkins Hosp. 4:17, 1893.

Harkins, H. N., Szilagyi, D. E., Brush, B. E., and Williams, R.: Clinical experiences with the McVay herniorrhaphy. Surgery 12:364, 1942.

Harkins, H. N.: The repair of groin hernias: Progress in the last decade. Surg. Clin. North Am. 29:1457, 1949.

Henry, A. K.: Operation for femoral hernia by a midline extraperitoneal approach: With a preliminary note on the use of this route for reducible inguinal hernia. Lancet 1:531, 1936.

Hesselbach, F. K.: Neuste Anatomisch-Pathologische Untersuchungen über den ursprung und das Fortschreiter der Leisten- und Schenkelbrüche. Würzburg, Bäumgartner, 1814.

Iason, A. H.: Hernia. Blakiston Co., Philadelphia, 1941.

Lotheissen, G.: Zur radikal operation des schenkel hernien. Zentralbl. Chir. 25:548, 1898.

Meade, R. H.: The history of abdominal approach to hernia repair. Surgery 57:908, 1965.

McVay, C. B.: An anatomic error in current methods of inguinal herniorrhapy. Ann. Surg. 113:1111, 1941.

McVay, C. B., and Anson, B. J.: A fundamental error in current methods of inguinal herniorrhaphy. Surg. Gynecol. Obstet. 74:746, 1942.

McVay, C. B., and Anson, B. J.: Inguinal and femoral hernioplasty. Surg. Gynecol. Obstet. 88:473, 1949.

Mikkelsen, W. P., and Berne, C. J.: Femoral hernioplasty: Suprapubic extraperitoneal approach (Cheatle-Henry). Surgery 35:743, 1954.

Morgagni, J. B.: The Seats and Causes of Diseases (translated by Benjamin Alexander, M.D.). New York, Hafner Publishing Co., 1960.

Moschcowitz, A. V.: Femoral hernia: A new operation for radical cure. N.Y. Med. J. 7:396, 1907.

Musgrove, J. E., and McCready, F. J.: The Henry approach to femoral hernia. Surgery 26:608, 1949.

Nyhus, L. M., and Harkins, N. H.: Hernia. Philadelphia, J. B. Lippincott Co., 1964.

Ruggi, G.: Metodo operativo nuovo per la cura radicale dell'ernia crurale. Bull. Scienze Med. ci Bologna 7(No. 3):223, 1892.

Zimmerman, L. M., and Veith, I.: Great Ideas in the History of Surgery (2nd rev. ed.). New York, Dover Publications, Inc., 1967.

## Supplemental Readings

Andrews, E.: A history of the development of the technic of herniorrhaphy. Ann. Med. Hist. 7:451, 1935.

Andrews, E., and Bisell, A. D.: Direct hernia: A record of surgical failures. Surg. Gynecol. Obstet. 58:753, 1934.

Billroth, T.: Clinical surgery: Reports of surgical practice between the years 1860–1876. London, New Sydenham Soc., 1881.

Burton, C.: The evolution and classification of hernial operations. Int. Abstr. Surg. 87:313, 1948.

Burton, C.: Rationale and factors for consideration in Cooper's hernioplasty. Surg. Gynecol. Obstet. 85: 1–8, 1947.

Bull, W. T.: Cited by Halsted. In The radical cure of inguinal hernia in the male. Bull. Johns Hopkins Hosp. 4:17, 1893.

Carlson, R. I.: The historical development of the surgical treatment of inguinal hernia. Surgery 39:1031, 1956.

Coley, W. B.: Review of radical cure of hernia during

the last half century (editorial). Am. J. Surg. *31*:397, 1936.

Cushing, H. W.: An improved method for the radical cure of femoral hernia. Boston Med. Surg. J. *119*: 546, 1888.

Fallis, L. S.: Direct inguinal hernia. Ann. Surg. *107*: 572, 1938.

Gallie, W. E., and Le Mesurier, A. B.: The use of living sutures in operative surgery. Can. Med. Assoc. J. *11*:504, 1921.

Halsted, W. S.: *Surgical Papers* (Vol. 1). Baltimore, Johns Hopkins Press, 1952, pp. 37–39.

Halsted, W. S.: The cure of the more difficult as well as the simpler inguinal ruptures. Bull. Johns Hopkins Hosp. *14*:208, 1903.

Harrison, P. W.: Inguinal hernia: A study of the principles involved in surgical treatment. Arch. Surg. *4*:680, 1922.

Hoguet, J. P.: Observations on two thousand four hundred and sixty-eight operations by one operator. Surg. Gynecol. Obstet. *37*:71, 1923.

Hoguet, J. P.: Direct inguinal hernia. Ann. Surg. *72*:671, 1920.

Keetley, C. B.: Radical cure of hernia. Ann. Surg. *1*:130, 1885. J. H. Chambers Co., 1885, St. Louis.

Keys, T.: *The History of Surgical Anesthesia*. New York, Schuman's, 1945.

Koontz, A. R.: Preliminary report on the use of tantalum mesh in the repair of ventral hernias. Ann. Surg. *127*:1079, 1948.

Koontz, A. R.: Historical analysis of femoral hernia. Surgery *53*:551, 1963.

Koontz, A. R.: *Hernia*. New York, Appleton-Century Crofts, 1963.

Lister, J.: On the antiseptic principle in the practice of surgery. Br. Med. J. *2*:246, 1867.

Lucas-Championnière, J.: Cure radicale des hernies; avec une étude statistique de deux cents soixante-quinze operations et cinquante figures intercalées dans le texte. Paris, Rueff et Cie, 1892.

Lytle, W. J.: *A History of Hernia*, Med. Press, *232*(No. 6034):1954.

Lytle, W. J.: Femoral hernia. Ann. R. Coll. Surg. Engl. *21*:244, 1957.

Marcy, H. O.: A new use of carbolized catgut ligatures. Boston Med. Surg. J. *85*:315, 1871.

Marcy, H. O.: The cure of hernia by the antiseptic use of animal ligature. Trans. Int. Med. Cong. *2*:446–448, 1881.

Marcy, H. O.: The cure of hernia. J.A.M.A. *8*:589, 1887.

Marcy, H. O.: *The Anatomy and Surgical Treatment of Hernia*. New York, Appleton-Century-Crofts, 1892.

Ponka, J. L.: The relaxing incision in hernia repair. Am. J. Surg. *115*:552, 1968.

Raaf, J. E.: Hernia healers. Ann. Med. Hist. *4*:377, 1932.

Ravitch, M. M., and Hitzrot, J. M., Jr.: *The Operations for Inguinal Hernia*. St. Louis, C. V. Mosby Co., 1960.

Richter, A. G.: Abhandlung von den Brüchen. Gottingen, J. C. Dieterich, 1778.

Sykes, S. W.: *Essays on the First 100 Years of Anesthesia* (2 vols.). London, E. S. Livingstone Ltd., 1961.

Tanner, H.: A "slide" operation for inguinal and femoral hernia. Br. J. Surg. *29*:285, 1942.

Taylor, F. W.: The evolution of herniorrhaphy. Am. J. Surg. *21*:131, 1933.

Watson, L. F.: *Hernia* (2nd ed.). St. Louis, C. V. Mosby Co., 1938.

Zimmerman, L. M.: Essential problems in the surgical treatment of inguinal hernia. Surg. Gynecol. Obstet. *71*:654, 1940.

Zimmerman, L. M., and Anson, B. J.: *Anatomy and Surgery of Hernia*. Baltimore, Williams & Wilkins Co., 1953.

Zimmerman, L. M.: A critique of the McVay operation for inguinal hernia. Surg. Gynecol. Obstet. *87*:621, 1948.

# 2

# Anatomy

## GENERAL CONSIDERATIONS

Accurate and detailed information concerning the anatomy of the abdominal wall is well documented in the excellent standard texts on anatomy currently available. Most of the illustrative material presented here has been obtained from the published reports of anatomists and surgeons, as recorded in the bibliographic references. Refinements in our knowledge of anatomy will continue, but much of the available information is not fully utilized even today. The purpose of this chapter is to present practical anatomic facts of importance to the surgeon.

Ordinarily, the normal structure of the musculofascial layers of the abdomen serves well in retaining its contents in place, and large areas of the abdominal wall remain free of abnormal protrusions throughout life. However, in spite of these facts, man does develop hernias, most of which occur in certain limited areas with recognizable deficiencies in the structure of the abdominal wall.

The surgeon should be aware of the direction of Langer's lines if, after abdominal section, the incision is to heal with minimal scarring (Fig. 2-1). Cox in 1941 studied the cleavage lines of the skin with precision and presented his findings clearly.

Vertical incisions across these lines produce widely gaping wounds, and although they do heal, with the passage of time there is a tendency for widening of the cicatrix. Generally speaking, there is far less spreading of the wound edges when transverse or oblique incisions are made.

The amount of subcutaneous fat be-

tween the skin and muscular layers is extremely variable. In the thin individual, the linea alba may be recognized as a slight depression in the midline and is usually more apparent above the umbilicus. The rectus muscles may be recognizable on either side of the midline. At the lateral margin of the rectus muscles, the linea semilunaris may be identified in thin, well-developed individuals.

Camper's fascia is the poorly developed, superficial fascial layer of the abdominal wall. Scarpa's fascia, which is an easily

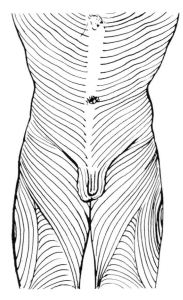

**Figure 2-1.** Subcutaneous elastic and connective tissue is arranged in predictable directions in various parts of the body, creating lines of tension in the skin. Langer's lines indicate the direction in which incisions may be made with minimal gaping of the wound so that it heals with the least possible scar formation.

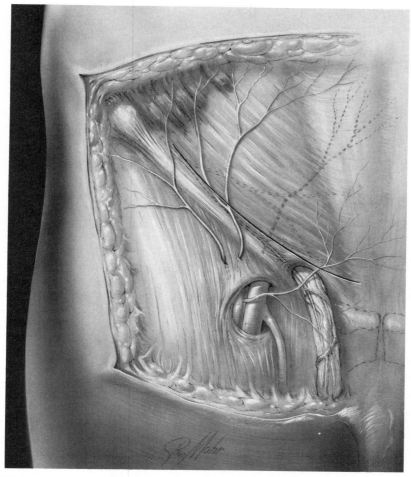

**Figure 2–2.** This composite view of the inguinal area suggests the direction in which an incision may be made for repair of a groin hernia. Location and identity of blood vessels and of other structures encountered in this area are also shown.

recognizable connective tissue structure, is situated more deeply and should be approximated during wound closure if the best cosmetic results are to be obtained postoperatively.

Upon making incisions into the abdominal wall, the surgeon encounters a fairly constant pattern of blood vessels. The subcutaneous tissue derives its blood supply from a number of arteries that make up a network. The intercostal arteries, the superior epigastric artery, and the musculophrenic arteries supply the area above the umbilicus. It should be recalled that the internal thoracic (internal mammary) artery arises from the subclavian artery and passes caudally posterior to the costal cartilages. The musculophrenic branch of the internal thoracic is given off at the costal margin and follows the costal

arch; it supplies the diaphragm and thoracic wall in the area. The superior epigastric artery, which is a continuation of the internal mammary, then passes downward on the posterior aspect of the rectus abdominis muscle.

The portion of the abdominal wall that we are concerned with also receives blood supply from the sixth to the twelfth intercostal arteries. In addition, the lumbar arteries supply the lower abdomen. The superficial epigastric, the superficial external pudendal, and the superficial circumflex iliac arteries arise from the femoral artery just below the inguinal ligament. The veins accompanying the arteries drain into the femoral vein at the saphenous opening. In a deeper plane, the lower abdomen just above the inguinal ligament also receives arterial supply via the deep inferior epigastric and the deep circumflex iliac arteries, which are given off by the external iliac artery.

In the inguinal area the external spermatic artery arises from the deep inferior epigastric artery. It joins the spermatic cord at the internal, or deep, inguinal ring. An arteriole called the superficial external pudendal artery arises from the femoral artery and supplies the area of the pubic tubercle. A composite view of important structures encountered in an inguinal incision is shown in Figure 2–2.

## MUSCLES OF THE ANTEROLATERAL ABDOMINAL WALL

### External Oblique

The muscles of the abdominal wall which are of prime interest to us include the external oblique, internal oblique, transversus abdominis, rectus abdominis, and the pyramidalis. Upon abdominal section lateral to the femoral sheath, the external oblique is the first musculofascial structure to be encountered (Fig. 2–3). It is an extensive flat muscle, which arises from the fifth to the twelfth ribs. Thus, this muscle actually covers a portion of the lower thorax. The muscle fibers then take an oblique course downward and toward the midline. The external oblique muscle is made up of muscular tissue superiorly and laterally, but it becomes aponeurotic in its medial and inferior extent. In other words, the external oblique muscle presents as an aponeurosis as it approaches the lateral margin of the rectus abdominis muscle, and then contributes its aponeurosis to the anterior sheath of the rectus abdominis. In the lower abdomen and inguinal area, the white, oblique fibers are

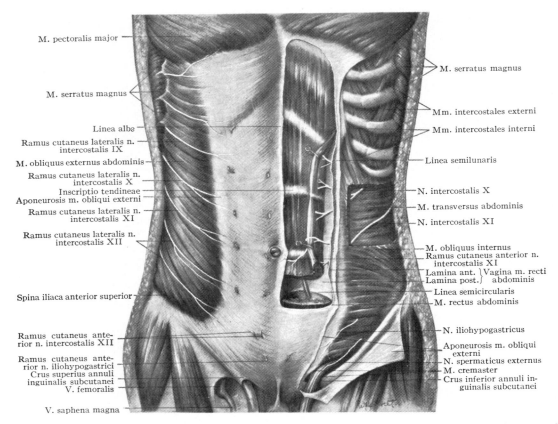

**Figure 2–3.** Muscles of the abdominal wall shown in this illustration include the external oblique, the internal oblique, and the transversus abdominis. Note that the external oblique becomes aponeurotic in its medial portion and in the inguinal area. The abdominal muscles take different directions from origin to insertion; this accounts for the great strength of the abdominal wall. (Reprinted with permission from Anson, B. J., and McVay, C. B.: *Surgical Anatomy*. Philadelphia, W. B. Saunders Co., 1971.)

readily seen after an oblique incision is made in the groin. The fibers of the upper portion of the external oblique are aponeurotic and form a portion of the anterior sheath of the rectus abdominis muscle. They then continue to decussate in the midline or linea alba. The aponeurosis of the external oblique in its lower extent may be easily separated from that of the internal oblique as it forms a portion of the anterior sheath of the rectus. The fibers from approximately the lower half of the external oblique muscle insert into the iliac crest. Those in the region of the groin form a free border known as Poupart's ligament. This ligament is no thicker than the aponeurosis of which it is a part. Some of the lowermost and medially displaced fibers, as the lacunar ligament of Gimbernat, curve posteriorly to the iliopectineal ligament.

Finally, as the cord passes through the external ring on its way to the testicle, it gains a covering, known as the external spermatic fascia, from the external oblique.

## Superficial Inguinal Ring

Located in the medial aspect of the inguinal canal, the aperture in the external oblique aponeurosis is recognized as the superficial, or external, abdominal ring (Fig. 2–3). It varies enormously in size, depending on the individual situation. In a simple congenital hernia it is small, whereas in a large direct hernia the ring may be greatly enlarged, and the fibers of the external oblique fascia may be spread apart. The shape of this opening also varies; it may be more triangular than oval. The aponeurotic fibers form the superior (medial) and inferior (lateral) crura, which makes definition of the ring a simple matter on digital examination. Lateral to the ring there may be seen a variable number of fibers running almost transversely between the crura; these are known as intercrural fibers. Beyond the superficial, or external, abdominal ring, the external oblique provides the cord with its external spermatic fascia. In this area the fascia is relatively thin.

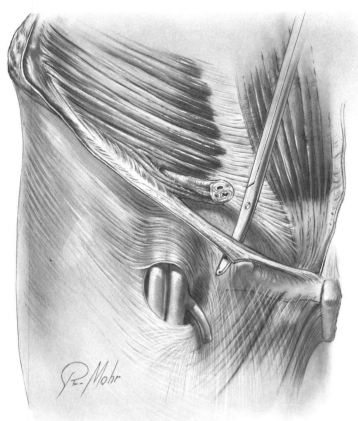

**Figure 2–4.** The inguinal ligament is poorly depicted in many illustrations; as a result, its structure is not well understood. Strictly speaking, it is not a ligament since it is a portion of the external oblique aponeurosis. It is no thicker than the aponeurosis of which it is an integral part. It is firmly attached laterally, but its edge is free medially where it can be separated easily from the transversalis fascia.

## Poupart's Ligament

The lowermost portion of the apo-neurosis of the external oblique muscle forms Poupart's ligament. It must be em-phasized that this ligament is no thicker than the structure from which it is derived, that is, the external oblique aponeurosis; McVay has repeatedly called attention to this fact. Gallaudet and McVay have pointed out that the medial lowermost margin of the inguinal ligament is free. It is attached firmly at the anterior superior iliac spine, and it is also attached to the fascia covering the iliopsoas muscle and the fascia lata of the thigh. The lateral portion of the inguinal ligament is firmly attached to bone and fascial structures, while the medial portion is comparatively easy to separate from the underlying transversalis fascia (Fig. 2–4). Lying la-terally under the inguinal ligament is the iliopsoas muscle, which is remarkably effective as a barrier to hernia formation; in fact, hernias are almost unheard of in this area.

The medial extent of Poupart's ligament lies over the femoral vessels. It is attached to the pubic tubercle; those fibers of the external oblique that insert into Cooper's ligament form the lacunar ligament of Gimbernat. The medial half of the inguinal ligament has a tenuous at-tachment to the transversalis fascia, which

it overlies. A portion of the ligament continues onto the lower portion of the rectus abdominis sheath, as the reflected inguinal ligament.

Since so many illustrators erroneously depict the inguinal ligament as a thick-ened ligamentous structure, it bears re-peating that this is not so. The inguinal ligament is as thick, but no thicker than the external oblique aponeurosis from which it is derived.

## Lacunar Ligament

The lacunar ligament of Gimbernat is a derivative of the inguinal ligament and, hence, of the aponeurosis of the external oblique muscle. The attachment of Pou-part's ligament to the pubic tubercle has been appreciated for some time, but the more complicated attachment of the la-cunar ligament to the iliopectineal line has been described relatively recently by Lytle, by McVay and Anson, and by Madden et al. (Fig. 2–5).

Lytle described the fan-shaped attach-ment of the lacunar ligament to the ilio-pectineal line as being fascial and ten-dinous. McVay has repeatedly stated that the lacunar ligament does not form the medial border of the normal femoral ring. Another important anatomic fact empha-sized by McVay is that the anterior margin

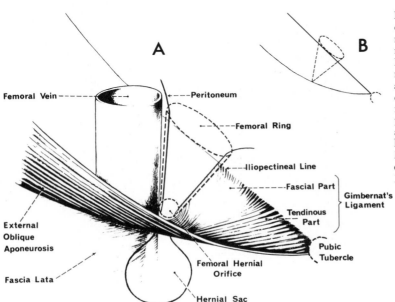

Figure 2–5. The relationship of the external oblique apo-neurosis and the lacunar liga-ment is clearly shown here. Note the attachment of the apo-neurosis to the pubic tubercle and the fan-shaped attachment of Gimbernat's ligament to the iliopectineal eminence. Re-printed with permission of author, W. J. Lytle, and of pub-lisher, In Nyhus, L. M.; and Harkins, N. H.: Hernia. Phila-delphia, J. B. Lippincott Co., 1964.

of the femoral ring is made up of the anterior femoral sheath—not the inguinal ligament, as noted in many textbooks. He also pointed out that the medial margin of the femoral ring is made up of the lateral attachment of the posterior abdominal wall to the iliopectineal ligament of Cooper. In the presence of herniation normal relationships are disrupted.

## Internal Oblique

The internal oblique muscle lies deep to the external oblique muscle. It arises from the iliac crest, the inguinal ligament, and the iliopsoas fascia. It inserts into the costal cartilages of the lower four ribs, the rectus sheath, and linea alba, and the pubis as the falx inguinalis. The internal oblique muscle appears largely as red muscle in the lateral portion of the in-

guinal area. The lowermost expanse of the muscle, taking its origin from the iliopsoas fascia, courses downward and obliquely above the cord toward the rectus sheath and pubis. In the lower abdomen the internal oblique continues onto the spermatic cord as the cremaster muscle. The general appearance of this muscle is illustrated in Figure 2–3. The strength and anatomic arrangement of the internal oblique are extremely variable in patients with groin hernias. This is generally true in individuals with direct inguinal hernias, where the interval between the lowermost fibers of the internal oblique and the inguinal ligament is wide.

## Transversus Abdominis

The transversus abdominis muscle originates from the lower six ribs, the lumbodor-

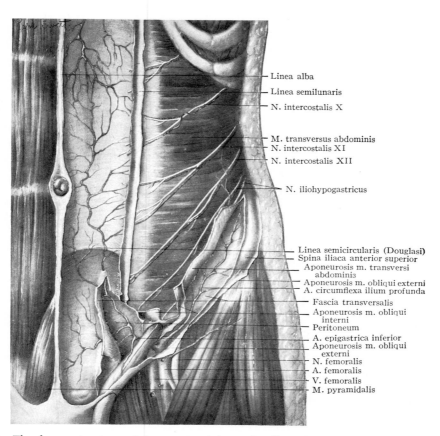

Linea alba
Linea semilunaris
N. intercostalis X

M. transversus abdominis
N. intercostalis XI
N. intercostalis XII

N. iliohypogastricus

Linea semicircularis (Douglasi)
Spina iliaca anterior superior
Aponeurosis m. transversi abdominis
Aponeurosis m. obliqui externi
A. circumflexa ilium profunda
Fascia transversalis
Aponeurosis m. obliqui interni
Peritoneum
A. epigastrica inferior
Aponeurosis m. obliqui externi
N. femoralis
A. femoralis
V. femoralis
M. pyramidalis

**Figure 2–6.** The deeper structures of the anterior abdominal wall include the posterior portion of the rectus sheath and the transversus abdominis muscle. The intercostal nerves are shown as they course over the muscle in a medial direction. Note the position of the linea semicircularis of Douglas. (Reprinted with permission from Anson, B. J., and McVay, C. B.: *Surgical Anatomy.* Philadelphia, W. B. Saunders Co., 1971.)

sal fascia, the iliac crest, the inguinal ligament, and the iliopsoas fascia (Fig. 2–6). From such a broad origin, the fibers pass in a transverse direction to the rectus sheath and the midline. The lower fibers of the transversus abdominis pass downward and medially and insert into the pubic crest, the tubercle, and the iliopectineal ligament of Cooper. Here the important anatomic detail is that the attachment of the transversus abdominis aponeurosis to Cooper's ligament forms the posterior inguinal wall in this area, and the lateral attachment forms the medial margin of the femoral ring.

The aponeurotic fibers of the transversus abdominis above the arcuate line (semicircular line, or fold of Douglas) pass posterior to the rectus abdominis muscle, while those below this level generally pass anteriorly and thus contribute to the anterior portion of the rectus sheath. The transversalis fascia and peritoneum usually comprise the posterior rectus sheath below the arcuate line. Variations in the precise location of the arcuate line are common, though it is frequently located midway between the umbilicus and symphysis pubis.

## Transversalis Fascia

The transversalis fascia is an extensive connective tissue layer that lines the entire abdominal cavity and lies just superficial to the peritoneum. It is not as easily recognized as, for instance, the external oblique fascia, but it is a distinct structure that varies in its appearance. The transversalis fascia forms a portion of the posterior sheath of the rectus abdominis muscle; it is contiguous with the fascia on the inferior surface of the diaphragm. It also lines the abdomen laterally and posteriorly, where it covers the psoas and quadratus lumborum. Furthermore, it is easily recognized in the pelvis, where it covers the levator ani muscles.

The transversalis fascia is one layer through which all hernias must pass; hence, the importance of this structure to the surgeon is clear. He must particularly appreciate the anatomy of the transversalis fascia in the inguinofemoral region. The great variation in its thickness, arrangement, and nomenclature accounts for the significant confusion and uncertainty as to the precise role the transversalis fascia plays in the genesis and repair of groin

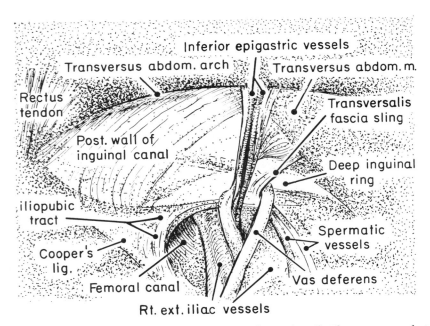

**Figure 2–7.** Posterior view of the lower right anterior abdominal wall. The important derivatives of the transversus abdominis are clearly shown. The strength and configuration of the fascial derivatives vary from patient to patient. (Reprinted from Condon, R. E.: Surgical anatomy of the transversus abdominis and transversalis fascia. Ann. Surg. 173:1–5, 1971. By courtesy of the author and with permission of J. B. Lippincott Co.)

hernias. Zieman emphasized that a strong, resistant transversalis fascia is essential to the avoidance of herniation.

It bears repeating that the transversalis fascia normally serves as a complete intact fascial lining for the entire abdominal wall. A number of terms are used to designate structures that are derivatives of the transversalis fascia (also called endoabdominal fascia). These structures include the transversalis fascial sling, a portion of the femoral sheath, the iliopubic tract (Thomson's ligament), the internal spermatic fascia, and the internal abdominal ring (Fig. 2–7).

The transversalis fascial sling is located at the internal abdominal ring. It may be considered a semicircular or curved condensation of the endoabdominal fascia on the medial aspect of the spermatic cord. The superior prolongation of this sling is known as the superior crus; the inferior crus of the sling lies just above the iliopubic tract.

The iliopubic tract may be recognized easily after division of the inguinal ligament. Its fibers actually parallel the inguinal ligament and become continuous with the anterior femoral sheath. There is a difference of opinion among surgeons as to the effective strength of the transversalis fascia in the repair of hernias. It is my opinion that the transversalis fascia and its derivative, the iliopubic tract, may be used in repair of small and moderate-sized indirect inguinal hernias, but they are not strong enough to contain a large direct hernia indefinitely in an individual who performs heavy work.

## Rectus Sheath and Rectus Abdominis

The rectus abdominis muscle and the rectus sheath are structures of paramount importance to the surgeon. They enter into the repair of ventral hernias located in the central abdomen, either above or below the umbilicus. Furthermore, the sheath of the rectus muscle is an important structure in that the relaxing incision, which is made in the anterior layer, is a basic adjunct in repair of direct, femoral, recurrent inguinal, and certain large indirect inguinal hernias.

The rectus abdominis muscle takes its origin from the lower thorax, specifically the fifth, sixth, and seventh costal cartilages as well as the xiphoid process. It attaches inferiorly to the superior pubic ramus and the symphysis. Three to five tendinous intersections, or inscriptions, cross the rectus muscle. They are attached to the anterior portion of the rectus sheath and, hence, serve to prevent retraction of the muscle in transverse incisions. The pyramidalis muscle is located medially within the lowermost portion of the rectus sheath.

The composition of the rectus sheath is variable, depending upon the level under consideration. Aponeurotic contributions from the three flat abdominal muscles that cross in the midline make up the powerful sheath.

If one were to select three different levels along the length of the rectus sheath, certain definite differences in the anatomic arrangement of the aponeurotic layers would become apparent (Fig. 2–8).

Midway between the xiphoid and the

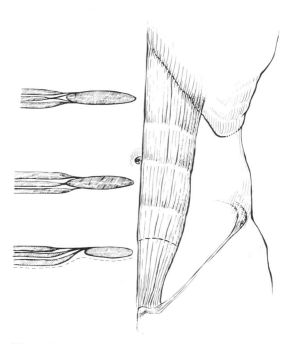

**Figure 2–8.** The rectus abdominis muscle extends from the thorax to the pelvis, where it inserts into the pubis. Contraction of the muscle causes forward flexion of the thorax toward the abdomen. The illustration shows the approximate disposition of the aponeuroses, derived from the flat abdominal muscles, as they form the rectus sheath at various levels.

umbilicus, the arrangement of the aponeurotic layers is such that the external
oblique aponeurosis passes in front of the
rectus abdominis muscle. The internal
oblique aponeurosis divides into two laminae at the lateral margin of the rectus
abdominis muscle. One layer passes in
front to form a portion of the anterior
sheath of the rectus, while the other layer
is contributed to the posterior rectus
sheath. Chouke found that the internal
oblique muscle splits into two parts from
its origin at the iliac crest to the linea
semilunaris.

Anson and McVay found the arrangement of the aponeurotic layers to be
somewhat different. They found that often
the external oblique and internal oblique
layers passed in front of the rectus without
the internal oblique dividing, while the
transversus abdominis aponeurosis actually provided a layer to the anterior sheath
and one to the posterior sheath as well.

Below the arcuate line, or the linea
semicircularis of Douglas, layers forming
the rectus sheath have yet another arrangement. Here the aponeurosis of the
external oblique, the internal oblique, and
the transversus abdominis muscles all pass
anterior to the rectus abdominis muscle.
The transversalis fascia forms the fascial
layer posterior to the rectus abdominis
muscles below the level of the arcuate
line. The arcuate line is found approximately midway between the umbilicus
and the symphysis pubis. As previously
noted, the posterior rectus sheath in this
area is composed of peritoneum, areolar
tissue, and transversalis fascia (Fig. 2-8).
Variations in the anatomic arrangement of
the laminae of the rectus sheath are common.

The blood supply to the rectus abdominis muscle is generous, coming from
above the muscle via the superior epigastric artery, which anastomoses with the
inferior epigastric. The inferior epigastric
artery takes origin from the external iliac
artery near the inguinal ligament. Upon
transverse section of the rectus abdominis,
two arterioles of considerable size are
encountered. These take origin from the
epigastric vessels and are found in the
medial and lateral portions of the rectus
abdominis muscle.

## NERVES

A knowledge of the nerve distribution is
of paramount importance to the surgeon
who performs abdominal operations. Sec-

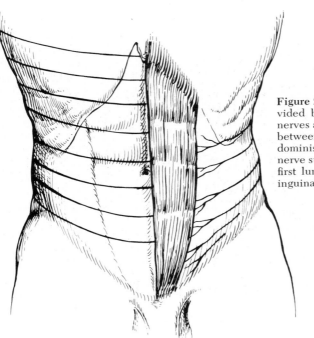

**Figure 2-9.** The nerve supply of the abdomen is provided by the ventral roots of the lower six thoracic
nerves and the first lumbar nerve. The main trunks run
between the internal oblique and the transversus abdominis muscles (see also Fig. 2-6). The tenth thoracic
nerve supplies the area about the umbilicus, while the
first lumbar nerve serves the groin through the ilioinguinal and iliohypogastric nerves.

tion of a single nerve results in little harm. Even the sensory functions are not greatly interfered with, since adjacent nerves overlap the area supplied. Division of two nerve trunks supplying the abdominal wall is not advisable, but the harm is not yet serious. If a third nerve trunk is divided, a particular type of hernia, or diffuse weakness, will result. Hence, the distribution of the intercostal nerves should be known to all who may incise the abdominal wall.

The segmental distribution of the intercostal nerves is well known (Fig. 2–9). The anterior rami are found between the internal oblique and the transversus abdominis muscles. These nerves run medially and penetrate the internal oblique muscle as they approach the rectus sheath. At the lateral margin of the rectus abdominis muscle, the nerves supply the muscle and its sheath. The sixth or seventh thoracic nerve supplies the epigastric area; the tenth innervates the area to the level of the umbilicus, while the twelfth thoracic nerve reaches the area just above the groin (see Fig. 2–6). The anterior rami of the first lumbar nerve complete the nerve supply to the inguinal area through the iliohypogastric and ilioinguinal nerves.

## HESSELBACH'S TRIANGLE

Every surgeon who may operate upon groin hernia must understand the boundaries of Hesselbach's triangle. This knowledge is basic to understanding direct and indirect inguinal hernias. Recognition and appreciation of the anatomic variants in this area are a necessity if disruptions here are to be repaired successfully.

The medial margin is made up of the lateral border of the rectus abdominis muscle and its sheath; at the inferior margin lies the inguinal ligament, and the lateral border of the triangle is marked by the deep inferior epigastric artery (Fig. 2–10). This artery arises from the external iliac artery just before it passes under the inguinal ligament. The cord lies anterior to the floor of this triangle after its egress from the abdomen just lateral to the deep inferior epigastric artery.

Indirect inguinal hernias arise lateral to the deep inferior epigastric artery. Such

hernias then continue in an oblique path along the cord from the internal abdominal ring, through the external ring, into the scrotum.

Direct hernias take an anterior path directly through the abdominal wall medial to the deep inferior epigastric artery.

Variations of the strength and configuration of the transversalis fascia, the transversus abdominis muscle, and the internal oblique muscle have much to do with the type of hernia seen in the groin. A clear understanding of the path taken by the various hernias as they protrude through the abdominal wall is essential if they are to be repaired successfully. An appreciation of the anatomy of Hesselbach's triangle leads to the correct differential diagnosis of direct and indirect inguinal hernias, and this, in turn, serves as a basis for effective repair.

## INGUINAL CANAL AND SPERMATIC CORD

The inguinal canal is not really a canal in the strict sense of the word. It should be thought of as an area, completely occupied by easily recognizable structures, that begins at the internal abdominal ring, which lies at a point approximately midway between the anterior superior iliac spine and the pubic tubercle, and the external abdominal ring, which is located just above and lateral to the pubic tubercle. The aponeurosis of the external oblique muscle lies anteriorly, and the inguinal ligament, as it curves posteriorly, forms the inferior boundary of the inguinal canal. Medially, the lacunar ligament forms a portion of the inferior boundary. Above, the internal oblique sweeps obliquely over the cord, thereby contributing the cremaster muscle to the spermatic cord. The transversus abdominis also contributes to the upper, or superior, wall of the canal. Transversalis fascia and a portion of the transversus abdominis arch are found posterior to the cord. The thickness of the cord in this area varies considerably. The cremaster muscle, contributed by the internal oblique, lies around the circumference of the cord except for the posterior aspect of the cord or that portion in contact with the transversalis fascia (Fig. 2–11).

In the male the spermatic cord traverses

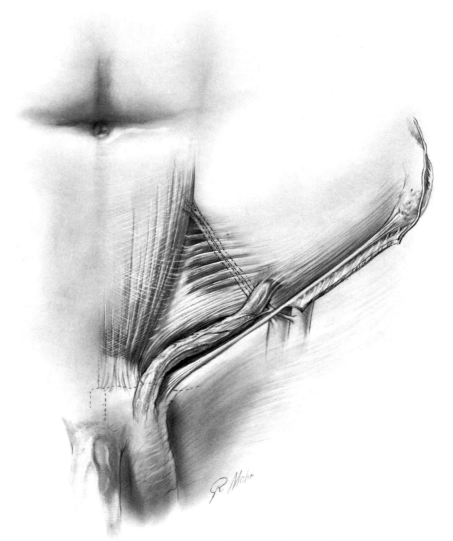

**Figure 2–10.**    Hesselbach's triangle is an important structure for the surgical anatomist, since it enables him to recognize fundamental differences between direct and indirect inguinal hernias. The boundaries include the margin of the rectus sheath medially, the inguinal ligament inferiorly, and the deep inferior epigastric artery laterally.

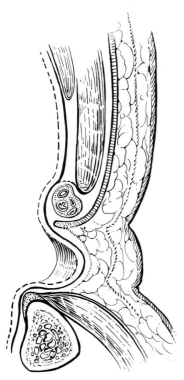

**Figure 2–11.** This parasagittal view shows the position of the cord anterior to the transversus abdominis layer. The external oblique aponeurosis lies anterior to the cord. This illustration is important because it clearly shows that the transversus abdominis layer, including the transversalis fascia, is anchored to Cooper's ligament.

the inguinal canal in an oblique direction, while in the female the smaller round ligament occupies the canal.

The spermatic cord in the inguinal canal is covered by the cremasteric muscle and fascia derived from the internal oblique muscle. In indirect inguinal hernias of long-standing duration, the cremaster muscle is greatly hypertrophied. On the other hand, in direct inguinal hernias, the cremaster muscle is usually poorly developed.

As the cord passes through the external abdominal ring, it acquires from the external oblique a fascial layer known as the external spermatic fascia.

The spermatic cord developmentally acquires its coverings as the testicle descends to its position in the scrotum. It retains a portion of the peritoneum as the processus vaginalis testis. If the processus vaginalis remains patent from the internal ring down to the testicle, a congenital

hernia results. After the peritoneum is traversed, the transversalis fascia is next encountered, and it provides the internal spermatic fascia to the cord.

Important structures composing the spermatic cord include the vas, or ductus, deferens; the artery to the vas; the venous, or pampiniform, plexus; the internal spermatic artery; the cremasteric, or external spermatic, artery; and the genitofemoral nerve and lymphatics. The remnant of the obliterated processus vaginalis is recognizable as an atrophic structure after full development of the infant (Fig. 2–12).

In the female the small round ligament is found in the area occupied by the spermatic cord in the male. The round ligament takes origin from the uterus, passes through the internal abdominal ring, down the inguinal canal, and finds its way through the external ring to the labia majora. The peritoneum that accompanies the cord is known as the canal of Nuck, but it becomes obliterated at approximately the sixth month of fetal life.

In adults, cysts in the inguinal canal may be the result of persistence of a portion of the canal of Nuck. If the entire peritoneal prolongation is patent, a congenital hernia results.

The spermatic cord in the male is recognizable at the internal ring, where the ductus deferens, together with the testicular artery and vein, forms a recognizable structure.

The ductus deferens, which passes upward from the testicle, is the most easily seen and palpated of all the structures within the cord. It feels very much like a thickened string or cord and usually measures approximately 2 mm in diameter.

The blood supply to the testicles is generous. The testicular, or internal spermatic, artery, which takes origin from the aorta, is an important source of blood supply to the testes. Another source of blood supply is the artery of the vas deferens, originating from the superior vesical artery. Blood may be supplied to the testicle via the external spermatic, or cremasteric, artery, which takes origin from the inferior epigastric at the medial aspect of the internal abdominal ring.

Venous drainage from the testicle is ample through the pampiniform plexus. Whereas the arteries are small and not

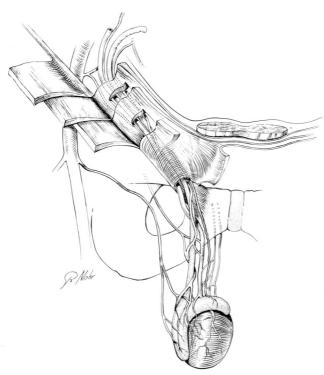

**Figure 2–12.** This schematic longitudinal view of the spermatic cord illustrates the contributions made to it by each abdominal wall layer. The external oblique muscle continues beyond the external abdominal ring as the external spermatic fascia; the internal oblique contributes the cremasteric muscle and fascia, and the transversalis fascia becomes the internal spermatic fascia.

easily seen, the venous plexus is easily seen upon division of the cremaster muscle. Should these veins become elongated, enlarged, and tortuous, a varicocele is the result. The plexus of veins ascends upward, forming the internal spermatic, or testicular, veins. The spermatic vein on the right usually empties into the inferior vena cava, while the one on the left empties into the left renal vein.

The important nerves closely related to the cord include the ilioinguinal and the genitofemoral nerves. The ilioinguinal takes origin mainly from the first lumbar nerve, passes through the internal oblique muscle medial to the anterior superior iliac spine, and usually passes downward with fibers of the cremaster muscle; it then courses through the external abdominal ring. It supplies sensory fibers to the anterior and lateral aspects of the scrotum. The ilioinguinal also serves as the motor nerve to the cremaster muscle.

The genitofemoral nerve takes origin from the first and second lumbar nerves. It passes downward on the psoas muscle and enters the cord at the internal ring. From this point, it continues downward with the cord to supply the base of the scrotum. The genital branch of the genitofemoral nerve serves as the nerve supply to the dartos musculature of the scrotum.

## INGUINOFEMORAL REGION

The structures of the inguinofemoral region deserve special consideration by the surgeon with specific interest in the hernia problem. This region becomes especially significant in cases of recurrent hernias where the inguinal ligament had been divided previously. Direct, indirect, and femoral hernias actually have their origins in the lower abdomen, but the femoral hernia finds its way into the upper thigh.

The area to be considered is bounded by Poupart's ligament above, the pectineus muscle medially, and the tensor fasciae latae laterally. Within this area is located the femoral triangle of Scarpa, which is bounded by Poupart's ligament above, the adductor longus muscle medially, and the sartorius muscle laterally (Fig. 2–13).

Superficial structures of importance in this region present in the region of the fossa ovalis. It is here that the greater or

Anatomy

31

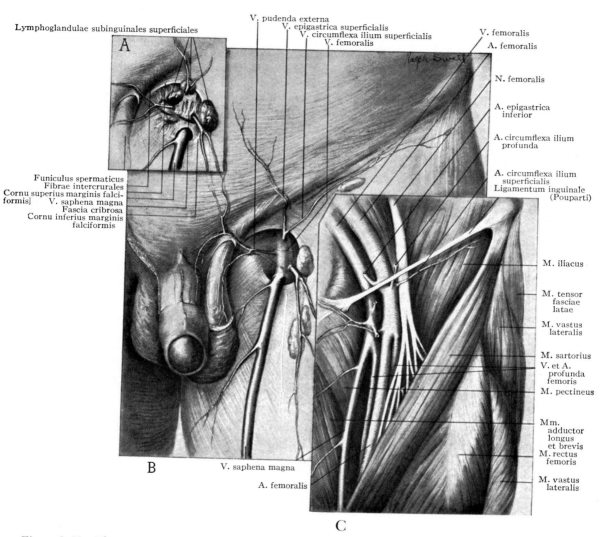

Lymphoglandulae subinguinales superficiales

V. pudenda externa
V. epigastrica superficialis
V. circumflexa ilium superficialis
V. femoralis

V. femoralis
A. femoralis

N. femoralis

A. epigastrica
inferior

A. circumflexa ilium
profunda

A. circumflexa ilium
superficialis
Ligamentum inguinale
(Pouparti)

Funiculus spermaticus
Fibrae intercrurales
Cornu superius marginis falci-
formis]
V. saphena magna
Fascia cribrosa
Cornu inferius marginis
falciformis

M. iliacus

M. tensor
fasciae
latae

M. vastus
lateralis

M. sartorius
V. et A.
profunda
femoris
M. pectineus

Mm.
adductor
longus
et brevis
M. rectus
femoris

M. vastus
lateralis

A

B

V. saphena magna

A. femoralis

C

**Figure 2–13.** The anatomic structures of the inguinofemoral are clearly presented in these illustrations. The superficial inguinal lymph nodes can be confused with a hernia, *A*. The superficial veins draining into the femoral vein at the fossa ovalis include the superficial external pudendal, the superficial epigastric, and the superficial circumflex iliac, *B*. After removal of the fascial coverings of the thigh, the femoral artery and its branches, the femoral vein, and the femoral nerve are seen, *C*. (Reprinted with permission from *Surgical Anatomy* by Anson and McVay, Philadelphia, W. B. Saunders Co., 1971.)

long saphenous vein passes through the fascia lata to empty into the femoral vein. A varicosity in this area may be confused with a femoral hernia. In addition, the external pudendal, the superficial epigastric, and the superficial circumflex iliac veins all empty into the femoral vein at the saphenous opening, or the fossa ovalis.

Several arteries take origin from the lower external iliac artery and the upper femoral artery in the region of the inguinal ligament. These vessels are the inferior epigastric, the deep circumflex iliac, and the superficial circumflex iliac arteries.

Lymphatics from the lower extremity, the perineum, the external genitalia, the anus, and the abdomen below the level of the umbilicus drain into the inguinal lymph nodes. The surgeon must be aware that an enlarged lymph node in the groin may be easily confused with a femoral hernia. There are two recognizable groups of lymph nodes, the superficial and the deep. The superficial nodes are related to the saphenous vein and the tributaries emptying into the femoral vein at the fossa ovalis. The deep inguinal lymph nodes are found beneath the fascia lata in the femoral triangle and are closely related to the femoral vein. The node of Cloquet is a large inguinal gland frequently found in the femoral canal beneath the inguinal ligament. It bears repetition that an enlarged and painful node of Cloquet or Rosenmüller may be confused with a femoral hernia.

The deeper structures of the upper thigh are covered by the deep fascia of the thigh. The saphenous opening, or fossa ovalis, is an anatomic defect in the deep fascia. It is covered with an attenuated connective tissue known as the cribriform fascia.

The important structures found in the upper thigh just distal to the inguinal ligament include the femoral vein, femoral artery, and femoral nerve.

## Femoral Sheath

After the subcutaneous tissues and fascia of the external oblique are removed, the deeper anatomic structures of the inguinofemoral region are seen. The iliopubic tract also may be seen. The relationship of the femoral sheath to the portion of trans-

versalis fascia designated as iliopubic tract is important (Fig. 2–14).

Within the upper and anterior portion of the thigh, posterior to the inguinal ligament, two distinct lacunae are easily recognized. The medial lacuna is known as the lacuna vasorum and contains the femoral canal medially and the femoral sheath just lateral to the potential femoral canal. From medial to lateral, the sequence of important anatomic structures in the lacuna vasorum include the femoral canal, the femoral vein, and the femoral artery (Fig. 2–15).

The lacuna vasorum is separated from the lacuna musculorum by a thickened fascia known as the iliopectineal arch. The iliopsoas muscle composes much of this lateral compartment, but the femoral nerve is an important component. It lies deep to the inguinal ligament and lateral to the femoral artery. To prevent injury of the femoral nerve, its position must be recalled by the surgeon operating upon complicated recurrent groin hernias.

The femoral sheath is largely a continuation of the transversalis fascia downward into the upper thigh for a distance of 3 to 4 cm. The anterior femoral sheath is a continuation of the transversalis fascia from the abdomen. The iliac fascia and the fascia covering the pectineus muscle form the posterior portion of the sheath. Inferiorly, the femoral sheath terminates at the profunda artery, where it combines with the adventitial layers of the femoral vessels. Connective tissue septa divide the sheath into arterial and venous compartments. The medial septum creates what amounts to a lymphatic compartment. Lymph nodes of variable sizes may be found in this area. Usually it amounts to a potential space.

In the medial aspect of the lacuna vasorum is the femoral canal. The femoral ring is the entrance to the canal. Its anterior margin is the anterior portion of the femoral sheath, a derivative of the transversalis fascia. The pectineus muscle and fascia, Cooper's ligament, and the superior ramus of the pubis make up the posterior aspect of the crural ring. The femoral vein and its connective tissue septum make up the lateral margin of the ring. The margin of the insertion of the transversus abdominis into Cooper's liga-

**Figure 2–14.** In this illustration, the external oblique aponeurosis has been ignored and the inguinal ligament divided. The continuity of the femoral sheath with the transversus abdominis layer is seen.

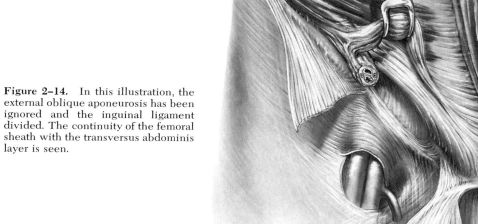

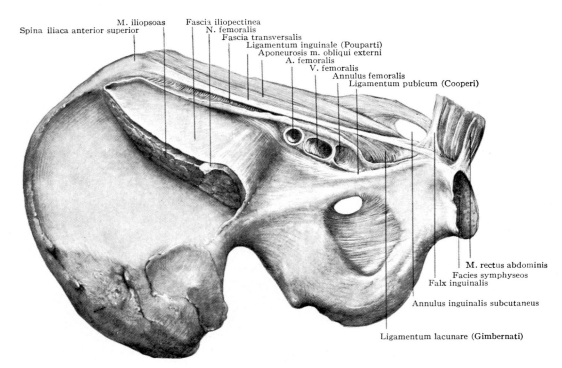

Spina iliaca anterior superior
M. iliopsoas
Fascia iliopectinea
N. femoralis
Fascia transversalis
Ligamentum inguinale (Pouparti)
Aponeurosis m. obliqui externi
A. femoralis
V. femoralis
Annulus femoralis
Ligamentum pubicum (Cooperi)

M. rectus abdominis
Facies symphyseos
Falx inguinalis

Annulus inguinalis subcutaneus

Ligamentum lacunare (Gimbernati)

**Figure 2–15.** The contents of the left femoral arch as seen from within the pelvis. The lacuna musculorum is seen laterally, with the important femoral nerve lying under the iliopectineal fascia. The precise location of the femoral ring can be seen in this view. (Reprinted with permission from *Surgical Anatomy* by Anson and McVay, Philadelphia, W. B. Saunders Co., 1971.)

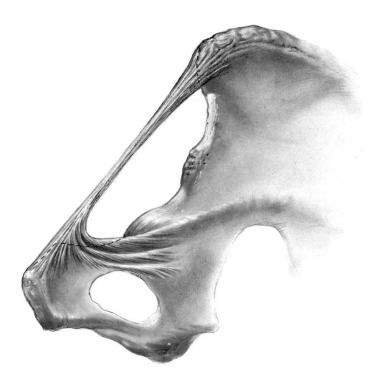

**Figure 2–16.** The angle between Cooper's ligament and the inguinal ligament may vary widely, as emphasized in this illustration. The distance between the inguinal ligament and Cooper's ligament will vary depending on whether example A, B, or C prevails. The anterior-posterior dimensions of the structures to be utilized in hernia repair must be considered by the surgeon.

ment comprises the medial boundary of the femoral ring.

Certainly, the inguinal ligament lies superficial to the transversalis fascia in the region of the femoral ring. Furthermore, in large femoral hernias Poupart's ligament is a firm, restraining structure. When a femoral hernia passes downward into the femoral canal and distends the ring, it then impinges upon the lacunar ligament as well. Thus, it is not difficult to understand why, for decades, the lacunar ligament was considered to be the medial limiting structure of a femoral hernia, and the inguinal ligament its anterior limiting structure.

Cooper's ligament is found on the superior ramus of the pubis. It consists of dense fibrous tissue of great strength and holding power when used in repair of hernias. This easily recognizable ligamentous tissue is always present and serves as a formidable anchoring structure to which the abdominal parities may be affixed. Its thickness is greatest medially, and then it decreases in size as it is traced laterally and posteriorly to the brim of the pelvis. It eventually becomes indistinguishable from the periosteum. In a few instances the lateral projection of Cooper's ligament is so attenuated that it can hardly be used in hernia repair. The transversalis fascia descends from above and is clearly and firmly attached to the ligament of Cooper.

The pectineus muscle arises from the superior pubic ramus and from Cooper's ligament. In the patient being operated for femoral hernia the whitish, glistening pectineus fascia is easily recognizable.

The direction taken by the iliopectineal eminence and its overlying Cooper's ligament varies considerably with the configuration of the individual pelvis. In some persons the course approaches the horizontal plane, whereas in others, the direction almost approaches the vertical plane. In other words, the angle between the inguinal ligament and Cooper's ligament is variable (Fig. 2–16).

In the female this angle is narrower than in certain male pelves. This is a matter of practical importance when considering the Moschcowitz repair of a femoral hernia whereby the individual inguinal ligament is approximated to Cooper's ligament.

## INGUINAL REGION

The surgeon must think of the inguinal area in a three-dimensional perspective. The angles and relationships of the inguinal ligament to Cooper's ligament and to the transversus abdominis arch are variable in different individuals, and particularly in patients with hernias. These structural or anatomic differences account for the variety of hernias seen in the groin. Furthermore, these same variations in anatomic relationships must be constantly kept in mind during attempts at repair of inguinal or femoral hernias.

The external oblique presents as an easily recognizable aponeurotic layer in the inguinal region. Its derivatives include the inguinal ligament and the lacunar ligament. The external oblique forms the anterior barrier to a hernia once it has developed, but it cannot prevent the formation or progression of a hernia. The hernia originating at the internal ring takes an oblique path toward the external ring.

The internal oblique muscle is muscular in its appearance in the upper and lateral aspects of the inguinal region. The red muscle mass, which is variable in amount, is seen above and lateral to the cord. Variation in the development and the insertion of the internal oblique and transversus abdominis muscles accounts for differences in structural integrity of the lower abdomen (Fig. 2–17).

Anson, Morgan, and McVay have shown that, in specimens in which there was no parietal defect, the internal oblique muscle was usually well developed and had its medial insertion low on the rectus sheath. The fibers of the lowermost portion of the internal oblique—those arising from the inguinal ligament and iliac crest—pass in an oblique direction toward the rectus abdominis and the pubis. The internal oblique contributes the cremaster muscle to the spermatic cord. Below the area, midway between the umbilicus and the symphysis, the aponeurosis at the internal oblique muscle passes as a single layer in front of the rectus, where it joins loosely with the aponeurosis of the external oblique to form the sheath of rectus abdominis muscle.

The specific development and arrangement of the internal oblique muscle and

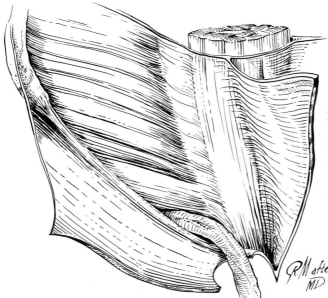

**Figure 2–17.** Variations in form and extent of the internal oblique muscle and the aponeurosis and its insertion account, in part, for various types of direct hernias seen by the physician. Reprinted with permission from Anson, B. J., and McVay, C. B.: Anatomy of the region inguinal hernia. Surg. Gynecol. Obstet. 66(2):186–191, 1938.

aponeurosis vary with the type of hernia seen. For instance, in the simple indirect inguinal hernia the internal oblique muscle is well developed and has its medial and inferior attachment near the inguinal ligament. The floor of Hesselbach's triangle is narrow.

On the other hand, in direct inguinal hernias the internal oblique muscle and aponeurosis are relatively poorly developed. In addition, the attachment medially is higher on the rectus sheath, or more cephalad; the result is a wide interval between the lowermost fibers of the internal oblique and the inguinal ligament. The resultant defect in the floor of Hesselbach's triangle is also wide as a consequence.

An important anatomic detail not fully understood by all surgeons is that the spermatic cord passes from the abdomen below or inferior to the lower border of the transversus abdominis muscle. It does, however, penetrate the internal oblique muscle from which it acquires the cremaster muscle. The portion of the transversus abdominis muscle in the inguinal region, like the internal oblique, takes origin from the iliopsoas fascia. Above the inguinal region, the aponeurotic fibers of the internal oblique join those of the transversus abdominis to form the rectus sheath. A most important detail in the anatomic

arrangement in the inguinal area is the insertion of the transversus abdominis into Cooper's ligament. Here the lowermost fibers of the transversus abdominis insert into the iliopectineal ligament from the pubic tubercle laterally to the point of formation of the medial margin of the femoral ring. The transversus abdominis muscle does not ordinarily appear as red muscle in the floor of Hesselbach's triangle. Here aponeurotic fibers are commonly seen, but their strength and attachment are variable. For instance, in direct inguinal hernia these fibers have a high insertion and are poorly developed. In such situations the aponeuroses of the internal oblique and the transversus abdominis are poorly developed in the inguinal region, and the transversalis fascia alone is insufficient to support the floor of the inguinal canal (Fig. 2–18).

An accurate description of the inguinal region as viewed from the posterior aspect was presented by Condon in the book on hernia by Nyhus and Harkins; it is reproduced here as Figure 2–7. The relationships and distribution of the derivations of the structures of the transversus abdominis lamina are very clearly shown. There remains some difference of opinion as to the precise anatomic arrangement and distribution of the transversalis fascia and that derived from the transversus

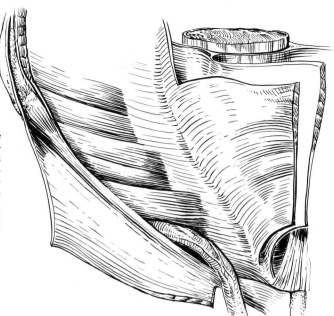

**Figure 2–18.** Variations also occur in the form, extent, and distribution of the transversus abdominis muscle. The insertion of its aponeurosis into Cooper's ligament is variable; when this insertion is narrow, it may result in not only direct hernias but also femoral hernias. Reprinted from Anson, B. J., and McVay, C. B.: Anatomy of the region inguinal hernia. Surg. Gynecol. Obstet.: 66 (2):186–191, 1938.

abdominis. Perhaps the most significant current advance in operative treatment of hernia comes from a full appreciation of the importance of the transversus abdominis and transversalis fascia in preserving the integrity of the abdominal wall. Groin hernias must pass through the transversalis fascia and its derivatives before they can displace, attenuate, or disrupt the internal and external oblique muscles and their aponeuroses.

## PELVIC PERITONEAL FOSSAE

The anatomic arrangement and significance of the peritoneal folds in the lower abdomen generally are poorly understood. The peritoneum lines the abdominal cavity and beneath it is a variable amount of adipose tissue. This is especially true in the lower abdomen. The surgeon encounters three peritoneal folds and certain fossae when operating in the lower abdomen. The surgical resident may find correct identification of these structures difficult.

The peritoneal fossae are significant because they are directly concerned in the formation of specific types of groin hernias. A middle, or midline, fold and two

lateral folds on each side are formed by surgically important structures which form fossae from lateral to the medial aspects as follows: the lateral inguinal fossa, the medial inguinal fossa, and the supravesical fossa (Fig. 2–19).

The lateral umbilical fold is composed of a fold of peritoneum, variable amounts of adipose tissue, and the deep inferior epigastric artery. The lateral inguinal fossa is situated in the region of the internal abdominal ring where the vas deferens and spermatic vessels converge to form a portion of the spermatic cord. The indirect inguinal hernia begins its egress at this point and therefore is sometimes called an external hernia. The middle, or medial, inguinal fossa is found medial to the deep inferior epigastric artery. This fossa occupies the interval between the inferior epigastric artery and the medial umbilical ligament. The medial umbilical ligament consists of a fold of peritoneum and the obliterated umbilical artery. This structure is atrophic and somewhat resembles a small artery, but in the adult it has no function. A depression in this fossa is situated in the area of Hesselbach's triangle. The direct or internal hernia takes origin from this fossa. The supravesical or internal inguinal fossa lies between the medial umbilical ligament

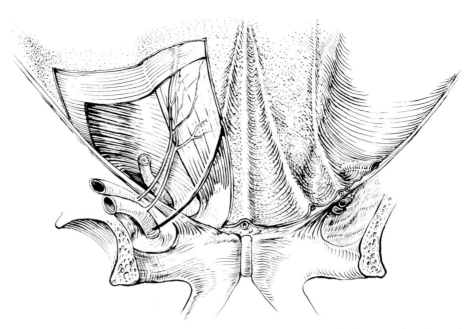

**Figure 2–19.**   The inferior epigastric artery, the obliterated umbilical artery, and the urachus form ridges on the posterior abdominal wall; this results in the formation of the external fossa, the middle fossa, and the internal, or supravesical, fossa. The indirect hernia finds its exit from the lateral fossa while the direct inguinal hernia passes through the middle fossa.

and the middle umbilical ligament, or fold, which is derived from the urachus and occupies the midline. In this region the abdominal wall has great strength due to the presence of the rectus abdominis muscle and rectus sheath. A variety of direct hernia may occasionally escape lateral to the rectus muscle and medial to the obliterated umbilical artery.

## REFERENCES

Anson, B. J., and McVay, C. B.: Inguinal hernia: I. The anatomy of the inguinal region. Surg. Gynecol. Obstet. 66:186, 1938.

Anson, B. J., Morgan, E. H., and McVay, C. B.: Surgical anatomy of the inguinal region based upon a study of 500 body halves. Surg. Gynecol. Obstet. 111:707, 1960.

Chouke, K. S.: The constitution of the sheath of the rectus abdominis muscle. Anat. Rec. 61:341, 1935.

Cox, H. T.: The cleavage lines of the skin. Br. J. Surg. 29:234, 1941.

Gallaudet, B. B.: A Description of the Planes of Fascia of the Human Body. New York, Columbia University Press, 1931.

Lytle, W. J.: The internal inguinal ring. Br. J. Surg. 32:441, 1945.

Madden, J. L., Hakim, S., and Agorogiannis, A. G.: The anatomy and repair of inguinal hernias. Surg. Clin. North Am. 15(6):1269, 1971.

McVay, C. B.: The normal and pathologic anatomy of the transversus abdominis muscle in inguinal and femoral hernia. Surg. Clin. North Am. 51(6): 1251, 1971.

McVay, C. B.: Preperitoneal hernioplasty. Surg. Gynecol. Obstet. 123:349, 1966.

McVay, C. B.: Hernia. The Pathologic Anatomy of the More Common Hernias and Their Anatomic Repair. Springfield, Ill., Charles C Thomas, 1954.

McVay, C. B., and Anson, B. J.: A fundamental error in current methods of inguinal herniorrhaphy. Surg. Gynecol. Obstet. 74:746, 1942.

McVay, C. B., and Anson, B. J.: The composition of the rectus sheath. Anat. Rec. 77:213, 1940.

McVay, C. B., and Anson, B. J.: Aponeurotic and fascial continuities in the abdomen, pelvis and thigh. Anat. Rec. 76:213, 1940.

McVay, C. B., and Savage, L. E.: Etiology of femoral hernia. Ann. Surg. 154(suppl. 25):14–57, 1961.

Nyhus, L. M., and Harkins, N. H.: Hernia. Philadelphia, J. B. Lippincott Co., 1964.

Zieman, S. A.: The fallacy of the conjoined tendon: The etiology and repair of inguinal hernia. Am. J. Surg. 50:17, 1940.

## Supplemental Readings

Basmajian, J. Y.: Grant's Method of Anatomy (8th ed.) Baltimore, Williams & Wilkins Co., 1971.

Chandler, S. B.: Studies on the inguinal region: II – The anatomy of the inguinal region (Hesselbach's) triangle. Ann. Surg. 124:156, 1946.

Chandler, S. B., and Schadewald, M.: Studies on the inguinal region: I. The conjoined aponeurosis versus the conjoined tendon. Anat. Rec. 89:339, 1944.

Fruchaud, H.: *Anatomie Chirugicale des Hernies de l'Aine.* Paris, C. Doin & Cie, 1956.

Hollinshead, W. H.: *Anatomy for Surgeons: Vol. 2. The Thorax, Abdomen and Pelvis* (2nd ed.). New York, Harper & Row, Publishers, Inc., 1971.

Hollinshead, W. H.: *Anatomy for Surgeons: Vol. 3. The Back and Limbs* (2nd ed.). New York, Harper & Row, Publishers, Inc., 1971.

Pick, J. W., Anson, B. J., and Ashley, F. L.: The origin of the obturator artery: A study of 640 body halves. Am. J. Anat. 70:317, 1942.

Tobin, C. E., Benjamin, J. A., and Wells, J. C.: Continuity of the fasciae lining of the abdomen, pelvis, and spermatic cord. Surg. Gynecol. Obstet. 83:575, 1946.

# 3

# Diagnosis of Hernia

*A protrusion of any viscus from its proper cavity is denominated a hernia.*

Sir Astley Cooper, 1804

In modern surgical practice, smaller and smaller hernias are being diagnosed and treated. In fact, such unsatisfactory terms as "pre-hernia" are creeping insidiously into the surgeon's vocabulary. By definition, if there is no protrusion, then the diagnosis of hernia is unwarranted. It is obvious that the protrusion is not necessarily continuous, since the contents may return to the abdominal cavity. A demonstrable protrusion is a useful and practical manifestation of herniation. In order for the swelling or protrusion to become manifest, there must be a pre-existing defect in the abdominal wall. X-ray examinations with radiopaque media are being employed by some physicians to demonstrate patency of the processus vaginalis. It should be recalled that simple patency of the processus without protrusion through the internal ring does not warrant the diagnosis of hernia. X-ray studies should be employed to obtain more accurate and detailed information in individual patients, but the diagnosis of hernia should remain largely clinical.

The erroneous idea prevalent among too many physicians and surgeons is that the diagnosis of hernia is simple and a differential diagnosis is unimportant. After having reviewed hundreds of medical records, I am convinced that there is a great need for reassessment of our diag-

nostic accuracy when dealing with hernias. The poorly developed clinical history and superficial physical examination lead to the noncommittal diagnosis of inguinal hernia. Too frequently the diagnosis may be recorded as "bilateral hernia" without further definition. How often have we seen "inguinal hernia" recorded in the medical record without further attempt at precise diagnosis? Incarcerated and strangulated femoral hernias may be overlooked completely, and an emergency memorandum may occasionally reveal the diagnosis of "intestinal obstruction." Rarely is the clinician willing to record the diagnosis of a sliding indirect inguinal hernia. Such a general attitude of indifference toward accuracy in diagnosis inevitably leads to improper operative treatment. We have seen more than one instance in which a femoral hernia was overlooked by the surgeon operating for an inguinal hernia.

The pelvic floor may be the site of an obturator hernia, a sciatic hernia, or a perineal hernia. There are a number of other areas in which protrusions occur through the confining structures of the abdomen and pelvis.

Hernias of the diaphragm are internal hernias and may be either congenital or acquired. The most commonly encountered diaphragmatic hernia is the acquired

## Table 3–1. CLASSIFICATION OF HERNIAS

### I. INGUINAL REGION

A. Indirect or Oblique Inguinal Hernias
  Congenital, incomplete, complete scrotal, or sliding
  Acquired, sliding
  Recurrent, sliding
  Any of these hernias may be incarcerated, obstructed, or strangulated.
B. Direct Inguinal Hernias (including diverticular type)
  Acquired, sliding
  Recurrent, sliding
  Direct inguinal hernias occur in the older age group and seldom become incarcerated or strangulated.
C. Femoral Hernias
  Acquired
  Recurrent
  *Femoral hernias are the most frequently overlooked hernia by clinicians and surgeons. The small femoral hernia is the most common variety, giving rise to obstruction and strangulation.*
D. Combination of Inguinal Hernias
  Direct-Indirect, the so-called pantaloon or saddlebag hernia.
  Direct-Femoral
  Indirect-Femoral
  Direct-Indirect-Femoral
  NOTE: The diagnostic possibility of a combination of defects is seldom recorded in the medical record at the time of physical examination. The surgeon is most likely to recognize the existence of a combination of defects *only after digital exploration at the time of operation.*

### II. ABDOMINAL WALL HERNIAS, OTHER THAN INGUINAL

A. Umbilical Hernia
  Congenital (neonates and children)
  Acquired (Adults)
B. Epigastric Hernia
C. Lumbar Hernia (through the inferior lumbar triangle of Petit)
D. Lumbar Hernia (through the superior lumbar triangle of Grynfelt-Lesshaft)
E. Lateral Ventral or Spigelian
F. Ventral-Postoperative or Incisional Hernias
  These hernias are largely iatrogenic in nature. In the groin, appendectomy incision may be the site of a ventral hernia resembling an inguinal hernia.

hernia protruding upward about the esophageal hiatus. Diaphragmatic hernias and eventration of the diaphragm may be secondary to trauma.

Congenital defects through the foramen of Bochdalek give rise to posterior and lateral diaphragmatic hernia, while a parasternal hernia may protrude through the foramen of Morgagni. Eventration of the diaphragm occurs when there is a congenital defect in the muscular development, or it may be acquired, for example, as a result of injury to the phrenic nerve.

There are a number of internal hernias that should be recalled for the sake of completeness. Hernias may occur about the paraduodenal fossae and through the foramen of Winslow into the lesser peritoneal cavity. They may protrude through the mesentery of the colon, about the cecum, in the region of the sigmoid colon, and above the bladder between the obliterated umbilical artery and the urachus. Such hernias are frequently seen in association with congenital anomalies.

Common varieties of abdominal wall hernias are listed in Table 3–1. This classification serves as a partial list of diagnostic possibilities that the surgeon must keep in mind if errors in diagnosis and treatment are to be avoided.

## PRINCIPAL ETIOLOGIC FACTORS

Before considering the history and physical examination presented by the patient with hernia, it is wise to discuss the various etiologic factors that lead to herniation. In every patient, the forces that cause protrusion are opposed by the restraining effect of the abdominal wall.

There are two mechanisms that protect man against hernia, to a greater or lesser degree. First, the oblique path taken by the cord through the abdominal laminae indirectly serves to protect the integrity of the abdominal wall. Second, the internal oblique muscles function much like a shutter over the internal abdominal ring. This is easily demonstrated when a hernia is being repaired under local anesthesia by simply requesting that the patient give a lusty cough.

It may be helpful to think of the various factors discussed under the following headings, as summarized in Table 3–2.

### Congenital Factors

The congenital factors that contribute to the formation of hernia are most readily recognized in indirect inguinal hernias and umbilical hernias.

### Table 3–2.  PRINCIPAL ETIOLOGIC FACTORS IN HERNIA

1. Congenital Factors
   a. Sex
   b. Descent of the testicle
   c. Maldevelopment of the abdominal wall
   d. Gastroschisis
   e. Subtle variants in the attachment and arrangement of abdominal muscles

2. Contributing Factors
   a. Aging
   b. Obesity
   c. Cardiac disease
   d. Pulmonary disease
   e. Prostatism
   f. Constipation, diverticular disease, and colonic carcinomas
   g. Genitourinary tract disease
   h. Pregnancy

3. Precipitating or Exciting Causes
   a. Sudden increase in intra-abdominal pressure
   b. Trauma

SEX has a great bearing on the variety and frequency of hernias seen. Inguinal hernias are seen more frequently in men than in women in a ratio of 9:1. Umbilical hernias are common in the female, whereas indirect and direct inguinal hernias are far more commonly seen in the male.

DESCENT OF THE TESTICLE.  The relationship of descent of the testes to indirect inguinal hernia is well recognized. As the testicle descends toward the scrotum, it carries with it a tubular projection of peritoneum known as the processus vaginalis. If, in addition to the patent processus vaginalis, there is an enlarged inguinal ring, the newborn infant may present a hernia promptly with the first cry. On the other hand, the peritoneal prolongation may be quite narrow; thus, in the presence of a well-developed internal ring, herniation may not appear until early adulthood when strenuous physical activity forces a viscus along the sac that had been present since birth.

MALDEVELOPMENT OF THE ABDOMINAL WALL AND GASTROSCHISIS.  I have seen indirect inguinal hernias occurring in three generations of several families. The anatomic configuration inherited by the son from the father and grandfather predisposes to herniation. In umbilical defects in neonates, abnormal development of the abdominal wall results in the prompt appearance of hernia. Rarely an abdominal wall defect may occur outside the umbilicus, with resultant gastroschisis.

SUBTLE VARIANTS IN THE ATTACHMENT AND ARRANGEMENT OF ABDOMINAL MUSCLES.  The female is peculiarly free of direct inguinal hernia. The narrowness of the interval between the transversus arch and the inguinal ligament is an important factor in protecting women against direct inguinal hernias. On the other hand, the configuration of the pelvis and the musculo-aponeurotic attachments in women is such that they frequently develop femoral hernias.

CONGENITAL ETIOLOGIC FACTORS IN THE DEVELOPMENT OF DIRECT INGUINAL HERNIA are more difficult to recognize. Direct hernias occur much later in life than do indirect hernias, and strenuous activity is often an important contributing factor to herniation. The evidence is convincing that the pattern of anatomic development in the inguinal area, including the disposition of the transversalis fascia and the transversus abdominis muscle, has a direct bearing on the eventual appearance of hernias through the floor of Hesselbach's triangle.

### Contributing Factors

A number of conditions and diseases should be considered as predisposing or contributing to hernia formation.

AGING is a factor in hernia formation, but its precise influence is difficult to state. With aging, a certain amount of atrophy of tissue occurs. This leads to a gradual weakening of the inguinal floor and the internal ring, with the result that direct and acquired indirect inguinal hernias appear. The geriatric patient suffers from certain conditions (such as pulmonary emphysema) that often result in an increase in intra-abdominal pressure. Direct and indirect sliding hernias are seen in increasing numbers as the age of the patient advances.

OBESITY is more difficult to assess as a factor in hernia formation. It is a well-recognized fact that umbilical and incisional hernias are commonly seen in obese women. There is no doubt that obesity increases intra-abdominal pressure. Fatty infiltration decreases the quality of abdominal musculature. The muscles become lax, and as they separate at the umbilicus herniation results.

CARDIAC DISEASE leads to congestive failure, with ascites and increased intra-abdominal pressure. Dyspnea may further aggravate the situation, with the result that a small direct or indirect sliding hernia becomes unmanageable with a truss.

PULMONARY DISEASES, including emphysema, bronchitis, and pneumonitis, also cause an increase in abdominal pressure. Coughing further aggravates the situation.

PROSTATISM causes obstruction to the flow of urine. In an attempt to overcome the obstruction, the patient must strain to void, so intra-abdominal pressure rises. Any point of weakness in the abdominal wall will permit a hernia to develop.

CONSTIPATION, DIVERTICULAR DISEASE, AND COLONIC CARCINOMAS result in bowel dysfunction. If the patient strains at stool repeatedly, a protrusion may result. Elderly patients with recently recognized hernias must be carefully examined for colonic disturbances.

GENITOURINARY DISEASES, such as cystitis, cystocele, and urethrocele, may cause serious voiding problems in women. The intra-abdominal pressure rises to overcome the resistance to the flow of urine.

PREGNANCY has been considered a factor in the development of umbilical and femoral hernias. Repeated pregnancies may cause separation and some atrophy of the rectus abdominis muscles. Furthermore, increased pressure within the abdomen causes protrusion to occur at the umbilicus or in the femoral area.

### Precipitating or Exciting Causes

Any of a number of other conditions causing ascites and increased pressure within the abdomen will contribute to the formation of a hernia in the patient with a weakened abdominal wall. Cirrhosis of the liver with ascites and abdominal tumors, both benign and malignant, can increase the intra-abdominal pressure significantly. Precipitating or exciting causes for herniation are comparatively few in number.

SUDDEN INCREASE IN INTRA-ABDOMINAL PRESSURE, when exerted upon an abdominal wall or inguinal area previously weakened by congenital defects or acquired abnormalities, will produce a visible or palpable protrusion. Coughing, straining, heavy lifting, sneezing, or crying may cause a hernia to appear.

TRAUMA, such as a severe, sudden blow to the abdomen or a crushing injury, may cause a disruption of the abdominal wall, resulting in hernia. Direct and severe trauma is not a frequent cause of hernia in my experience.

### THE HISTORY

The patient is most helpful in arriving at the correct diagnosis if he is able to describe the presence of a "swelling," "knot," or "lump" in the inguinal area. Infants, of course, cannot communicate their problems, but in such situations, the parents are helpful. The swelling or protrusion appears after heavy lifting, straining or coughing or simply after prolonged standing. The mother may describe a protrusion in the groin when the infant cries. Most adult patients will report that the swelling disappears after cessation of activity or after reclining. Some curious patients will recognize that pressure applied over the mass causes it to disappear. It is truly remarkable that a number of elderly patients have been able to tolerate the discomfort and embarrassing physical deformity due to large scrotal hernias for as long as 40 years. The average patient seen in modern practice, however, has a relatively small hernia, which has been present for several weeks or months.

While the protrusion due to hernia is related to activity and physical exertion, the swelling due to tumor shows no such relationship. A tumor appears as a small swelling initially; then, it becomes progressively larger and never disappears. It may cause little or no discomfort.

The enlarged inguinal lymph node appears rather rapidly, is tender to palpation, and occurs in the presence of infection or dermatitis of the lower abdomen, groins, buttocks, perineum, and lower extremities. The swelling due to lymphadenitis is persistent and does not disappear upon reclining.

Pain attributable to the presence of an uncomplicated hernia is ordinarily not severe. Even large hernias may cause the stoic patient very little discomfort. A burning type of pain is frequently described by the patient. Other individuals describe a sensation of pressure over the area or a dragging or pulling sensation. Severe, constant pain in the region of an irreducible mass suggests incarceration. Cramping abdominal pain associated with nausea and vomiting is seen in patients with obstruction. If the incarcerated mass persists for periods of 48 to 72 hours, strangulation is a strong possibility.

Attention should be paid to the severity of the pain and its pattern of distribution. If the patient complains bitterly of pain while demonstrating a small, uncomplicated hernia, the surgeon must seek other possible explanations. Although not common, pain in the groin may be due to low back problems and disorders of the hip as well as prostatic disease.

Few patients seen today attempt to control their hernias by wearing trusses. Such appliances frequently fail to maintain reduction in those individuals who need help the most. I have seen patients in congestive heart failure and in severe respiratory difficulty due to emphysema who could not maintain reduction of herniations by wearing appliances

Infants cannot describe the swelling due to hernia, but the mother's account of a swelling in the groin must be taken seriously. Babies often cause a hernia to appear while crying.

Details of previous operative treatment of hernia should be carefully recorded. It is advisable to obtain the previous operative note if possible. Such information will be useful if the recurrent hernia is to be repaired with greater ease. For example, it is advantageous for the surgeon to know the location of the cord and the type of repair previously attempted.

Complications occurring after initial surgical treatment should also be carefully detailed. Wound infections and postoperative bleeding or hematomas are of particular interest.

Furthermore, the length of time elapsing from repair to recurrence should be noted. A few patients insist that the recurrence was observed while in the hospital or shortly after discharge from the hospital.

These more than likely are examples of overlooked hernias.

A few patients with exaggerated symptoms will complain of sexual impotency. On occasion, they may attribute their loss of sexual powers to the presence of a hernia. The simple truth must be carefully explained to such individuals before embarking upon a surgical misadventure.

Finally, from time to time, a patient is seen with a history of orchitis that has led to testicular atrophy. The importance of recording such details is obvious.

## PHYSICAL EXAMINATION

A thorough physical examination must be performed on every patient with hernia. This is especially true of aged patients who are so often afflicted with degenerative, cardiac, pulmonary, renal, and metabolic diseases. Infants are likely to have congenital anomalies associated with their hernias.

In order to avoid an operation on the wrong side, it is most important that the operating surgeon be the one who performs the physical examination that leads to the diagnosis of hernia in the first place.

Prior to examination, the patient must remove all clothing so that the entire abdomen is seen. The patient is asked to point out the site of swelling or location of his discomfort. The precise location of the hernia and the direction it follows are important details to be noted. The indirect inguinal hernia commences its egress at the internal ring above Poupart's ligament and continues obliquely toward the external ring (Fig. 3–1). Its path of protrusion is characteristically oblique, hence, the term "oblique" hernia. The direct hernia appears somewhat more medially and takes a direct path through the abdominal wall in an anterior direction (Fig. 3–2). It does not reach the scrotum, as does the indirect inguinal hernia. Furthermore, only the largest direct hernias reach the upper scrotal area.

The femoral hernia is easily diagnosed in many patients, but at times, it may cause difficulties in diagnosis. A small hernia in an obese patient may easily be overlooked. This is especially true of the small incarcerated femoral hernia in the senile patient whose ability to communicate has been impaired. The femoral hernia may take an upward course, in which case, it can be misinterpreted as a direct inguinal hernia (Fig. 3–3). At the other times it may project somewhat medially toward the scrotum, suggesting an indirect inguinal hernia (Fig. 3–4). Note that the hernia lies below a line from the anterior superior iliac spine to the pubic tubercle. If the femoral sac is thin, with a bulbar expansion in the upper thigh, the presence of an enlarged lymph node may be suspected (Fig. 3–5).

Since a large saphenous varix may appear at the fossa ovalis, it too may be confused with a femoral hernia. There is little excuse for confusing a hydrocele with a femoral hernia.

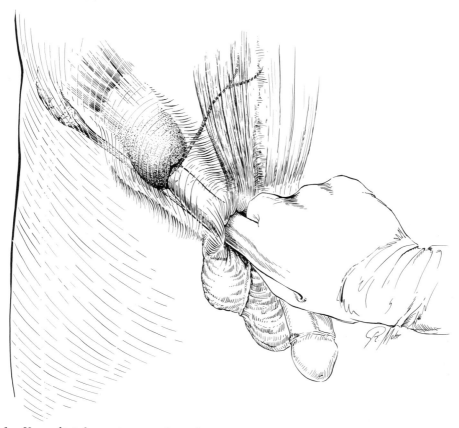

**Figure 3–1.** Upon digital examination, the indirect inguinal hernia can be seen to protrude through the abdomen at the internal ring, lateral to the deep inferior epigastric artery. The floor of Hesselbach's triangle is intact.

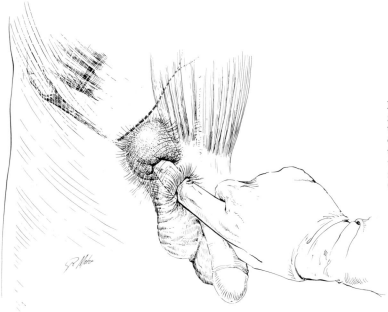

**Figure 3–2.** In a direct inguinal hernia, the mass protrudes directly through the floor of Hesselbach's triangle, medial to the deep inferior epigastric vessels. The weak inguinal floor may permit palpation of Cooper's ligament.

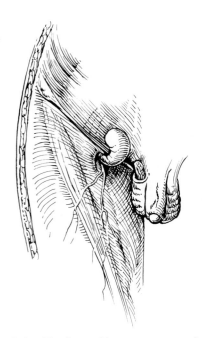

**Figure 3–3.** The femoral hernia may extend upward after passing through the fossa ovalis; thus, it may be confused with a direct inguinal hernia.

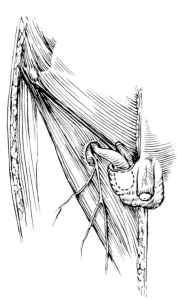

**Figure 3–4.** If the femoral hernia, after passing through the fossa ovalis, takes a path towards the scrotum, it may be confused with an indirect inguinal hernia.

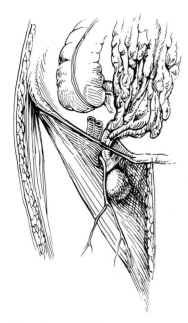

**Figure 3–5.** If a small femoral hernia protrudes through the fossa ovalis and remains unchanged for some time, it may lead to the diagnosis of inguinal lymphadenopathy.

After inspection, gentle and considerate palpation must be carried out in a methodical fashion. The hands must be warm to avoid reflex contraction of the abdominal musculature. The size, shape, consistency, and mobility of the testes must be noted. Atrophic testicles may be present prior to any operative treatment as a result of antecedent mumps orchitis.

It is essential to examine the patient both in the standing and in the reclining decubitus positions if diagnostic errors are to be avoided.

On digital examination, the indirect hernia sac will be noted to egress at the internal ring and to follow the index finger in an oblique path to the external ring (see Fig. 3–1). If the hernia is large, I prefer to reduce it prior to digital examination. The indirect hernia is located above a line from the anterior superior iliac spine to the pubic tubercle. In such hernias, the inguinal floor is strong, and Cooper's ligament and the iliopectineal eminence cannot be reached.

On digital examination, the direct inguinal hernia presents through the floor of Hesselbach's triangle (see Fig. 3–2). Again, this type of hernia lies above the inguinal ligament. The examining index finger may be inserted deeply so as to identify the size of the defect, and it may be possible to reach the area of Cooper's ligament. This maneuver cannot be performed when an indirect hernia is present in a patient with an intact inguinal floor.

Only thorough palpation will reveal the presence of small femoral hernias in obese women, or obese men, for that matter. Again, the relationship of the protrusion to the inguinal ligament is essential. There is ordinarily no protrusion above the inguinal ligament in femoral hernias, but it may reach the area after passing through the fossa ovalis. The groin must be thoroughly palpated for a mass below the inguinal ligament deep in the inguinal crease. Femoral hernias are commonly associated with incarcerated preperitoneal fat; hence, after a determined search, the mass, though small, may be recognized.

In a patient with obstructive symptoms, a small Richter's hernia may be deceptive to the clinician. Hyperactive bowel sounds, the absence of marked abdominal distention, and the presence of a small mass in the groin should suggest the possibility of a Richter's hernia or a partial enterocele.

Of obvious importance is the presence of an incarcerated mass in the inguinofemoral area. Associated symptoms of nausea, vomiting, abdominal cramps and the presence of distention suggest intestinal obstruction. Marked tenderness in the area suggests the presence of strangulation as well.

Ordinarily, hydroceles are easily diagnosed. The swelling may be limited to the scrotal area in a patient found to have an intact inguinal floor. Confusion arises in diagnosing obese patients with associated hernias. Transillumination of the scrotal mass, conducted in a dark room with a flashlight, will help make the differential diagnosis. The choice of flashlight is important, since one equipped with a large lens has been found to be inferior to the small, pocket-type flashlight.

## HERNIAS IN INFANTS

Infants and children with hernias present special problems, since they are not able to communicate their complaints clearly, if at all. Therefore, the physical examination assumes a greater importance. The surgeon should carefully consider the observations made by the child's parents. The protrusion may be seen by the obstetrician at the time of the baby's delivery. Often the mother will observe a new swelling in the groin. Crying, straining, walking, and onset of strenuous physical activity are events that can cause the swelling to appear in infants and children. The mother will observe that, after a bath or a good nights sleep, the swelling will subside. With protrusion of the hernia, the infant may become irritable and fretful. Obstruction will lead to the refusal of feedings and to vomiting.

By the time the physician sees the infant or child, there may be no swelling at all. The infant may cause the hernia to reappear upon crying. Older children may be able to cooperate in the effort to demonstrate the hernia by coughing, jumping, or walking about. On the other hand, when incarceration exists the mass is easily seen and palpated.

If the internal ring is small and the external ring is tight, it may be impossible to cause the hernia to protrude on short notice. In this event, the patient may be asked to return when the swelling appears. If the mother is a stable, reliable individual, her history may be depended upon in arriving at the diagnosis. The frequency with which mothers are capable of making a correct diagnosis is truly remarkable.

Palpation must be gentle in infants, since reflex contraction of the abdominal muscles makes examination impossible. Furthermore, in infants and small children, ordinary digital examination of the groin is inadvisable. Palpation over the internal ring may reveal an enlarged ring. Light palpation over the inguinal canal and cord may suggest the sensation of silk being rubbed over silk. The cord may be palpably enlarged and thickened.

Every attempt should be made to differentiate hydroceles from hernias in infants, since operation for hydroceles may be deferred for several months without danger or inconvenience. The hydrocele is a persistent soft mass that transmits the light from a small flashlight. The hernia may recede after the baby has had its nap

and will recur after the baby cries or becomes active.

Femoral hernias and direct hernias are rarely seen in infants; however, since they do occur, every infant should be examined and treated with those possibilities in mind.

## DIAGNOSIS OF SLIDING HERNIAS

The greatest aid in the proper diagnosis of sliding hernia is a high index of suspicion, which leads the surgeon to a thorough examination. Although there are no pathognomonic clinical signs differentiating large sliding hernias from incarcerated inguinal hernias, there are certain features that are helpful in distinguishing one from the other. The surgeon must make every attempt to arrive at the correct diagnosis in every patient he is to treat. In merely suspecting the possible existence of a sliding hernia in a given patient, operative injury to a viscus may be avoided.

Sliding hernias are far more common in males of advancing years. Adult females are rarely found to have sliding hernias. Any male over the age of 50 years who is obese and has a large hernia that has been present for many years should be suspected of having a sliding hernia. A truss may have been worn with decreasing effectiveness over the years. Such hernias are reducible, but reduction is difficult to maintain. Not infrequently patients with sliding hernias will have bowel dysfunction or urinary tract disturbances. In an ordinary reducible indirect inguinal hernia, one gains the impression that the contents have literally "fallen out" of the sac into the peritoneal cavity; whereas in sliding hernias, under the same circumstances, the examiner gains the impression that something remains at the large, lax internal ring. Reappearance of the hernia is prompt after the pressure over the inguinal area is released.

It is well recognized that a sliding hernia may be seen in an infant as a congenital abnormality and in aged patients as an acquired defect.

Female infants are more likely to have sliding hernias than are small boys. In a baby, the presence of a congenital hernia that contains an undetermined viscus should be suspected as possibly being a sliding hernia.

In male infants, the bladder might comprise a portion of the sac.

X-ray studies, including flat abdominal films and those employing contrast media, are useful in providing detailed diagnostic information regarding certain types of hernias. Since so little information has been available on roentgen studies in relation to hernia, Chapter 5 will deal exclusively with the subject.

## DIFFERENTIAL DIAGNOSIS OF HERNIA

Besides differentiating the various types of hernias, the surgeon must consider a number of other conditions that may appear similar to hernias.

**LIPOMAS** are not infrequently encountered in the groin or lower abdomen. Swelling produced by fatty tumors does not vary in size with changes in activity. They are of a soft consistency and do not enlarge when the patient coughs or strains. There is a common type of lipoma which accompanies the cord along with a small indirect inguinal hernia. This combination deserves surgical correction, since with passage of time these hernias continue to

enlarge. I have seen a moderate-sized lipoma resemble a hernia of the lumbar triangle of Petit (Fig. 3–6).

**LYMPHADENITIS,** in my experience, is most often confused with femoral hernia but may be difficult to differentiate from an inguinal hernia. It must be recalled that there are two groups of nodes in the groin, the superficial and the deep. Furthermore, it is not possible to palpate the deepest nodes in the area. The superficial nodes communicate with the lymphatics of the lower extremity, the lower abdomen below the umbilicus, the genitalia, the buttocks, the perineal area, and the distal part of the anal canal.

The deepest nodes in the area are located medially to the femoral vein. They communicate with the deep lymphatics of the lower extremity, the glans penis, the spongy urethra, and the urethra. Why detail the above anatomic details? If the differential diagnosis between hernia and lymphadenitis is to be made, the area of lymphatic drainage must be carefully examined and inspected for inflammatory or neoplastic lesions. Dermatologic conditions, folliculitis, and fungous infections of the feet and perineal areas may cause an inguinal lymph node to become enlarged.

Characteristically, the enlarged lymph node is quite firm and tender and may be

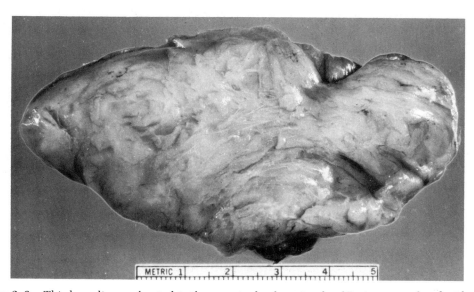

**Figure 3–6.**   This large lipoma, located in the superior lumbar triangle of Petit, was confused with a hernia.

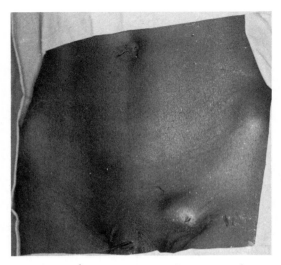

**Figure 3–7.** Lymphadenitis in the groin produces a painful swelling, which is of relatively short duration. Redness and induration may also be present locally in this type of patient.

fairly well delineated upon palpation (Fig. 3–7). Coughing and straining cause no change in its size. Upon lying down, there is no change in its size. Smaller satellite lymph nodes may be present in the groin as well.

The patient may be found to have an elevated temperature, and a leukocyte count must be obtained.

**HYDROCELE.** Other than hernia, the hydrocele is the most common cause of swelling in the inguinoscrotal area (Fig. 3–8). However, in the average patient it is easily differentiated from hernia. The swelling due to hydrocele remains, regardless of the state of activity. Patients with large hydroceles are remarkably free of pain. The hydrocele has a characteristic firmness, and palpation elicits little or no discomfort. Often the upper and lower poles of the hydrocele may be identified (Fig. 3–8). Transillumination of the hydrocele in a totally dark room results in the transmission of a reddish light, which is strongly suggestive of the diagnosis. In a thin patient with dilated intestine in a hernia sac, it may be possible to see a similar phenomenon, but the symptoms would probably vary.

Palpation and digital examination must be carefully carried out in every patient with a hydrocele. The abdominal wall should be checked for defects at the internal ring. Digital examination is often helpful. By this method, it is possible to establish the relationship, if any, between the hernia and the hydrocele.

When considering the differential diagnosis between hernia and hydrocele, it is important that neither one be overlooked, since both conditions may be corrected safely in one operative endeavor.

**SAPHENOUS VARIX.** When performing an examination for hernia, it is important

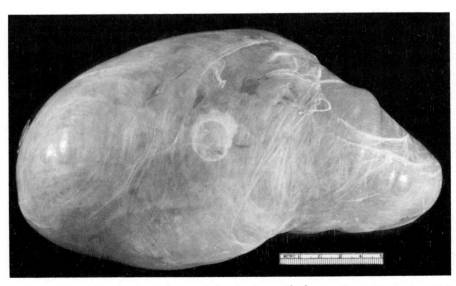

**Figure 3–8.** This large hydrocele showed no variation in size, with changes in position or in activity. It transmitted light and was diagnosed as hydrocele.

to inspect the extremities for varicose veins. An enlarged varix at the fossa ovalis may be confused with a reducible femoral hernia. The skin in a thin patient may have the bluish color seen in varicosity elsewhere. It will recede when the patient lies down and reappear with coughing or straining. It is nontender to palpation and may be easily "reduced." It also has a characteristic quality of softness to palpation. Furthermore, no continuity can be established between the varix and the femoral canal just above the varix.

**VARICOCELES** are far more common on the left side than on the right. The left spermatic vein empties into the left renal vein; whereas on the right side, the vein empties into the vena cava. The left testicle normally hangs lower than the right, and the valves of the veins become incompetent, leading to dilatation and elongation of the veins of the pampiniform plexus. Varicosities of the pampiniform plexus seldom cause a problem in differential diagnosis of hernia. The swelling due to varicocele may be visible through the skin and recedes when the patient reclines. Palpation of the varicocele pro-

vides a characteristic sensation, which has been compared to that of feeling a "bag of worms."

**TUMORS.** Periodically, the surgeon will encounter a patient with an inguinal mass that had been considered to be a hernia. It should be recalled that primary tumors may arise from any tissue in the area, such as fibrous tissue, muscle, or bone. Furthermore, these tumors, although more often benign, may be malignant in rare instances.

Tumors tend to grow slowly, and once the swelling appears it remains permanently. The mass ordinarily is not at all painful and increases slowly in size. On palpation the benign mass may be firm, whereas malignant tumors are likely to be hard. These growths do not transmit light.

When secondary tumors appear in the groin area, they may cause confusion as to the correct diagnosis. These are more common than primary tumors in this region. Carcinomas from any of the abdominal organs may appear in the groin as secondary foci (Fig. 3–9). Such masses are hard and permanent; they increase in size

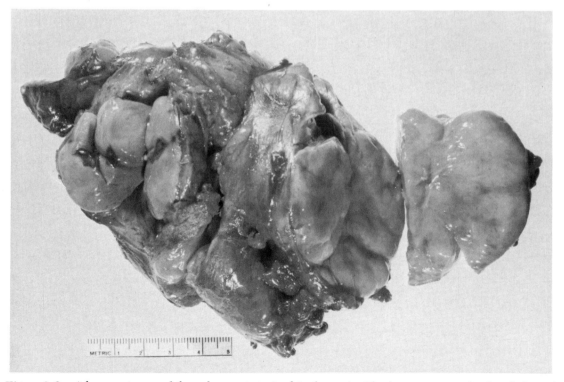

**Figure 3–9.** Adenocarcinoma of the colon, metastasized to the groin. The large mass was hard and showed progressive enlargement.

with the passage of time and cause little or no pain. These groin masses will not be confused with hernia if the clinician thinks of the possibilities in the particular case.

Malignant melanoma may be seen to metastasize to the inguinal lymph nodes and lead to some confusion as to the proper diagnosis.

**ABSCESS.** In former years, the cold abscess, or tubercular abscess, extended along musculofascial planes into the groin. In this situation, the differential diagnosis between femoral hernia and cold abscess had to be made. In modern practice the cold abscess is rarely seen. Where it is suspected, x-ray studies of the spine and pelvis are obviously indicated.

**CYSTS.** The most common cyst in the inguinal canal of the male or female, in my experience, is that arising from the processus vaginalis. The processus may be obliterated at the internal ring, but farther down in the inguinal canal, an encysted hydrocele may remain. Such cysts may communicate with the processus vaginalis testis, or they may simply remain as small cysts in the inguinal canal or canal of Nuck. They are commonly designated as hydroceles of the cord. Rarely such cysts may be multiple.

In the female, a cyst of Bartholin's gland may be confused with an indirect labial hernia. In such situations the internal inguinal ring will reveal no weakness, and the canal itself will appear normal to inspection. No inguinal mass will be present. Cysts of Bartholin's gland are translucent.

**ENDOMETRIOSIS.** Endometrial tissue may find its way into the inguinal region and lead to periodic discomfort and swelling in the groin. The pain is most severe at the onset of the menstrual period and then regresses later in the cycle. With the pain, swelling appears in the area.

## REFERENCES

Burton, C. C.: The embryologic development and descent of the testis in relation to congenital hernia. Surg. Gynecol. Obstet. *107*:294–302, 1958.

Condon, R. E., and Nyhus, L. M.: Complications of groin hernia and of hernial repair. Surg. Clin. North Am. *51*:1325–1336, 1971.

Keith, A.: On the origin and nature of hernia. Br. J. Surg. *11*:455–475, 1923–1924.

Light, H. G., and Routledge, J. A.: Intra-abdominal pressure. Arch. Surg. *90*:115–117, 1965.

Moorhead, J. J.: The relation of trauma to inguinal hernia. An analysis of 1,376 herniotomies. Am. J. Surg. *47*:312–327, 1940.

Patten, B. M.: *Human Embryology* (3rd ed.). New York, McGraw-Hill Book Co., 1968.

Potts, W. J., Riker, W. L., and Lewis, J. E.: The treatment of inguinal hernia in infants and children. Ann. Surg. *132*:566–576, 1950.

Read, R. C.: Observations on the etiology of spigelian hernia. Ann. Surg. *152*:1004–1009, 1960.

Watson, L. F.: *Hernia* (2nd ed.). St. Louis, C. V. Mosby Co., 1935.

Zimmerman, L. M.: Pitfalls in the management of inguinal hernias. Surg. Clin. North Am. *38*:189–195, 1958.

# 4

# Preoperative Evaluation

## INTRODUCTORY COMMENTS

Preoperative assessment of the patient with hernia is exceedingly important and must be thorough. Hernias, unless complicated, do not cause death of the patient, whereas hidden coexisting systemic disease may endanger the patient's very life if overlooked and untreated. Elective operations should be undertaken with each patient at an optimal level of health. This does not mean that the patient is otherwise in perfect health.

In our experience, deaths and complications are uncommon in infants, children, and young adults following hernia repair. Neonates and children tolerate surgical repair of hernias very well. We see more complications in infirm, aged patients.

### Surgery and the Aged

According to Ziffren (1960), the average duration of life for the white male has increased by 19 years during the past 50 years. Such favorable survival statistics are due to better control of infant mortality and improved treatment of infectious diseases. Nevertheless, the individual life span has changed but little in the recorded history of man. It is well known that increasing numbers of people live to old age.

In view of the above facts, surgeons have studied the physiology of the aged patient and his response to surgery. Beal (1959) demonstrated that in geriatric patients the amount of body water is decreased. He has also documented the fact that both cardiac output and renal function are impaired. Clinicians had suspected that respiratory function in the elderly is less than optimal; but Beal showed that ventilatory capacity and oxygen consumption are decreased. These considerations should guide the surgeon in his management of the elderly patient and in the choice of anesthetic agents.

I have consistently observed that a number of degenerative and metabolic diseases afflict the older patient. Clowes (1967), Ziffren (1960), and Glenn (1963) found that arteriosclerosis, arteriosclerotic heart disease, hypertension, hypertensive cardiovascular disease, malignancies, diabetes, benign prostatic hypertrophy, pulmonary and genitourinary tract diseases, malnutrition, and bronchitis plague the aging individual. This formidable list of disorders is documented so that it may be recalled during the clinical evaluation of the older patient.

### Surgery and the Infant or Neonate

Infants and children are often the victims of various types of hernias. In 1950 Gross reported that nearly one-fifth of the operations performed at Boston Children's Hospital were for repair of inguinal and umbilical hernias. The significant incidence of such abnormalities demands that the surgeon be aware of certain events that occur in neonates and infants. The common occurrence of multiple congenital anomalies in the same individual is well known. The great importance of psychologic needs of the child must not be minimized during the clinical appraisal. Time must be taken to reassure the child that his welfare, comforts, and needs are not being overlooked.

The physiologic peculiarities of the infant should be recalled. The metabolic rate is higher; hence, the need for adequate ventilation is clear. The heart rate is rapid, varying from 120 to 200 beats per minute at times, and the systolic blood pressure is well under 100 mm. Hg. The kidneys and liver must develop further before reaching functional maturity. The infant cannot tolerate excessive amounts of sodium. The adrenal gland does not become functionally effective until some three to four weeks after normal delivery (Klein, 1954). This might be one reason neonates tolerate major and prolonged surgery poorly.

Finally, surgeons must be alert to the fact that infants have little control over their body temperatures. The central regulatory mechanisms unfortunately permit rapid and severe changes toward hyperthermia or hypothermia. I wish to stress the importance of this instability insofar as thermoregulation is concerned, since operating rooms may be too cold as a result of air conditioning. Furthermore, the infant may remain exposed too long with little or no protective clothing.

Excellent publications on the physiology of infants and children are available. The surgeon who would operate upon newborn infants and children should study the works of Smith (1951) and of Klein (1954). The physiology of the infant varies significantly from that of the adult. Whenever a newborn infant presents with a complicated hernia requiring urgent repair, the assistance of a pediatrician and an anesthesiologist should be sought.

## CLINICAL APPRAISAL OF THE PATIENT

The patient with hernia must be carefully and thoroughly evaluated. A casual approach may lead to inaccurate diagnosis as to the type of hernia present, and serious systemic disease may be overlooked. The operation is considered by some to be of a minor nature—one that carries little danger. It is important to remember that no operative procedure, no matter how trivial, can be performed with a zero mortality rate. The patient's problem must never be taken lightly, for other diseases may well be present. The modern surgeon is expected to operate upon patients who are in less than vigorous health, with a mortality rate approaching zero and a negligible complication rate. In order to achieve a more rapid and accurate assessment of patients about to undergo hernia repairs, I find it convenient to divide them into three broad categories based on age. Such a grouping gives us a clue as to the type of hernia that requires repair and alerts us to any possible concurrent diseases or anomalies. The three categories are as follows:

1. Neonates and infants and children
2. Vigorous adults
3. Geriatric patients

This breakdown of patients with hernias has great practical merit, and yet, it is simple.

**Neonates and Infants** most commonly are found to have indirect inguinal and umbilical hernias; nervertheless, the infant must be examined systematically. Are there anomalies about the oral cavity and upper respiratory tract? Cardiac anomalies, genitourinary anomalies, and gastrointestinal abnormalities must be carefully excluded. It is well known that an infant with one anomaly may very possibly have others. The need for careful examination of the genitalia and the opposite groin is obvious. Female infants often have bilateral indirect inguinal hernias, and sliding components are not rare. An umbilical hernia causes such a prominence of the navel that it is seldom overlooked. When dealing with infants and children, the assistance of a pediatrician is highly desirable.

**Adults.** Indirect inguinal hernias are more likely to be found in healthy young adults; however, as age increases, direct inguinal hernias appear in increasing numbers, particularly in those individuals doing heavy work. Female patients rarely appear with direct inguinal hernias. In this group of patients a complete history and physical examination are necessary. Chest x-ray examination, urinalysis, blood counts, and serology are advisable in all patients. In the presence of a completely negative history and normal physical examination, special studies, such as barium studies of the gastrointestinal tract and barium and intravenous pyelography, are not obtained in young and healthy adults.

THE ELDERLY. Since many hernias occur in patients over the age of 50 years, the question arises as to how detailed the preoperative evaluation should be. I feel that these patients deserve thorough evaluation, since arteriosclerosis, arteriosclerotic heart disease, and pulmonary, renal, metabolic, and neoplastic diseases appear in increasing numbers in patients who have reached their fifth, sixth, seventh, and eighth decades. Even if the discovery of concurrent diseases does not alter the plan to proceed with operative treatment, it will serve to alert the surgeon as to the possible type of postoperative complications that may arise. For example, patients with prostatism not infrequently develop urinary retention. Local anesthesia and early ambulation may obviate the need for catheterization and thus diminish the hazard of a urinary tract infection. The rectal examination is essential not only to evaluate the condition of the lower rectum but also to check the size and consistency of the prostate.

All patients must be examined for concurrent dermatologic conditions in the operative area before incisions are made if postoperative wound infections are to be avoided.

Serious errors in diagnosis are fortunately uncommon, but there is still room for improvement in the care of patients with hernias. This chapter will include a few brief, but interesting, examples illustrating certain diagnostic problems and their management.

## HISTORY

Chapter 3 dealt at length with the clinical history and diagnosis of hernia. An accurate diagnosis of the particular type of hernia present is absolutely necessary if the proper operative procedure is to be attempted. The clinical history other than that referring to the hernia must be accurately recorded as well if embarrassing errors are to be avoided.

THE NEONATE OR INFANT HISTORY may be obtained from the obstetrician, pediatrician, or mother of the patient. Inquiries should be made as to the earlier recognition of other congenital anomalies or defects.

THE YOUNG ADULT who is in excellent general health will usually report that he has observed a swelling in the groin, particularly after vigorous activity. The protrusion is likely to be of the indirect variety. In older adults who perform heavy work, the direct inguinal hernia is seen in increasing numbers.

THE HISTORY OBTAINED FROM THE AGED PATIENT must be interpreted individually. The older patient with complete control of his faculties gives an excellent history. It must be stressed that many geriatric patients will tend to minimize their problems. They are able to endure discomfort and are hopeful that their pain will subside again as it has so many times in the past. Such patients may conceal a Richter's hernia until strangulation occurs.

We are seeing more aged and senile patients with chronic brain syndrome due to cerebrovascular arteriosclerosis. These individuals are often brought to the hospital from nursing homes. They are relatively feeble, disoriented, and more or less confused. Hernias that have been present for a quarter of a century now become unbearable to the patient and, perhaps more important, to his family. I advise thorough clinical and laboratory investigation of all such patients before embarking upon elective surgical procedures. I recommend repair even in the poor-risk patients, since incarceration of a hernia may lead to gangrene of the intestine. Once obstruction develops, vomiting leads to dehydration. If the incarcerated bowel becomes gangrenous, sepsis and dehydration may follow; hence, these complications must be avoided.

Patients who have reached old age should be managed a bit differently than their younger counterparts. They must be given an opportunity to discuss their problems slowly with the physician. This takes some time, but the advantage of having a cooperative patient is enormous. Specific questions that help clarify the status of the cardiovascular, pulmonary, renal, and central nervous systems must be directed to the patient. Metabolic diseases, anemia, and infectious diseases must be suspected. Malignancy is an ever-present threat to the elderly.

It is always necessary to ask specific questions regarding medication that the patient is taking. Is he on anticoagulant or antihypertensive medications? In modern practice, patients may be seen with both pacemakers and cardiac valve replacements. I have repaired hernias successfully on such patients. When dealing with older patients, more information regarding physical work, eating, smoking, and health habits is desirable. Is he physically active, or is he feeble with atrophy of his musculature? Is there a history suggestive of malfunction in other organ systems? If so, the patient must be studied thoroughly.

**Arteriosclerosis and arteriosclerotic heart disease** are the leading causes of death in older patients. Furthermore, atherosclerosis contributes greatly to the infirmity of aging patients. Parkinsonism and cerebrovascular arteriosclerosis leading to stroke are other disabilities encountered in the aged. Chronic brain syndrome due to cerebrovascular arteriosclerosis is not rare. Does the patient complain of weakness, shortness of breath, and swelling of the ankles? Does he have difficulty breathing? Chest pain following minimal activity may be due to coronary arteriosclerosis.

A history of unexplained fever, productive cough, and hemoptysis requires thorough investigation of the chest. Emphysema, chronic bronchitis, asthmatic bronchitis, and carcinoma of the lung are too often seen in older patients. **Pulmonary disease** contributes directly to hernia formation and leads to postoperative complications in a significant number of cases. Nevertheless, hernias in such patients should be repaired, since with the passage of time, the hernia becomes more of a problem while the patient's general health further deteriorates.

**Genitourinary tract disorders** are seen in increasing numbers as the patient exceeds his fifth decade of life. Prostatism is a progressively annoying problem to the aging patient. Difficulty in voiding causes the patient to strain, with the result that intra-abdominal pressure rises. Direct hernias appear in increasing numbers as the age of the patient population increases. Prostatic enlargement must be recognized before the patient is operated upon, since it may interfere with voiding postoperatively. Symptoms of burning on urination, more frequent urination, dysuria, chills, and fever indicate urinary tract infection. Patients with such histories should undergo a thorough urologic examination and appropriate treatment before surgery is advised. Local anesthesia permits operation upon certain borderline problems, since the patient retains his reflexes and mobility.

After the age of 50, **diseases of the digestive tract** are seen with increasing frequency. Rectal bleeding, increase in constipation, and change in bowel habits constitute indications for investigation of the colon and rectum. Rectal polyps are relatively common; I have also been impressed with the frequency of colon and rectal neoplasms in elderly patients with hernia and can recall having seen three such patients in the past 18 months. The combination of hernia and carcinoma of the colon and rectum is more common in aged patients than is generally recognized. It is important that the possible existence of neoplasms be at least considered, since as patients advance in years, combinations of disorders increase steadily in frequency.

Metabolic disturbances such as diabetes may be responsible for symptoms of weight loss and frequent and excessive urination. Gout occasionally causes joint pains in some patients. Osteoporosis may result in collapse of vertebral bodies, leading to a radicular type of pain.

Symptoms of weight loss, anemia, weakness, chills, and fever obviously call for thorough laboratory and radiologic studies.

## PHYSICAL EXAMINATION

A general impression of the patient's health is gained from his appearance. Does the patient look chronically ill? Does he appear to be older than his actual age?

The patient must be disrobed completely for examination purposes. A partially clothed patient may easily conceal a femoral hernia.

**The vital functions** must be observed,

and the results recorded. The temperature, pulse, respirations, and blood pressure should be taken, and several readings should be entered in the patient's medical record. Fever is not due to the presence of a hernia unless complications are present. Therefore, other explanations for an elevated temperature course must be sought. If the respiratory rate is increased, pulmonary or cardiac disease should be suspected. The blood pressure should be recorded several times throughout the day in order to detect significant variations.

**The weight of the patient** should be recorded. Such an observation will reveal any recent unsuspected weight loss. Physical inspection will reveal significant weight loss, for example, if the skin appears loose and wrinkled over the torso and arms. Again, the weight loss must be explained. Very few patients will lose weight voluntarily and maintain such a loss. Does the patient have diabetes? Is a malignancy present?

**Mouth, ears, eyes, nose, and throat examinations** should be carried out systematically lest some disease, unrelated to the hernia, be overlooked. Is oral sepsis a problem? Sclerae should be examined under good illumination if icterus is to be detected. Pallor of the conjunctivae may suggest anemia. Is there evidence of malignancy in the nasopharynx?

**THORAX.** Physical examination of the chest must be methodic and thorough. We have had two patients referred for hernia repair with active pulmonary tuberculosis. Carcinoma of the lung is all too commonly found in elderly men. Emphysema is characterized by the so-called barrel chest, with enlargement in the anterior-posterior diameter. The diaphragm shows somewhat limited excursions and remains low in the thorax. Emphysema predisposes the patient to serious pulmonary complications postoperatively (Fig. 4–1). Poor ventilation is becoming an increasing problem to many patients in the postoperative state.

On percussion the hyperresonance is easily demonstrated in emphysematous patients, and on auscultation the breath sounds in the periphery are diminished. If bronchial infection is present, rales may be heard. In asthma the breath sounds are musical or wheezing in character; if active pulmonary disease is discovered, it is treated with postural drainage, antibiotics, and positive pressure assisted breathing as indicated, especially in older individuals. Chronic pulmonary disease does not preclude the repair of bothersome hernias,

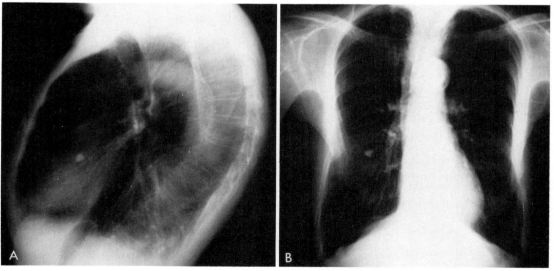

**Figure 4–1.** This patient, aged 72 years, had severe respiratory difficulty. The lateral view (*A*) shows dorsal kyphosis, osteoporosis, compression of dorsal vertebra, and increased anterior-posterior diameter of the chest. On fluroroscopic examination there was diminished excursion of the diaphragm. The anterior-posterior view (*B*) shows the diaphragmatic leaves to be flattened. Repair of this patient's hernia under local anesthesia and early ambulation resulted in an uneventful recovery.

but optimal health should be gained before an operation is recommended.

Examination of the breasts is extremely important in view of the frequency of carcinoma of the breast.

**HEART.** The blood pressure is noted, and several readings should be recorded during a period of hospitalization. It is not rare to discover hypertension and hypertensive cardiovascular disease for the first time during preoperative examination. The heart rate and rhythm are observed, and findings recorded. Disturbances in the rate and rhythm are seen in patients with arteriosclerotic cardiovascular disease and rheumatic fever and after myocardial infarction. Arteriosclerotic heart disease is the most common type of disturbance found in aged patients (Fig. 4–2). Of course, any evidence of cardiac decompensation is noted, so that it can be treated promptly. The patient with decompensated cardiac disease is preferably treated by an internist or cardiologist. Decompensation is treated before any elective procedures are performed.

**ABDOMINAL EXAMINATION.** The groins, umbilical area, and femoral areas are carefully inspected and palpated. In every instance, the patient is examined for hernia in the standing and decubitus positions. The condition of the testes is noted. Mumps in childhood may have caused an orchitis, which occasionally leads to an atrophic testicle. Less frequently, the testicle is congenitally hypoplastic. These findings should be recorded accurately. Details concerning diagnosis of hernia are presented more completely in Chapter 3.

The strength, or lack of strength, of the abdominal wall is noted. The size of a ventral hernia defect must be recorded in centimeters. It is important to remember that a large, protuberant hernia may find its egress through a relatively small abdominal wall defect.

Palpation of the abdomen for masses must always be done methodically and thoroughly. The patient with a hernia may be found to have a colonic tumor.

The size and position of the kidneys and liver are noted, if palpable. In obese individuals, little can be felt.

**RECTAL EXAMINATION AND VAGINAL EXAMINATION** should not be omitted in aging patients. In male patients the prostate must be examined, since an enlarged prostate may cause postoperative urinary retention. Carcinoma of the prostate is not rare in patients above the age of 60 years. Pelvic neoplasms and masses may be discovered in older women if the gynecologic examination is properly performed.

**EXTREMITIES.** I strongly urge prompt ambulation in postoperative patients, provided their vital functions are capable of supporting such ambulation. Therefore, the condition of the patient's legs must be ascertained. Is the circulation adequate? Are large varicosities present? If the medical record describes the preoperative state accurately, complications such as postoperative phlebothrombosis can be more easily recognized and consequently better treated.

## CLINICAL STUDIES FOR FURTHER ASSESSMENT

**PROCTOSIGMOIDOSCOPIC EXAMINATIONS** are performed on patients over 50 years of age, with few exceptions. The patient with constipation, rectal bleeding, diarrhea, anemia, and change in bowel function should have a sigmoidoscopic examination.

**LABORATORY EXAMINATIONS.** No matter how astute the clinician, there are times when the laboratory uncovers essential information for the surgeon. Hence, a complete blood count and urinalysis are required for every patient. Anemia, blood dyscrasias, diabetes, and urinary tract infections may be uncovered. Patients suspected of being diabetics are given glucose tolerance tests. We have identified a number of diabetics through the methodic examination of the urine for sugar in patients referred for repair of a hernia.

**CHEST X-RAY EXAMINATIONS** are obtained on all adult patients. It may not be necessary to subject the healthy infant, child, or young adult to a routine chest x-ray, but certainly all patients with symptoms suggestive of pulmonary disease require chest x-ray studies. Chest x-rays are indicated in all babies with recogniz-

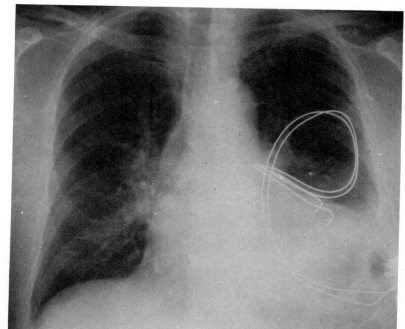

**Figure 4–2.** The presence of arteriosclerotic heart disease and resultant disabling brady-cardia did not preclude repair of an annoying direct inguinal hernia.

Note the cardiomegaly on the top chest x-ray. After the pace-maker was inserted, the effu-sion cleared and heart size de-creased greatly after treat-ment, as seen in the film on the bottom. Repair was accom-plished under local anesthesia and satisfactory recovery fol-lowed.

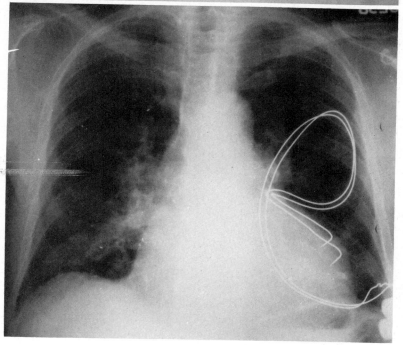

able anomalies, since other conditions may be present as well (Fig. 4–3).

ELECTROCARDIOGRAMS are useful in patients over the age of 50 years. The EKG is also obtained in patients with symptoms suggestive of heart disease, such as precordial pain that may radiate into the upper extremities. Patients with cardiac arrhythmias should have an electrocardiogram and consultation with an internist or cardiologist if there is any question of active heart disease. If there is evidence of cardiac decompensation, medical consultation should be obtained.

SPECIAL EXAMINATIONS. By no means are all patients subjected to a number of unnecessary special examinations. How-

ever, in individual cases, a more thorough investigation may be necessary because of certain findings unrelated to the hernia. Urologic examinations, gastrointestinal x-rays, and radiologic studies of the skeletal system are indicated in particular patients.

UROLOGIC EXAMINATION is requested when there is definite clinical and laboratory evidence of genitourinary tract disease. All elderly patients should have a digital rectal examination, and if an enlarged prostate or a firm suspicious nodule is discovered, the help of a urologist should be sought. Cystograms can document significant prostatic enlargement (Fig. 4–4). If there is definite hematuria,

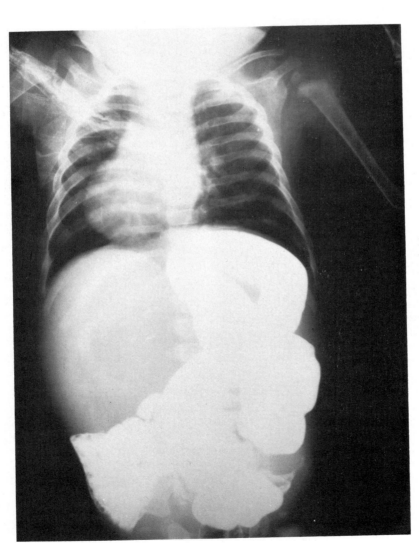

**Figure 4–3.** This x-ray film demonstrates the presence of multiple anomalies in the same infant. Dextrocardia, omphalocele, and malrotation of the colon are well demonstrated in the same infant.

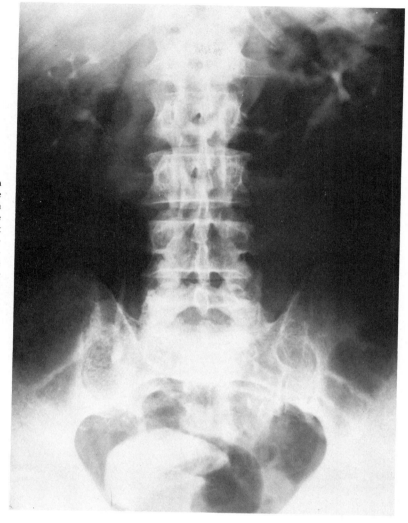

**Figure 4–4.** In patients with complaints referable to the urinary tract, drip infusion pyelography is a worthwhile examination. In this patient the intrarenal collecting systems and ureters were unremarkable, but the prostatic elevation of the bladder floor was prominent. Use of local anesthesia and prompt ambulation helped to avoid postoperative urinary retention.

cystoscopic examination and intravenous or retrograde pyelography are indicated, and a urologist should be consulted.

Impotence as a complaint may be very important in a few patients with hernia. In such situations, the patient may have the erroneous impression that repair of a hernia will also correct his sexual problem. This type of patient may be troublesome to manage postoperatively, since he may feel that the repair was a failure. I have found that a clear explanation of the facts does much to avoid such problems postoperatively. Consultation with a urologist prior to surgical repair of hernias in impotent individuals is worthwhile assistance.

**GASTROINTESTINAL STUDIES**, including cholecystograms, barium enemas, and upper gastrointestinal studies, are ordered in symptomatic patients. The obese patient with an umbilical hernia may have cholelithiasis. The patient with fever, leukocytosis, and a painful hernial mass may have diverticulitis. The patient with a large sliding hernia may have a carcinoma of the colon (Fig. 4–5).

Although not common, such combinations of disease entities can prove embarrassing to the unsuspecting surgeon. The magnitude of special investigations employed should be suggested by the number and severity of symptoms presented by the individual patient.

**ORTHOPEDIC EVALUATION** is occasionally indicated. Some patients complain bitterly of pain in the lower abdomen,

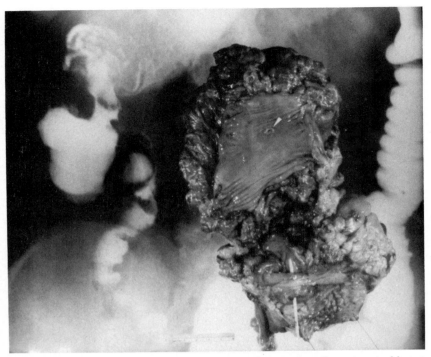

**Figure 4–5.** This 55-year-old male was referred for repair of a large right indirect inguinal hernia. He showed evidence of weight loss and looked pale. The presence of anemia was confirmed. Barium enema examination revealed a large irregular fungating lesion in the ascending colon. Right colectomy was performed for the carcinoma before hernia repair was recommended.

groin, upper thigh, hip, and back. They may relate such pain to an incisional hernia, when in fact, the discomfort is due to a disease of the hip or low back (Fig. 4–6). X-rays of the back, pelvis, and hips are strongly recommended. I also suggest orthopedic consultation in patients who complain bitterly of widespread pain in the upper thigh, lower abdomen, and hip.

OBESITY. One of the most annoying and complicating factors in patients with hernia is obesity. Experience teaches us that patients with a thick layer of adipose tissue and fatty infiltration of the abdominal wall often do poorly after hernia repair. Hence, I insist upon some reduction in the amount of excess weight. Reaching the ideal weight for a given patient is not a necessity, but a substantial reduction in the mass of adipose tissue is desirable. In some instances, the assistance of experts in the field of metabolism should be sought.

DERMATOLOGIC LESIONS should be treated prior to surgical treatment, since dermatitis increases the possibility of postoperative infection. Eradication of folliculitis is required before an incision can be made safely in such an area. Fungous infections about the groin and genitalia may require the assistance of a dermatologist.

I have attempted to indicate a reasonable approach to the clinical and special investigation of the patient being considered for hernia repair. I can conceive no plan that will cover all situations; hence, the surgeon must individualize his management of each patient.

## REFERENCES

Beal, J. M.: Basic principles in the surgical management of the aged. Geriatrics 14:269, 1959.
Benson, C. D., et al.: *Pediatric Surgery* (Vol. I). Chicago, Year Book Medical Pubs., Inc., 1962.
Clowes, G. H. A., Jr.: Surgical problems in the aged

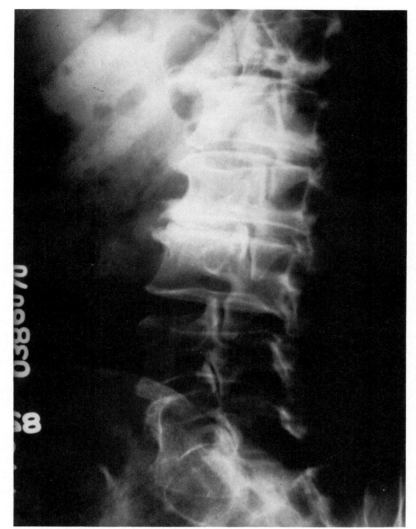

**Figure 4–6.**   This patient underwent successful emergency repair of an incarcerated right indirect inguinal hernia. Recovery was uneventful. After discharge from the hospital, he complained of lower abdominal pain following activity. X-rays revealed evidence of severe degenerative disc disease at the L2/3 interspace.

patient. *In* American College of Surgeons: *Manual of Preoperative and Postoperative Care.* Philadelphia, W. B. Saunders Co., 1967, pp. 240–251.

Glenn, F.: Physiologic principles in surgery of the elderly. J. Am. Geriatr. Soc. *11*:622, 1963.

Gross, R. E.: *The Surgery of Infancy and Childhood.* Philadelphia, W. B. Saunders Co., 1953.

Klein, R.: Neonatal adrenal physiology. Pediatr. Clin. North Am. *1*:321–334, 1954.

Ponka, J. L., and Brush, B. E.: Experiences with repair of groin hernias in 200 patients aged 70 years and older. J. Am. Geriatr. Soc. *22*(1)18–24, Jan. 1974.

Smith, C. A.: *The Physiology of the Newborn Infant* (2nd ed.). Springfield, Ill., Charles C Thomas, 1951.

Ziffren, S. E.: *Management of the Aged Surgical Patient.* Chicago, Year Book Medical Pubs., Inc., 1960.

# 5

# X-ray Studies in Patients with Hernia

I have decided to include a chapter on x-ray studies in patients with hernia, since such information is uniformly absent in other publications on the subject. More important is the fact that useful, but often overlooked, information may be obtained through the thoughtful use of roentgen studies (Table 5–1). Coexistent diseases sometimes play an important part in the etiology of direct hernias in particular.

As stated previously, the diagnosis of hernia is essentially a clinical matter. Pain and demonstrable protrusion are commonly found; therefore, the generic diagnosis of hernia is simple. On the other hand, additional useful information can be easily obtained with judicious use of x-ray. I have been critical of the attitude expressed by those physicians who are satisfied with the simple and noncommittal diagnosis of "hernia." It is essential to pinpoint the exact type of hernia or hernias present and to employ those adjuncts which may add to the accuracy of the diagnosis. Proper diagnosis helps in avoiding operative complications and leads to the selection of an effective operative procedure.

It is not my intention to suggest that every patient with hernia should be subjected to unnecessary and useless diagnostic tests An indirect inguinal hernia in a young male is a case in point. However, should a large indirect inguinal hernia be discovered in an elderly male with a history of bowel dysfunction, we have an entirely different situation. In such patients, a rectal examination, proctoscopic examination, and barium enema study of the colon are performed. If a sliding hernia is suspected, its presence may be confirmed preoperatively, and as a result, the colon may be spared injury at operation.

It is the purpose here to draw attention to those studies applicable to selected patients with hernia. Excellent works on roentgen diagnosis are available, and recent texts by Paul and Juhl and by Meschan have been consulted. The indications for such examinations and their

### Table 5–1. ROENTGEN STUDIES OF VALUE IN PATIENTS WITH HERNIA

I. *Three-dimensional Views of the Abdomen (Scout films or flat films)*
   Intestinal obstruction
   Incarcerated hernia
   Richter's hernia
II. *Barium Enema Examination*
   Sliding hernia; ileocecal segment on right
   Sliding hernia; sigmoid colon on left
   Sliding inguinal or femoral hernia; bladder
   Carcinoma of the colon
   Diverticular disease
III. *Upper Gastrointestinal Studies*
   Hiatal hernia
   Ventral postoperative hernias
   Internal hernias
IV. *Cystograms and Intravenous Pyelograms*
   Sliding hernia, bladder
   Femoral hernias
   Bladder diverticula
V. *Herniography in the Diagnosis of Hernia*

usefulness will be described and illustrated. The clinical material and roentgenograms presented here are selected from the files of Henry Ford Hospital.

## FLAT FILMS OF THE ABDOMEN

In the evaluation of the patient with acute abdominal disease, I prefer x-ray studies to be made initially without contrast material. Three-dimensional films are particularly useful in patients with ventral hernia and obstructive symptoms. It should be emphasized that three separate views are preferred: prone, or supine; lateral; and vertical, with the patient standing or sitting. Specifically, certain abnormalities should be recognized. Dilated loops may vary in the degree of distention and the number of loops involved, but in the adult they must always be taken seriously (Fig. 5–1). The pattern of intestine involved may be identified by the pattern of the distended segment.

Air-fluid levels may be present, indicating obstruction (Fig. 5–2). In some cases, there may be a stepladder-like pattern of arrangement, and in rare instances, a single closed loop obstruction may be seen. Free air under the diaphragm should be looked for lest a perforation of a strangulated portion of bowel be overlooked. Fortunately, such a complication is rarely seen in hernia.

In thin individuals, much of the information can be obtained by a physical examination, but in the obese patient, additional useful information may be obtained by x-ray studies. In the lateral view, one may recognize the presence of intestine in the hernial sac prior to incising the abdominal wall and, thereby, avoid injury to the intestine, Flat films of the abdomen are useful in patients with large ventral hernias when it is difficult to decide whether large bowel, small bowel, omentum, or some combination of viscera is present in the sac.

The usefulness of flat abdominal films in

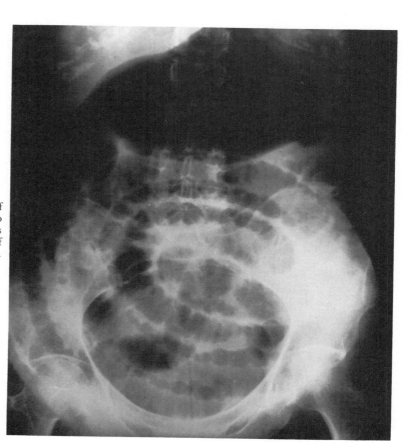

**Figure 5–1.** Dilated loops of small intestine, secondary to obstruction due to Richter's hernia. Correct diagnosis of such cases is too often delayed.

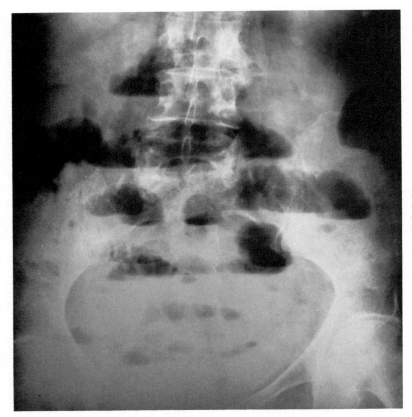

**Figure 5–2.** Air-fluid levels, secondary to entrapment and obstruction of small bowel in a femoral hernia.

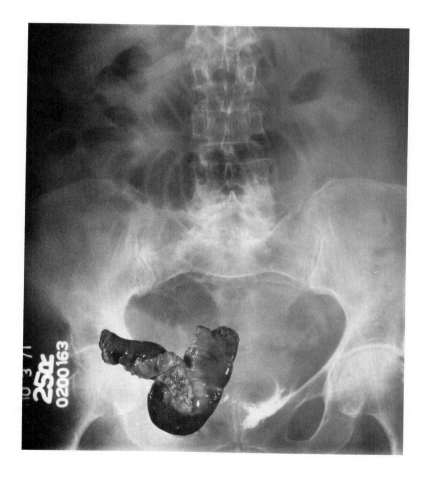

**Figure 5–3.** In this x-ray the distended small intestine was caused by a Richter's type of femoral hernia.

the diagnosis of Richter's type of hernia has been largely overlooked in modern publications on the subject (Fig. 5–3). Evidence of intestinal obstruction should lead to careful inspection of the femoral ring region. A small pocket of air trapped in the femoral canal in a symptomatic patient should never be taken lightly. I have seen many films that failed to include the groins and lower abdomen.

## BARIUM ENEMA EXAMINATION OF THE COLON

Contrast studies of the colon are particularly useful in aged patients with symptoms of colonic dysfunction and large hernias. Although carcinoma of the colon is not common, it occurs frequently enough in older patients to warrant consideration. I have noted that patients are inclined to assign all of their symptoms of bowel disorders to the presence of a hernia. The physician must not do the same, however, without carefully weighing the facts in the particular case.

Contrast studies of the colon are most helpful in identifying the ileocecal sliding hernia on the right (Fig. 5–4). Avoidance of injury to the colon and proper repair of sliding hernias are easily achieved objectives if the abnormality present is fully understood. In a number of patients the sigmoid colon may be partially obstructed as a result of partial volvulus, secondary to a sliding type of hernia (Fig. 5–5).

I have seen patients with acute diverticulitis in combination with inguinal hernias (Fig. 5–6). Injury to the bowel must be avoided, since the hazard of infection is great. Repair of the hernia is not ordinarily advised during the period of acute inflammation, nor do I advocate contrast studies during the acute inflammatory phase of the disease.

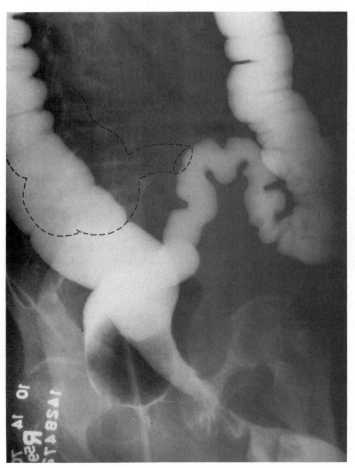

**Figure 5–4.** A barium enema examination shows the great displacement of the ileocecal segment in this patient with an indirect sliding inguinal hernia. The broken line indicates an approximately normal position for the cecum.

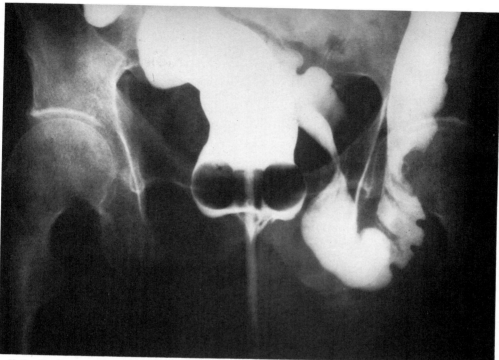

**Figure 5–5.** In this contrast study, the sigmoid colon forms a portion of the sac of the indirect sliding hernia. Note the partial volvulus, which often accounts for bowel dysfunction in these patients.

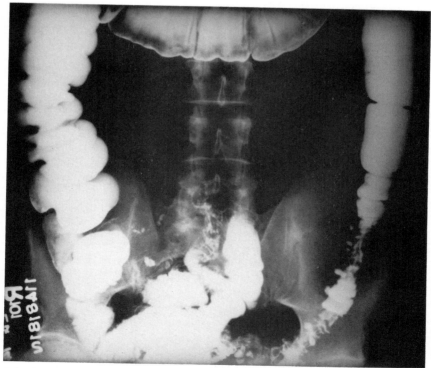

**Figure 5–6.** A barium enema examination revealed diverticulitis in this patient with prolonged and severe postoperative pain following herniorrhaphy.

Colonic polyps are a serendipitous discovery of x-ray contrast studies of the colon. The colonic polyps may be treated electively after repair of the hernia. Carcinoma of the colon is occasionally discovered in older patients.

## UPPER GASTROINTESTINAL AND SMALL BOWEL SERIES

Although this text does not consider the problem of diaphragmatic hernia, it should be emphasized that X-ray examination of the stomach in such cases is a necessity.

In selected patients, x-ray examination of the small intestine in a hernial sac may be precisely identified. These examinations, of course, are not performed in the presence of intestinal obstruction. Barium is never administered orally to the patient with intestinal obstruction for obvious reasons. On the other hand, contrast studies may reveal such worthwhile information as the partial obstruction of both ileum and colon in a patient with a large incisional hernia (Fig. 5–7).

## INTRAVENOUS PYELOGRAMS

When there is an absence of urologic complaints and a negative urinalysis, we, of course, do not carry out x-ray studies of the genitourinary tract. In selected patients we have been able to obtain additional helpful information. For instance, an enlarged prostate can be demonstrated easily (see Fig. 4–4, Chapter 4). In other patients, the bladder may be seen as a sliding component in a femoral hernia (Fig. 5–8). Obviously, important information is obtained about the status of the urologic tract.

## CYSTOGRAMS

Contrast studies of the urinary bladder are useful in some patients. The presence of bladder in certain sliding hernias in adults may be clearly demonstrated. At times a femoral hernia may be found to contain a surprisingly large segment of bladder. The value of a cystogram can be illustrated with the following case. A male

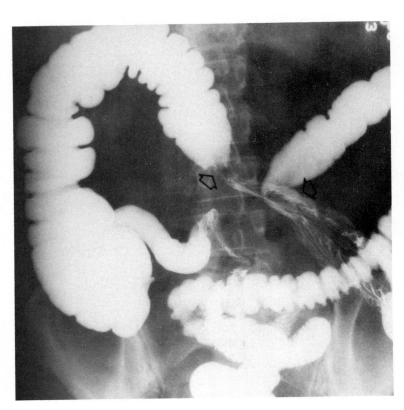

**Figure 5–7.** This barium enema examination in a patient with a large incisional hernia shows partial obstruction of the ileum and transverse colon. Arrows show site of constriction at point of herniation.

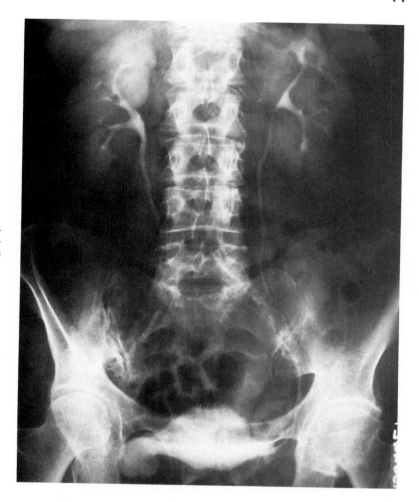

**Figure 5–8.** Intravenous pyelograms reveal bilateral femoral hernias in a patient with numerous complaints.

patient 78 years of age had repair of an inguinal hernia 25 years earlier. He had a recurrent but reducible mass in the left groin and experienced increasing difficulty in voiding. The cystogram showed a huge portion of the bladder to be present in the large, recurrent indirect inguinal hernia (Fig. 5–9A). At the time of the operation he was found to have a large indirect sliding inguinal hernia. The bladder was reduced, and a McVay repair was performed because of weakness in the inguinal floor. The postoperative cystogram showed that the bladder has been returned to its normal position (Fig. 5–9B). He has remained asymptomatic for two years and continues to do well.

We have recently had an elderly female with symptoms suggestive of a femoral hernia, the presence of which could not be demonstrated convincingly on physical examination. Cystograms revealed bilateral femoral hernias (Fig. 5–10A). Repair of the hernias through a midline incision by the Cheatle-Henry-Nyhus technique corrected the defect (Fig. 5–10B). In my experience, the preoperative cystogram has proved extremely useful in selected patients with problem hernias.

## HERNIOGRAPHY AND PERITONEOGRAPHY

In 1967 Ducharme, Bertrand, and Chacar described their attempt at diagnosis of inguinal hernias by injection of radiopaque medium into the peritoneal cavity and then obtaining x-ray films of the abdomen. In their first attempts, diatrizoate meglumine (Renografin-60) was used in amounts of 2 to 4 cc, depending upon the weight of

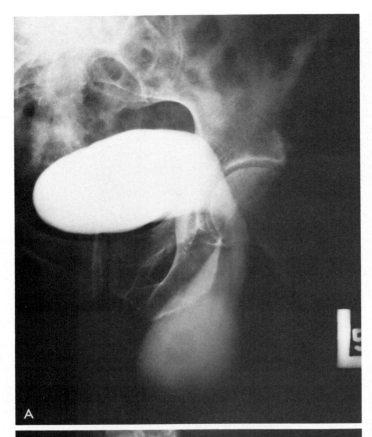

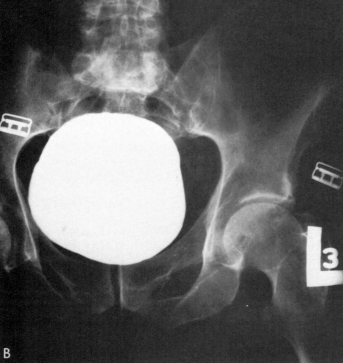

**Figure 5–9.** *A,* This cystogram reveals a huge sliding indirect inguinal hernia. The hernial sac contains almost as much of the bladder as the pelvis does. *B,* Postoperative cystogram shows a normal-appearing bladder.

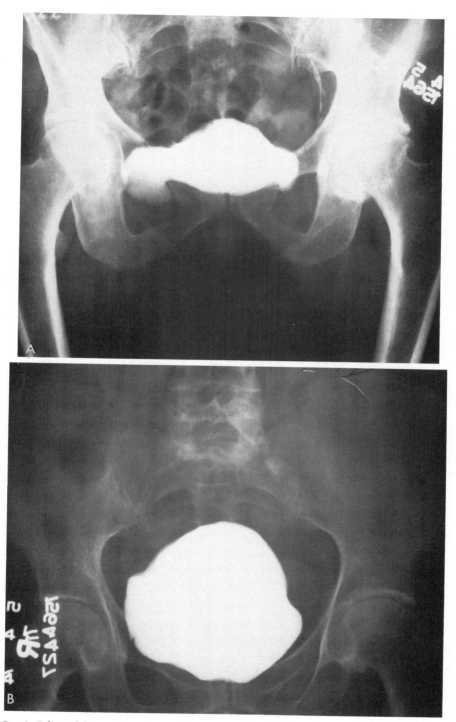

**Figure 5–10.** *A*, Bilateral femoral hernias are demonstrated in this eystogram. The patient was operated upon by Dr. Jorge Gomez of the Henry Ford Hospital Staff. *B*, The bladder appears normal in the postoperative cystogram following repair of both femoral hernias via the preperitoneal approach.

the patient. Using aseptic technique, the material was injected into the peritoneal cavity through an area that had been anesthetized. They listed no serious complications, but they admitted that injections had been made inadvertently into the abdominal wall, small bowel, and colon. They were unable to demonstrate three hernias known to be present. In 60 satisfactory herniographies, 17 unsuspected hernial sacs were discovered. Since the publication by Ducharme et al., other reports have appeared in the literature.

In a most interesting report by Griscom et al. (1970) in the journal *Radiology*, patency of the male processus vaginalis was demonstrated as a normal finding during intrauterine transfusion in the last trimester of pregnancy. Fetal peritoneograms were performed by injecting 3 to 10 ml of diatrizoate meglumine (Renografin-60). The purpose of the peritoneography was for localization prior to injection of packed red blood cells into the peritoneal cavity of fetuses with erythroblastosis. Films obtained from 142 pregnancies were available for review. Of nine survivors with probable or definite patent processus vaginalis, only one developed a hernia. This report reaffirms the observation made by Mitchell that the processus vaginalis is usually patent in late fetal life. Even in early infancy, it is quite common to find that the processus vaginalis is patent. Griscom et al. point out that the mere presence of a patent processus vaginalis does not justify the diagnosis of hernia. It is well known that most of these peritoneal prolongations will close shortly before birth or in early infancy. Even if obliteration should not occur into adulthood, the occurrence of hernia is not assured. From 15 to 37 percent of adult males have been found to have some degree of patency of the processus vaginalis without hernia. In no case did Griscom and his colleagues produce filling of the processus vaginalis in the female, and yet such patency is often demonstrable at surgery.

James and Hunsicker in 1972 performed herniograms on 166 children while searching for the best approach to the problem of contralateral hernia repair. They included those children with a history of hernia, those manifesting the "silk sign," and those with cryptorchidism.

They even performed such examinations postoperatively, when recurrence was suspected or when a newly discovered mass was present in the inguinal region. Only 18 of their patients were females. They reported no deaths or serious complications. The contrast medium was injected into the bladder of one patient and into the colon of a second. In two other patients, the complications included hematoma and injection of the contrast material into the abdominal wall. In two patients the abdominal pain was considered serious enough to warrant exploration, but no visceral perforation was found. They reported three false negative results, but in two of these, obvious incarcerated inguinal hernias were present. James and Hunsicker recommend herniograms for children with a history suggestive of hernia but in whom the hernia cannot be demonstrated. When a unilateral hernia is found, they feel a herniogram is helpful in detecting a hernia on the opposite side. They also perform the examination in cryptorchidism and in certain postoperative cases if a recurrence is suspected. They have not reached a final conclusion as to what is to be done with infants less than one year of age in whom a small patent processus vaginalis has been demonstrated. They plan to re-evaluate such cases in five years.

White et al. in 1970 reported their technique and experiences with herniography. They were particularly interested in the contralateral side when a hernia had been diagnosed. Their report concerns 100 patients, 84 male and 16 female, in whom bilateral explorations were performed. In this study, herniography returned 3 percent false negative and 2 percent false positive diagnoses. Haller and his colleagues found that herniography was 95 percent accurate in demonstrating a patent processus vaginalis. Complications of the procedure were considered minor. Even though injections of the contrast material were made into the bladder twice and into the bowel lumen several times, no serious sequelae were noted. Because accuracy of the herniogram exceeds that of the best physical examination, the authors feel that the decision to operate is reasonably based on both methods of examination. The examination is particularly appropriate for those children in whom a hernia is suspected but not proved on physical examination. The radiation dosage is considered to be low enough so that it does not represent a hazard.

Guttman, Bertrand, and Ducharme modified their procedure in 1972 and currently used diatrizoate sodium (Hypaque-M), which has been found less irritating. Their current technique is described in detail. They have discontinued performing the examination in children older than 10 years of age because of poor distribution of the contrast material. In this report, the authors performed herniography in 562 patients and found a definite contralateral sac in only 22.9 percent of their patients, a significantly lower figure than that found by many surgeons who perform routine contralateral exploration. Published reports indicate that when the side opposite a clinically demonstrable hernia is explored, a sac is found in 40 to 90 percent of the cases. Guttman et al. state that minor complications occur in 11 percent of their examinations.

### Comments on Herniography

The technique of herniography has been described in detail by several authors listed in the references. From the available reports, it is evident that the procedure can be done with relative safety. Patent vaginal processes can be demonstrated with a high degree of accuracy.

My attitude toward the examination of herniography is not one of enthusiastic endorsement. This is because I do not equate the presence of a small patent processus vaginalis with hernia. By definition, until the protrusion of some viscus occurs, the diagnosis of hernia is not justified. It is well known that patent vaginal processes are found in adult males without hernia. On the other hand, once a hernia becomes manifest, repair is the proper treatment. At this time, I prefer to repair recognizable hernias, and I do not feel that the mere demonstration of a patent processus vaginalis requires operative closure.

### REFERENCES

Ducharme, J. C., Bertrand, R., and Chacar, R.: Is it possible to diagnose inguinal hernia by x-ray? J. Can. Assoc. Radiol. 18:448, 1967.

Griscom, N. T., Cochran, W. C., Harris, G. B. C., Easterday, C. L., Umansky, I., and Frigoletto, F. D.: The processus vaginalis of the third trimester fetus with comments on inguinal hernias in childhood. Radiology 96:107–109, 1970.

Guttman, F. M., Bertrand, R., and Ducharme, J. D.: Herniography and the pediatric contralateral inguinal hernia. Surg. Gynecol. Obstet. 135:551–555, 1972.

James, P. M., and Hunsicker, R.: Is herniogram the answer to routine bilateral hernia repair? Am. Surg. 38:43–48, 1972.

Meschan, I.: Analysis of Roentgen Signs in General Radiology (Vol. III.) Philadelphia, W. B. Saunders Co., 1973.

Paul, L. W., and Juhl, J. H.: The Essentials of Roentgen Interpretation. Hagerstown, Md., Harper & Row, Publishers, Inc., 1972.

White, J. J., Haller, J. A., and Dorst, J. P.: Congenital inguinal hernia and inguinal herniography. Surg. Clin. North Am. 50:823–837, 1970.

# 6

# Premedication, Preoperative Orders, and Preoperative Preparation for Anesthesia*

## Introduction

The anticipation of surgery and anesthesia by the patient about to be introduced to the strange sights, sounds, and aromas of the operating room often provokes apprehension and actual fear. Contemplation of surgery and anesthesia by the surgical team should consider all of the foregoing and much that is to follow.

### CONSIDERATIONS BEFORE SURGERY AND ANESTHESIA

Whenever possible, the surgeon should acquaint the anesthesiologist with any special problems posed by the patient, his disease, or the proposed surgical procedure and its planned accomplishment. The ability to tolerate the adverse effects of anesthetics and operation depends largely on the functioning of the respiratory, circulatory, and neuromuscular systems

*Much of this chapter is reproduced from the *Surgical Procedures of the Henry Ford Hospital* (6th ed.), 1971, a publication of the Henry Ford Hospital. Reproduction and modification is possible through the courtesy of Dr. Paul R. Dumke, member of the Department of Anesthesiology, and with permission of the Editor, Joseph L. Ponka, M.D.

and on homeostasis of liver, kidneys, and endocrine glands. Occasionally, elective operations should be delayed because the patient has developed an intercurrent respiratory tract infection, has been inadequately digitalized or requires further study because of an abnormal laboratory finding. It is important not only from a medical point of view but also from the medicolegal standpoint for all patients to have essential laboratory tests performed and data recorded before proceeding to the operating suite. The minimum data required are a recent hemoglobin test and a urinalysis. The oxygen transport system requires that not less than 10 gm of hemoglobin per 100 ml of blood be present for acceptable safe standards in elective surgery.

The obtaining of last-minute consultations or the placing of tubes in various orifices at the time of the preoperative sedation immediately prior to surgery often defeats the entire purpose of preoperative sedation. There is no substitute for talking to a patient, listening to his problems, knowing of previous reactions to sedatives or anesthetics, looking at his earlier anesthetic records, and acquainting him with the planned procedure. The probable duration of the surgery, the amount of time the patient might reasonably be expected to remain in the postanesthetic recovery room, and the communication available between relatives in the surgical lounge and the operating room staff should be explained carefully to the patient and his relatives. With all the above goals accomplished in a satisfactory manner, the amount of preanesthetic medication needed to allay apprehension often may be reduced considerably. Exposure of improperly premedicated patients to the preparations for anesthesia and surgery not infrequently precipitates undesirable responses. Unpleasant memories retained by patients may influence later decisions they may have to make about surgery. The anesthesiologist may inadvertently overdose the patient with an anesthetic in order to compensate for ill-advised dosages or improperly timed amounts of preoperative sedation. A preoperative visit by the anesthesiologist to the patient with an explanation of the contemplated anesthetic procedure does much to allay the patient's fear as well as to allow selection of preoperative medication on the basis of need of the individual patient. When this is not possible, a member of the anesthesiology staff or surgical staff should perform this function and transmit his findings to the person who will give the anesthetic.

Preoperative preparation for anesthesia should include close questioning of the patient regarding previous experiences with anesthetics and sensitivity or "allergies" to various medications. Hypertensive patients should be especially questioned regarding a history of antihypertensive medication. Patients with rheumatic disease should be questioned in regard to steroid therapy within the past year. A history of nausea and vomiting after use of opiates should be sought but should not be confused with undue sensitivity to the substance, since these reactions occur as a common phenomenon. If there is doubt as to the history or if the history suggests untoward reactions with opiates, it is best to avoid the opiate.

The surgical or medical personnel writing orders that require either severe limitation of fluid intake or the use of supplemental fluids in the immediate preoperative period should consider the effects on the patient's physiology as well as the potential interference with the administration of the anesthetic; that is to say, patients who are not to be operated on until late afternoon and who have had fluids withheld from the previous midnight are potential candidates for serious dehydration. This is especially true in pediatric surgery. Furthermore, patients with diabetes mellitus or those receiving intravenous infusions immediately prior to leaving their rooms for the operating room should have infusions begun with large enough needles in suitable veins, so that these infusions can be properly continued during surgery. In patients with upper intestinal tract disease in whom gastric retention is likely or in whom large amounts of barium from recent ingestion may be present at the time of anesthetic administration, consideration should seriously be given to eliminating such retention with appropriate drainage tubes. It is important to emphasize that gastric emptying is delayed with pain and with sedative drugs and that vomiting and aspiration following the induction of general anesthetic with the use of barbiturates and relaxants can be a serious problem.

### Physical Status Versus "Risk"

In the preparation for anesthesia and surgery, especially with reference to preoperative sedation and planning for surgery, one is familiar with the once commonly used term "risk"—a term involving an estimate of prognosis from the standpoint of either mortality or morbidity. There is considerable feeling in anesthesiology that this is a poor term, which should perhaps be abandoned, since to evaluate "risk" completely would necessitate prior knowledge of such variables as reliability of the suture, adequacy of sterilization, availability of drugs, responsibility of those in charge of the postoperative nursing care, and so forth. Too frequently, a patient is characterized in retrospect as a "poor risk" only after a catastrophe has occurred. The following is a classification of physical status as approved by the American Society of Anesthesiologists:

 I. A normal healthy patient.
 II. A patient with a mild systemic disease.
 III. A patient with a severe systemic disease that limits activity but is not incapacitating.
 IV. A patient with an incapacitating systemic disease that is a constant threat to life.
 V. A moribund patient not expected to survive 24 hours, with or without surgery.

In the event of emergency operations, the above number should be preceded by the letter "E." It is desirable that all patients about to receive anesthesia and surgery be evaluated and classified in respect to physical status.

## Emergency Versus Routine Preparation for Surgery and Anesthesia

True surgical emergencies requiring *immediate* operation are rare. As stated by Greene (1963):

The vast majority of cases listed as "emergencies" are in reality urgent or emergent and as such benefit by a certain amount of time devoted preoperatively to full evaluation of the patient's condition, to institution of corrective and supportive measures, and to the organization of an appropriately skilled operative team with a rational plan of action commonly sought out in advance of surgery.

Patient safety is based upon well-established physiologic and pharmacologic facts. It is not based upon the ability to get away with a "calculated risk." The management of the full stomach is but one example. The mere fact that one has been successful with a given technique one hundred times in a row often indicates nothing except coincidence. Such a past record is of no consolation to the widow of the hundred and first case. In the emergency patient, one should always suspect a full stomach and act accordingly. This often is true up to 24 hours after the time of

initial trauma or disturbed physiologic process. Another example of difficulty in determining optimal time of urgent surgery is the patient with active bleeding internally. On the one hand, one hesitates to anesthetize a patient in hemorrhagic shock for fear of altering an already precarious cardiovascular state so that cardiac arrest develops. On the other hand, continued but futile transfusions leave the patient in shock while exposing him to all the risks of repeated transfusions. Currently available data indicate that enough blood should be replaced to cause either the blood pressure to rise or the pulse rate to decrease. This is the moment that is most propitious for the start of anesthesia and surgery.

Whether the anesthesia is to be provided for an emergency or "routine" elective surgery, the anesthesiologist should never be induced into starting an anesthetic, regardless of how extreme the emergency, without having all of his equipment immediately at hand and in functioning order. In many instances, preparing to give a proper and safe anesthetic takes more time than its actual administration. In the true emergency case, the overall physical status of the patient is often poor. By virtue of this fact, most premedicant drugs can be omitted, with the exception of a belladonna drug. In all cases, it is wise to consider the opinions of the Department of Anesthesiology in this regard.

In order to accommodate members of the hospital staff and their friends – whether they be patient or servant, many so-called "emergencies" that are truly urgent in nature are brought to the operating room with no premedication, or premedicant drugs have been given in elevators or clinics a few minutes before surgery. It is important to reiterate that premedicant drugs serve two basic functions: (1) to allay the apprehension of the patient and (2) to create a better physiologic status of the patient preparatory to the induction of anesthesia. For premedicant drugs to have these effects, they should be administered in quiet surroundings and the patient not disturbed or moved to the operating room or anyplace else for a minimum of 30 minutes after the injection.

## AMBULATORY SURGERY

### Preanesthetic Sedation

The type, quantity, and timing of preanesthetic drugs ordered depends upon the anesthesiologist's goal. This accounts for the preference in some institutions for the avoidance of narcotic drugs in all cases, in other institutions for the frequent use of ataractic and tranquilizing drugs, in other cases for the high dosage schedules for belladonna, and in other institutions for the liberal use of narcotics. We prefer our patients to come to the operating room in a semi-awake state, drowsy, free of apprehension, but cooperative in moving to the operating table. We believe that the routine use of phenothiazine and related compounds for the prevention of postanesthetic and postoperative nausea and vomiting is not warranted. The price is persistent sleep, serious pre-, intra-, and postoperative hypotension, and respiratory embarrassment, which frequently accompany these drugs. Irrespective of claims made for them, they are not (in our opinion) warranted for routine use. If pain is a prominent feature, analgesic and narcotic drugs must, of course, be used. If pain is not a part of the preoperative picture, one may then consider principally the use of sedative drugs. With the use of inhalation drugs, such as halothane and cyclopropane, it is beneficial to have adequate dosages of a belladonna drug employed. This is especially true for the apprehensive child, black children, and others receiving open-drop ether anesthesia. While large doses of preanesthetic drugs (especially narcotics) diminish the amount of general anesthetic required, it is preferable, in our opinion, to take a halfway position and reduce the overall anesthetic requirement only in part. A practice that is reasonable for the young adult may be hazardous in the elderly patient; likewise, it must be remembered that muscular and physically active patients require larger doses than the frail, obese, or sedentary patient. It is our opinion that, whenever in doubt, it is better to use less rather than more drugs. It is unlikely that apprehension per se is ever fatal, while depression caused by excessive amounts of narcotics may be a threat to life in the presence of such additional stresses as shock or hemorrhage.

When writing orders for preoperative sedation, one should withhold food and liquids by mouth in adults for a minimum of 8 hours prior to the induction of anesthesia. Infants may be fed a liquid diet within 4 hours of induction of anesthesia, the last formula being withheld and pure water substitution often being additionally advisable. Certain additional generalizations may be made. Weight is a fairly good guide for the determination of dosage, except when the weight is largely fat. Premedication of infants and children is of great importance for successful and uncomplicated anesthesia and should not be omitted because they are young patients. The geriatric patient likewise needs preoperative medicants; however, if some doubt is expressed regarding its effect on the cardiovascular system, it is wise to omit the opiate.

Patients who are to have nerve block field block, or extensive local infiltration should be given one of the relatively short-acting barbiturates in addition to opiate derivatives. This tends to counteract the central nervous system stimulating effect of local anesthetics. It provides additional analgesia and tranquility while the patient is being operated upon under an "awake" condition. While there is no routine dose schedule for any patient, it is, however, essential to proper premedication to know under what conditions a "standard" dose may be altered.

**A.** Time of Administration. Medication which is properly timed in sequence and is given following an adequate night's rest usually may be reduced in overall amount. Therefore, the order for sedation in the evening should usually specify that, for the average adult pentobarbital (Nembutal) or secobarbital (Seconal), 100 mg, may be ordered for 10 P.M., with orders to repeat in one hour if not effective in producing sleep. In general, this is better than ordering one capsule at bedtime, or when in doubt, two capsules. The timing of the orders for the operative day should generally require a barbiturate sedative 1½ hours prior to the time the patient is to be sent to the operating room and a hypodermic of belladonna drug and perhaps a narcotic to be administered at least 45 minutes prior to being sent to the operating room. While "on call" orders are frequently written for the sake of convenience, they are mentioned only to be *avoided*. Medication given too late has little psychic effect on the patient facing operation and often will reach its maximum effect when the patient is most depressed from the anesthesia itself. Those writing preoperative sedation orders should make an educated guess at all times as to the approximate time the patient is likely to arrive in the operating room.

B. THE "STANDARD" DOSE may be

1. *Increased* in the presence of
   a. Increased metabolic rate
   b. Fever
   c. Pain
   d. Robust habitus
   e. Marked apprehension
2. *Decreased* in the presence of
   a. Decreased metabolic rate
   b. Debilitation
   c. Old age

An average healthy adult male or female can use 10 mg of morphine or 100 mg of meperidine as a standard dose. This should be coupled in the average patient with 0.4 to 0.6 mg of atropine or 0.4 to 0.6 mg of scopolamine. *Scopolamine* is preferred in children and adults because it is superior to atropine in all of its pharmacologic properties except for a block of the cardiac vagus. It is superior in its drying effect and has the added advantage of retrograde amnesia, which is highly desirable for postanesthetic and surgical patients. It is said that scopolamine should be avoided in the aged, but with the increasing geriatric population, it seems unlikely that one should consider age 60 as the cut-off age for a patient. We believe that scopolamine can be used in patients older than this. Larger doses of belladonna derivatives are required for blacks and patients with chronic or recent upper respiratory infections. The latter two categories of patients show a significantly greater tendency to form secretions in the upper respiratory tract.

The dosage schedule (Table 6–1) for children has been adequate in most cases.

## Preoperative Orders

As already noted in this chapter by Dr. Paul Dumke, orders are written individually for each patient. I am summarizing the basic orders that I feel are important and useful in the average, healthy adult patient.

1. Nothing by mouth is permitted after midnight.
2. Cleansing enema is given at bedtime. Soapsuds or a small saline type enema may be used.
3. On the evening prior to operation, a tub bath with one of the surgical soaps is insisted upon.
4. Sedation at bedtime if needed. Secobarbital, 100 mg, may be given, and repeated once if necessary.
5. On the morning of operation, the abdomen is shaved from the nipple line to, and including, the pubes, groins, and upper thighs. The entire area is then cleansed with a surgical soap.
6. The patient should void just prior to departure for the operating room.
7. Early morning sedation may be given if the operative procedure is to be performed later in the day.
8. On call medication is given intramuscularly at least one-half hour, and preferably one hour, before the operative procedure is to begin and may include

   Meperidine hydrochloride (Demerol, 100 mg) (or morphine sulfate 10 mg)
   Atropine sulfate, 0.4 to 0.6 mg

9. When local anesthesia or regional anesthesia is contemplated and the patient is to remain conscious, it is not necessary to medicate the patient with atropine or scopolamine. The discomfort of dry mouth and cracked lips may be the biggest complaint during or after surgery.

   If the anesthesiologist must, for any reason, use general anesthesia and thinks atropine is necessary, he can easily administer the drug intravenously just prior to induction of general anesthesia.

Orders for aged patients are modified on an individual basis. Narcotics may be

Table 6–1. PREOPERATIVE MEDICATION FOR CHILDREN

| Age | Average Weight (kg) | Pentobarbital (Nembutal) (mg) | Morphine (mg) | Atropine (mg) |
|---|---|---|---|---|
| Newborn | 3.3 | — | — | 0.15 |
| 6 months | 8.1 | 30 pr | — | 0.2 |
| 1 year | 10.6 | 45 pr | 1.0 | 0.2 |
| 2 years | 14.0 | 60 pr | 1.5 | 0.3 |
| 3 years | 15.0 | 60 pr | 2.0 | 0.3 |
| 4 years | 17.1 | 90 pr | 3.0 | 0.3 |
| 5 years | 19.4 | 90 pr | 3.0 | 0.3 |
| 6 years | 22.0 | 90 pr | 4.0 | 0.4 |
| 7 years | 24.7 | 90 pr | 5.0 | 0.4 |
| 8 years | 27.9 | 100 po | 6.0 | 0.4 |
| 9 years | 31.4 | 100 po | 6.0 | 0.4 |
| 10 years | 35.2 | 100 po | 7.0 | 0.4 |
| 11 years | 39.6 | 100 po | 7.0 | 0.4 |
| 12 years | 44.4 | 100 po | 7.0 | 0.4 |
| 13 years | 49.1 | 100 po | 8.0 | 0.4 |
| 14 years | 54.4 | 100 po | 8.0 | 0.4 |
| 15 years | 58.8 | 100 po | 8.0 | 0.4 |
| 16 years | 61.9 | 100 po | 8.0 | 0.4 |

1. This table is a guide to be followed for average, well-developed patients. Increases or reductions in medication must be made for patients who do not fall into the guidelines, i.e., hyperactive, obese, or poor-risk patients.
2. Nembutal should be given at least 90 minutes before surgery.
3. Morphine should be given 30 to 45 minutes (IM or SC) before surgery.
4. Suggested guide for pentobarbital when followed by morphine is 4.0 mg/kg for rectal use (maximum dose, 120 mg) and 3.0 mg/kg for oral use (maximum dose, 100 mg).
5. Suggested guide for morphine is 0.75 mg/year of age.

From Smith, R. M.: *Anesthesia for Infants and Children* (4th ed.). St. Louis, C. V. Mosby Co. (in preparation).

omitted in feeble patients, since they require much less sedation; apprehension is not a common reaction in older patients.

## REFERENCES

Greene, N. M.: *Clinical Anesthesia for Emergency Surgery.* Philadelphia, F. A. Davis Co., 1963.
Smith, Robert M.: *Anesthesia for Infants and Children* (4th ed.). St. Louis, C. V. Mosby Co., (in preparation).

## Supplemental Readings

Dripps, R. D.: The pharmacological basis for preoperative medication. Surg. Clin. North Am. *24:* 1377, 1944.
Dripps, R. D., Eckenhoff, J. E., and Vandam, R.: *Introduction to Anesthesia* (5th ed.). Philadelphia, W. B. Saunders Co., 1977.
Nicholson, M. J.: Preoperative preparation and premedication. Surg. Clin. North Am. *30:*635, 1950.

# 7

# The Hernia Problem in the Female

## INTRODUCTION

A statistical study of the overall incidence of the more common hernias in males and females was undertaken in order to establish a basis for a discussion of the hernia problem as it relates to the female. In order to accomplish this, I selected at random the years 1965 and 1967 and included only those patients operated on at our institution. A compilation of the incidence of direct, indirect, femoral, and combinations of the three, and incisional, esophageal, hiatal, umbilical, and epigastric hernias has resulted in some interesting and, I hope, worthwhile observations concerning the sexual predisposition toward the development of certain types of hernias.

In general, hernias of the abdominal wall occur far less frequently in women than in men. The greatest disparity is seen in the incidence of indirect and direct inguinal hernias, which occur so often in men. During the years 1965 and 1967, 1340 direct and indirect hernias were operated upon in men, while only 112 were operated upon in women, producing a male-female ratio of 12:1 (Table 7–1).

## ANATOMIC CONSIDERATIONS

The inguinal region in the male is such that it permits development of groin hernias following excessive increase in intra-abdominal pressure. However, the abdominal wall in the female is surprisingly resistant to the development of hernias, in spite of the regular testing of its strength by three factors: obesity, pregnancy, and surgical operative procedures. Obesity is a

Table 7–1. HERNIAS IN MALES AND FEMALES, HENRY FORD HOSPITAL (1965 and 1967)

| | Males | | | Females | | |
|---|---|---|---|---|---|---|
| | NUMBER | % | | NUMBER | % | |
| Indirect | 887 | 53.6 | | 107 | 32.9 | |
| Direct | 453 | 27.4 | | 5 | 1.5 | |
| Combination direct-indirect-femoral | 126 | 7.6 | | 10 | 3.1 | |
| Incisional | 57 | 3.4 | | 57 | 17.5 | |
| Femoral | 47 | 2.8 | | 36 | 11.1 | |
| Umbilical | 38 | 2.3 | | 54 | 16.6 | |
| Hiatal | 36 | 2.2 | | 48 | 14.8 | |
| Epigastric | 11 | 0.7 | | 8 | 2.46 | |
| Total | 1655 | | | 325 | | |

frequent accompaniment of hernia in women. Multiple pregnancies often precede the development of femoral and umbilical hernias. Operative procedures, especially if multiple, can cause abdominal wall weakness that, sooner or later, may result in herniation.

Important anatomic differences between the sexes account for the variations in type and incidence of hernias in males and females. These include: (1) descent of the testes and ovaries, (2) anatomic differences in the relationship of musculofascial layers of the lower abdomen, (3) anatomic differences in the bony pelvis, and (4) differences in etiologic factors.

The effect of the descent of the testicles on the incidence of hernias is discussed in detail in Chapter 10. The embryologic events whereby the testes reach, or attempt to reach, the scrotum result in a definite weakness in the groin of the male. Failure of obliteration of the processus vaginalis is directly implicated in the formation of indirect inguinal hernias in males and females. In the female, just as in the male, the gonads arise retroperitoneally. During the developmental process, the pelvic organs move caudally and laterally so that the ovaries and fallopian tubes eventually reach the pelvis. The cephalic part of the inguinal ligament of the mesonephros becomes the round ligament of the ovary, while the caudal part becomes the round ligament of the uterus. The distal portion of the round ligament normally reaches the labium majus, just as the gubernaculum does in the male. An evagination of the peritoneum related to the round ligament is known as the canal of Nuck. This structure is obliterated at about the eighth month of fetal life. Should it persist, an indirect inguinal hernia could result. Arnheim and Linder (1956) believe that the broad ligament plays an important role in the development of sliding hernias in females. Since this structure is proximate to the internal ring, traction upon it and, consequently, upon the genital organs results in sliding hernias, which may include the ovary, fallopian tubes, and even the uterus. The round ligament and the internal ring are smaller structures in females than the corresponding spermatic cord and internal ring are in males.

From the anatomic point of view, the transversalis fascia and transversus abdominis layers are well developed in the female. These layers are of such strength that direct hernias through the floor of Hesselbach's triangle are rare indeed. McVay (1961) has repeatedly pointed out that the broad attachment of the transversus abdominis arch onto Cooper's ligament further adds to the strength in this area and gives protection against direct and femoral hernias. In the male, the high insertion of the internal oblique and transversus abdominis muscles to the sheath of rectus abdominis and the comparatively narrow attachment of the transversus abdominis arch to Cooper's ligament predispose him to direct and femoral herniation.

The bones of the female are more slender, the iliac fossae shallower, and the true pelvis wider. The angle between Cooper's ligament and the inguinal ligament is not as great or acute in the female as it is in the male. However, the interval between the medial aspect of the femoral ring and the femoral vein is somewhat larger in the female when examined during operative procedures.

Pregnancy, obesity, and operative procedures are factors that commonly contribute to the formation of hernias in women. These events often occur in the same woman and result in umbilical, femoral, or postoperative incisional hernias.

Developmental anatomic differences in the male and female account for the incidence and variety of hernia seen in each. There are few differences insofar as exciting causes are concerned.

## INCIDENCE

The precise incidence of hernias in males and females will vary somewhat among studies, but approximate values are useful. The incidence in any series will vary greatly with age, sex, and occupation of individuals studied (Table 7–2). Any analysis containing large numbers of infants and children will show a preponderance of indirect inguinal hernias. Series

Table 7–2.  INCIDENCE OF VARIOUS TYPES OF HERNIAS

| | Male and Female (Collected Cases) Zimmerman | | Female Only (Personal Cases) Glasgow | |
|---|---|---|---|---|
| | NUMBER | % | NUMBER | % |
| Inguinal | 82,467 | 81.4 | 1,243 | 53 |
| Incisional | 1,724 | 1.7 | 353 | 15 |
| Femoral | 5,320 | 5.3 | 384 | 17 |
| Umbilical | 8,419 | 8.4 | 284 | 12 |
| Epigastric | 2,037 | 2.0 | 45 | 2.0 |
| Miscellaneous | 147 | 0.1 | 16 | 1 |
| Total | 100,114 | | 1,725 | |

emanating from industrial centers will show indirect inguinal hernias, but as the population age increases, so will the incidence of direct inguinal hernias. Studies limited to direct inguinal hernias alone will include few females indeed.

Most statistical studies show that men incur hernias nine times as often as women. In 1893 Macready, in a collected series of 21,795 patients with hernia, found that 18,223, or 84 percent, occurred in men, while 3572, or 16 percent, occurred in women. Massive statistics are available in the literature to further substantiate the fact that hernias are far more common in men. Watson in 1938 collected the statistics from the publications of Malgaigne, Berger, Macready, and Coley, in which 104,641 hernias were amassed. Of these, 80,870, or 77 percent, occurred in males and 23,771, or 23 percent, in females. In the two years that I selected to study, 84 percent of 1980 hernias occurred in males, while 16 percent occurred in females.

Armentrout (1936) reported that of 37,472 working men examined, 1837, or 4.9 percent, were found to have hernias. Keith (1923) found that 20 of every 1000 men in Great Britain had hernias. He estimated the male-to-female ratio of hernias to be approximately 6:1. Zimmerman and Anson (1967) found that inguinal hernias were seen nine times more often in men than in women. Hagan and Rhoads (1953) studied 1082 inguinal herniorrhaphies and found that 86 percent of the total occurred in males. McClure and Fallis in 1939 found only 36 females with femoral hernias out of 241,037 hospital admissions, producing a ratio of one femoral hernia per 6700 admissions. Koontz (1952) found 93 femoral hernias in women in 316,525

patients, giving a ratio of one femoral hernia per 3400 hospital admissions.

## STATISTICAL ANALYSIS

In order to better understand the problem of hernia as it affects the female, I have personally reviewed our operating room ledgers for the years 1965 and 1967. In cases in which the diagnosis was incomplete or suspected of being inaccurate, the medical record was reviewed. Such an analysis provides us with the types and number of hernias seen in males and females. Although several varieties of hernia were encountered, a practical classification demands simplification; therefore, general types of hernias were listed. For instance, sliding hernias were listed as direct, indirect, or femoral. No attempt was made to list incarcerated or strangulated hernias, since the purpose of this analysis was simply to view the overall problem of herniation as it occurs in the female. Complications, such as strangulation and incarceration, are dealt with separately in other chapters.

In this study, I found that for every female with a hernia at least five men required treatment of some type of hernia. This observation, that nearly 85 percent of hernias occurred in men, seemed almost unbelievable until the statistics were scrutinized further. Indirect, direct, and combinations of such hernias are seen far more frequently in men. The male-to-female ratio of such hernias is somewhat better than 12:1. The incidence of the common types of groin and abdominal wall hernias seen in the studies of Zimmerman and Glasgow is shown in Table 7–2.

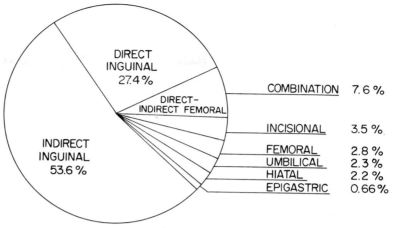

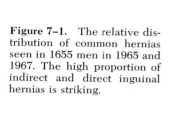

**Figure 7-1.** The relative distribution of common hernias seen in 1655 men in 1965 and 1967. The high proportion of indirect and direct inguinal hernias is striking.

## Indirect Inguinal Hernias

During the years 1965 and 1967, 887 men and 107 women were treated for indirect inguinal hernias at the Henry Ford Hospital. Indirect inguinal and recurrent indirect inguinal hernias made up 53.6 percent of hernias in males (Fig. 7–1) and nearly 33 percent of all hernias in females (Fig. 7–2). The significantly greater frequency of indirect inguinal hernias in men has been noted many times in the literature. It is confirmed again in this study, in which eight times as many men as women appeared with indirect hernias. The inguinal canal from the internal abdominal ring to the external abdominal ring is a smaller structure in the female. The descent of the testicle is directly

implicated as a factor in the etiology of indirect inguinal hernias in the male. Differences in anatomic configuration are additional factors.

While 32 recurrent inguinal hernias were encountered in men, four such hernias were seen in women. Although far more recurrent indirect inguinal hernias were seen in men, the relative incidence of recurrent indirect inguinal hernias was identical for both sexes. The incidence ratio of both indirect inguinal hernias and recurrent indirect inguinal hernias, males to females, is approximately 8:1. From this study, there is no evidence to suggest that repair of indirect inguinal hernias in men is followed by a greater incidence of recurrence. Since only one-eighth as many indirect inguinal hernias were seen in

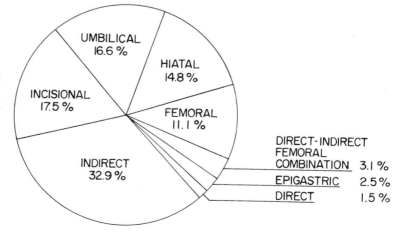

**Figure 7-2.** The distribution of common hernias in 325 females in 1965 and 1967. Note the relatively greater frequency of incisional, umbilical, hiatal, and femoral hernias in the female.

women, recurrent indirect inguinal hernias likewise will be seen rarely in females.

One feature not apparent from this study is the frequency of bilateral indirect inguinal hernias and sliding hernias in infants. Bilateral indirect hernias in infants are not at all rare and may contain ovaries, fallopian tubes, and even the uterus as sliding components. These observations were made after studying hernias in infants and children and are recorded in greater detail in Chapters 10 and 18. It has long been known that indirect inguinal hernias occur with much greater frequency in the male. Coley (1924) studied the incidence of different types of hernias found in 3000 operations. He had a mixed patient population insofar as age and sex are concerned. He found that a total of 2168 operations, or 72 percent of the total, were performed for indirect inguinal hernias in males, while only 237, or 7.9 percent, were performed upon females. Of all indirect inguinal hernias in this study, 90 percent occurred in males. In a study of 1600 operations for inguinal hernia, McClure and Fallis (1939) found that only 1.1 percent were performed in females. This is the lowest incidence in women that I have found in the literature for studies carried out in hospitals treating male and female patients of all ages.

Hagan and Rhoads (1953) found that the indirect inguinal hernia was the most common hernia encountered in females, occurring in 51 percent of the cases studied.

Glassow (1965) reported that of 2374 consecutive hernia repairs in women, 1784 were inguinal and 590 were femoral. In his experience, groin hernias occurred 25 times more often in men than in women. Of the total, 1548 repairs were carried out for primary indirect inguinal hernias in females. In reviewing data for the two years, I found that indirect inguinal hernias composed approximately one-third of the total number of hernias occurring in females (Fig. 7–2). Just as in the adult female, less than 15 percent of hernias occurred in female infants.

Ljungdahl analyzed his personal experience with inguinal and femoral hernias in 1973. He found that the primary indirect type accounted for 64.9 percent of the hernias in men. His incidence of primary indirect inguinal hernia in women was 61.5 percent.

Some comment is necessary pertaining to the important subject of indirect inguinal hernias and sliding inguinal hernias in female infants, since such hernias not at all rarely contain adnexa, which may become incarcerated and even strangulated. Watson (1938) cited a gynecologist and obstetrician with the unlikely name of Soranus as the first to describe a hernia of the ovary in the second century A.D. By 1948, Watson was able to collect 469 cases in which some combination of ovary, fallopian tube, and uterus was found in hernial sacs in females of all ages. Although several authors had referred to the existence of such hernias, Arnheim and Linder in 1956 reported on 29 cases of inguinal hernia of the pelvic viscera in 28 female infants. Ovary and fallopian tubes were present in 14; ovary, fallopian tube, and uterus in nine; fallopian tube in three; fallopian tube and uterus in two; and the uterus alone was present in only one of the 28 infants. Bilateral inguinal hernias are not at all uncommon in female infants. The subject of infantile hernias is considered in greater detail in Chapter 10.

## DIRECT INGUINAL HERNIAS IN FEMALES

The direct inguinal hernia, so often seen in men (Fig. 7–2), is rarely seen in women. The type that I have seen most often is a diverticular type located medially to the deep inferior epigastric artery. The defect in the transversalis fascia is usually small, and the sac has a finger-like configuration. The transversalis fascia in the floor of Hesselbach's triangle is so strong that it rarely permits a large diffuse disruption such as seen in males.

The remarkable preponderance of direct inguinal hernias in men can be appreciated when the statistics are considered. In the years 1965 and 1967, 453 direct and direct recurrent inguinal hernias were seen in males, while only five such hernias were seen in females. The male-female ratio of direct inguinal hernias was found to be approximately 90:1.

My observations lead me to the opinion that the absence of the spermatic cord and the more effective and lower attachment of the transversalis fascia, the transversus abdominis, and the internal oblique to Cooper's ligament and rectus sheath are responsible for the stronger inguinal floor in the female. Only one recurrent direct inguinal hernia was found in a female.

Hoguet (1923) encountered only seven direct inguinal hernias in women and 252 in men while repairing 2468 hernias.

Coley (1924) repaired 284 direct inguinal hernias among 3000 operations performed on men, but only three direct inguinal hernias were seen in females during the same period.

Hagan and Rhoads studied 1082 herniorrhaphies and found that 95 percent of direct inguinal hernias occurred in males. In their series, 10 women were treated for direct inguinal hernias. Combining the statistics of Hoguet, Coley, and Hagan and Rhoads, we have a total of 6550 operations for abdominal and inguinal hernias. These statistics are somewhat open to criticism, since the patient populations are not identical; nevertheless, it is noteworthy that only 20 direct inguinal hernias were seen in females.

Glassow, during a 26-year period from 1945 to 1970, reported an experience derived from operating upon 1548 primary indirect inguinal hernias and 124 primary direct inguinal hernias in females. His experience again confirms the rarity of direct inguinal hernias in females.

Ljungdahl found that direct inguinal hernias were present in 33.5 percent of the males in his series, but only 7.7 percent of his female patients had such hernias.

During the two years of our study, 325 abdominal hernias were seen in women, but only five, or 1.5 percent, were of the direct variety (Fig. 7–2).

The abdominal wall in the female is well endowed by nature to resist the development of direct inguinal hernias. The surgeon who repairs groin hernias in females should be cognizant of this important fact. Indirect hernias should be repaired by techniques that close the transversalis fascia completely at the internal ring. Any techniques that might disrupt the floor of Hesselbach's triangle should be avoided.

## COMBINATIONS OF DIRECT, INDIRECT, AND FEMORAL HERNIAS

Hernias in which an indirect sac and a direct protrusion occur simultaneously in the same groin are not rare. Such hernias are known as pantaloon or saddle-bag hernias for obvious reasons. Occasionally, a femoral hernia may be present as well. The possibility of such combinations makes it mandatory for the surgeon to consider their existence whenever any type of hernia is being repaired.

Combinations of defects in the groin, as might be expected, are more common in males. For the two years in my study, I found combinations of direct, indirect, and femoral herniation in 127 males but in only 10 females (Table 7–1). Direct and indirect combined hernias were seen in 93 men but in only four women. In general, for every female with some combination of an indirect, direct, and femoral hernia, I found that at least 12 males will develop such hernias. The preponderance of both indirect inguinal and direct inguinal hernias in men is again confirmed here.

Coley (1924), in analyzing 3000 operations for hernia, found that 100 operations for combined direct and indirect inguinal hernias were performed in males, while only one such operation was performed on a female. Furthermore, he found 22 instances of bilateral direct and indirect hernias in men, but none in women.

Clearly, the female seldom develops more than one type of groin defect simultaneously, and when she does, it is more likely to be indirect and femoral.

### Femoral Hernias

Whereas the incidence of indirect and direct inguinal hernias in males greatly exceeds their occurrence in females, femoral hernias are somewhat more equitably distributed between the sexes. In a study at Henry Ford Hospital covering a two-year period, 36 femoral hernias were seen in 325 females, while 47 femoral hernias were seen among 1655 males. Converting these figures into percentages, 11 percent of the hernias in females were femoral, while only 3 percent of the hernias in males were of the femoral variety (Figs. 7–1 and 7–2). The incidence of femoral hernias for both male and female patients was somewhat more than 4 percent.

Coley found the incidence of femoral hernia in both males and females to be 3.37 percent in 3000 operated cases. Of the 3000 operations, 43 were for repair of femoral hernias in males, and 53 were for repair of femoral hernias in females.

Glassow, in a study of 1101 primary operations for femoral hernia, found that 687 operations, or 62.4 percent, were performed upon males, and 414, or 37.6 percent, were performed upon females. Thus, the distribution of femoral hernias was again found to be more equitable for males and females than is the case with indirect and direct inguinal hernias, which are so common in males.

Glassow, in a separate study of 2325 abdominal hernias, found the incidence of femoral hernias to be 17 percent, while inguinal hernias made up 53 percent of the total.

In an analysis of inguinal and femoral hernias in males and females, Macready found that femoral hernias comprised 5.9 percent in females but only 2.1 percent in males.

Zimmerman and Anson compiled supporting statistics to show that the incidence of femoral hernia is from 5 to 7 percent of all hernias. These figures are, I believe, valid. They also concluded that femoral hernias make up approximately 2 percent of all hernias in men, but they constitute 34 percent of all hernias in females.

The studies of Ljungdahl were of interest insofar as femoral hernias are concerned. He found that femoral hernias accounted for 1.6 percent of the hernias in males and 30.8 percent of the hernias in females. He did find, however, that there were almost as many men as women with femoral hernias.

Femoral hernias are occasionally difficult to diagnose in elderly females and can lead to incarceration and strangulation of the bowel. I have investigated the problem of complicated femoral hernias and have been impressed with the common delay in diagnosis and treatment; this delay too often results in intestinal stran-gulation and the need for resection. The resultant postoperative course is stormy and prolonged. The problem of the femoral hernia is further discussed in Chapter 15.

## INCISIONAL HERNIAS

Postoperative incisional hernias were seen relatively more frequently in women. In the study discussed in this chapter, I examined the incidence of postoperative hernias at Henry Ford Hospital for the years 1965 and 1967. Thirty-six, or 11.08 percent, of 325 females were found to have incisional hernias (Fig. 7–2). During this same period, 57, or 3.44 percent of 1655 men underwent repair of incisional hernias. The total number of incisional hernias for both sexes was 93, or 4.7 percent of all hernias in the study.

The incidence of incisional hernias has been found to vary considerably among hospitals. McVay found the incidence to range from 5.7 percent to 11.5 percent in various series.

In most studies, the high incidence of incisional hernias in females has been attributed to hysterectomy, a common operation in females. Branch (1934) reported that females were found to have 71.6 percent of incisional hernias. The experience with postoperative ventral hernias at Henry Ford Hospital is discussed in greater detail in Chapter 21.

## UMBILICAL HERNIAS

In this study, umbilical hernias occurred in 92 of a total 1980 patients, for an incidence of 4.65 percent.

Umbilical hernias in females constitute 16.62 percent of the hernias studied in a two-year period (Fig. 7–2). Among 325 females, 54 were found to have such hernias. During the same period of time, only 38 of 1655 males were found to have such hernias, for a percentage incidence of 2.3 percent. The preponderance of umbilical hernias in females is striking.

Many patients will attribute the onset of umbilical herniation to pregnancy. Furthermore, multiple pregnancies often precede the development of umbilical hernia.

Obesity is another common finding in females with this type of hernia.

## EPIGASTRIC HERNIAS

Epigastric hernias were not commonly encountered in either sex. In 1980 patients, 8 females and 11 males were found to have epigastric hernias or hernias of the linea alba. The incidence of epigastric hernia was found to be nearly 1 percent among our patients. The relative incidence of epigastric hernias in females was 2.46 percent, whereas the incidence in males was 0.66 percent. This experience with epigastric hernias is further described in Chapter 22.

## ESOPHAGEAL HIATAL HERNIA

Although they are not dealt with in this book, hernias at the esophageal hiatus are fairly common. I found the statistics related to the incidence of such hernias to be of interest. Hiatal hernias were found in 48, or 14.77 percent, of 325 women and in 36, or 2.18 percent, of 1655 men. The incidence of esophageal hiatal hernia for both men and women was 4.24 percent. Thus, the problem of esophageal hiatal hernia is considerably greater in females.

## SUMMARY

Although groin hernias occur far more frequently in males, they present a common problem in females as well. Certain facts regarding the incidence of hernias in females are becoming increasingly clear. The female is afflicted with indirect inguinal hernias far less often than the male. In any large series, the male will be found to have such hernias seven to ten times more often than the female. In our experience, the male-to-female ratio of indirect inguinal hernias was 8:1.

Direct inguinal hernias also are more commonly seen in males. The fact that direct protrusions through the floor of Hesselbach's triangle are most unusual in females has been confirmed by many observers. The ratio of direct to indirect inguinal hernias in females has been reported to be as high as 1:557. To look at the matter from another perspective, I found the female-to-male ratio of direct inguinal hernias to be 1:90. The implication of such statistics is that the inguinal floor in the female is unusually strong and seldom requires repair. Any attempt at strengthening the floor of the inguinal canal without good indication is ill founded.

Combinations of direct, indirect, and femoral hernias occurred 12 times more often in males than in females in our experience.

Femoral hernias have been found to account for slightly more than 5 percent of all hernias in both men and women. The incidence of femoral hernias in the female was found to vary from 11 to 17 percent. In a study of our cases, femoral hernias occurred in 11 percent of the females but in only 2.84 percent of the males.

Incisional hernias have shown an increase in incidence in the past 50 years. Abdominal operative procedures have increased in frequency and magnitude. Knowledge as to how operative wounds heal is well documented, but the application of such principles to the operative wound shows a distressing time lag. With improved technique in wound management, the incidence will decrease. The incidence of incisional hernias has ranged from 2 to 17 percent in various reported series. I found that postoperative incisional hernias accounted for 3.5 percent of hernias in men and 17.5 percent in women. Gynecologic procedures have accounted for the statistical preponderance of such hernias in females.

Umbilical hernias account for 12 to 16 percent of the hernias in females. I found that umbilical hernias accounted for only 2.3 percent of the hernias in males but 16.6 percent of the hernias in females. Obesity and pregnancy were common factors in the etiology of umbilical hernias in adult females.

Epigastric hernias have been found to account for approximately 2 percent of all hernias in both males and females. The incidence was less than 1 percent of all hernias in females and nearly 2.5 percent of those in males.

Because esophageal hiatal hernias represent a substantial number of all hernias occurring among males and females, I recorded their incidence during the years 1965 and 1967. In males, hiatal hernias accounted for 2.18 percent of the total, while in females they accounted for nearly 15 percent. Thus, hiatal hernias were significantly more common in females.

## REFERENCES

Armentrout, C. R.: Hernia and its effect on the industrial worker. South. Med. J. 29:630, 1936.

Arnheim, Ernest E., and Linder, Jerome M.: Inguinal hernia of the pelvic viscera in female infants. Am. J. Surg. 92:436, 1956.

Branch, C. D.: Incisional hernia: Analysis of three hundred cases. N. Engl. J. Med. 211:949, 1934.

Coley, B. L.: Three thousand consecutive herniotomies. Ann. Surg. 80:242, 1924.

Glassow, F.: Inguinal and femoral hernia in women. Int. Surg. 57(1):34, 1972.

Glassow, F.: Femoral hernia in the female. Can. Med. Assoc. J. 93:1346, 1965.

Hagan, W. H., and Rhoads, J. E.: Inguinal and femoral hernias: A follow-up study. Surg. Gynecol. Obstet. 96:226, 1953.

Hoguet, J. P.: Observations on two thousand four hundred and sixty-eight hernia operations by one operator. Surg. Gynecol. Obstet. 37:71, 1923.

Keith, A.: On the origin and nature of hernia. Br. J. Surg. 11:455, 1923.

Koontz, A. R.: Femoral hernia: Operative cases at the Johns Hopkins Hospital during a twenty-one year period. Arch. Surg. 64:298, 1952.

Ljungdahl, I.: Inguinal and femoral hernia. Personal experience with 502 operations. Acta Chir. Scand. Suppl.:1, 1973.

Macready, J. F. C. H.: A Treatise on Ruptures. London, Griffin & Co., 1893.

McClure, R. D., and Fallis, L. S.: Femoral hernia: Report of 90 operations. Ann. Surg. 109:987, 1939.

McVay, C. B., and Savage, L. E.: Etiology of femoral hernia. Ann. Surg. 154:25, 1961.

Watson, L. F.: Hernia (2nd ed.). St. Louis, C. V. Mosby Co., 1938.

Wiley, J., and Chàvez, H. A.: Uterine adnexa in inguinal hernia in infant females. West. J. Surg. 65:283, 1957.

Zimmerman, L. M., and Anson, B. J.: Anatomy and Surgery of Hernia (2nd ed.). Baltimore, Williams & Wilkins Co., 1967, pp. 15–43.

## Supplemental Readings

DeBoer, A.: Inguinal hernia in infants and children. Arch. Surg. 75:920, 1957.

Donovan, E. J., and Stanley-Brown, E. G.: Inguinal hernia in female infants and children. Surg. Gynecol. Obstet. 107:663, 1958.

Gans, Stephen, L.: Sliding inguinal hernia in female infants. Arch. Surg. 79:109, 1959.

Glassow, F.: An evaluation of the strength of the posterior wall of the inguinal canal in women. Br. J. Surg. 60(5):342, 1973.

Glassow, F.: Bilateral hernias in the female. Can. Med. Assoc. J. 101:540, 1969.

Glassow, F.: Inguinal hernia in the female. Surg. Gynecol. Obstet. 116:701, 1963.

Goldstein, I. R., and Potts, W. J.: Inguinal hernia in female infants and children. Ann. Surg. 148(5):819, 1958.

McVay, C. B.: Christopher's Textbook of Surgery (7th ed.). Philadelphia, W. B. Saunders Co., 1960, pp. 524–569.

Pender, R., Lucas, J., and McAteer, G. H.: Report on inguinal hernias in female children. Clin. Proc. Child. Hosp. Wash. 7(4):113–115, 1951.

Ponka, J. L.: Incarcerated femoral hernia. Henry Ford Hosp. Med. Bull. 15(3):203, 1967.

Ponka, J. L., and Brush, B. E.: Problem of femoral hernia. Arch. Surg. 102:417, 1971.

Wakaley, C. P. G.: Hernia of the ovary and fallopian tube, 25 cases. Surg. Gynecol. Obstet. 51:256, 1930.

# 8

# Local Anesthesia for Abdominal Wall Hernias

## INTRODUCTION

There are operative procedures that lend themselves anatomically and technically to accomplishment under local anesthesia. Safety and minimal morbidity are benefits that offset the slight inconvenience to the surgeon and some temporary discomfort to the patient. Local anesthesia will be used with increasing frequency as more surgeons and anesthesiologists learn of its advantages, particularly in feeble, aged patients with serious cardiac, pulmonary, and renal diseases. Furthermore, the young surgeon can learn gentleness and precision in the safe performance of a common procedure.

## HISTORICAL BACKGROUND

The earliest contributors who introduced the first local anesthetic drugs, invented the necessary armamentarium, and initiated the technique of local anesthesia needed foresight, a keen sense of observation, and courage. Certain historical events in the development of local anesthesia should be of interest to every surgeon. The texts on the subject by Allen (1918), Sherwood-Dunn (1920), Labat (1922), Bonica (1953), and Southworth and Hingson (1946) were consulted for much of the information in this section.

Discovery of the hypodermic syringe is attributed to F. Rynd of Edinburgh in 1845. There is a difference of opinion as to who first made use of the syringe, since Keys (1945) gives credit to Pravaz for having employed this device in 1853. Also in 1853, another important contribution was made by Wood, who is credited with having invented the modern metallic hollow needle. The availability of this device led to the injection of various concoctions beneath the skin.

Nevertheless, the syringe and the hollow needle were not enough. A safe drug capable of producing anesthesia was necessary. In 1855 Gadecke isolated a substance from the leaves of the coca plant, *Erythroxylon* coca. In 1860, Niemann isolated the pure alkaloid from coca leaves. Wöhler, in whose laboratory Niemann made his discovery, noticed the numbing effect on the tongue and the bitter taste of the drug. He is credited with naming the new agent "cocaine."

In a most remarkable oversight, the investigations of von Anrep in 1879 were not appreciated at that time. He observed that following a subcutaneous injection of a weak solution of cocaine, one first experienced warmth, followed by numbness that lasted approximately 35 minutes. His suggestion that the drug be used as a local anesthetic was ignored until six years later.

The clinical usefulness of cocaine was made clear in 1884, when Karl Koller demonstrated that complete anesthesia followed instillation of a 2 percent solution into the eye of a rabbit. His observations were presented at the Ophthalmological Congress in Heidelberg. This discovery reached revolutionary proportions within various surgical specialities, and within one year its effectiveness was tested in many clinics. Anesthesia was available upon local application of cocaine to mucous membranes.

Surgeons are, no doubt, more directly concerned with the next milestone in anesthesia. In 1885 William Stewart Halsted demonstrated that cocaine could block impulses through nerve trunks. Nerve block anesthesia became a reality for the first time.

The fact that dilute anesthetic solutions were effective was not always appreciated. Reclus in 1885 vigorously and continuously advocated the use of solutions no stronger than 1 percent because of greater safety. Schleich introduced infiltration anesthesia in 1892.

The development of the science of anesthesiology is one of the strange events in the progress of medicine. General anesthesia had been discovered and well developed within the years 1842–1847. This was approximately 38 years before the science of local anesthesia reached a comparable level of development.

Although the discovery of cocaine was a great gift to mankind, certain undesirable effects unfortunately appeared. According to Farr (1922), death had been reported from doses as small as 16 and 40 mg. Toxicity of the agent was manifested by nervousness, tachycardia, deepened respirations, and vertigo. Convulsions were not rare. Addiction to the drug created serious social problems and, even worse, an occasional death.

The search for safer, nonaddictive effective drugs was being carried on vigorously. Today's problem of drug addiction is hardly new. One of the most dramatic incidents in the history of medicine occurred as a result of Halsted's research into the pharmacologic effects of cocaine. Unaware of its addicting properties, he fell victim to the drug, probably in 1885. He was hospitalized and, fortunately, had the strength of character and will to overcome its devastating effects. His subsequent achievements as a teacher and surgical scientist made him one of the greatest surgeons of all time.

Early enthusiasm for cocaine was replaced by respect for this useful, yet dangerous, drug. Dissatisfaction with it led to determined efforts to discover an effective and safer drug. Einhorn and his associates searched for such an agent, and in 1905 procaine became available. Interest in developing new, safe, long-acting stable agents has continued since that time.

This chapter would be incomplete without reference to the use of epinephrine. In 1903 Professor Heinrich Braun of Zwickau, Germany published his observations on the effects of epinephrine in *Die Lokal Anesthesie*. He noted that the desirable effect of epinephrine produced vasoconstriction, resulting in longer duration of anesthesia, even when dilute anesthetic solutions of 1 percent or less were used. The toxic effects of the drug were found to be both annoying and serious. Substernal oppression, palpitation of the heart, tachycardia, and increased depth of respirations due to epinephrine injection were also described by Braun in 1903.

In reviewing the historical development of the technique of local anesthesia, it becomes evident that many of the common technical procedures were developed by the French and German contributors. Sherwood-Dunn (1920) acknowledges the contributions of Professor Reclus of the Paris Faculté. His method was one of local infiltration, which he had used in 1890. Schleich used the same method two years later. Professor Victor Pauchet was an early advocate of regional anesthesia. Sourdat and Laboure were others who recommended regional anesthesia. The various basic techniques are well illustrated in the text by Sherwood-Dunn. Braun and Kocher of Germany also perfected techniques that produced effective anesthesia about the head and neck.

Southworth and Hingson (1946) expressed vigorous and justifiable criticisms of certain procedures advocated by the French school. For instance, they referred to the limitations of abdominal wall infiltration anesthesia when attempting intraabdominal procedures. They pointed out the need for blocking the sympathetic fibers to the organs concerned in a given operation. In spite of such criticisms, it is possible in aged, debilitated patients to carry out extensive procedures under abdominal wall block anesthesia together with local infiltration of the sympathetic branches to the specific organs if necessary. We have been pleased with the effectiveness of abdominal wall block in poor-risk patients with ventral hernias.

In 1900 the internationally known neurosurgeon, Dr. Harvey Cushing, described the neuroanatomy of the inguinal region as well as his experiences with local anesthesia in repair of hernias.

From 1884 through 1905, tremendous progress was made in the field of local anesthesia. A suitable but dangerous drug, cocaine, became available. A variety of techniques for local infiltration and nerve block anesthesia were developed. In 1905, the first of the synthetic agents, procaine, was made available. Newer agents, less toxic and more rapidly active, were forthcoming. During this period of 21 years (1884–1905), useful drugs were discovered, and local anesthesia had become of age.

## PRACTICAL ANATOMY FOR LOCAL ANESTHESIA

Knowledge of certain simple basic anatomic facts is indispensable if local anesthesia is to be used effectively. The free nerve endings are distributed throughout the epidermis, and effective anesthesia is less than perfect if a skin wheal is not produced during the injection.

The distribution of the cutaneous nerves to the abdominal wall, groin, and upper thigh must be familiar to the surgeon who would use local anesthesia. The anterior rami of the seventh to ninth nerve trunks pass posterior to the costal cartilages, while those of the tenth, eleventh, and twelfth trunks pass behind the ribs themselves. The intercostal nerves then come to lie in the plane between the internal oblique and transversus abdominis muscles. Branches pass through the internal oblique, the rectus abdominis, and the rectus sheath, subcutaneous tissues and supply the skin as anterior cutaneous nerves. In considering the anatomy of the

**Figure 8–1.** Sensory nerve supply to the anterior abdominal wall. Note that the tenth intercostal nerve supplies the area about the umbilicus. (Modified from Sherwood-Dunn, B.: *Regional Anesthesia (Victor Pauchet's Technique)*. F. A. Davis Co., London, Stanley Phillips, 1920.)

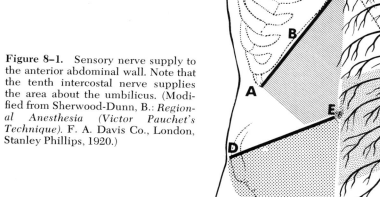
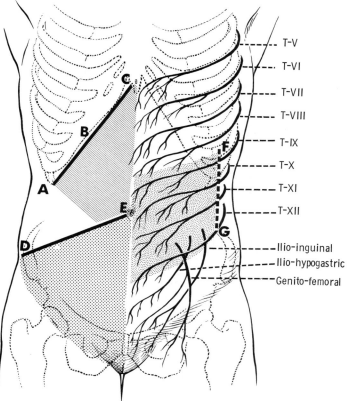

anterior abdominal wall, it is important to remember that the seventh thoracic intercostal nerve supplies sensory fibers to the epigastrium, the tenth supplies the umbilicus, and the twelfth supplies the lower abdomen just above the groin (Fig. 8–1).

The ilioinguinal nerve, which is derived from T-12 and L-1, and the iliohypogastric, derived from T-12 and L-1, supply the lower abdomen. It is well known that there are anastomosing branches between the intercostal nerves in this area. The genitofemoral nerve takes origin from L-1 and L-2. The genital branch enters the inguinal canal at the internal ring and lies posterior to the spermatic cord. It supplies the scrotal skin in the male and the labia majora in the female with sensory nerve fibers. The femoral branch of the genitofemoral nerve passes deep to the inguinal ligament and supplies sensory innervation to the cutaneous area of the upper thigh known as Scarpa's triangle (Fig. 8–2).

Knowledge of the detailed anatomy of a typical intercostal nerve is of paramount importance if the surgeon or anesthesiologist is to achieve effective nerve block. If an intercostal nerve block is to be effective, injection must be made near the posterior axillary line. The reason for selecting this site for injection is obvious from Figure 8–3. If the intercostal nerve is blocked too far anteriorly, the anterior branch of the lateral cutaneous portion of the intercostal nerve is not blocked (Fig. 8–3).

Furthermore, when performing intercostal nerve block, it should be recalled that the intercostal nerve is located nearer the rib in the posterior one-third and almost in the middle of the intercostal space as the nerve courses anteriorly (Fig. 8–4).

Direct abdominal wall infiltration is sometimes useful in producing adequate anesthesia in certain geriatric patients with relaxed abdominal walls. Ventral hernias can often be successfully repaired under local anesthesia. This technique is,

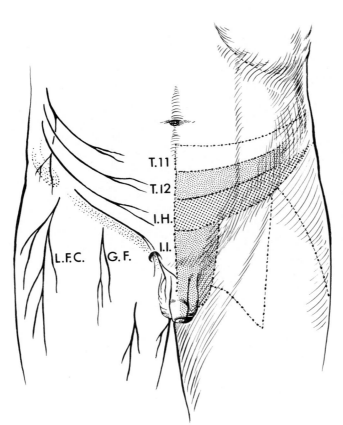

**Figure 8–2.** Cutaneous nerve distribution to the lower abdomen and upper thigh. I.H. refers to the iliohypogastric nerve. I.I. refers to the ilioinguinal nerve. G.F. refers to the genitofemoral nerve, and L.F.C. refers to the lateral femoral cutaneous nerve.

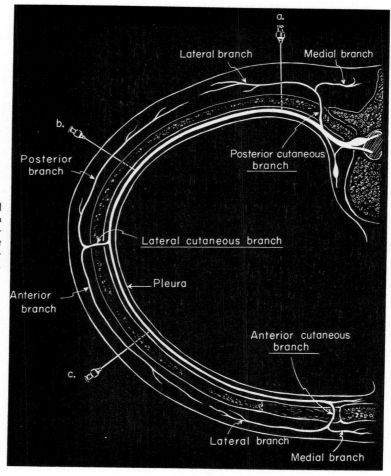

**Figure 8–3.** A typical intercostal nerve with its main branches. In order to block the lateral cutaneous branch, the intercostal nerve must be blocked at a point posterior to the posterior axillary line.

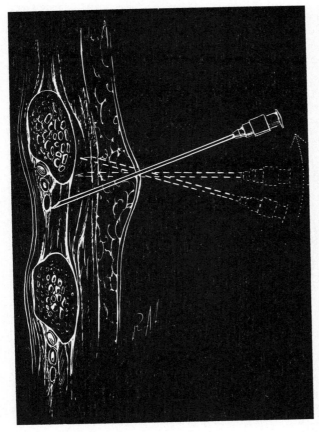

**Figure 8–4.** · The relationship of the intercostal nerve to the intercostal space varies with the position. For example, posterior to the axilla, the intercostal nerve is found inferior to the rib. Farther anteriorly, the nerves are found near the middle of the intercostal space. The method of locating the proper site for injection is shown.

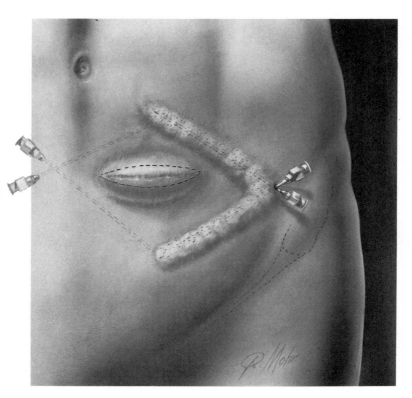

**Figure 8–5.** A satisfactory method of direct infiltration of the abdominal wall for repair of a small defect.

unfortunately, too frequently overlooked (Fig. 8–5).

Detailed knowledge of the neuroanatomy of the groin is also necessary if femoral hernias are to be repaired under local anesthesia. The sensory distribution of the eleventh and twelfth spinal nerves to the lower abdomen is well known to surgeons. The first and second lumbar nerves supply the area nearer the inguinal ligament. However, there are other nerve fibers providing sensory innervation to the upper thigh that perhaps are not as well known. The distribution of the lateral femoral cutaneous nerve and the ilioinguinal and femoral branches of the genitofemoral nerves is of special interest to the surgeon attempting repair of femoral hernias under local anesthesia (See Fig. 8–2).

Finally, the points of perforation of the abdominal wall by the iliohypogastric and ilioinguinal nerves are of particular interest to anyone using local anesthesia. Jamieson, Swigart, and Anson (1952) have carefully studied this anatomic detail, which has practical application in the field of local anesthesia. The illustrations

of Jamieson et al. have been modified to emphasize that in over 90 percent of the cases perforation of the abdominal wall by the ilioinguinal and iliohypogastric nerves occurs slightly posterior to the anterior superior iliac spine. This observation supports the opinion that injection of local anesthetic solution should be made just posterior to and slightly above the anterior superior iliac spine if the surgeon wishes to achieve effective anesthesia (Figs. 8–6 through 8–9).

## ARMAMENTARIUM

The equipment needed to accomplish local anesthesia is remarkably simple. Sterile physiologic solution, which serves as a diluent, is readily available in the operating room at all times. More concentrated solutions of the various anesthetics are easily available. A stainless steel cup with a capacity of 150 to 180 cc serves as a mixing basin (Fig. 8–10).

Three 10 cc Luer-Lok syringes have been found ideal for the purpose of local injection. One syringe is filled while

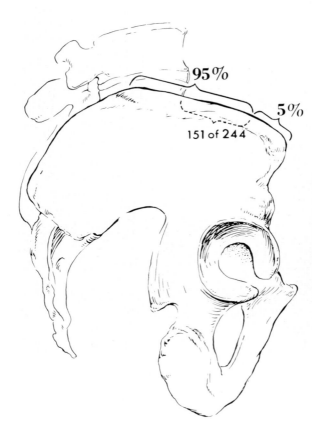

**Figure 8–6.** The iliohypogastric nerve perforates the transversus abdominis muscle posterior to the anterior superior iliac spine in 95 percent of the instances. The practical application of this information in local anesthesia is obvious.
(Fig. 8–6 through 8–9 modified with permission from Jamieson, R. W., Swigart, L. L., and Anson, B. J.: Points of parietal perforation of the ilioinguinal and iliohypogastric nerves in relation to optimal sites for local anesthesia. Q. Bull. Northwestern Med. Sch. 26:22–26, 1952.)

**Figure 8–7.** Area of perforation of the internal oblique muscle by the iliohypogastric nerve. In two-thirds of the instances, the site of penetration is shown in the area enclosed in the darker lines.

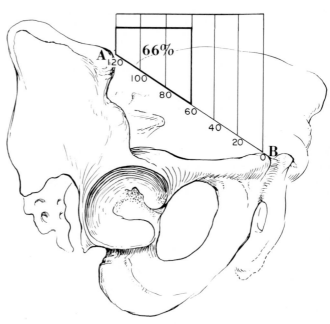

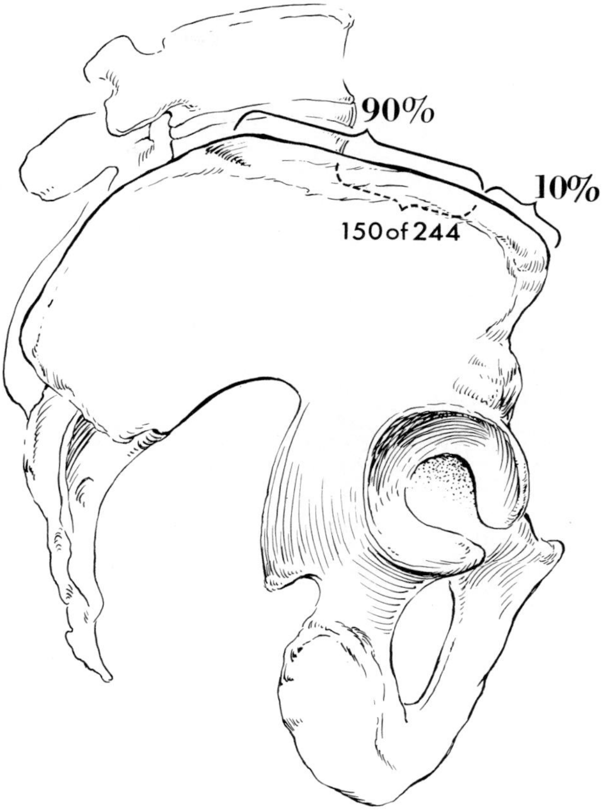

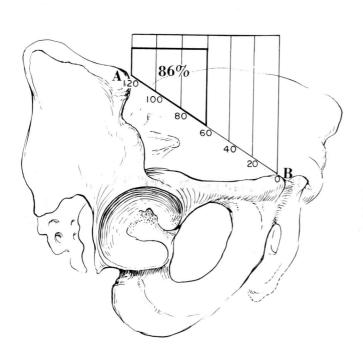

**Figure 8–8.** The ilioinguinal nerve penetrates the transversus abdominis muscle posterior to the anterior superior iliac spine above the iliac crest in 90 percent of the instances.

90%

10%

150 of 244

86%

120
100
80
60
40
20

A

B

**Figure 8–9.** The ilioinguinal nerve penetrates the internal oblique muscle in a relatively limited area, outlined in dark lines, in approximately 86 percent of 116 body halves examined.

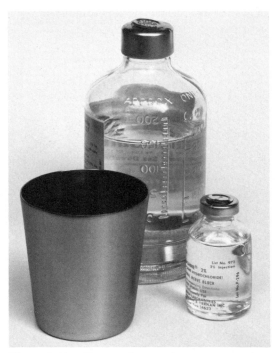

**Figure 8–10.** The stainless steel mixing cup, saline solution, and concentrated solutions of anesthetic drugs are readily available in the well-supplied operating room.

another is in use, thus minimizing loss of time. Breakage or malfunction of a single syringe is less annoying if a third syringe has been provided. The single 1 cc tuber-

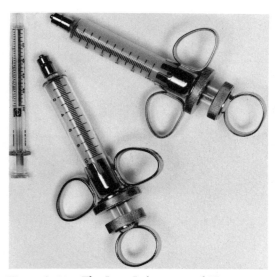

**Figure 8–11.** The Luer-Lok syringe of 10 cc capacity is ideal for injections of local anesthetic solutions. The tuberculin syringe permits accurate measurement of epinephrine if it is to be used.

culin syringe is important, since it is graduated to 0.01 cc, permitting accurate measurement of the epinephrine to be added (Fig. 8–11).

The needles vary in caliber and length, depending upon their specific uses. The short 25 gauge needle is suitable for the initial intradermal injection. The blunt 19 gauge needle, 8 cm in length, is suitable for the injection made laterally near the anterior superior iliac spine. As the large-bore needle penetrates the fascia, a sudden loss of resistance suggests that the aponeurosis has been penetrated. The long 20 and 22 gauge needles are suitable for lengthy intradermal and subcutaneous injections (Fig. 8–12).

## PHARMACOLOGIC CONSIDERATIONS

The agent or agents to be used for local anesthesia must possess certain desirable qualities. Safety is a prime consideration. Otherwise, it would be difficult to justify the use of local anesthetic drugs. Complete absence of toxicity is the ideal, but practically, we accept a low incidence of drug toxicity. Needless to say, the drug must be effective as an anesthetic agent, and it must maintain anesthesia for adequate periods of time. The need for repeated injections greatly reduces the usefulness of drugs that might otherwise be acceptable. The agent must not have a necrotizing effect on tissues, and its effect must be completely reversible. Finally, the drug must be nonaddicting. Cocaine is extremely dangerous because of its addictive quality.

Physical characteristics desirable in local anesthetic drugs are not numerous but important. The drug must be easily soluble in water; it must remain stable in solution for a reasonable period of time, and it must lend itself to autoclave sterilization. Compatibility with other drugs is yet another desirable characteristic.

An exhaustive treatment of the nature of local anesthetic agents will not be attempted here. It is far better to become familiar with a few of these drugs and to use them regularly than to change from drug to drug. Nevertheless, a brief introduction to the pharmacology of local

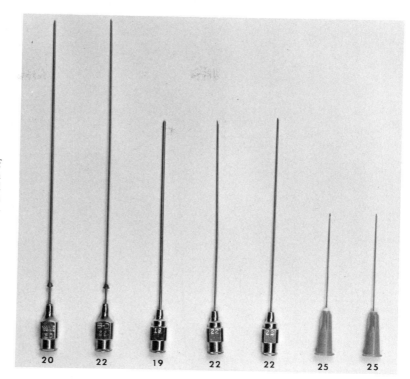

**Figure 8–12.** A variety of needles should be included in the equipment; the length and diameter of the needle varies with the technique to be performed.

anesthetic drugs is important to those who would use them.

The exact method by which local anesthetics act has been studied extensively. The important practical fact is that they are able to block initiation and conduction of impulses in a nerve.

A great variety of compounds have been found by Hirschfelder (1932) and by Adriani (1960) to possess local anesthetic qualities; however, toxicity, tissue injury, and unacceptably short periods of effectiveness are undesirable qualities that are too frequently found.

Anesthetics that have proved clinically useful are usually nitrogen-containing compounds made up of an amino group connected to an aromatic residue by an intermediate group. The link between the aromatic residue and the intermediate group may be an ester or an amide bond (Table 8–1). The type of bond is important, for it is at this point that hydrolysis and inactivation occur. I have listed a few of the more desirable local anesthetic agents in Table 8–1, which includes information from Moore (1975) and Goodman and Gilman (1975).

Accurate comparison of the drugs is extremely difficult, since desirable quali-

ties are offset by certain limitations. For example, chloroprocaine is relatively nontoxic, but its duration of anesthesia is short, being expended in 30 to 60 minutes. The addition of epinephrine, 1:200,000, will prolong the effect for up to 2 hours. On the other hand, tetracaine is much more toxic than procaine but it may be used in a much more dilute solution. Furthermore, lengthy operations of up to 6 hours may be performed without the use of epinephrine.

My personal choice of a local anesthetic drug is bupivacaine (Marcaine), but chloroprocaine and lidocaine continue to be useful. Ponka and Sapala (1976) have conducted a study in which bupivacaine and chloroprocaine were used in comparable groups of patients undergoing hernia repair. Bupivacaine provided anesthesia consistently lasting longer than 6 hours. It has proved to be safe in a 0.25 percent solution, and as a result of its prolonged effect, the need for postoperative medication is greatly reduced. Chloroprocaine has proved to be a safe anesthetic agent, and its action is prolonged up to 2 hours with the addition of epinephrine, 1: 200,000.

These compounds which have been

**Table 8–1. CHEMICAL STRUCTURE OF SEVERAL CURRENTLY POPULAR LOCAL ANESTHETIC DRUGS**

| Ester Linkage | | | Amide Linkage | | |
|---|---|---|---|---|---|
| AROMATIC RESIDUE | INTERMEDIATE CHAIN | AMINO GROUP | AROMATIC RESIDUE | INTERMEDIATE CHAIN | AMINO GROUP |

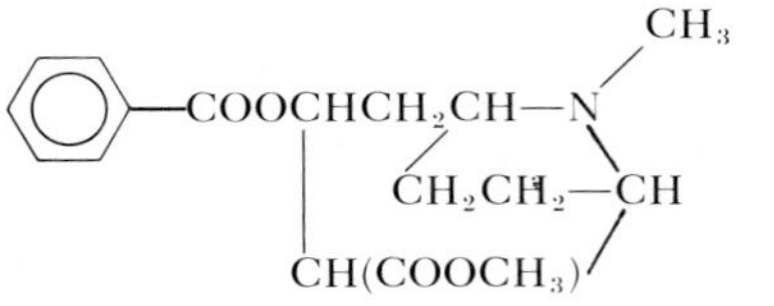

Cocaine

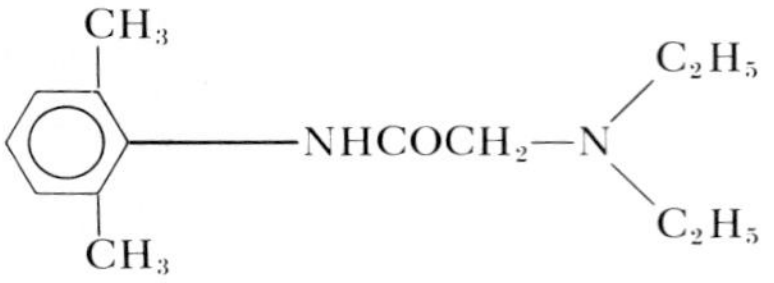

Lidocaine
(Xylocaine)

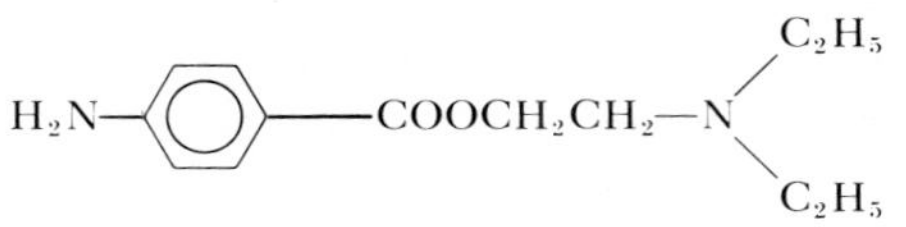

Procaine
(Novocaine)

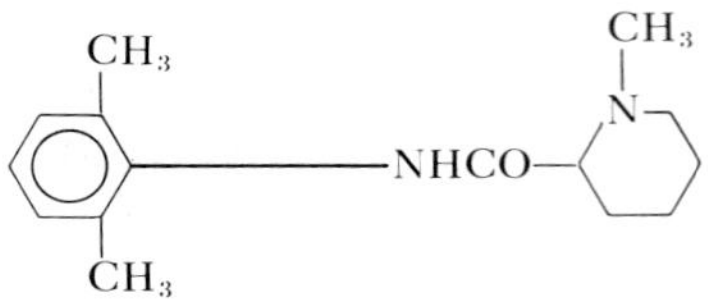

Mepivacaine
(Carbocaine)

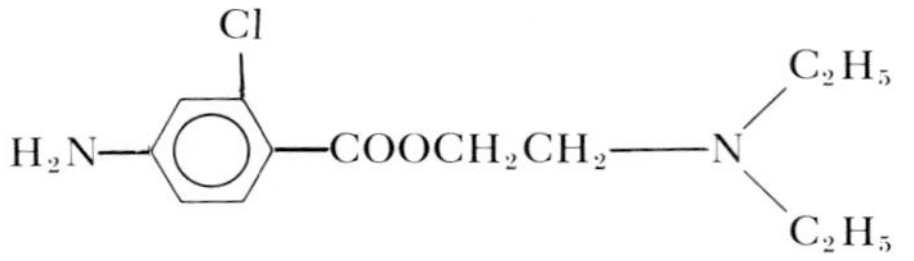

Chloroprocaine
(Nesacaine)

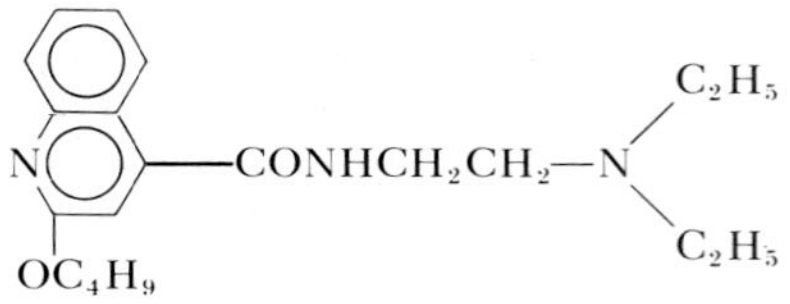

Dibucaine
(Nupercaine)

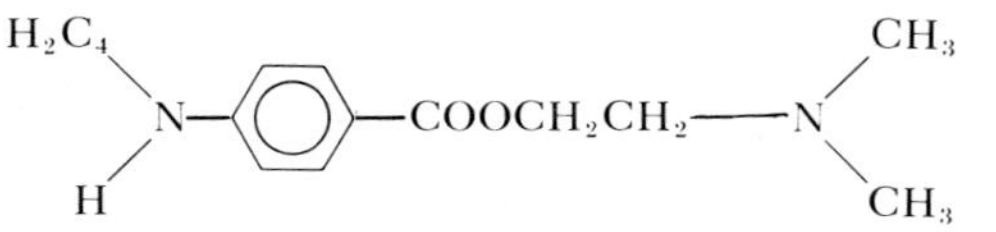

Tetracaine
(Pontocaine)

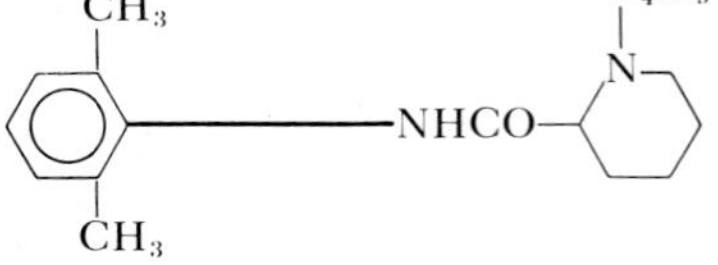

Bupivacaine
(Marcaine)

Modified with permission from Goodman, L. S., and Gilman, A.: *The Pharmacological Basis of Therapeutics* (5th ed.). New York, Macmillan Publishing Co., Inc., 1975, p. 373.

found effective and relatively safe for clinical use are generally esters and amines. Table 8–1 is produced and modified from Goodman and Gilman's textbook, *The Pharmacological Basis of Therapeutics*. The table clearly shows that the currently popular local anesthetics are made up of three components—the aromatic residue, the intermediate chain, and the amino group. The hydrophilic amino group is connected to a lipophilic aromatic residue by an intermediate group. The amino group is either a secondary or tertiary amine. To reiterate, the linkage between the intermediate chain and the aromatic residue may be an amide bond. The ester link between the aromatic acid and alcoholic intermediate is important because it is at this point that hydrolysis and inactivation occur. Those agents possessing the ester linkage (procaine and chloroprocaine) are rapidly hydrolyzed by the esterases in the tissues, plasma, and liver. Since they are rapidly hydrolyzed and inactivated, their duration of action is short. Local anesthetics possessing the amide linkage (lidocaine, bupivacaine) are destroyed in the liver in reactions involving N-dealkylation and hydrolysis. These actions proceed slowly, even in a normal liver. Hence, the choice of agent and the dosage administered to patients with liver disease should be given consideration. Changes in any constituent of the molecule affects the potency and toxicity of the new agent. Lengthening the alcohol group increases the anesthetic potency and the toxicity as well. It can be seen from the table that the number of possible variations is enormous.

In recent years a number of safe and effective local anesthetic drugs have appeared; their chemical formulas show considerable uniformity in structure. A number of chemists, pharmacologists, and anesthesiologists have made important contributions toward the development of new drugs. Their chemical variations, actions, clinical effects, and effectiveness have been investigated. Toxicity of these drugs and treatment of respiratory, cardiovascular, and neurologic complications will be considered. Table 8–2, which lists a few of the more popular drugs used for local analgesia, has been

## Table 8–2. PRACTICAL INFORMATION ON DRUGS FREQUENTLY USED TO ACHIEVE LOCAL ANESTHESIA

| Chemical Name and Trade Name | Suggested Maximum Dosage for Injection | °Onset of Anesthesia in minutes | °Duration of Anesthesia in minutes | Relative Toxicity | Relative Potency |
|---|---|---|---|---|---|
| Procaine (Novocaine) | 200 cc of 0.5% = 1000 mg<br>100 cc of 1.0% = 1000 mg<br>50 cc of 2.0% = 1000 mg | 3–5 | 45 90 | 1 | 1 |
| Tetracaine (Pontocaine) (Amethocaine) | 1 mg per lb body weight<br>Do not exceed 200 mg<br>Concentration 0.25% | Slow 10–15 | 150–360 (2½–6 hrs) | 10–12 | 10 |
| Lidocaine (Xylocaine) | 100 cc of 0.5% = 500 mg<br>50 cc of 1.0% = 500 mg<br>25 cc of 2.0% = 500 mg | 1–3 | 60–180 | 1.5 | 1.5–2 |
| Mepivacaine (Carbocaine) | 100 cc of 0.5% = 500 mg<br>50 cc of 1.0% = 500 mg<br>25 cc of 2.0% = 500 mg | 1–3 | 60–180 | 1.5 | 1.5 |
| Chloroprocaine (Nesacaine) | 200 cc of 0.5% = 1000 mg<br>100 cc of 1.0% = 1000 mg<br>50 cc of 2.0% = 1000 mg | At once 1–2 | 30–60 | 0.5 | 2 |
| Bupivacaine (Marcaine) | 200 cc of 0.25% = 500 mg | 3–5 | 360–720 Ponka & Sapala | 10–12 | 10+ |

°Time given is approximate.

Modified from Moore, Daniel C.: *Regional Block* (4th ed.). Springfield, Ill.: Charles C Thomas, 1975, pp. 13 and 14.

prepared after consulting the books on the subject by Moore and by Goodman and Gilman.

## REACTIONS ATTRIBUTED TO LOCAL ANESTHETICS

It has long been known that anesthetic solutions pass from the site of injection into the circulatory system. The more vascular the tissue, the more rapid the absorption. The body tissues are the site of partial or complete detoxification of specific agents. Hydrolysis occurs in the liver, other tissues, and the blood. Toxicity depends not only upon the nature of the drug but also upon its rate of absorption and speed of detoxification. Epinephrine, by delaying absorption, results in prolonged anesthesia and lessens the possibility of drug reaction. Commonly used local anesthetic drugs are esters and, hence, they are detoxified by hydrolysis, which occurs in the plasma as well as the liver where the enzyme esterase is active. In patients with severe liver disease, the use of local anesthetics might be hazardous. If such agents are used, they must be employed in the most dilute solutions and in the smallest amounts necessary.

Some local anesthetic agents are excreted in the urine, particularly those slowly detoxified in the liver.

Steinhaus experimented on the comparative toxicity of several local anesthetic agents. Severe reactions to local anesthesia are remarkably infrequent in patients. It should be recalled that epinephrine itself may result in anxiety, excitement, and restlessness. The patient may complain of substernal oppression and palpitation. The heart rate may be rapid, and cardiac irregularities may occur. The blood pressure may become elevated. Other reactions include hypotension, convulsions, and respiratory embarrassment.

A number of pharmacologists and anesthesiologists, including Geddes, Hirschfelder, and Steinhaus, have studied the untoward responses to the injection of local anesthetic drugs. Many physicians and surgeons tend to lump all reactions to local anesthetics into the broad category of "reactions" or "allergic reactions." In truth, such reactions are rare indeed. In my 30 years of experience, I cannot recall

seeing a single instance in which a patient suffered an anaphylactic reaction. Local reaction at the site of injection characterized by redness, induration, and significant edema is seen occasionally. When procaine was used, convulsions were not rare. I saw more convulsions due to this agent than to any other. Chloroprocaine, Xylocaine, and bupivacaine have proved to be safe, effective drugs in practice.

Sandove et al. (1952) provide us with a simple, yet remarkably complete, classification of the various manifestations of toxicity following local anesthesia.

I. Toxic responses in normal individuals
  A. Central nervous system effects— stimulation
    1. Cerebral cortex
    2. Medulla
      a. Respiratory
      b. Vasomotor
      c. Others
  B. Peripheral effects
    1. Cardiovascular
      a. Direct action on the heart
      b. Action on the vascular bed
    2. Respiratory tract
II. Abnormal responses
  A. Allergic responses
  B. Hypersensitivity
  C. Idiosyncrasy
III. Reactions not due to local anesthetic agent
  A. Psychomotor
  B. Vasopressor

Steinhaus (1957) has studied the effects of local anesthetic drugs on the central nervous system. He was of the opinion that following initial overstimulation, depression and respiratory arrest occur. Stimulation of the nervous system may be manifested by nervousness, excitement, disorientation, apprehension, or of course, convulsions. Such reactions due to chloroprocaine must be rare. The untoward effects of the local anesthetic drug on the medulla may result in increased blood pressure and pulse rate. The respiratory center in the medulla may be stimulated, resulting in increased respirations. Vomiting may also occur as a result of undesirable effects on the vomiting center.

## MANAGEMENT OF REACTIONS

A thorough knowledge of the anesthetic drugs used by a surgeon or anesthesiologist is perhaps the greatest factor in preventing or minimizing untoward reactions from their use. It is helpful to become thoroughly acquainted with the use of one or two local anesthetic drugs.

It is well recognized that reactions are due to high blood concentrations of the anesthetic agent. This may occur following an injection of large amounts of solution, following an injection made too rapidly, or following an injection made directly into the blood stream. Rapid absorption of the drug or delayed detoxification may lead to an unusual reaction. Liver diseases may impair detoxification, and elimination may be slow as well. Assessment of the patient who shows an unusual reaction to local anesthetic drugs should be promptly made by an experienced surgeon or anesthesiologist. First and foremost, it is always sound practice to expose the patient to the least possible amount of drug. This implies using the drug in dilute solutions in carefully measured amounts. In patients with normal blood pressure epinephrine in the ratio of 1:200,000 will result in delayed absorption and prolonged action of the anesthetic agent.

Convulsions do not occur frequently, but they may cause a variety of serious problems. Vomiting might result in aspiration and serious respiratory tract injury. This in turn may lead to cerebral anoxia and insufficient oxygenation of the heart, with the hazard of myocardial infarction or cardiac arrest. The various reactions may occur with remarkable speed and severity.

Moore and Bridenbaugh (1960) found oxygen to be an effective antidote for systemic reactions due to toxic effects of local anesthetic drugs. Every attempt must be made to provide the patient with oxygen promptly. The airway must be cleared of secretions and vomitus. If convulsions are severe, it may be necessary to resort to a muscular relaxant such as succinylcholine. Two cc, or 40 mg, of succinylcholine may be given intravenously. This is preferably administered by an anesthesiologist if the need for artificial respiration becomes mandatory. The same care should be exercised in the use of barbiturates; at times up to 50 mg or 100 mg of thiopental sodium may be helpful. Barbiturates should be given cautiously, since they may add to the depression.

In the event of hypotension, measures to restore the blood pressure include the use of intravenous fluids and vasopressors. A number of effective vasoconstrictor drugs are currently available. Some thought should be given to the particular agent employed. Methoxamine (Vasoxyl) may be given in amounts of 2 mg intravenously. Intramuscular injection of 10 mg will result in sustained action. The pharmacologic effect of methoxamine is peripheral vasoconstriction. Metaraminol (Aramine) and levarterenol (Levophed) are more powerful vasoconstrictor drugs and are to be used in selected patients. It is recommended that the anesthesiologist be consulted whenever hypotension is a continuing or acute problem.

If cardiac arrest has occurred, cardiac massage is mandatory. Again, ventilation of the patient must be assured. If acidosis is suspected, sodium bicarbonate is given as necessary. Electrocardiographic monitoring of the patient is advisable. Ventricular fibrillation requires defibrillation with a direct electric current.

Although severe toxic reactions are rare, the need for the assistance of a competent anesthesiologist is never greater than in such situations. Hence, local anesthesia should be carried out with the supervision of a competent anesthetist.

## ADVANTAGES AND DISADVANTAGES OF LOCAL ANESTHESIA

During the past 30 years, I have gained substantial experience in the use of local anesthesia for hernia repair. Local anesthetic can be quickly administered; it is safe, effective, and satisfactory to the patient. Initially, I employed such anesthesia for elderly poor-risk patients. As I gained greater experience, I found that over 90 percent of my patients accepted this method.

The use of local anesthesia does not eliminate the need for a competent anesthesiologist. It is just as important to have skillful monitoring of the patient under local anesthesia as it is when other forms of analgesia are used. We have had the excellent support of Dr. Paul R. Dumke, Chairman of the Department of Anesthesiology of the Henry Ford Hospital. He has recommended agents for our use and

**Table 8–3. SUMMARY OF ADVANTAGES AND DISADVANTAGES OF LOCAL ANESTHESIA**

| *Advantages* | *Disadvantages* |
|---|---|
| 1. Greater safety for poor-risk patient. | 1. Rejection by the patient. |
| 2. The patient is conscious. | 2. Unsuitable for neurotic, psychotic, or very young patients. |
| 3. Adequacy of repair may be tested by having the patient cough at the time of operation. | 3. Requires more time. |
| 4. Less urinary retention, since voiding reflexes are functional. | 4. Anesthesia is not always ideal; may require supplementation. |
| 5. Earlier ambulation decreases hazard of phlebothrombosis and pulmonary embolism. | 5. Some patients "want to be asleep"; hence, they may demand supplementation. |
| 6. Less danger of aspiration. | 6. Greater incidence of wound complications, such as skin necrosis, seroma, and wound infection. |
| 7. Better respiratory exchange; hence, less atelectasis. | 7. If there is a complicated problem, it cannot be managed as easily as it could under general anesthesia. |
| 8. Headaches are less frequent. | 8. Drug toxicity. |
| 9. Backaches are less frequent. | 9. Drug sensitivity. |

has given the procedure encouragement. It should be stressed that the anesthesiologist is a most important member of the surgical team, providing support and supplementation of sedatives and analgesics as necessary for the individual patient.

Local anesthesia, like other modes of treatment, has its advantages as well as its undesirable aspects. I have been impressed with the great difficulty in trying to support the commonly listed advantages or disadvantages with objective evidence. Perhaps, the greatest single limiting factor is that certain patients are specifically selected for local anesthesia. They are, as a group, aged, not infrequently with decompensating cardiac, pulmonary, renal, or metabolic disease. The younger, healthier patient may be given spinal or general anesthesia. The advantages and disadvantages of any anesthetic procedure must be considered for each patient and the appropriate method selected for the individual patient (Table 8–3).

## REFERENCES

Allen, C.W.: *Local and Regional Anesthesia*. Philadelphia, W. B. Saunders Co., 1918, pp. 17–35, 359.

Bonica, J.J.: *The Management of Pain*. Philadelphia, Lea & Febiger, 1953.

Cushing, H.: The employment of local anesthetics in the radical cure of certain cases of hernia with a note on the nervous anatomy of the inguinal region. Ann. Surg. 31:1, 1900.

Dumke, P.R.: Personal communication to the author.

Farr, R.E.: *Practical Local Anesthesia*. Philadelphia, Lea & Febiger, 1923, p. 33.

Geddes, I.C.: A review of local anesthetics. Br. J. Anaesth. 26:208, 1954.

Goodman, L.S., and Gilman, A.: *The Pharmacological Basis of Therapeutics* (5th ed.). New York, Macmillan Publishing Co., Inc., 1975, pp. 371–389.

Hirschfelder, A.D., and Bieter, R.N.: Local anesthetics. Physiol. Rev. 12:190, 1932.

Jamieson, R.W., Swigart, L.L., and Anson, B.J.: Points of parietal perforation of the ilioinguinal and iliohypogastric nerves in relation to optimal sites for local anesthesia. Q. Bull. Northwestern Med. Sch. 26:22, 1952.

Keys, Thomas E.: *The History of Surgical Anesthesia*. New York, Schuman's, 1945, pp. 106–110.

Labat, G.: *Regional Anesthesia: Its Technique and Clinical Application*. Philadelphia, W. B. Saunders Co., 1922.

Moore, D.C.: *Regional Block. A Handbook for Use in the Clinical Practice of Medicine and Surgery* (4th ed.) Springfield, Ill., Charles C Thomas, 1975.

Moore, D.C., and Bridenbaugh, L.D.: Oxygen: The antidote for systemic toxic reactions for local anesthetic drugs. J.A.M.A. 173:842, 1960.

Ponka, J.L.: Seven steps to local anesthesia for inguino-femoral hernia repair. Surg. Gynecol. Obstet. 117:115, 1963.

Ponka, J.L., Welborn, J.K., and Sanchez, S.M.: Local anesthetic technics in geriatric surgery. J. Am. Geriatr. Soc. 12(11):1022, 1964.

Ponka, J.L., and Sapala, J.A.: Bupivacaine as a local anesthetic for hernia repair. Henry Ford Hosp. Med. J. 24:31, 1976.

Sandove, M.S., Wyant, G.M., Gittelson, L.A., and Kretchmer, H.E.: Classification and management of reactions to local anesthetic agents. J.A.M.A. *148*:17, 1952.

Sherwood-Dunn, B.: *Regional Anesthesia (Victor Pauchet's Technique).* F.A. Davis Co., London, Stanley Phillips, 1920.

Southworth, J.L., and Hingson, R.A. *In* Pitkin: *Conduction Anesthesia.* Philadelphia, J.B. Lippincott Co., 1946.

Steinhaus, J.E.: Local anesthetic toxicity: A pharmacological re-evaluation. Anesthesiology *18*:275, 1957.

Steinhaus, J.E.: A comparative study of the experimental toxicity of local anesthetic agents. Anesthesiology *13*:577, 1952.

## Supplemental Readings

Adriani, J.: The clinical pharmacology of local anesthetics. Clin. Pharmacol. Ther. *1*:645, 1960.

Adriani, J., and Zepernick, R.: Some recent studies on the clinical pharmacology of local anesthetics of practical significance. Ann. Surg. *158*:661, 1963.

Anson, B.J., and McVay, C.B.: *Surgical Anatomy.* Vol. I (5th ed.). Philadelphia, W.B. Saunders Co., 1971.

Campbell, D., and Adriani, J.: Absorption of local anesthetics. J.A.M.A. *168*:873, 1958.

MacCallum, W.G.: *William Stewart Halsted.* Baltimore, Johns Hopkins Press, 1930.

# 9

# Seven Steps to Local Anesthesia for Inguinal and Femoral Hernia Repair

## INTRODUCTION

The technique of local anesthesia currently being employed has been slowly evolving over a period of 20 years. Approximately 90 percent of the hernias being repaired on the Fourth Surgical Division of the Henry Ford Hospital are done under local anesthesia. It has been learned that it is impossible to achieve effective local anesthesia with haphazardly placed injections of a "little local." It has been found that a total of 150 to 200 cc of a 1 percent solution of chloroprocaine or a 0.25 percent solution of bupivacaine is adequate and safe for most patients undergoing hernia repair. Failure to administer adequate amounts of drugs as premedication accounts for some unsatisfactory results. Another error lies in not allowing a sufficient time interval between the premedication and the operative procedure. The premedication drugs should be given at least one-half hour before the incision is to be made (see Chapter 6).

Bupivacaine and chloroprocaine are the drugs that I prefer at present. A solution of 1 percent chloroprocaine is prepared with epinephrine in a dilution of 1:200,000 if there are no cardiac or circulatory contraindications to its use. Other effective drugs for use as local anesthetics are listed in Chapter 8.

## STEP ONE

After the skin has been well prepared with an antiseptic, the first injection is made into the epidermis 2 to 3 cm above and slightly lateral to the anterior superior iliac spine (Fig. 9–1). The patient is always informed when the injection is to be made. The first pinprick must never come as a surprise to the patient. This anesthetized area is then used for subsequent injections. The free nerve endings in the epidermis are thus anesthetized. Repeated injections through unanesthetized skin must be avoided. The common error of placing the wheal too far medially or too high results in poor anesthesia. Throughout the procedure, gentleness is of paramount importance. Neither the surgeon nor the assistants are to lean heavily upon the patient.

## STEP TWO

The injections are next made in three directions. At least 5 cc of anesthetic solution are injected superiorly, horizontally, and inferiorly, as indicated in Figure 9–2. This injection must be made above and just lateral to the anterior superior iliac spine.

The purpose of injection at this site is to

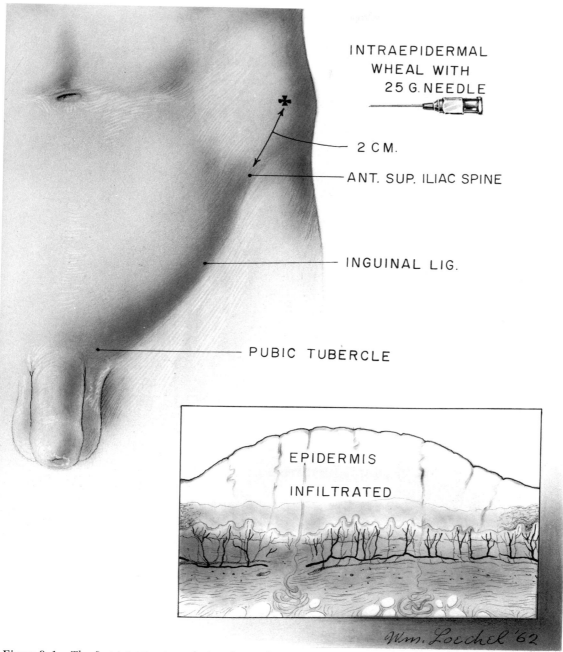

**Figure 9–1.**   The first injection is made into the epidermis, slightly lateral to and just above the anterior superior iliac spine.

(Figs. 9–1 through 9–7 are from Ponka, J. L.: Seven steps to local anesthesia for inguinofemoral hernia repair. Surg. Gynec. & Obst. 117:115-20, 1963. By permission. Surgery, Gynecology and Obstetrics.)

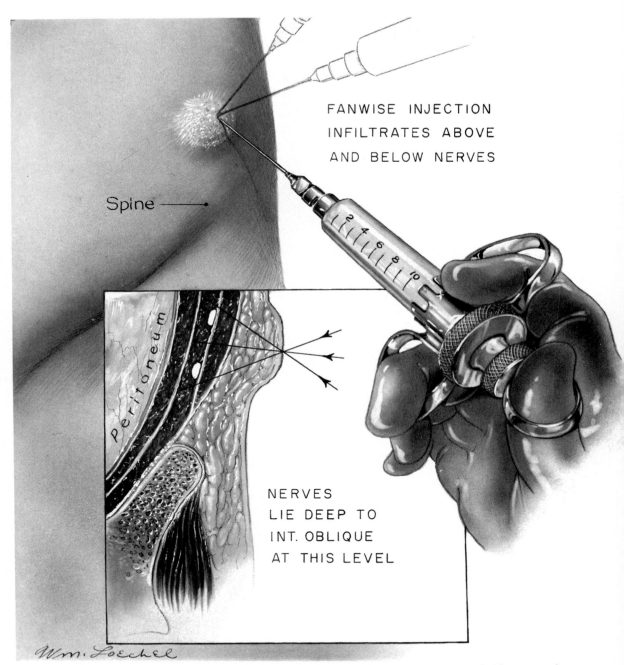

FANWISE INJECTION
INFILTRATES ABOVE
AND BELOW NERVES

Spine →

NERVES
LIE DEEP TO
INT. OBLIQUE
AT THIS LEVEL

**Figure 9–2.**   The injections are now made in three directions deep to the external oblique muscle.

anesthetize the ilioinguinal and iliohypogastric nerves, which lie deep to the internal and external oblique muscles at this level (see Figs. 8–6 through 8–9). The penetration of the needle through the external oblique can be perceived as a sudden loss of resistance to the advancing needle. The surgeon must be certain to inject the anesthetic solution under the external oblique at this point if the best results are to be achieved. A common error is a failure to inject the anesthetic solution far enough laterally.

### STEP THREE

Additional injection of the anesthetic solution is then made medially toward the umbilicus to anesthetize the area supplied by the eleventh thoracic nerve. Next, the injection is made toward the anterior superior iliac spine. Intradermal injection of the anesthetic solution is necessary if the skin incision is to be made painlessly. The injection is continued above the inguinal ligament in the direction of the proposed incision (Fig. 9–3). Injection must be carried across the midline if the patient is to remain free from pain, since no anesthetic agent is injected into the opposite side.

The skin incision is made above and parallel to the inguinal ligament in the direction of Langer's lines. All bleeding vessels are clamped and ligated with fine 4–0 silk. The dissection is carried through the fascia to the aponeurosis of the external oblique. Heavy pressure on the patient by any of the staff must be avoided. Excessively vigorous retraction is not only unnecessary but highly undesirable.

### STEP FOUR

The external oblique fascia is not an insensitive structure, as some surgeons believe. Injections of approximately 2 cc of anesthetic solution are made at intervals of 2 cm. The entire field is injected in this manner, as illustrated in Figure 9–4.

The fascia of the external oblique is incised at the level of the superior crus. The ilioinguinal and iliohypogastric nerves are identified and preserved.

The spermatic cord in the male, or the round ligament in the female, is dissected out of the floor of Hesselbach's triangle. Gentleness here means avoidance of traction. The autonomic fibers in the cord are not blocked by any of the procedures just described. Many surgeons overlook this important and simple step. Palpable relaxation of the abdominal wall occurs after effective accomplishment of this step.

### STEP FIVE

Injections must be made into the cord about the internal ring so that the visceral type of pain, which results from traction on the sympathetic nerve fibers present in the cord, is avoided.

The hypertrophied cremaster muscle seen in patients with indirect inguinal hernia is excised, and the peritoneal sac is identified. Even if the hernia is direct or femoral, we identify the prolongation of peritoneum at the internal ring.

The detail of injecting the base of the cord is indeed important but, unfortunately is omitted by many surgeons. When using local anesthesia, there is no other technique by which the sympathetic fibers in the cord can be blocked.

### STEP SIX

Using a 20 gauge needle, 3 to 5 cc of anesthetic solution are injected into the iliopectineal eminence and the pubic tubercle (Fig. 9–6). This is necessary if a Cooper's ligament (McVay) repair is to be performed. I have observed that no matter how well the preceding steps have been carried out, the periosteum about the pubic tubercle and Cooper's ligament requires individual injection. These areas are supplied by the sacral plexus. It is interesting and surprising to note that many texts on the subject make no reference to this step.

### STEP SEVEN

Anesthetization of the peritoneum may be accomplished through the use of two techniques. The peritoneum may be in-
*Text continued on page 117*

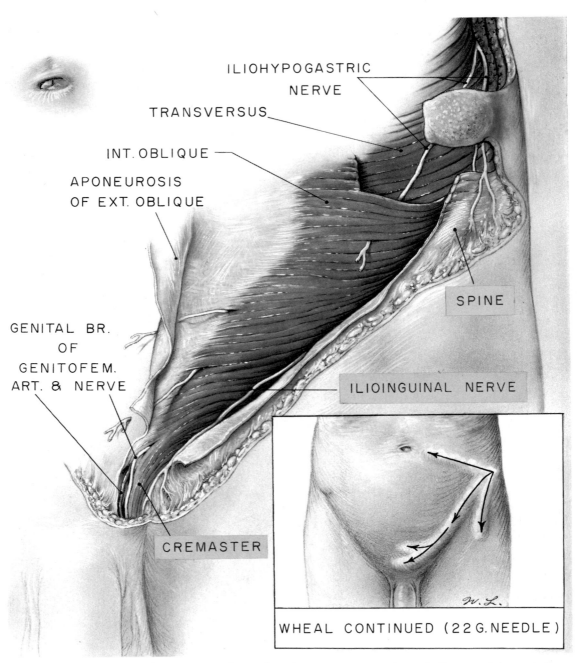

ILIOHYPOGASTRIC NERVE

TRANSVERSUS

INT. OBLIQUE

APONEUROSIS OF EXT. OBLIQUE

SPINE

GENITAL BR. OF GENITOFEM. ART. & NERVE

ILIOINGUINAL NERVE

CREMASTER

WHEAL CONTINUED (22 G. NEEDLE)

**Figure 9–3.** *Step 3.* Subcutaneous and intradermal injections are made medially toward the umbilicus, inferiorly toward the anterior superior iliac spine, and obliquely in the direction of the proposed injection.

POINTS OF INJECTION ✠

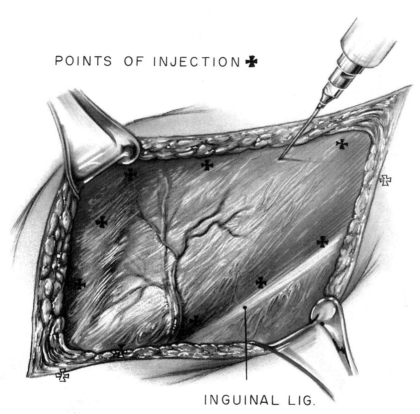

INGUINAL LIG.

**Figure 9–4.** *Step 4.* Multiple injections of small amounts of local anesthetic solution are placed just under the external oblique fascia.

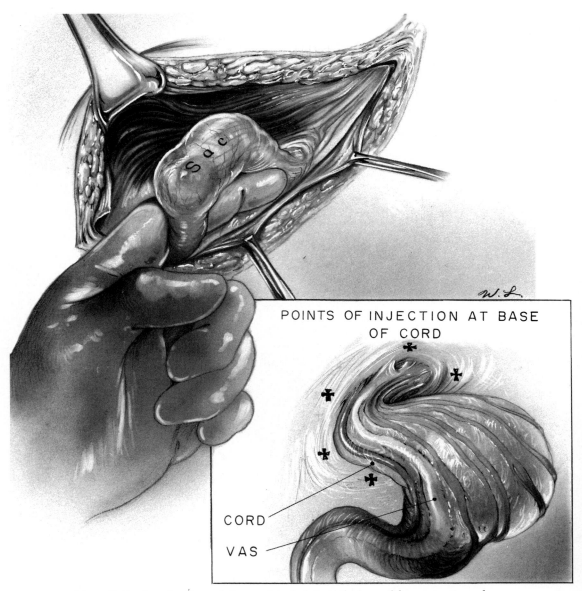

**Figure 9–5.** *Step 5.* Several sites are injected about the base of the spermatic cord.

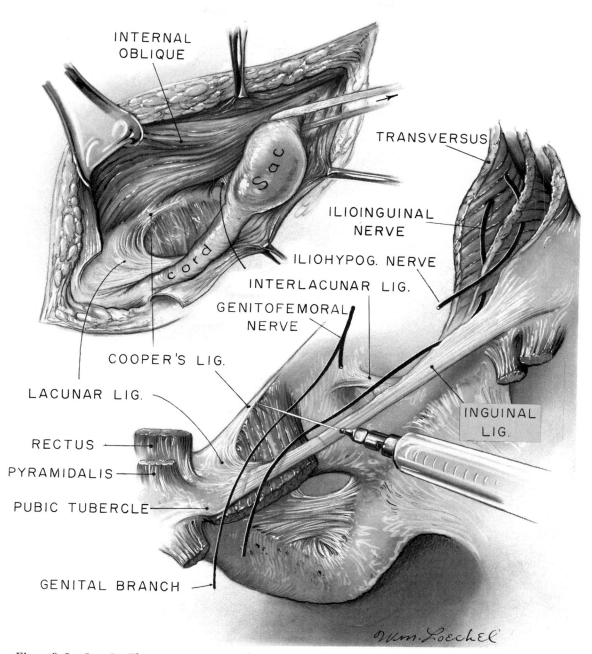

**Figure 9–6.** *Step 6.* The area in proximity to Cooper's ligament is being anesthetized with multiple injections of small amounts of local anesthetic solution.

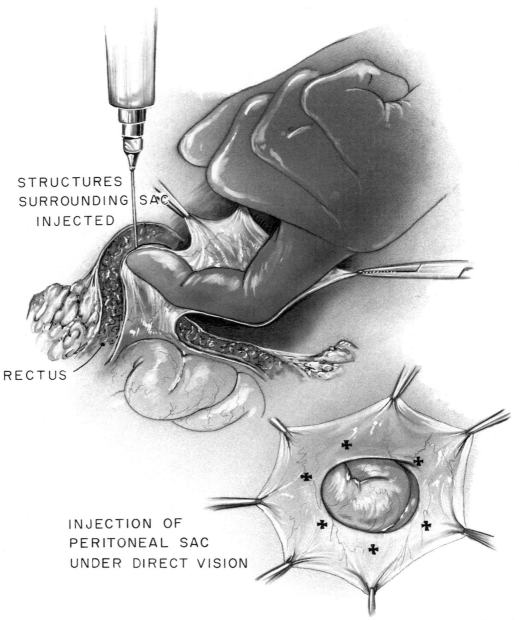

STRUCTURES
SURROUNDING SAC
INJECTED

RECTUS

INJECTION OF
PERITONEAL SAC
UNDER DIRECT VISION

**Figure 9–7.** *Step 7.* The peritoneum may be anesthetized by direct injections or by infiltration through the thickness of the abdominal wall (shown here).

jected directly with 3 to 5 cc of anesthetic solution, as shown in Figure 9–7. In the second method, also shown in Figure 9–7, the index finger is placed into the peritoneal cavity through the internal ring. The needle is inserted through the thickness of the abdominal wall down to the peritoneum. As the peritoneum is approached with the needle at a distance from the internal ring, the injection is made at different points about the internal abdominal ring. Some surgeons prefer to instill large amounts of anesthetic solution directly into the peritoneal cavity.

If each detail described has been carefully carried out, the hernia repair may be performed with remarkable ease and comfort for the patient. Further injections during the reconstruction are rarely needed. The patient may actually sleep through the operative repair.

It is suggested that the young surgeon should have an opportunity to observe the physiology of the lower abdomen by having the patient cough before, during, and after repair. This is possible under local anesthesia. Occasionally, he will see a sudden unexpected break occur in an improperly placed suture, an unforgettable sight.

The need for local infiltration of additional local anesthetic solution in repair of femoral hernias will be apparent if the illustration showing cutaneous nerve distribution in the groin is studied carefully (see Fig. 8–2). This is particularly true if the operation is performed through an incision in the upper thigh.

## REFERENCES

Ponka, J.L.: Seven steps to local anesthesia for repair of inguino-femoral hernia. Surg. Gynecol. Obstet. *117*:115–120, July 1963.

Ponka, J.L., Welborn, J.K., and Sanchez, S.M.: Local anesthetic techniques in geriatric surgery, J. Am. Geriatr. Soc. *12*(11):1022–1036, November 1964.

# 10

# Congenital Indirect Inguinal Hernia and Related Abnormalities

## INTRODUCTION

Hernia repair is one of the most common of all operative procedures performed on pediatric patients. The purpose of this chapter is to present a practical discussion of congenital inguinal hernia and related abnormalities, such as hydrocele and cryptorchidism, that are often inseparable components of the total problem of congenital herniation.

A review of the repair technique for congenital inguinal hernia, as practiced over a period of 20 years, revealed a trend toward a more conservative operative approach. Although the surgeons varied considerably as to the exact technique of repair, the majority followed sound, broad principles of repair and, in general, agreed that hernias in infants and children should be repaired promptly and simply.

For statistical data included in this chapter, the available records of those patients at the Henry Ford Hospital with a recorded diagnosis of congenital inguinal hernia, between the years 1947 and 1975, were reviewed. Attention was directed largely to those indirect inguinal hernias, in infants and children, where the underlying cause was a patent processus vaginalis.

Normally, the peritoneal processus vaginalis is obliterated; the resultant fibrous structure is known as the vaginal ligament. The remaining portion of the peritoneal pouch, overlying and partially surrounding the testicle, is called the tunica vaginalis testis and consists of visceral and parietal layers. The congenital inguinal hernias so often seen in neonates and children are defects in the inguinal area. They are associated with abdominal visceral protrusion due to failure of the processus vaginalis to undergo obliteration. Since a substantial number of young individuals fail to undergo herniorrhaphy, it is not unusual to see an adult with a complete indirect inguinal hernia dating back to infancy. It must be recalled, however, that even though a patent processus vaginalis does exist in an individual, a diagnosis of hernia is not justifiable unless there is actual protrusion of some viscus through the patent processus. This event may occur with the first cry after birth or may not be evident until young adulthood, when strenuous activity forces the omentum or intestine through the preformed peritoneal sac.

### Incidence of Patency

How often is a patent processus vaginalis found in neonates? This question requires a statistical answer, with appropriate discussion. In statistics cited by Snyder and colleagues (1962) from three sources in German literature, the processus was open in 80 to 94 percent of neonates at birth. Even at one year postpartum, the processus was patent, or at least partially so, in 57 percent of those babies studied. It was remarkable that according to a number of studies, some degree of patency of the vaginal process was found in adulthood in a significant number of individuals. Morgan and Anson (1942) found some degree of patency of the vaginal process in 20 percent of 100 examinations, whereas Engle (1857) found patency in 37 percent.

Two important and practical conclusions must be drawn from the preceding observations: first, patency of the processus vaginalis is not synonymous with a diagnosis of hernia; and, second, the vaginal process remains patent to some degree in a substantial number of individuals into adulthood. Clinical experience supports these conclusions.

## Incidence of Congenital Inguinal Hernias

Many studies have attempted to provide information as to the frequency of congenital indirect inguinal hernias, but the precise incidence of hernias in children is difficult to determine. Snyder and Greaney found the incidence to vary from 0.8 percent to 13 percent, depending on the type of patient studied. For instance, in studying the experience in an out-patient pediatric clinic, Herzfeld (1925) reported an incidence of 13 percent. This study, in my opinion, represents a highly selected patient population—the figure is too high.

Experience at the Henry Ford Hospital has shown that indirect inguinal hernias are far more common a problem of the early postnatal period than of late childhood. In my personal experience, the congenital indirect inguinal hernia was most commonly seen in male infants during the first year of life. Congenital indirect inguinal hernias occur more frequently on the right side—an incidence consistent with the observation that descent of the right testicle proceeds more slowly and, therefore, obliteration of the processus vaginalis occurs somewhat later. According to Keeley (1973), 60 percent of hernias in infants and children occur on the right side, 25 percent on the left, and 15 percent are bilateral.

Prematurity has a predictable effect on the incidence of inguinal hernia as well as other abnormalities. Clatworthy and colleagues (1957) found that 37.7 percent of premature infants had bilateral inguinal hernias; however, the incidence of such hernias in mature, or nearly mature, infants was only 17 percent.

My observation, which has been corroborated by other studies, was that congenital indirect inguinal hernias occurred nearly nine times more frequently in boys than in girls. Also, when congenital indirect inguinal hernias did occur in female infants, sliding components (consisting of fallopian tube and ovary) were very often present; such hernias were likely to be bilateral.

## RELATED ABNORMALITIES

### Hydrocele

Hydrocele may be defined as an endothelial-lined sac, occurring in the inguinoscrotal or inguinolabial area and containing serous fluid. One variety, which may be considered congenital, is seen in infants and is directly related to patency of a greater or lesser portion of the processus vaginalis. Keeley (1973) found hydroceles of this type to be present in 15 percent of the infants and children he studied. The other type, which appears during adulthood or even old age, may be considered acquired; in this type, irritation may be recognized about the tunica vaginalis testis.

In my experience, the hydrocele is the second most common cause of swelling in the inguinoscrotal area. By far, most of the hydroceles I have seen have been scrotal in location and have involved the tunica vaginalis testes. It must be recalled that when the entire processus vaginalis remains patent, a communicating hydrocele may be present along with an indirect inguinal hernia. A great variety of abnormalities can occur as a result of variable and incomplete obliteration of the vaginal process. At times, the hydrocele may occur as a cystic mass in the inguinal canal; such a cystic mass is designated as a hydrocele of the cord. Less often, the lesions may appear as multilocular cysts along the path of the cord. When such congenital cysts occur in the female along the course of the round ligament in the inguinal canal, they are known as cysts of the canal of Nuck; these cysts may extend as far down as the labia majora. Congenital cysts in the canal of Nuck in females are rare, when compared to the incidence of hydroceles in males.

### Mislocated Testis

It is important to consider the situation of "out-of-pocket" testicles from at least four aspects: (1) retractile, or "bashful," testicle; (2) ectopic, or maldescended, testicle; (3) cryptorchidism—an anomaly

that is almost uniformly accompanied by an indirect inguinal hernia; and (4) bilateral anorchia.

RETRACTILE, OR "BASHFUL," TESTICLE. This situation is one in which the testicle occupies a position high in the scrotum, near the external abdominal ring. The cremasteric reflex in infants presenting with this condition is strong and easily activated by the stimulus of a cold hand or as a result of an overenthusiastic examination. The testicle will find its way to a position in the scrotum if the infant is given a warm tub bath or is wrapped in a warm blanket. Gentle palpation with warm hands also may settle

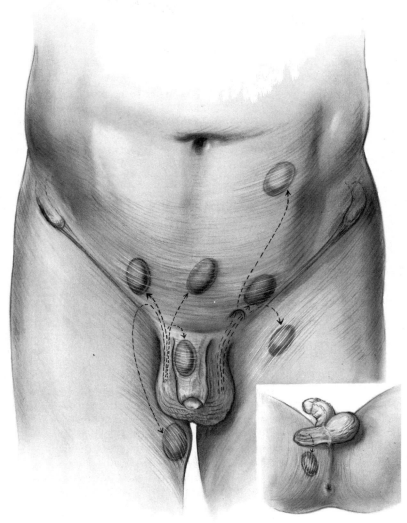

**Figure 10–1.**   Ectopic testicles. (Modified from Alyea, E. P.: Dislocation of the testis. Surg. Gynecol. Obstet., 49:601, 1929. Reproduced by permission of *Surgery, Gynecology & Obstetrics* and the author.)

the question of nondescent. Since the testes are normal, treatment is unnecessary in such patients.

ECTOPIC TESTICLE. In ectopia, or "out-of-place" testis, the spermatic cord has more than sufficient length to reach the scrotum, and the testicle is likely to be normal. It might be said that the testis descended and then wandered, for it is outside the external abdominal ring. Ectopic testicles have been found at the base of the penis, in the perineum, in the femoral region, and even in the opposite side of the scrotum (Fig. 10–1). Treatment consists of mobilization of the testicle, then its replacement in the scrotum. The prognosis for normal testicular function is far better in cases of testicular ectopia than in those of cryptorchidism.

CRYPTORCHIDISM. Cryptorchidism may be defined as a developmental defect in which the testicle fails to descend into its normal position in the scrotum and remains hidden from view in the abdomen or in the inguinal canal. The word is derived from Greek: the prefix *crypt-* may be translated as "hidden" and the word *orchis,* as "testis" — hence, the term *cryptorchidism,* or "hidden testicles." Another term that applies to this situation is undescended testicle.

Browne (1938) very clearly emphasized the need for recognition of the specific type of abnormality present when the testicle is not located in its usual position.

In the individual with true cryptorchidism, the testicle may be arrested in its abdominal position or may reach the inguinal canal; however, it does not pass through the external ring. A representation of the incidence of undescended testes arrested at various levels of descent is shown in Figure 10–2. A considerable number of testes in cryptorchidism are found in the abdomen. Campbell (1951) reports the incidence of abnormal testes to be 26 percent of 275 infants with undescended testes. In 8 percent, the arrest in descent occurred at the internal ring; in 62 percent, in the inguinal canal; and in 4 percent, the testicles reached the external ring (see Fig. 10–2). In 40 infants, the testes could not be identified and were considered to be completely absent or ectopic.

A testicle that can be seen through the skin, and that is located in a position

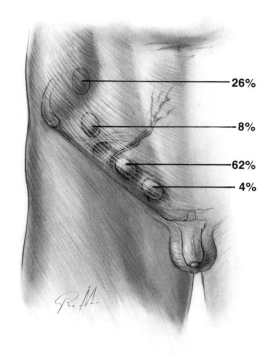

**Figure 10–2.** In most patients with undescended testicles, the testis is found in the inguinal canal. The distribution of the testes in 275 infants seen by Campbell is shown in this illustration.

other than the scrotum is ectopic. The differentiation between an ectopic testicle and cryptorchidism is important; in the former, the cord structures are of sufficient length to permit relatively easy placement of the testicle in the scrotum. Browne stated that a testicle in the inguinal canal could not be palpated through the skin and that the cremaster cannot actually withdraw the testis into the inguinal canal. Even when influenced by an active cremasteric reflex, the testis remains external to the abdominal muscles. Browne further noted that if the testicles can be pushed downward over the pubic bone, descent will occur by the time full growth is attained. Hormonal treatment, according to Browne, would not cause the descent of any testicle that would not have descended without treatment; however, he felt that descent could be accelerated with such therapy.

Reasons for the failure of normal testicular descent may be listed briefly as follows: inadequate production of androgenic hormones, mechanical factors, abnormalities in testicular development, and inflammatory reactions.

Perhaps more important than the abnormal location of the testicle in cryptorchidism is the abnormality in the structure of the testicle itself. Many undescended testicles, Hinman (1955) pointed out, are so abnormal that neither operative nor hormonal therapy would restore normal function. He stated that if the testes are potentially normal, they must be restored to the scrotal location before they are damaged by the intra-abdominal temperature. Hinman found that in cryptorchid boys, few changes occur in the testes from birth to six years of age. However, from age six years to puberty, tubular growth takes place in normal boys but not in those with cryptorchidism. In boys of 9 to 12 years of age, immaturity of the tubules is more striking. Such tests show disorganization and regression at puberty. According to Hinman, if both testes are retained in the abdomen, spermatogenesis does not occur. The increased intra-abdominal temperature is responsible for sterility; and once the testes have been injured, subsequent orchidopexy does not restore spermatogenesis.

Androgenic hormonal secretion continues in the cryptorchid individual but in decreased amounts; nevertheless, libido and potency are reported to be normal. Engberg (1949) has shown that individuals with bilateral undescended testicles daily produce approximately one-half as much androgenic hormones as do normal individuals. Androgen production in boys with cryptorchidism is only slightly less than that in normal boys. It can be said that endocrine function remains fairly satisfactory in the individual with bilateral cryptorchidism, but spermatogenesis is compromised.

**BILATERAL ANORCHIA.** When the location of testicles is uncertain, endocrine function tests must be utilized to rule out anorchia. Martin (1977) advised to proceed by determining the initial blood plasma testosterone level. Then, 2000 units of human chorionic gonadotropin (HCG) are given intramuscularly for 5 consecutive days. The plasma testosterone level is measured again. Patients with anorchia will show little or no elevation of plasma testosterone, but those with nondescent of testicles will show an early and significant elevation of this hormone.

## EMBRYOLOGY

### Origins and Development of the Testis and Ovary

The testis and ovary originate far from the positions they assume in normal adulthood. The ovary travels the shorter distance to the pelvis; the testicle has a more complicated journey to reach its scrotal position. Burton (1958) referred to the earliest developmental phase as the intra-abdominal phase. As early as the third or fourth week of gestation, the urogenital fold arises from invagination of the posterior wall of the coelomic cavity. By this time, degeneration of the pronephros has occurred. At approximately the fourth week of development, the urogenital fold becomes the genital fold medially and the mesonephric fold laterally. These folds have an attachment to the posterior abdominal wall. The mesorchium and the mesovarium are derivatives of mesentery of the genital fold. The grooves of the genital fold move or press inwardly, narrowing the mesenteric attachment.

In the embryo of eight weeks, the mesonephros extends from the fifth cervical to the fourth lumbar segment. By this time, the upper five-sixths of the mesonephros has undergone atrophy. According to Burton, the caudal portion of the mesonephros remains and extends from the first to the third segments. The mesonephros contains the mesonephric tubules, the excretory mesonephric duct, and the müllerian duct. The distal one-sixth of the mesonephros eventually divides into epigenitalis tubules, which connect the testis to the epididymis (the paragenitalis tubules do not have such a connection). Subsequently, the urogenital folds of the two sides meet and fuse to form the genital cord. In the male, it unites with the posterior portion of the bladder. This does not occur in the female; the genital cord remains separate from the bladder. Sex differentiation commences at about the eighth week of gestation. By the third

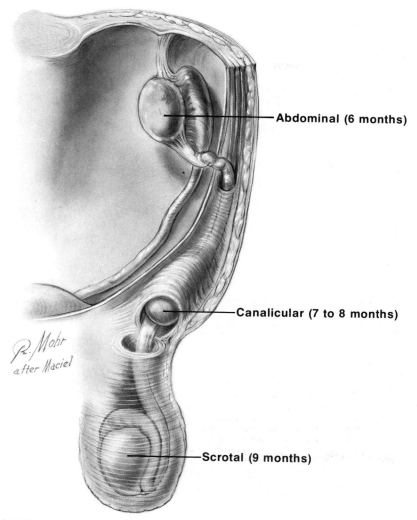

Abdominal (6 months)

Canalicular (7 to 8 months)

R. Mohr
after Maciel

Scrotal (9 months)

**Figure 10–3.** Artist's interpretation, showing the position of the testicle and gubernaculum at various stages of development. (Modified from Burton, C. C.: The embryologic development and descent of the testis in relation to congenital hernia. Surg. Gynecol. Obstet. *107*:296, 1958. Reproduced by permission of *Surgery, Gynecology & Obstetrics.*)

month, the müllerian ducts of the male fetus undergo atrophy; and upon close inspection, sexual differentiation is recognizable.

Important structures derived from the mesonephric duct include the epididymis, the paraepididymis, the seminal vesicles, and the vas deferens. The ureter develops as a diverticulum of the mesonephric duct. The uterus, fallopian tubes, and broad ligaments develop from the müllerian ducts in the female.

The gubernaculum, which is composed of fibrous and muscular tissue, affects the descent of the testicle in some mysterious way. There is some argument as to whether the gubernaculum has a contracting and pulling effect or merely serves as a path for descent. In any event, for the first six months, the testicle is in an intra-abdominal position; during the seventh and eighth months, the testes may be found at a location from the internal abdominal to the external abdominal ring (Fig. 10–3). The gubernaculum is of considerable length during this time. At term, the testes have reached the scrotal position, and the gubernaculum is quite short.

**THE TESTES.** The intimate association of the gonads and the nephric systems from the developmental aspect is well known. In the 10-mm embryo, Patten described the gonads as ridgelike thickenings on the ventral border of the mesonephros. In a 13-mm embryo (six weeks), the sex cords are assuming a characteristic shape; by the fourteenth week, the testicle becomes recognizable. Patten (1968) has shown that the vas deferens, rete testis, seminiferous tubules, and interstitial cells may be identified in the testicle of a 14-week-old embryo. By midpregnancy, the testicle has developed to a point where its structure can be appreciated. The testicle originates in the retroperitoneal tissues and remains technically a retroperitoneal structure. It does not normally become an intra-abdominal or pelvic organ in the sense that the ovary does.

**THE OVARY.** The gonad that is to become an ovary, in its very earliest developmental phase, cannot be differentiated from the testicle. The sex cords develop somewhat as they do in the testes. Eventually, the cords assume the shape of more or less separate masses of cells.

As Patten (1968) has shown, in an embryo of ten weeks the gonadial cords in the ovary are hardly recognizable. The potential germ cells are distributed diffusely in the stroma. As already noted, sex differentiation starts at about the eighth week when the sex cords develop into seminiferous tubules. In the female, the sex cords regress. The architecture is of a diffuse type, and primary follicles appear at about the fourth month. The tunica albuginea is a prominent structure in the testicle. There is much less connective tissue formation just under the germinal epithelium in the ovary, compared to a similarly developing testicle. In an eight-month-old fetus, the ovary shows the presence of primary ovarian follicles, which are easily identified under the microscope.

**DESCENT OF THE TESTIS.** The process whereby the testicles and ovaries reach their normal anatomic position is usually orderly and remarkably accurate. The testes and ovaries usually reach their proper destinations on time; however, in a small percentage of individuals, this orderly chain of events fails to materialize. The testicle may be maldeveloped, or it may be detained in the abdomen or the inguinal canal. Wells has reviewed in de-

tail the anatomic and hormonal factors that are involved. His excellent review (1943) includes 160 references on embryologic, hormonal, and experimental studies that dealt with testicular descent. He concluded that chorionic, gonadotropic, and androgenic hormones are involved in the descent of the testis in man. Estrogens did not appear to influence descent favorably. Wells felt that the gubernaculum probably did not pull the testis into the scrotum.

Campbell in 1942 collected and published statistics regarding nondescent of the testicle in 12.5 million recruits and found the incidence to be 0.28 per cent ($\pm$ .0015). In reviewing the literature, Snyder and Greaney (1962) found the reported incidence of undescended testicle to vary from .28 to 4.2 percent; however the latter figure, in my opinion, is too high for large numbers of males. Scorer (1956) examined 1700 newborn male infants and found the incidence of incomplete descent to be 3.4 percent in full-term infants and 30.3 percent in prematurely born infants.

Sonneland (1925) felt that a number of factors accounted for the progressive change in location of the testes and ovaries. According to him, the following mechanisms were important:

1. intraabdominal pressure;
2. intramuscular pressure due to contraction of muscles draped around the canal; and
3. guidance and active contraction of the smooth muscle of the cord.

It should be recalled that certain primitive structures atrophy and other structures (such as the kidney) enlarge; still others (as a portion of the bladder) come to occupy unique positions in the genitourinary systems. According to Woodburne (1973), "It would be incorrect to say that the gubernaculum draws the testis downward, for inequality in development and growth rates is probably fundamental to the apparent migrations of embryonic organs, but the net effect is much the same."

**DESCENT OF THE OVARY.** The ovary is not found as often in abnormal locations as is the testicle, but it has a less complicated route to follow in its descent. In the female, the primitive guber-

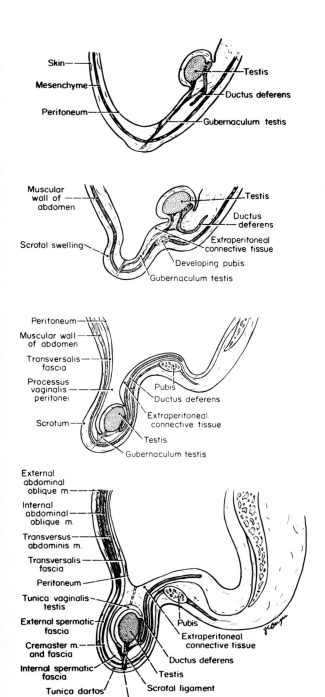

**Figure 10-4.** Location of the testicle: in the iliac fossa at the third month and fifth month, in the inguinal canal during the seventh and eighth months, and reaching the scrotal position at term. (From Woodburne, R. T. (ed.): *Essentials of Human Anatomy* (5th ed.) London, Oxford University Press, 1973, Reproduced with permission of the author and the Oxford University Press.)

naculum attaches to the ovary and to the müllerian ducts — the structures from which the uterus develops. Because of this attachment to the uterus, the ovary does not ordinarily descend below the uterus. The ovarian ligament is a derivative of the gubernaculum between the ovary and uterus, while the portion of the gubernaculum leading from the uterus into the inguinal canal and the labium majus remains as the round ligament and passes through the abdominal wall. Obliteration occurs much earlier in the female, and at term the processus vaginalis is obliterated. The fact that the processus vaginalis is patent at birth in the female not nearly as often as it is in the male bears repeating.

It is useful to summarize the position assumed by the testes and ovaries at various stages of fetal development. In a fetus of approximately seven weeks, the gubernaculum testis is recognizable; this structure is derived from connective tissue in the inferior fold from the testis and the connective tissue from the abdominal wall. At about the fourth month, an evagination of the body cavity begins at the caudal site of attachment of the gubernaculum and eventually becomes the scrotum. During the fifth and sixth months, the scrotal pouch enlarges. The peritoneum becomes evaginated, and it is now simple to recognize the processus vaginalis. According to Woodburne (1973), by the third month the testis is in the iliac fossa; and in a fetus of five months, it has reached the vicinity of the internal inguinal ring. During the sixth month, the testis remains in this location; during the seventh and eighth months of gestation, the testis passes through the inguinal canal and inguinal ring and normally reaches its position in the scrotum by the ninth month. The right testicle will reach its scrotal position somewhat later than the left (Fig. 10-4).

**THE PROCESSUS VAGINALIS.** The nature and significance of the vaginal process of the peritoneum, as it concerns the surgeon, should be well understood. It is interesting to note that although the testicles are retroperitoneal in origin, they exert a profound influence on the peritoneal lining of the lower abdomen (Fig. 10-5; *A, B,* and *C*).

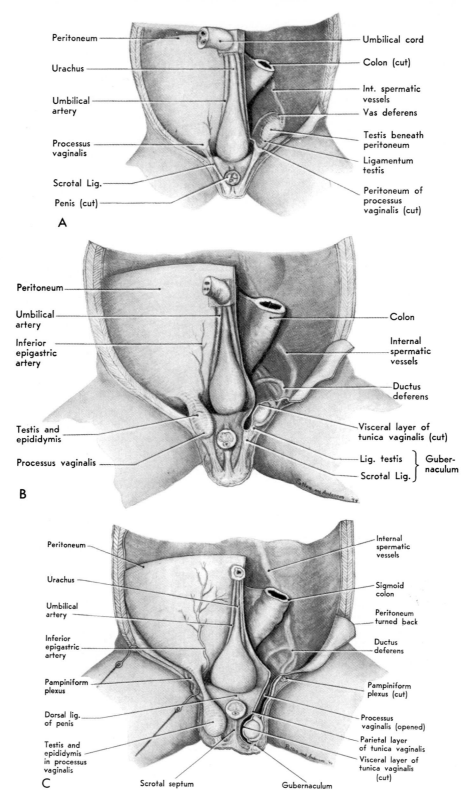

**Figure 10–5.** *A*, Dissection to show formation of the processus vaginalis and descent of testes. Fetus is approximately 20 weeks gestation. *B*, Similar view to *A* — the fetus is now in the seventh month of development. The processus vaginalis is beginning to develop. *C*, The dissection shows the position of the testis in a fetus at term. In this instance, the processus vaginalis is opened. (From Patten, Bradley M.: *Human Embryology*, 3rd ed. Copyright 1968, The Blakiston Division. By permission of McGraw-Hill Book Company. Courtesy of Bruce M. Carlson, Department of Anatomy, University of Michigan, Ann Arbor, Michigan.)

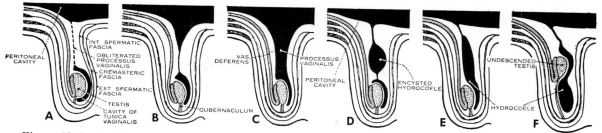

**Figure 10–6.** A, The processus vaginalis has undergone obliteration normally. B and C, Infantile type of hernia. D, Encysted hydrocele of the cord. E, Elongated congenital hydrocele of the cord. F, The infant with cryptorchidism almost always has an associated hernia; a hydrocele is also present. (Reproduced from Hamilton, W. J., and Mossman, H. W.: *Human Embryology* (4th ed.). By permission of the authors and the Macmillan Press, Ltd., London.)

A swelling or protrusion known as the inguinal bursa develops in a fetus of three or four months' gestation and occurs at the site that is to become the scrotum. The gubernaculum, which is quite large and elongated, extends from the lower or caudal pole of the testis to the scrotum. The gubernaculum probably does not exert traction on the testicle but merely provides a path for the testicle to follow. Evagination of the coelomic cavity occurs in the inguinal region, and the peritoneally lined protrusion becomes the processus vaginalis. Figure 10–5, A, depicts an intact peritoneum on the right, while the anterior abdominal wall has been removed from the left side. The fetus is approximately five months old. In B, the processus vaginalis has enlarged, and the testicle is in the lower position of the inguinal canal. The fetus is in the seventh month of gestation. At birth the processus vaginalis has obliterated, and the testicle has reached the scrotum (C). Only the tunica vaginalis testis remains, since the portion in the inguinal canal has undergone obliteration. Thus, the testis remains in its extraperitoneal position. Normally, the inguinal portion of the processus vaginalis becomes obliterated during early infancy or the first year of life. The resultant fibrous structure is known as the vaginal ligament. The portion of the peritoneal pouch overlying and partially surrounding the testicle is known as the tunica vaginalis testis. As already noted, it consists of visceral and parietal layers.

Precisely when does the processus from the internal abdominal ring to the testis become obliterated? The answer to this question is of great importance to surgeons; since opinions vary, some discussion of this point will be included here. Woodburne (1973) stated that the processus vaginalis remains patent in 50 percent of newborn babies for a period of one month postpartum.

Illustrations can best help to clarify the ultimate fate of the processus vaginalis in a number of situations. In A of Figure 10–6, normal obliteration of the processus is shown. In B, an infantile hernia is illustrated; and C, a complete scrotal type of congenital hernia is shown. The vaginal process is widely patent. Also shown are other abnormalities in which incomplete obliteration occurs (Fig. 10–6, D, E, and F). In D of Figure 10–6, a portion of the vaginal process persists as an encysted hydrocele. Hydroceles may vary in their configuration, depending on the degree of obliteration of the processus vaginalis (E and F).

**THE PROCESSUS VAGINALIS IN THE FEMALE.** In the female, the processus vaginalis develops in much the same way as it does in the male. The peritoneal prolongation extends along the round ligament and may communicate with the peritoneum at the internal ring, and it may extend through the external abdominal ring to the labium majus. At approximately six months, the vaginal process is obliterated. The great difference between the male and female in the time of obliteration of the processus vaginalis is striking and significant. In the female, the time of obliteration is six months; however, in 50 percent of male newborn infants, it remains patent for up to one month postpartum. Should the processus vaginalis fail to obliterate in the female, a persistent canal of Nuck remains; and congenital hernia may result. At other times, cystic remnants in the inguinal canal may be the result of incomplete obliteration of the peritoneal prolongation.

## DIRECT INGUINAL HERNIA IN INFANTS AND CHILDREN

Although admittedly rare, direct inguinal hernias do occur in infants and children. As with femoral hernias in infancy, direct inguinal hernias often go unreported; and authoritative textbooks on surgery and pediatric surgery have little or no information on the subject.

In reading the report by Fonkalsrud and colleagues (1965), I found that several patients were excluded from their study because the anatomic defect had not been clearly described in the operative note. I have also made the same observation about several of our records; unfortunately, I found that poor descriptions and inaccuracies were most often evident when an unusual or difficult problem had been encountered. Fonkalsrud and his colleagues treated 13 patients with direct inguinal hernias over a period of 17 years. In four patients, the direct hernia followed repair of an ipsilateral indirect hernia. Eleven of the children were boys, and six of them were less than two years of age. In three patients, large pantaloon hernias were present.

Isolated reports of individual cases of direct inguinal hernia in infants can be found in the literature. I suspect that there are more of these case records lost in other medical records departments, just as occurred at our institution.

The exact incidence of direct inguinal hernias in infants has not yet been determined. An indifferent attempt at diagnosis, both preoperatively and at the time of operation, leads to a less than precise description of the problem at hand. For instance, once the infant or child is seen to have a hernia, it is concluded by many, almost automatically, that an indirect inguinal hernia is present. No further attempt is made at differential diag-

nosis. I would make a plea for an accurate description of the hernia. Where does the sac originate? What is its relationship to the deep inferior epigastric artery? What is the size of the internal ring? What is the anatomic structure and arrangement of the internal oblique and transversus abdominis muscles? What is the condition of the transversalis fascia? If the hernia is recurrent, what type of repair was done initially? It is true that in infants and children, the common hernia is the indirect inguinal hernia; nevertheless, when unusual findings are encountered, other diagnostic possibilities must at least be entertained.

## FEMORAL HERNIAS IN INFANTS AND CHILDREN

It is noteworthy that discussions of femoral hernias in infants and children have not as yet found their way into most books written on the general subject of hernia. Even some outstanding works on pediatric surgery deal only briefly with such hernias occurring in infancy and childhood. Surgeons are becoming increasingly aware of the fact that femoral hernias, although uncommon, do occur in very young patients and that a differential diagnosis is therefore important. The incidence of femoral hernias in infants and children has been reported to be between 0.3 and 0.5 percent.

Mestel and colleagues in 1959 compiled a collective review of femoral hernias in infants and children and found 29 such hernias among 6,416 herniotomies in children. Mestel reported two additional cases he had encountered. In children, the differential diagnosis includes: lymphadenopathy, hydrocele, lipoma, cystic hygroma, ectopic testis, psoas abscess, obturator hernia, and even saphenous varices. Mestel and his coworkers found that femoral hernias were more common in the 6- to 15-year age group than in the 1- to 5-year age group and that more cases occurred in males. He recommended a McVay or Cooper's ligament repair. Fifteen references were cited, dealing with the problem of femoral hernia in infants and children.

Cherry in 1963 recognized two children with bilateral femoral hernias; the ages were 20 months and 3 years. In both patients, Cooper's ligament repairs were performed successfully; and short-term follow-up observations revealed no recurrence.

Ingall in 1964 also called attention to the rarity of femoral hernia in children. He found that the differential diagnosis should include the pathologic entities listed previously by Mestel and his coworkers and added inguinal hernia and cysts of the canal of Nuck to the list of diagnostic possibilities. He advocated the type of repair performed by Lotheissen in 1898.

Fosburg and Mahin in 1965 reviewed in detail the literature on femoral hernia in children from 1880 to 1964 in their report, which included 74 references. They amassed a total of 400 femoral hernias in infants and children under 15 years of age. Fosburg and Mahin further pursued the subject of femoral hernia in children by sending out a questionnaire to 30 general and pediatric surgeons, seeking their opinions as to treatment. Fosburg and Mahin stated that femoral hernias represent less than one percent of all hernias in children, and the incidence in children under five years of age is low. They referred to the fact that strangulation of a femoral hernia in a child is extremely rare. They concluded that repair of femoral hernias in children should be performed through an incision above the inguinal ligament and should utilize Cooper's ligament. Several surgeons favored the McVay repair.

Fonkalsrud and colleagues in 1965 reported on their experiences with femoral and direct inguinal hernias in 25 pediatric patients. Twelve femoral hernias and thirteen direct inguinal hernias were treated, but the correct preoperative diagnosis was made in only eight patients. The authors correctly pointed out that success in repair is attainable if the correct diagnosis is made preoperatively. Fonkalsrud and his coworkers found that femoral hernias occurred generally in older children. Nine of the twelve were eight years of age or older, and only one was six weeks of age. Nine of the twelve underwent Cooper's ligament repair; in two the pectineus fascia was sutured to the inguinal ligament, and in one a Bassini repair was performed.

Burke in 1966 encountered seven femoral hernias in seven children previously subjected to inguinal hernia repairs. It is obviously impossible to decide whether or not the femoral component was present at the original repair. In only one of Burke's seven patients was the possibility of femoral hernia considered at the time of inguinal herniorrhaphy. Burke also found nine femoral hernias in infants and children with no previous history of surgery for groin hernias. His incidence of femoral hernias for all patients with hernia was 0.3 percent. The correct diagnosis was made preoperatively in only four of his patients. The McVay repair—the method most frequently used—was performed on eight patients; the second most frequently used method was one utilizing the inguinal ligament and pectineus fascia in the repair.

Immordino reported his observations on six children with femoral hernias in 1972. He advised that the diagnosis of femoral hernia should be considered, particularly in recurrent hernias when the operative findings do not confirm the clinical impression. Immordino recommended the Cooper's ligament repair for both direct and femoral hernias.

## Comment

The infrequent occurrence of femoral hernias in infants does not justify the attitude that all hernias in infants and children are indirect inguinal hernias. I enthusiastically support those surgeons who urge that a differential diagnosis be made preoperatively for each infant. The correct diagnosis should lead to the proper surgical corrective procedure. Most surgeons prefer the McVay or Cooper's ligament repair of femoral hernia in infants; however, in selected patients, other procedures may be employed.

## HISTORICAL NOTES ON REPAIR OF CONGENITAL INDIRECT INGUINAL HERNIAS

Banks is often cited as a surgeon who advised high ligation of the peritoneal sac as a method of hernia repair in 1882 and, later, in 1884. He stated (1884): "The sac having been thoroughly separated and opened, and its contents having been disposed of, should be well pulled down and tied as high up as possible, whether at the femoral or inguinal apertures." He then continued his repair and described his procedure as follows: "Turning next to the pillars of the ring I employ two, three or four silver wire sutures to pull them together, inserted with a curved needle in a handle." He added, "Room must, of course, be left at the lower part of the ring for the spermatic cord to pass through." Banks was a pioneer in the field of hernia surgery, and he showed great respect for the importance of adequate closure of the external ring. This procedure is not currently considered an adequate repair by many surgeons.

Probably the next most significant observation came from Mr. Hamilton Russell of Melbourne. In 1899 he recognized that inguinal hernias in infants were due to a congenital structure, the patent funicular process. He also thought (erroneously) that direct inguinal hernias have a similar origin.

Turner in 1912 pointed out that high ligation of the peritoneal sac at the internal ring was effective in curing hernia in children. He felt that it was unnecessary to open the external oblique aponeurosis through the external ring in order to gain access to the hernial sac. He advocated use of a small incision in the external oblique to expose the internal ring. This procedure limits exposure of the rest of the inguinal area.

Gertrude Herzfeld, surgeon to the Royal Edinburgh Hospital for Sick Children, wrote a substantial paper on the subject of hernia in infancy in 1925 (Fig. 10–7). She fully understood the pathology of hernias: "It should be noted that there is no interference [*during repair*] with the canal for in children this structure is not at fault, the presence of the sac being the main causal factor in the production of a hernia." She recommended high ligation of the peritoneal sac as follows: "The proximal portion is now carefully isolated by dissection and pulled upon until on the inner side the extraperitoneal bladder fat comes into view showing that the neck of the sac has been reached." The proximal sac was transfixed with number one chromic catgut and ligated. However, her convic-

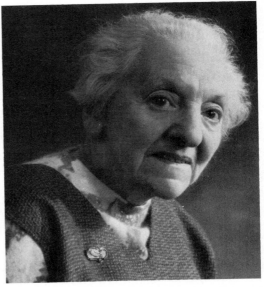

**Figure 10–7.** Miss Gertrude Herzfeld, whose inquiries into the problem of infantile hernia led her to the conclusion that such hernias should be treated by high ligation of the peritoneal sac.

tions as to the effectiveness of high ligation of the sac alone were less than absolute. She added, "The operation is completed by one stitch across the region of the pillars of the ring."

Hamilton Russell of Melbourne, Australia, again described his technique of repair in 1925. He classified hernias simply as being saccular and nonsaccular. Oblique hernias, femoral hernias, and certain direct inguinal hernias were nonsaccular. He pointed out that oblique (indirect) inguinal hernia is never caused by muscular weakness. He then logically insisted that the muscles are perfectly capable of preventing return of a hernia once the sac is removed. As a technical detail in repair of indirect inguinal hernias, he strongly recommended that high ligation of the sac is of paramount importance.

In 1945 Coles described his technique for the operative cure of inguinal hernia in infancy and childhood in a report from the Children's Surgical Service of Bellevue Hospital in New York. Coles recognized that the congenital type of hernia in the infant was not due to any weakness or deficiency in the abdominal muscles and aponeuroses. The presence of the preformed sac—the patent peritoneal processus—accounted for the infantile hernia. With this concept as a background, Coles then began utilizing an operative procedure that requires definition of the sac and its proximal closure at the internal ring. He preserved the normal anatomic relationships, omitting all attempts at suture of the musculoaponeurotic structures about the internal ring.

Potts, Riker, and Lewis presented a significant paper at the 1950 meeting of the American Surgical Association. They reported their results of 600 operations for hernia in infants and children. Potts emphasized the well-known embryologic and anatomic fact that most hernias in infants are due to a patent processus vaginalis rather than a weakness in the abdominal wall. Continuing with simple logic, he insisted that all that is necessary to cure such hernias is high ligation of the peritoneal sac. Decrying any attempts at repairing the inguinal floor, Potts complained, "The inguinal region is the lawful domain of the surgical resident. He has learned from his predecessors the Bassini technique and many of its modifications, and continues to use them indiscriminately on every hernia he can commandeer."

Besides those noted above, a number of surgeons today accept the principle that high ligation of the peritoneal sac cures infants and children of congenital indirect inguinal hernias. Snyder and Greaney (1962), Clatworthy and colleagues (1957), and DeBoer (1957) all feel that ordinarily nothing more need be done towards repair of the hernia once the sac is properly closed.

Surgeons are unanimous in the opinion that high ligation of the peritoneal sac is essential in the repair of congenital indirect inguinal hernias. I have referred to the opinions of Turner (1912), Russell (1925), Herzfeld (1925), Coles (1945), and Potts and his coworkers (1950), who felt that high ligation of the peritoneal sac is all that is required.

On the other hand, there are a number of surgeons who prefer to assess the size of the internal ring, then perform an appropriate repair of any defect encountered. The late Dr. Amos Koontz (1963) of Johns Hopkins University believed that closure of the transversalis fascia at the internal ring could be achieved with from one to three sutures of fine silk. Koop (1957) adds a modified herniorrhaphy after high liga-

tion of the sac. James (1971) places two cotton sutures about the internal ring, if it is enlarged. One suture is placed about each side of the cord as it passes from the internal ring. Gross (1955) advises a more extensive repair after high ligation of the sac, and he describes a modification of the Ferguson repair in his book. Swenson (1969) also feels that a modified repair is indicated. After the transversalis fascia is approximated with number 4–0 silk, the internal oblique and conjoined tendon are sutured to the shelving portion of the inguinal ligament. Kieswetter (1961) does not ordinarily advise a formal herniorrhaphy for the average pediatric patient, but he does recommend inspection of the size of the internal ring before deciding on its repair. If it is enlarged, he places several nonabsorbable sutures between the fibers of the internal oblique muscle, the transversalis fascia, and Poupart's ligament, near the internal ring. Zimmerman decides upon his precise procedure after he has had the opportunity to inspect the internal ring (Zimmerman and Anson, 1967). An enlarged ring is repaired with a single suture of fine silk. Lynn (1961) also employs a single suture to repair a patulous internal ring.

## SUMMARY

There is a strong and well-justified trend today toward early operation for inguinal hernia in infants. Effective methods of preparation and excellent anesthesia make it possible for surgeons to operate upon small infants and even premature neonates when necessary. Most surgeons feel that the time for repair should be when the hernia is discovered, allowing the necessary time for preparation.

Since Potts and colleagues (1950) — and others as well — took a strong position for simple high ligation of the sac as treatment of choice for congenital indirect inguinal hernia, a number of pediatric surgeons and general surgeons have followed suit.

Well-known surgeons, however, hold to a slightly different opinion. While they agree on the importance of high ligation of the sac, they advise that the internal ring merits individual inspection; furthermore, when indicated, one to three sutures may be placed in the transversalis fascia at the internal ring. A number of surgeons still feel that the Bassini repair has a place in repair of congenital hernias in older children and young men, particularly when the internal ring is enlarged or when a weakness in the floor is evident. The Ferguson repair appears to be losing its popularity.

I feel that each hernia should be assessed individually. If the internal abdominal ring is small and if no other abnormality exists, high ligation of the peritoneal sac only is performed. Extensive reconstruction not only is unnecessary but also may be meddlesome. If the internal ring is large, it is repaired with nonabsorbable sutures. In older children and young men, the Bassini repair may be employed.

## PRINCIPLES OF MANAGEMENT

### Congenital Indirect Inguinal Hernia

It obviously is necessary for each patient to have a careful history and physical examination, as well as a urinalysis and blood count. As a rule, children with other complicating congenital abnormalities should be admitted to the hospital. Furthermore, I always discuss the plan and procedure to be followed with the parents. If the parents are unintelligent or irresponsible or both, admission to the hospital is insisted on.

At the Henry Ford Hospital, we have favored general anesthesia in the repair of hernias in infants and children. While local anesthesia is preferred in aged and high-risk patients, it is rarely used in infants and children. At the present time, ketamine hydrochloride is fairly popular as the anesthetic of choice. We also are permitting increasing numbers of infants and children to return home on the afternoon or evening of surgery.

I heartily agree with the admonition by a number of surgeons who advocate gentleness and precision when operating upon infants and children. Infants and children, as well as adults, deserve every refinement in technique and instrumentation currently available to all well-trained surgeons. Halsted (1924), a general surgeon, was a foremost exponent of careful technique in all operations. He insisted on asepsis, gentleness, meticulous dissection, and careful hemostasis, and on the use of fine, nonabsorbable suture material. His influence on surgical technique has been unmatched. In his practice, fine silk was a popular suture material; and Halsted recognized the importance of fine-pointed hemostats, designing such instruments personally.

Preparation of the skin is somewhat simpler in the infant because of the relative absence of hirsutism. The abdomen, pubes, upper thighs, and scrotal areas are bathed with soaps containing hexachlorophene and rinsed with warm water. The area of preparation must be generous, since the distances from the anterior superior spine to the pubic tubercle and from the umbilicus to the groin are so small. The scrotum and upper thigh are carefully cleansed, if either a hydrocele or cryptorchidism complicates the picture. Some surgeons prefer preparation of the skin with povidone-iodine compounds, such as Betadine or Isodine.

**OPERATIVE TECHNIQUE** (Fig. 10–8, A–J). After anesthesia is achieved, restraints are applied. The skin is prepared by bathing the abdomen, upper thighs, and scrotum with a surgical soap or any preferred surgical antibacterial agent. The skin incision in infants should be made somewhat more transversely than it is in adults, and it should be made in line with a transverse abdominal skin crease that often is present (Fig. 10–8, A). Some infants are obese, with a thick layer of "baby fat." The incision is placed so that it will reach from the internal to the external ring—a distance of three to five centimeters. Small skin towels are clipped in position to protect the wound edges. Bleeding points are grasped with tiny hemostats and ligated with number 4–0 or 5–0 silk.

The incision is deepened with a scalpel until an identifiable layer of fascia is encountered. Those with limited experience will have difficulty recognizing it as Scarpa's fascia, for it is well developed in infants and may be confused with the aponeurosis of the external oblique. This superficial layer of fascia is divided in the direction of the incision and deepened to the next layer, which is the fascia of the

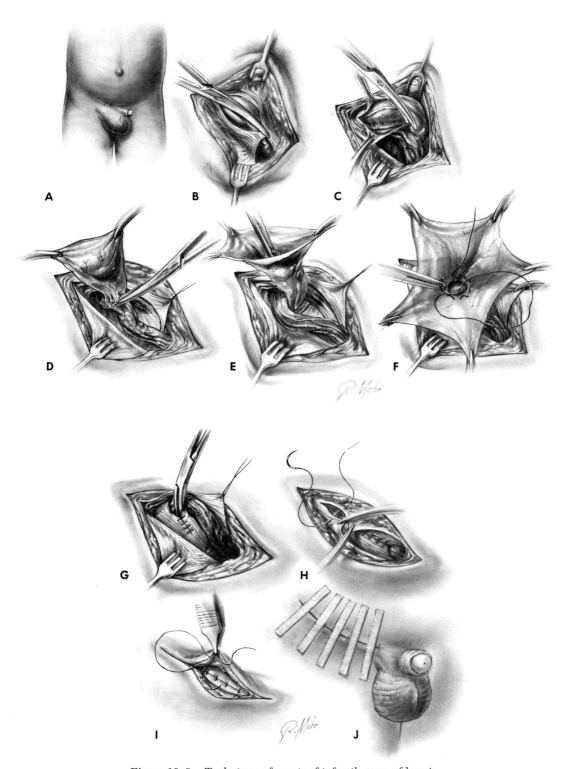

**Figure 10–8.** Technique of repair of infantile type of hernia.

external oblique. Although the dissection at this level is limited, the external ring and the area of Poupart's ligament should be identified.

The fascia of the external oblique is opened at the level of the superior crus of the external ring (Fig. 10–8, *B*). The small, threadlike ilioinguinal nerve should be recognized here. The purpose of incising the external oblique is to gain access to the region of the internal ring. Some surgeons do not open the external oblique through its length to the external ring. I favor opening the external oblique, so that inspection of the spermatic cord can be performed easily and safely.

With elevation of the superior leaflet of the external oblique fascia, the internal oblique muscle and cremasteric muscle are seen. The cremaster muscle fibers are separated longitudinally by careful dissection with a small hemostat. The dissection is performed in the direction of the fibers of cremasteric muscle at the internal ring (Fig. 10–8, *C*). The peritoneal sac is a thin, delicate, whitish membranous structure located in the anteromedial portion of the internal ring (Fig. 10–8, *D*). The peritoneal sac lies on the vas deferens, with which it is intimately related. Since the hernial sac is quite thin in infants, careful dissection is essential. Separation of the sac from the surrounding tissues is completed with blunt and sharp dissection, while the cord and vas deferens are protected (Fig. 10–8, *E*). The vas deferens, though small, is easily identifiable.

I prefer to open the peritoneal sac and complete its dissection under direct vision. The peritoneal sac must be freed of all attachments to the abdominal wall. Omental adhesions are not a problem in infants, since the omentum has not developed to a point where it reaches the sac. In females, after dissection of the sac is completed, a fair amount of adipose tissue may be seen medially. At this point, dissection is discontinued lest the bladder be injured. In female infants, the tube and ovary are often found in the peritoneal sac as a sliding component. The technique of management of such hernial sacs is illustrated in Chapter 18 (Fig. 18–23, *A–C*). In this clinical study, seven female infants had sliding inguinal hernias, most often involving the tube and ovary. Bilateral sliding inguinal hernias were present in four of the seven.

The next important and basic requirement is high ligation of the peritoneal sac (Fig. 10–8, *F*). I prefer to place a purse-string suture of number 4–0 silk proximally to achieve high ligation of the sac. A number of techniques may be used, but the basic requirement still is effective high ligation of the peritoneal sac without injury to the cord. Any excess peritoneal sac is excised. At this point, the ligated sac will be seen to withdraw to a point under the transversus abdominis and internal oblique muscles. No attempt is made to transplant the proximally ligated sac. The transversalis fascia and transversus abdominis muscles remain free to function as restraining structures.

I inspect the internal abdominal ring and the floor of Hesselbach's triangle. Although they are rare in infants and children, femoral and direct hernias are considered as diagnostic possibilities. If the ring is large, one or two sutures of fine silk or two synthetic nonabsorbable sutures are inserted between the elements of transversalis fascia at the site (Fig. 10–8, *G*). If the floor of the inguinal canal is considered to be weak (as occurs in the occasional growing child), a Bassini repair is performed with number 3–0 silk. In repair of infantile hernias, it is rarely necessary to do more than dissect the peritoneal sac cleanly and perform high ligation.

The external oblique fascia has been closed with number 4–0 silk; and the subcutaneous tissues, including Scarpa's fascia, are approximated with number 4–0 plain catgut (Fig. 10–8, *H*). Subcuticular sutures of number 4–0 absorbable sutures are placed so as to approximate the wound edges (Fig. 10–8, *I*). Finally, small strips of nonallergenic adhesive tape are placed to approximate the epidermis (Fig. 10–8, *J*). This technique avoids a painful experience for the small patient and a distressing out-patient visit for the surgeon, since suture removal is unnecessary. The child can be given a warm tub bath in four or five days, and the adhesive strips will fall away. Dispensing with suture removal in infants and children (and in some adults, too) is substantial progress in the care of postherniorrhaphy patients.

## Hydrocele

The best method of disposing of the distal hernial sac and coexisting hydrocele merits a brief discussion, since hydroceles are second only to hernia as a cause of inguinoscrotal swelling. Occasionally, such fluid-filled cysts are found in the canal of Nuck in females.

A number of surgeons specifically warn against the dangerous practice of aspiration of hydroceles in infants. These surgeons do not feel that complete excision of the hydrocele sac is necessary, nor do they recommend the bottle procedure. Clatworthy and colleagues (1957), Potts and his coworkers (1950), and Snyder and Greaney (1962) all share the opinion just mentioned. Small hydroceles in infants under one year of age do not, alone, warrant hasty surgical treatment. The hydroceles may subside and disappear; however, those which enlarge and become symptomatic will require operative treatment.

A word of caution is in order regarding hydroceles in infants. If a hydrocele is observed to persist and even to increase in size, then the likelihood of a communicating hydrocele is overwhelming. Needle aspiration is never recommended in children, nor is transscrotal hydrocelectomy indicated. I have never aspirated a hydrocele in an infant or child. I advocate the same surgical approach as in repair of inguinal hernia in infants, since the hydrocele may be associated with a patent processus vaginalis.

I have seen a hydrocele result from failure to deal with the distal sac in complete congenital indirect inguinal hernias in children. The objective should be to eliminate the possibility of a complete, serosal sac forming from the remaining distal processus vaginalis. Small to moderate serosal sacs are usually drained operatively and the sac partially removed. Larger peritoneal sacs should be partially dissected and a sufficient amount of the serosal membrane excised, so that only a portion of the peritoneal surface remains. Certainly, no determined effort is made to completely excise the entire sac near the testicle, though a portion of the parietal layer of the processus vaginalis testis is excised. Eversion and suture of the peritoneum about the cord and testicle—the so-called bottle procedure—is unnecessary and may even be dangerous, if performed improperly. Small hydroceles in infants and children should be observed, since many will regress spontaneously.

## THE QUESTION OF CONTRALATERAL REPAIR

If there is one aspect of the surgery of hernia that provokes a difference of opinion, it is the proper management of the groin opposite a demonstrable hernia that requires repair. A number of more or less valid arguments based on truths that may not apply to the problem have been advanced as reasons for supporting whatever position the author may assume. Sparkman contributed a significant review and appraisal of the subject of contralateral exploration in 1962. A great number of the articles published on this subject favor the procedure, but this does not mean that the procedure of contralateral exploration is either universally practiced or endorsed. I will review here some of the opinions expressed on this matter in the literature.

A number of authors have offered evidence in support of contralateral exploration. Rothenberg and Barnett (1955), Mueller and Rader (1956), McLaughlin and Kleager (1956), Gilbert and Clatworthy (1959), Kieswetter and Parenzan (1959), and Lynn and Johnson (1961) have advocated exploration of the contralateral side in certain patients.

Rothenberg and Barnett in 1955 published their findings on 50 infants and children in whom only a unilateral hernia was diagnosed preoperatively. The study was conceived when the authors discovered indirect inguinal hernias in six children who had already undergone operations for hernia on the opposite side three years earlier. They found that 100 percent of the infants under one year of age had bilateral hernias; but in children over one year of age, only 65.8 percent had bilateral hernias. Here I must interject the observation that 27 infants and children upon whom these observations were made had sacs measuring two to three centimeters in length. The authors then stated that bilateral exploration seemed to be justified, since the procedure permitted the cure of "undiagnosed indirect inguinal hernias." The procedure in their hands did not lengthen the period of hospitalization, nor did it result in increased operative morbidity. They encountered no wound infections or operative complications.

In 1956 Mueller and Rader reported their experiences with surgical treatment of inguinal hernia in 90 children. They found the incidence of unsuspected or potential hernia to be 65 percent and recommended bilateral exploration for all children under the age of seven years.

McLaughlin and Kleager repaired 298 hernias in 240 infants and children and presented their report in 1956. They performed contralateral repairs in 48 infants under three years of age and found a definite hernia on the second side in 25 (52 percent). McLaughlin and Kleager also found a higher incidence of hernia on the explored side when the presenting hernia was on the left side.

In 1959 Gilbert and Clatworthy presented their views on the subject of bilateral repairs in infancy and childhood. They studied 164 patients admitted for unilateral herniorrhaphy. These authors were among the few who described their technique of exploration and their operative criteria for a positive exploration. According to Gilbert and Clatworthy:

If the processus vaginalis was patent below the internal ring and could be demonstrated to communicate with the peritoneal cavity by observing a free flow of fluid into the patent sac by passing a probe through the opened sac into the peritoneal cavity. . .

— only then was the exploration considered to be positive. They recognized that by traction the surgeon could produce a pseudosac. Gilbert and Clatworthy found that 60 percent of their patients with unilateral hernias had had a patent processus vaginalis on the second side. These authors, unlike others, felt that family history, age, history of prematurity, and side explored had no influence on the total incidence of positive explorations. They advocated bilateral herniotomy for healthy infants with unilateral hernia.

In 1959 Kieswetter and Parenzan were still trying to answer the question: "When should hernia in the infant be treated bilaterally?" They studied two groups of patients: in one group, 100 bilateral repairs were performed in infants under two years of age; in the other group, 237 patients (also under two years of age) had unilateral repair. The two researchers were contacted subsequently by mail or in person to determine if a contralateral hernia had developed. Kieswetter and Parenzan defined their limits of what was considered to be a hernial sac. They felt that if a sac of one centimeter or greater was present below the ring when no tension was exerted on the cord, then the exploration was considered positive. Based on the preceding criteria, they found bilateral hernias in 60 percent of the 100 infants on whom they performed bilateral explorations. Of the 237 infants and children under the age of two years with previous unilateral repairs, 31 percent later underwent contralateral hernia repair. Kieswetter and Parenzan advocated bilateral herniorrhaphies on all children under the age of two years.

Lynn and Johnson in 1961 presented a critical analysis of 1000 herniorrhaphies in children. They diagnosed a peritoneal protrusion, of 1.5 cm in length and without any traction on the cord, as a hernia in their series. Based on this definition, they were able to demonstrate 180 additional hernias in 198 selected explorations. Lynn and Johnson consequently recommended contralateral repair in selected cases. For instance, they advocated bilateral repair in healthy boys with an evident hernia on one side.

In a discussion of the presentation by Lynn and Johnson, Ryan of Toronto felt that not all small peritoneal protrusions demonstrated during contralateral exploration would eventuate into hernias. He believed that as many as 75 percent of these patients were operated upon unnecessarily.

On the other hand, a number of distinguished general surgeons as well as pediatric surgeons do not advise routine contralateral repair or exploration when a unilateral hernia is found. This group of surgeons felt that the advantages gained by exploring the second side were hardly justified because of the high incidence of negative explorations. They pointed out that although the complication rate is not high, some injuries to the testes and vas deferens do occur. Surgeons who do not perform routine contralateral exploration include: Packard and McLauthlin (1953); Gross (1955); McVay (1965); Fischer and Mumenthaler (1957); Clausen, Jake, and Binkley (1958); Ryan; Santulli and Shaw (1961); Snyder and Greaney (1962); and Swenson (1969).

Packard and McLauthlin in 1953 reported their observations on 681 hernias in infants and children at Denver Children's Hospital. In their experience, only 23 patients returned later for repair of a hernia on the opposite side; consequently, they did not feel that contralateral exploration was justified when a unilateral hernia was repaired.

Clausen and colleagues (1958), in surveying ten large children's hospitals, found that bilateral exploration was carried out routinely in one, while in three hospitals, the second side was explored upon specific indication.

Gilbert and Clatworthy (1959) questioned 46 members of the surgical section of the American Academy of Pediatrics and found that 37 percent explored the opposite side routinely. Other members were selective and considered the age, sex, initial side of the hernia, and presence of other evidence of hernia (such as the "silk sign" or thickening of the cord).

Gross (1955) practiced exploration of both sides for a period of time; however, because the number of negative explorations was too great, he abandoned the procedure. He stated that "at present we open the second side only when there is something in the history or physical examination which suggests that a hernia might be present on the second side."

McVay (1965), in a discussion of the paper by Mueller and Rothenberg, cited a figure of 14.3 percent as the rate of bilateral hernia in all age groups. He indicated that an additional six percent had undergone previous repair on the opposite side. He did not feel that routine bilateral exploration was warranted if a hernia was diagnosed on one side only. He also pointed out the need for careful examination of the inguinofemoral region. As a result, in one infant, a direct inguinal hernia was recognized and repaired.

McVay in 1965 restated his position against routine contralateral exploration when one hernia is clinically recognizable. He emphasized that the presence of a persistent processus vaginalis alone does not justify the diagnosis of a hernia. He cited odds of 80 percent against a second hernia occurring when a unilateral hernia is repaired in infants.

In a candid report from Switzerland by Fischer and Mumenthaler in 1957, the authors found that a contralateral hernia developed in 11 percent of 625 patients after previous unilateral hernia repair. They acknowledged that testicular atrophy occurred in 1 percent and a decrease in size of the testicles was noted in 2.7 percent. Since the incidence of a second hernia after unilateral repair was only 11 percent, they felt the additional exploration of the contralateral side was not justified.

Clausen, Jake, and Binkley examined in depth the matter of contralateral exploration in 1958. Besides analyzing their results critically, they made inquiries into the practice of bilateral repair at ten large pediatric hospitals. In six institutions, contralateral explorations were not performed. It was interesting that in only one institution was contralateral exploration a routine matter. In three institutions, the surgeons performed operations on the opposite side where there was specific indication, such as prematurity, left-sided hernia, hydrocele, cryptorchidism, and evidence on physical examination that a hernia might be present.

Clausen and colleagues studied four groups of infants and children: 708 consecutive patients with hernia, admitted over a period of three years; 164 patients in whom contralateral exploration was performed; 1000 adult patients with indirect inguinal hernia; and 97 patients who had had one side repaired and were followed for 10 to 28 years. As a result of their observations, the authors found that among the 708 patients admitted for hernia repair, 36 (or 7.6 percent) were admitted for repair of the second side. They found upon contralateral exploration that the sac was demonstrable in 73.2 percent of infants less than six months of age. But, at two years of age, this number dropped to 37.5 percent. In analysis of 1000 records of adult patients, Clausen and coworkers found that 242 of the hernias were bilateral; and in a 10- to 28-year follow-up of 97 infants, they found that 16, or 16.5 percent, subsequently required repair of the opposite side. The authors indicated that in infants less than two years of age, a high incidence of patent processus vaginalis alone does not justify routine exploration of the contralateral side. They advised that the exploration of the opposite side should be performed in selected cases—for example, if no technical or anesthetic problems had been encountered in repairing the original hernia. Ryan of Toronto, in his discussion of Lynn and Johnson's paper (1961), pointed out that a patient with a unilateral hernia has a maximum chance of approximately 25 percent in developing a hernia of the contralateral side; this observation includes the life span from childhood to death. Ryan does not advocate routine contralateral exploration and advises parents that the chances of their child's developing a second hernia are only one in four.

Santulli and Shaw continued their studies of hernia in infants and children and published their report in 1961. They examined the records of 359 patients aged 5 to 14 years following unilateral hernia repair and found that a contralateral hernia appeared in 12 percent. They also explored the contralateral side in a second group of 175 patients with unilateral hernia. They found positive explorations in 56 percent, or 98 patients. Their definition of a positive exploration is interesting: "Positive exploration was defined as a projection of the peritoneum well below the internal ring in the absence of traction on the spermatic cord." Because of the discrepancy between the incidence of actual hernias found (12 percent) and the incidence of positive explorations (56 percent), routine exploration was not advised. Santulli and Shaw felt that a reliable history compatible with hernia, and such findings as thickening of the cord, justified contralateral exploration.

Snyder and Greaney in the book on pediatric surgery by Benson and his coauthors (1962) advocated repair of the recognizable hernia. They emphasized that finding a patent processus vaginalis did not necessarily mean a hernia would develop in the future.

Swenson (1969) does not practice routine exploration of the contralateral side. But if there is thickening of the cord or the presence of a positive "silk sign," the second side is explored and repaired, when necessary.

## Personal Comments on Contralateral Exploration for Hernia in Infants

In principle, I am opposed to routine operations that can be considered successful in perhaps only 25 percent of all cases. Surgeons are well aware that the diagnosis of hernia is warranted only when a protrusion can be visualized or palpated or both. Occasionally, though, strong suspicion based on clinical experience justifies surgical correction of a defect that is not easily evident. The presence of a patent processus vaginalis alone does not justify the diagnosis of hernia.

Even greater confusion is generated in the literature because of the failure of surgeons to agree upon what constitutes a positive exploration. I could not make a valid comparison of statistics among the various authors, since there were considerable variations in the age of the patients and in the criteria of what constituted a positive exploration on the contralateral side. It is well known among surgeons experienced in hernia repair that some peritoneal sac can be produced in every patient whose groin is explored. The size of the fabricated sac, in such cases, will vary directly with the determination of the surgeon to produce a "contralateral hernial sac." It would be helpful if a number of surgeons adopted the same technique for determining the size of the sac and patent processus vaginalis, in the case of an asymptomatic hernia. Various surgeons have elected to call an exploration positive if it extends 1 cm, 2 cm, 3 cm, or more below the internal ring without traction on the cord structures. Other surgeons record no measurements at all, relying upon estimates at the time of operation. Obviously, then, *the frequency of positive explorations reported by different surgeons will be influenced by their individual criteria of what constitutes a positive exploration.*

What is the actual significance of a small peritoneal prolongation of the processus, discovered during contralateral exploration? There is no doubt that some of them would eventually become recognized as hernias; however, it is also known that some adults may have patent vaginal processus without clinically recognizable hernias. Morgan and Anson (1942) found some portion of the processus to be present and patent in 20 percent of 100 body halves without clinically recognizable hernias. In examination of 200 adults, Clausen and colleagues (1958) reported that incomplete closure of the processus vaginalis was found in 47 instances. Engle (1857) found incomplete closure of the processus vaginalis in 37 percent of 100 bodies he studied.

Those surgeons who advocate contralateral repair point out the high incidence of positive findings in the very young. However, as the infants grow into childhood, the incidence of positive explorations decreases, as does the frequency of indirect inguinal hernias; this is consistent with the known fact that the mere presence of a small processus vaginalis does not mean that a hernia exists, nor does it mean that one will necessarily develop. A number of such vaginal processes close during the first year of life without surgical intervention.

## Inguinal Hernia and Cryptorchidism

In their excellent book entitled *Embryology for Surgeons*, Gray and Skandalakis (1972) stated that hernias can be found in about 90 percent of patients with undescended testicles. In my clinical experience (which largely deals with adults), when presented with a patient with undescended testicle, I would expect to find a congenital hernia due to the patent processus vaginalis that accompanies failure of descent of the testicle.

Snyder and Greaney (1962) have presented statistics that were gathered from several sources in the literature and that demonstrated cryptorchidism and hernia to be present simultaneously in from 66 to 97.7 percent of the cases studied. The precise incidence need not provoke serious debate, since the surgeon who operates to correct cryptorchidism can easily close the processus vaginalis and repair any coexisting defect.

CONSEQUENCE OF CRYPTORCHIDISM. The undescended testicle is an abnormality that must be reckoned with for the following reasons:

1. In almost every patient I saw, inguinal hernia accompanied the undescended testicle; and such hernias require treatment, sooner or later.
2. The danger of malignancy exists, but its magnitude is debated in the literature. The testicle is positioned out of reach and out of sight; a tumor of some size could grow on the testicle before being detected.
3. In most, if not all, undescended testicles, spermatogenesis is seriously impaired. Orchiopexy may preserve this function, if done in time.
4. In some boys, the absence of testes in the scrotum could result in social maladjustments and psychologic problems.
5. The testicle in the groin may be subject to mechanical trauma in sports or in other types of physical activity.
6. Torsion of the testicle is not at all rare in cases of cryptorchidism.

It is beyond my objectives here to examine the preceding list in detail, but a brief discussion of each item will serve to form a practical basis for the management of cryptorchidism, when encountered in a hernia patient.

MALIGNANCY OF THE TESTES AND CRYPTORCHIDISM. The literature on malignancy of the testes in cryptorchidism is controversial and abundant. Campbell (1959), who felt that the abdominal testicle is more vulnerable to malignant changes than is the inguinal, stated that one abdominal testicle in approximately 20 shows malignant change, whereas one inguinal testicle in 80 shows evidence of malignancy. Yet, Carroll (1949) questioned 662 American Urological Association members and 76 per cent reported that they had never seen a malignancy in an undescended testicle! On the other hand, Martin assembled a total of 13,089 patients with testicular tumors and found that 1,288, or 9.8 percent, had cryptorchidism. It can be concluded that even though malignant tumors of the undescended testicle are rare, they are more difficult to demonstrate in undescended testicles than in normal ones.

FAILURE OF SPERMATOGENESIS IN CRYPTORCHIDISM. It is a well-known fact that men with bilateral testicular nondescent are uniformly sterile. In fully grown men with undescended testicles, the appearance of the retained testes is much like that found in a child. Rea in 1942 studied 46 retained testes from postpubertal patients aged 15 to 73 years. Atrophy was observed histologically in all specimens, and in none were spermatozoa seen.

Robinson and Engle (1954) studied 150 testicular biopsies taken from undescended testes. On measuring the diameters of seminiferous tubules in both normally descended and cryptorchid testes, they identified a failure of tubular growth in the undescended testicle of boys over five years of age.

It is being recognized that in the early years, there is growth and development of the seminferous tubules. Martin (1977) noted the undescended testis fails to mature and differs from a normal scrotal testicle after the child reaches the age of two years.

Scorer and Farrington (1971) identified such abnormalities in cryptorchidism as the following: partial obliteration or absence of the vas, obstruction of the vas, and various abnormalities of the epididymis. Such identifiable abnormalities could interfere with the passage of spermatozoa and, hence, contribute to sterility in patients with testicular nondescent.

Hand (1955) studied testes extirpated from individuals with cryptorchidism, and the microscopic sections of testes obtained from 22 patients aged 18 to 73 showed degeneration of germinal elements in all. Prepubertal tubules were found in five, indicating congenital defectiveness. The cells of Leydig were well preserved in 19 of 22 such examinations. Spermatogenesis is indeed seriously interfered with in the cryptorchid individual. Given an individual with bilaterally undescended testicles, the likelihood of sterility is overwhelming. The surgeon performing orchidopexy should be extremely cautious in giving a favorable prognosis insofar as the reproductive function is concerned. Occasional cases of fertility reported after surgical correction of bilaterally undescended testicles should be considered on an individual basis.

Atkinson (1975) studied 32 patients who had undergone surgical correction of unilateral cryptorchidism and found the paternity rate to be 42.1 percent. In 8 patients with bilateral undescended testis, the paternity rate was 22.2 percent.

**PSYCHOLOGIC ABNORMALITIES AND CRYPTORCHIDISM.** When the patient is an infant or a small boy with cryptorchidism, the mental distress falls upon the parents who, understandably, want to know if the child will grow and develop into a normal male. If true cryptorchidism is present bilaterally, the parents should be informed that fertility upon reaching adulthood is unlikely. They can be told that the secondary sex characteristics will develop satisfactorily. If one testicle has descended to its normal position, then fertility is to be expected.

As the boy grows and develops, he becomes conscious of the fact that his testes are missing. Furthermore, the anatomic abnormality may be observed by his friends. Thus, he may develop a shy, withdrawn personality because he is physically unlike his male friends.

**CRYPTORCHIDISM AND TRAUMA.** The undescended testicle is occasionally somewhat fixed in its position in the inguinal canal and over the pubes. It is true that such a testicle may move up and down the canal for short distances; nevertheless, it is relatively fixed when compared to the mobile normal testicle. In such situations, the undescended testicle may be subject to trauma during physical work or athletic participation.

**CRYPTORCHIDISM AND TORSION OF THE TESTICLE.** The occurrence of torsion of the testicle in individuals with cryptorchidism has long been appreciated. Scorer (1962) points out that torsion of the testicle can only occur when the mobile testicle is suspended by a kind of mesentery called the mesorchium. The epididymis may be lengthy, and the tunica vaginalis is capacious. Hand (1955) found torsion of the spermatic cord in only 3 of 153 patients, but Smith (1957) found this complication in 5 out of 31 patients with cryptorchidism. Gross (1955) also confirms the increased incidence of torsion of the testicle in cryptorchidism.

**MANAGEMENT OF CRYPTORCHIDISM.** The surgeon who repairs congenital indirect inguinal hernias must be prepared to deal with the undescended testicle.

James (1971) found that 6 percent of males with hernias have associated cryptorchidism. Concerning the problem of cryptorchidism, my personal experience has been largely limited to its occurrence in boys and young men rather than in neonates. It has been necessary to draw upon the experience of other surgeons, urologists, and pediatricians in order to complete this chapter authoritatively.

It has been my experience that cryptorchidism is uniformly associated with the congenital indirect type of hernia. If the hernia has failed to appear (as occurs in some infants), the processus vaginalis is, nevertheless, usually patent. Thus, the surgeon about to perform an orchidopexy is also faced with the problem of hernia repair in the same individual. The repair of a hernia in conjunction with cryptorchidism is obviously more complicated than that of a simple indirect inguinal hernia.

A difference of opinion exists in the literature as to the effectiveness of hormonal therapy in causing descent of the testicle. Part of the confusion arises from a difference in the selection of cases. For instance, an infant with retractile testicles may be described as having undescended testicles; however, this is not, strictly speaking, true. Given a sufficient amount of time, such testes will descend to their normal position. Yet, if such a patient had been given gonadotropic hormones, the good result would have been attributed to the therapy rather than to a natural cause.

Some comment should be made about experimental work performed on macaque monkeys in which Engle (1857) found that descent could be induced by hormones from the anterior pituitary and from pregnancy urine. The results that he obtained cannot be disputed, but application of this information to the treatment of infants and children with cryptorchidism merits discussion. In many individuals with cryptorchidism, it is the abnormal anatomy rather than a hormonal deficiency that prevents testicular descent.

Rajfer and Walsh (1977) have studied hormonal regulation of testicular descent in rats. They concluded that testicular descent is mediated by androgenic hormones regulated by pituitary gonadotropic hormones. As others have indicated, the inguinal canal must be normal. Structural abnormalities in the area can interfere with descent of the testicle into the scrotum.

Gross (1955) and the group at the Children's Hospital in Boston have had extensive experience with cryptorchidism. They feel that hormonal therapy offers little permanent value when true cryptorchidism is present. Excessive stimulation might be followed by testicular atrophy, with discontinuance of treatment. Gross believes that if hormonal therapy is attempted, it should be administered for a short period of time and then discontinued.

According to Clatworthy and colleagues (1957), if the testicle is either ectopic or truly undescended, hormonal therapy cannot penetrate an obstructing dartos fascia, which mechanically obstructs the path of descent. Clatworthy and his coworkers depend upon hormone therapy for only a few patients who have hypoplastic genitalia, bilateral cryptorchidism, and other evidences of hormonal imbalances; they elect to operate when these children are five or six years old (in the preschool period). Benefits of early operation include freedom from psychic trauma to the child, optimal conditions for tubular growth, and cure of the hernia in the preschool period.

Scorer (1962) studied the anatomy of testicular descent with great care and reported his operative findings on 100 cases of undescended testicles. He did not use hormones preoperatively. He felt that the age group from 5 to 14 years was most suitable for operation. Scorer noted that in infants and small children, the operation was difficult and should be delayed if possible. Anatomic findings at operation reported by Scorer are interesting, indeed. In 9 patients, the anatomy was considered to be normal. In such patients, the retractile, or "bashful," testicle would probably have descended by puberty. Such observations form the basis for the recommendation that surgical treatment of undescended testicles be delayed until later childhood. In 42 instances of undescended testicles, Scorer found normal anatomy with completely or partially patent processus vaginalis. Significantly, in these cases he found a fascial barrier or sheet, which was located just below the pubic tubercle and which prevented descent. The severing of this barrier made it possible to bring the testicle into the scrotal position. More serious problems were found in the remaining 49 cases, ten of which revealed such gross anomalies as absence of the testicle or severe abnormalities of the epididymis.

Gross (1955) feels that the optimal age for placement of the testicle into the scrotum was between the ages of 9 and 12 years. At that time, the structures to be dealt with are more easily recognized; and there is less likelihood of operating upon those patients whose testes might have reached the scrotal position without surgical intervention. (I am referring here to the patient with the retractile testicles or active cremasteric reflex.)

Hinman (1955) recommends earlier corrective treatment for cryptorchidism because of the fear that after six years, irreversible damage may occur. He also advocated hormonal therapy initially to determine the possible effect that the onset of puberty might have on the undescended testicle — without waiting for permanent testicular damage to occur. If hormonal therapy fails to bring the testes down, so will puberty; hence, operative correction is advisable.

Clatworthy and coworkers (1957) have discontinued the routine administration of gonadotropic hormones to achieve descent, since such therapy cannot eliminate the congenital hernial sac nor can it alter the obstructing dartos fascial layer found in so many of these cases. They advocate orchidopexy and hernia repair at about five or six years of age. The child is then free to attend school without interruption.

Swenson (1969) feels that the optimal age range for orchidopexy is between 9 and 12 years of age. If a hernia becomes troublesome in an individual with cryptorchidism, he recommends that the hernia be repaired and orchidopexy performed. Swenson does not advise routine use of hormonal therapy, but he feels that hypopituitarism and hypogonadism justify such therapy.

Surgeons agree that in infants in whom the testicle is absent from the scrotum, a correct diagnosis is of paramount importance. The retractile testicle will descend in time. The ectopic testicle can be replaced in the scrotum with relative ease because the cord is of sufficient length. On the other hand, when true cryptorchidism is present, orchidopexy will be necessary in order to place the testicle in the scrotum.

Hormonal therapy is not endorsed with enthusiasm, though some surgeons will administer such therapy on a short-term trial basis. Hormonal therapy is looked upon more favorably when there is evidence of hypogonadism and hypopituitarism.

I have detected a strong trend toward earlier operation for cryptorchidism. Surgeons generally agree that whenever a hernia becomes troublesome in an infant or child with cryptorchidism, the hernia should be repaired and an orchidopexy performed.

Until rather recent times, there were two distinct schools of thought on when orchidopexy should be performed. However, the group that formerly advocated deferring orchidopexy until the age of 9 to 12 years is rapidly losing support. The argument advanced for delay in surgical treatment was that growth and development of the child permitted greater ease in the identification of structures.

Although the ideal time for performance of orchidopexy is unknown, there is a definite trend toward corrective surgery at a much earlier age. It is accepted that the undescended testicle cannot be expected to mature normally. Studies by Robinson and Engle (1954) have shown that after the age of five years, there is a failure in growth of seminiferous tubules in the undescended testicle. In fact, it has been shown by Scorer and Farrington (1971) and by Mengel et al. (1974) that after two years of age, the undescended testicle fails to develop normally. As a result of such observations, correction of cryptorchidism by two years of age is being recommended by an increasing number of surgeons.

## FUNDAMENTAL PRINCIPLES IN ORCHIDOPEXY

Certain historical facts pertaining to the development of the technique of orchidopexy are of interest. Benson and Lotfi (1967) cited certain fundamental principles in performing orchidopexy. These include:

1. Freeing and high ligation of the patent processus vaginalis.
2. Thorough mobilization of the vas, internal spermatic vessels, and venous channels to insure adequate length; thus, the testis may be placed in the scrotum without undue tension, thereby facilitating its viability and function.
3. A technique for maintenance of the testis in its scrotal position, by some temporary method of fixation, until healing occurs.

Bevan in 1899 described an operation for undescended testicle and congenital inguinal hernia. He freed and mobilized the cord structures and testis. He was then able to place the testis in the scrotum without fixation sutures.

Cabot and Nesbit in 1931 introduced the principle of fixation of the testicle in the scrotum by means of a testicular suture placed through the scrotum, attached to a rubber band, and fixed to the thigh with adhesive tape.

To further aid in the effort to achieve adequate length of the cord structures, Davison in 1911 added sectioning of the deep inferior epigastric vessels. This maneuver permitted the internal spermatic vessels to reach the scrotum more directly. The need for greater mobilization in some patients led LaRoque in 1931 and Rosenblatt in 1945 to add retroperitoneal dissection of the cord structures. Gross and Jewett in 1956 recommended extensive retroperitoneal dissection in which the internal spermatic arteries were dissected up to the kidney and the vas dissected down to the bladder.

### Technique of Orchidopexy

There are a number of modifications of the technique of orchidopexy as noted by Benson and Lotfi. Torek's technique (1909) called for fixation of the testis to the fascia of the thigh for up to three months. A second procedure was needed to place the testis in its scrotal position. The procedure lost its popularity because of the high incidence of atrophic testicles. Benson and

Lotfi (1967) also presented a method of fixation, the "pouch technique," in which a space was developed between the skin and dartos muscle low in the scrotal pouch. Regardless of the method chosen for orchidopexy, it must achieve adequate length of the cord structures to permit the testis to reach a scrotal position. Fixation must be of sufficient duration to permit healing.

The technique of orchidopexy that I had formerly used has been well described in the literature. It is essentially the technique described by Bevan but greatly modified and improved by Gross and Jewett. The currently used technique of orchidopexy is illustrated in Figure 10–9, A–G.

It is important to prepare the skin of the abdomen, upper thighs, genitalia, and scrotum with hexachlorophene liquid soap. It is essential that the area described be bathed for ten minutes in order to reduce the bacterial count in the area to a minimum. Drapes are applied, permitting access to the scrotum.

The skin incision is made approximately one or two centimeters above and parallel to the inguinal ligament. The incision is much longer than that through which a hernia is ordinarily repaired. It extends from a position lateral to the internal ring to a point just above and slightly lateral to the pubic tubercle. The incision is enlarged even further laterally, if the testicle is intra-abdominal. Branches of the superficial epigastric and of the superficial external circumflex iliac arteries and veins are clamped with fine-pointed hemostats and ligated with suture material no heavier than number 4–0 (a finer gauge may be used in small infants). The incision is developed through Scarpa's fascia to the aponeurosis of the external oblique muscle.

The opening in the external oblique is made in the direction of the muscle's fibers, commencing at the level of the superior crus. The incision must be made beyond or lateral to the internal ring. The lower leaflet is freed to the shelving edge of Poupart's ligament. The upper or medial leaflet is elevated so that the internal ring can be well visualized. The cord is then easily identified, and it is freed from the floor of the inguinal canal. If the

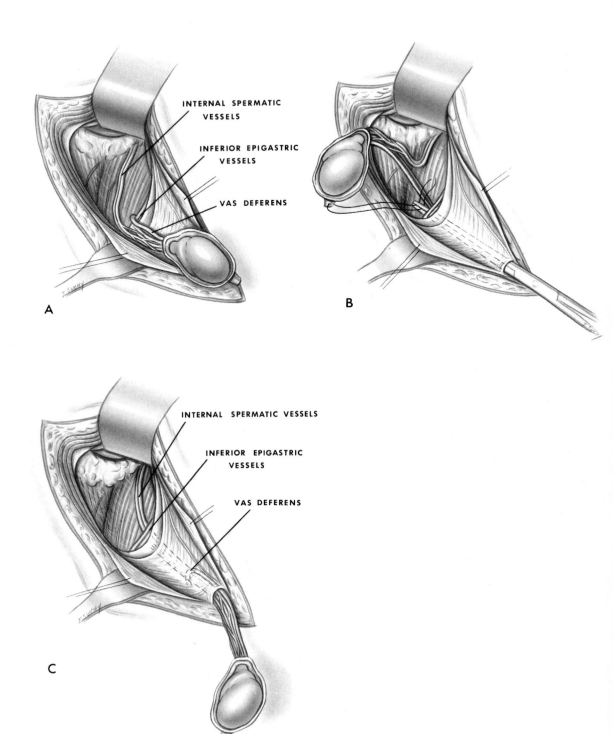

**Figure 10–9,** *A–C.* Access may be gained to the important cord structures by extending the incision laterally to the retroperitoneal space. The cord is delivered through a small incision near the pubic tubercle.

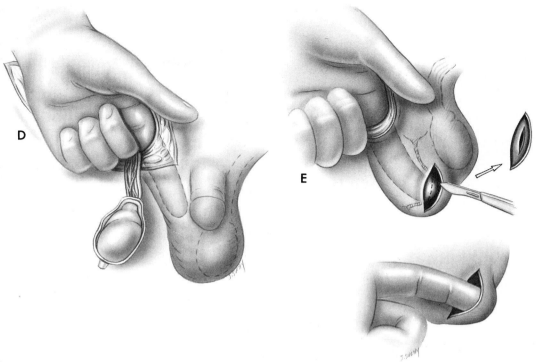

**Figure 10–9,** *D–E.* A scrotal pouch is created by insertion of the index finger firmly into the scrotum (*D*), and then an incision is made through the scrotal septum (*E*).

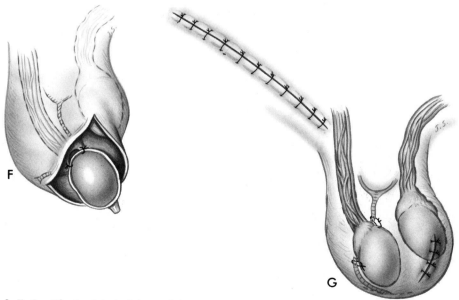

**Figure 10–9,** *F–G.* The testicle is delivered through the scrotum to the new scrotal pouch on the opposite side (*F*). The tunica albuginea is sutured to the surgical defect in the scrotal septum.

testicle is at the internal ring, then, of course, the cord would be absent from its normal position in the canal. The gubernaculum is identified in the canal, dissected free, and divided in its distal or scrotal portion.

I have found the anatomy in cryptorchidism to be variable, but most cases have a number of features in common. Along with the undescended testicle, the processus vaginalis is usually patent; and an indirect inguinal hernial sac is present. The cremaster is often hypertrophied and foreshortened. There is present a certain amount of fibrosis that interferes with mobility of the testicle. It becomes necessary to sacrifice most, if not all, of the cremasteric muscle fibers and connective tissue in order to gain mobility of the cord structures and testicle. It is often necessary to divide a portion of the internal obliques lateral to the internal ring as well as the transversalis fascia in the inguinal floor in order to gain optimal exposure. When careful dissection is completed, the testicle, vas deferens, internal spermatic artery, and branches of the pampiniform plexus of veins remain (Fig. 10–9, A–C). Only after the dissection of all but these essential structures can a respectable degree of mobility of the testicle be gained. At times it may be necessary to carry the dissection, in the retroperitoneal plane, up toward the kidney. It is essential that the amount of traction used is not so great as to compromise the blood flow to the testes when the testicle is replaced in the scrotum.

It may be necessary to divide the deep inferior epigastric artery and vein to permit medial displacement of the internal spermatic artery. This technique was described by Gross and is used in selected cases by a number of surgeons.

Once sufficient length has been achieved, the scrotal pouch is prepared. Digital exploration is performed, and then the fascia is incised to the subcutaneous plane. The scrotum is usually quite small in infants and boys with cryptorchidism; hence, some effort is required to stretch the scrotal sac to an optimal size. The index finger is insinuated into the scrotum through the groin incision, and a small incision is made transversely through a portion of the scrotum in its most dependent part. A pouch is made between the skin and the dartos (Fig. 10–9, D and E).

The testicle is attached to the dartos, care being taken to avoid torsion of the testicle. The testicle is placed in the contralateral scrotal pouch, the scrotal septum having been divided (Fig. 10–9, F and G). The scrotal skin is closed with fine subcuticular absorbable sutures. Currently, the fixation of the testicle in its new location by attaching it to the thigh via a rubber band is used infrequently, and many surgeons think that the procedure is counterproductive. If good position of the testicle is achieved without undue tension, then the hernia is repaired. Care must be taken to avoid twisting the cord during the orchidopexy. It is always essential to close the transversalis fascia from the region of the internal ring to the pubic tubercle. If there is no encroachment in the repair, I then suture the transversus arch to the iliopubic tract and inguinal ligament (as in a Bassini repair).

The external oblique is then closed anterior to the spermatic cord. Subcutaneous tissues are approximated with number 4–0 plain catgut, and the epidermis is approximated with small strips of non-allergenic adhesive tape.

## CLINICAL STUDY

In order to evaluate our experience at the Henry Ford Hospital with congenital inguinal hernias, 255 records of patients with such hernias were available for review. These were randomly selected from the period, 1948 through 1972. The purpose was twofold—to evaluate the effectiveness of treatment and to note any significant changes in our approach.

### Age

Infants and children with hernias are generally seen early in the postpartum period. The first group to be diagnosed includes premature infants as well as others in the immediate postdelivery period, since the physician readily recognizes the defect. The second group is somewhat larger than is generally appreciated. The nurse, parents, or grandparents often report unusual swelling in the groin.

A consistent observation among several authors is that groin hernias present the

Table 10-1. AGE AT TIME OF REPAIR: 255 INFANTS AND CHILDREN WITH GROIN HERNIAS

| Age in Yrs. | No. Patients | Percent |
|---|---|---|
| 0 to 1 | 97 | 38 |
| 1 to 2 | 35 | 14 |
| 2 to 3 | 28 | 11 |
| 3 to 4 | 22 | 8 |
| 4 to 5 | 18 | 7 |
| 5 to 6 | 15 | 6 |
| 6 to 7 | 8 | 3 |
| 7 to 8 | 5 | 2 |
| 8 to 9 | 4 | 2 |
| Above 9 | 23 | 9 |
| Total | 255 | 100 |

greatest problem in neonates. Furthermore, the incidence of such hernias is even greater in small premature infants. Lynn and Johnson (1961) found the age incidence to be less than six months in 37.1 percent of their patients requiring surgical treatment. McLaughlin and Coe (1960) found that 31.6 percent of their infants who required surgery were younger than six months of age. Clatworthy and coworkers (1957) found that almost one-half of 637 infants with inguinal hernias required operative procedures in the first year of life.

This study also showed that congenital hernias are commonly seen as problems in the very young (Table 10-1). Thirty-eight percent of hernias requiring surgical correction were encountered in infants up to one year of age.

## Sex Distribution

There were 225 males with groin hernias (88 percent) and 30 females (12 percent). Statistics from various sources show the incidence of inguinal hernias to be seven to nine times greater in young males than in young females. Gross (1955) reported the sex incidence among 3,874 children to be 90.6 percent male and 9.4 percent female. The incidence in De-Boer's study (1957) of 2,110 cases was 86.3 percent male and 13.7 percent female.

## Clinical Picture

The correct diagnosis of congenital indirect inguinal hernia is ordinarily not difficult. The physician will be the first to recognize the nature of the protrusion, either at birth or during a subsequent visit. The presence of a swelling in the groin is regularly noted for the first time by a parent, grandparent, or nurse. Parents may comment that the bulge can be seen when the baby cries or strains at stool. (The infant's family as a source of important information should not be taken lightly, for parents and grandparents have a vested interest in their offspring.) Other infants will demonstrate the hernia following coughing or sneezing. Infants, not infrequently, will cause the hernia to manifest itself during an asthmatic attack or following a severe respiratory tract infection. Of all the clinical clues to the presence of a hernia in an infant, the mother's account of a groin swelling, which appears following some type of exertion, must be given serious consideration. Once incarceration occurs, pain and irritability become important symptoms. The sudden appearance of a firm, tender mass in the groin will lead to the correct diagnosis of incarcerated hernia, in the great majority of cases. With the onset of colicky pain and vomiting, a strangulating obstruction must be considered. The longer the incarcerated mass persists, the greater the risk of strangulation.

In a number of cases, the complaint will be registered by the parents that the testicle is absent from the scrotum. In such infants, cryptorchidism is the probable diagnosis; and the condition is accompanied with a congenital indirect inguinal hernial sac in almost every instance.

Finally, whenever an infant is seen with other congenital anomalies, the additional diagnosis of hernia should be considered.

On physical examination, the swelling in the groin is ordinarily demonstrable, although in some cases the mass may be absent while the examination is being conducted. Furthermore, the mass may be present during the day and disappear at night. Examination of infants and children is complicated by the fact that these patients cannot cough upon request as do adults, and matters are further complicated because of the small inguinoscrotal area, prohibiting digital exploration by invagination of the skin. Children usually rebel at any attempts at such examinations; hence, they should be avoided. But it is possible, after some experience, to gain an impression of thickening of the cord by an examination of the area from the internal ring to the external ring using one or two fingers. The "silk sign" is helpful, if it can be demonstrated; it is elicited when the two serosal surfaces of the processus vaginalis are rubbed against each other.

Infants and young children can produce a hernia bulge if they react to the surroundings by crying. Older children can be encouraged to jump up and down or to attempt lifting a relatively heavy object. Such measures increase intra-abdominal pressure, thereby causing the hernia to become evident.

Hydroceles must be considered in the differential diagnosis of hernias in infants, since the condition is so common. Hydroceles are not usually tender. They may be quite soft and do not cause distress on palpation. Their configuration will depend upon the effectiveness of the obliteration of the vaginal process, as it occurs in the particular case. The shape of hydroceles is usually somewhat oblong but may be oval or elongated in some infants. Transillumination is a helpful aid in the diagnosis of hydroceles; but thin-walled, intestine containing fluid may at times cause confusion.

The condition and location of the testicles must always be noted. The fact that the testicle may be located high in the scrotum or even in the lower inguinal canal should not contribute to a diagnosis of cryptorchidism. Such testicles may reach the scrotum when the infant relaxes at sleep or in a warm tub bath.

### Operative Experience

Over a 25-year period, a variety of congenital inguinal hernias and associated abnormalities were seen in 255 randomly selected patients (Table 10–2). Of 255 patients, 44 were found to have bilateral indirect inguinal hernias, for an incidence of 17 percent bilaterality. In 211 patients with unilateral hernias, 126 (60 percent) were found on the right side, and 85 (40 percent) were found on the left.

Incarceration was described as being present in 35, or 14 percent, of the total of 255 patients. Unfortunately, details of the exact nature of the incarceration were occasionally missing. For instance, the incarcerated mass was consistently well

**Table 10–2.  CONGENITAL INDIRECT INGUINAL HERNIA: OPERATIVE FINDINGS IN 255 PATIENTS**

| Findings | No. of Patients | Percent |
|---|---|---|
| Congenital indirect inguinal hernia | 255 | 100 |
| Incarceration | 35 | 14 |
| Hydroceles | 47 | 18 |
| Undescended testicles | 15 | 6 |

described in the initial notes, but the subsequent course was not always well documented. Some incarcerations were reduced in the emergency room; others reduced spontaneously after patients were given sedatives or after the onset of anesthesia. (A dosage schedule for premedication is detailed in Chapter 6.) Various techniques were used to achieve reductions — i.e., sedation, warm tub baths, and use of gravity (achieved by lowering the head of the bed). Manual reduction was used, but applied with gentleness and discretion. Excessive pressure was particularly avoided. Operative repair is generally recognized to be safer if the incarcerated mass can be reduced and if surgical treatment can be delayed for a day or two until the child or infant is in a more stable condition. The edema at the site of incarceration will subside, making identification of structures simpler during the operative procedure. On the other hand, if conservative measures fail to achieve reduction, operative correction is necessary. Resection of gangrenous bowel was necessary in only two patients, both of whom survived.

### Anesthesia

General anesthesia was selected for nearly all infants and children. The occasional seriously ill infant is a suitable candidate for local anesthesia.

In the 1940's open drop ether was the anesthetic agent of choice; it was remarkably safe and served its purpose well. A number of agents were later used in combination — such as ether-ethylene, halothane–nitrous oxide, and cyclopropane–nitrous oxide. Spinal anesthesia was infrequently used in young adults.

The anesthesiologist was consulted regarding choice of anesthetic agent in the individual case. In our current practice, the preferred agent for repair of hernias in pediatric patients is ketamine hydrocloride.

### Suture Material

The suture material of choice was silk in over 90 percent of the operations. More surgeons on our staff are using synthetic nonabsorbable sutures. Silk has proven to be a very effective suture material for repair of congenital indirect inguinal hernias.

### Operative Procedures

In this study of 299 operations performed upon 255 patients, it is seen that there is some difference of opinion among the staff members as to the best operative procedure for repair of congenital inguinal hernias (Table 10–3).

At the Henry Ford Hospital, there has been a consistent trend toward the more conservative operative procedure for correction of congenital indirect inguinal hernias in infants and children. We have not, however, employed the technique of repair whereby the congenital sac is identified at the external ring and dissected free from the cord at this vantage point.

In my opinion, it is essential to open the external oblique from the external to the region of the internal ring. As a result of a comparatively small incision, it becomes possible to visualize the anatomic abnormalities clearly. The argument that the external ring is in close proximity to the internal ring in infants only strengthens the position of those of us who prefer to open the external oblique aponeurosis, for only a small incision in this structure

makes optimal exposure possible. Complete dissection of the processus vaginalis at and through the internal abdominal ring is an essential detail. If the internal ring is small, it is not disturbed; if there is moderate enlargement, one or two sutures of numbers 3–0 or 4–0 silk or synthetic nonabsorbable material are used to decrease the size of the ring by approximation of transversalis fascia. More extensive repair of the inguinal floor is infrequently indicated. In two-thirds of the repairs included in this study, the conservative repair of the internal ring—as advocated by Gross (1955), Swenson (1969), Kieswetter (1961), McVay (1965), Lynn (1961), and Benson and coworkers (1962)—was employed. "Potts Procedure" is the term used to denote the repair of indirect inguinal hernias in infants and children by simply performing high ligation of the peritoneal sac at the internal abdominal ring.

In 75 infants and children, the Potts procedure was considered appropriate and was utilized. The peritoneal sac was dissected free through the internal ring, and high ligation achieved. No further reconstruction was necessary.

The Ferguson repair was popular following its enthusiastic introduction by Ferguson of Chicago in 1899. The method has slowly fallen from favor and is now infrequently used. The dissection is similar to that utilized in other methods, and the peritoneal sac is ligated at the internal ring. The internal oblique and transversus abdominis are sutured to the inguinal ligament anterior to the spermatic cord. This method was used to repair congenital indirect inguinal hernias in 36 patients, or in 12 percent of the operations performed on 255 patients.

The Halsted operation in this report refers to the transplantation of the cord to the subcutaneous position—that is, the

Table 10–3.  **OPERATIVE PROCEDURES IN CONGENITAL INDIRECT INGUINAL HERNIAS IN 255 PATIENTS**

| Procedure | No. Operations | Percent |
|---|---|---|
| Closure internal ring with partial repair of floor of inguinal canal | 178 | 60 |
| Potts procedures | 75 | 25 |
| Ferguson repair | 36 | 12 |
| Halsted repair | 10 | 3 |
| Total | 299 | 100 |

spermatic cord comes to lie upon the external oblique aponeurosis. The procedure was utilized in only 10 of 255 patients; thus, it was used in only 3 percent of the patients studied. I believe that the Halsted repair is unnecessarily complicated for use in repair of congenital indirect inguinal hernias, and I do not use the method. I see no reason for removing the cremaster, which usually presents no problem in infants and children. Placing the spermatic cord in the subcutaneous position offers no promise of increase in integrity of the repair.

### Other Procedures

In our experience with congenital hernias, other conditions requiring surgical correction—for example, hydroceles and undescended testicles—are often encountered. Occasionally, the atrophic testicle is in such an unfavorable location that orchidectomy is desirable. Whenever associated anomalies are present, it is prudent to review the possible consequences of abnormal testicular development and descent with the family. The parents should be informed that even if atrophic testicles are delivered into the scrotum, effective spermatogenesis is not to be expected. When bilateral undescended testicles are present, the likelihood of later procreation is remote, if not exactly nonexistent. The cells of Leydig provide a source of androgenic hormones; hence, for this reason, we preserve the testes. Functioning endocrine activity of the cells of Leydig is influential in the development of masculine features (such as the male body habitus, growth of beard, and masculine voice). Statisticians have argued over the exact incidence of malignancy in undescended testes. Some insist that neoplasms develop in undescended testes, while others refuse to recognize any correlation. The results of these arguments have made it possible to take either stand on the matter. Obviously, it is not possible to visualize or easily palpate an intra-abdominal or canalicular testicle; whereas one in a scrotal position can be easily examined. Where the possibility of malignancy developing in a malpositional testicle does exist — no matter how remote — it must be brought to the parents' attention.

I have already reviewed the various opinions as to when orchidopexy should be performed. I advise the family to have the operation completed before the child enters school. Younger children tolerate the procedure remarkably well; however, as the youngster approaches puberty, problems of social adjustment and scholastic performance may arise.

Hydrocelectomy was performed in 47 of 255 patients, for an incidence of 18 percent. Small asymptomatic hydroceles will often disappear spontaneously after a few weeks and should simply be observed. In principle, when dealing with larger hydroceles, no attempt is made to remove the entire sac. When a communicating hydrocele is present (Fig. 10–6, E), the easily accessible anterior portion of the sac is dissected free and partially excised. As a rule, we have found that in the larger persistent hydroceles, a hernial sac is present as well. For this reason, I advocate a groin, rather than scrotal, incision through which the hernia is repaired. The so-called Bottle procedure (in which the sac is everted and sutured about the testicle and spermatic cord) is obsolete. Experience has taught us that more conservative management is effective.

Orchidopexy was performed in 15 (6 percent) of the cases studied. A careful period of observation is essential in some instances to determine the true nature of the problem. Not infrequently, given a period of observation, those testes low in the inguinal canal or upper scrotum will descend on their own; these are the so-called bashful testes and are not examples of cryptorchidism. Operative treatment for this condition is unnecessary. The ectopic testicle is abnormally located but usually has a spermatic cord which permits normal placement of the testicle into the scrotum (Fig. 10–1). Since the undescended testicle is so often accompanied by a patent processus vaginalis, the surgical approach is similar to that used in repair of an inguinal hernia; in addition, a longer incision provides more adequate exposure.

Orchidectomy is, unfortunately, an occasional necessity. In some instances, the atrophic testicle is stubborn in its insistence to remain within the abdomen. In other instances, the testicle resides in a position over the bony pelvis. If it cannot be better positioned, removal is indicated, provided that a normal testicle is present in the opposite side. The possibility of and need for orchidectomy should be discussed with relatives of the patient before proceeding with the operation. Orchidectomy was performed in five patients, and in each instance the pathologist found the testicle to be hypoplastic.

## Complications

### *Mortality*

Repair of a groin hernia and other anomalies of the area in infants and children can be carried out with remarkable safety. There were no deaths in this series of 255 patients.

One infant experienced respiratory arrest but was easily and safely resuscitated. It is my opinion that the danger of anesthetic complications is as great as, if not greater than, the possibility of serious surgical complications following hernia repair in infants and children.

The fact that congenital inguinal hernias can be repaired with uniform success is well documented in the literature. A mortality rate of "zero" has been reported by many surgeons, and one may consult any of the references cited here for confirmation; nevertheless, deaths do occur in infants with complications resulting from strangulation obstruction.

### *Recurrences*

Congenital indirect inguinal hernias are relatively simple to repair, but attendant details are extremely important. There were two recurrences in this series; one at 17 months following a Bassini repair, the other at 24 years following a Ferguson repair. In the first case, there was a failure to achieve snug closure of the internal ring. The cord was left in situ, and the internal ring was not inspected. This would be a technical failure. With reoperation, the small peritoneal sac was thoroughly freed, and high ligation of the peritoneal sac achieved. In addition, repair of the internal ring through snug closure of the transversalis fascia was effective.

The second recurrence was seen 24 years following a Ferguson repair. The hernia recurred as an indirect protrusion, and a Bassini repair was successful. This case would not appear in most series as a recurrence because of the time factor. It did not present until after the operating surgeon had been deceased for several years. Nevertheless, statistics have a relative value that promotes critical analysis and favors progress. A recurrence rate of 0.67 percent is tolerable but can be further improved.

### *Other Complications*

Infants and children tolerate repair of groin hernias remarkably well. They adjust quickly to the result of an operative procedure.

Certain complications, which are common in adults, are almost nonexistent in infants. I have never seen urinary retention in an infant. They experience no difficulty in voiding as a rule. Since there is a rare need for catheterization, urinary tract infection does not follow. Phlebothrombosis and pulmonary embolism must be considered in every aged patient, and especially in those who are immobile. These complications must be exceedingly rare in infants. Infants are inclined to develop respiratory tract infections rather easily. They are exposed to the bacterial flora of other infants and contract infections rather easily. Three infants developed rather severe respiratory tract infections requiring antibiotic therapy and a lengthened period of hospitalization.

Wound complications included seromas in four infants, scrotal swelling in five, and infection in three. The seromas represented minor complications and subsided spontaneously. Scrotal swelling occurred in those infants with large complicated hernias and was treated expectantly. Tub baths, given twice daily after the second postoperative day, were thought to be beneficial.

Atrophic testicles were recognized in two infants, both of whom had undergone orchidopexies. I suspect that this complication is more common than is generally recognized and reported. This observation is made from a clinical experience in which adults are found with atrophic testicles after having had hernias repaired in infancy. Since our patient population is constantly on the move, complete and accurate long-term statistics are difficult to acquire. It might be worthwhile to add that the danger to the testicle is greater when incarceration and strangulation are present. Rowe and Clatworthy (1970) found evidence of vascular compromise to the testicle in 11.76 percent of 68 patients requiring emergency operative reduction of hernias.

Wound infections occurred in 3 of 255 patients with congenital hernias. In one infant the infection was of a minor nature, being confined to the wound margins. The other two infants required drainage and treatment for the infection due to staphylococci. One of these infants had a strangulated hernia requiring small bowel resection.

## SUMMARY

Congenital inguinal hernias in infants and children can be repaired with a mortality rate approaching "zero." Hernias should be repaired when discovered, allowing the time needed for good preoperative preparation. If easily accomplished, reduction of incarcerated hernias is prudent. Elective repair, in the presence of minimal edema and a well-prepared infant, leads to better results.

The actual repair should be directed at high ligation of the patent processus vaginalis. Any additional surgical effort should be directed at an anatomically demonstrated defect.

Concomitant conditions, such as hydroceles and cryptorchidism, should be recognized and treated at the time of hernia repair.

Complications that do occur following hernia repair in infants and children include wound seromas, scrotal swelling, testicular atrophy, and wound infection. Their frequency has been steadily reduced with the improvement of knowledge and technique.

## REFERENCES

Alyea, E. P.: Dislocation of the testes. Surg. Gynecol. Obstet. 49:600, 1929.
Atkinson, P. M.: A follow-up study of surgically treated cryptorchid patients. J. Pediatr. Surg. 10:115, 1975.
Banks, W. M.: Notes on radical cure of hernia. Med. Times Gaz. (London) 2(1777):71, 1884.
Benson, C. D., and Lotfi, M. W.: The pouch technique in the surgical correction of cryptorchidism in infants and children. Surgery 62:967, 1967.
Benson, C. D., Mustard, W. T., Ravitch, M. M., Snyder, W. H., Jr., and Welch, K. H.: Undescended Testes, Pediatric Surgery. Chicago, Year Book Medical Pubs., Inc., 1962, pp. 1041–1061.
Bevan, A. D.: Operation for undescended testicle and congenital inguinal hernia. J.A.M.A. 33:773, 1899.
Browne, D.: Diagnosis of the undescended testicle. Br. Med. J. 2:168, 1938.
Burke, J.: Femoral hernia in childhood. Ann. Surg. 166:287, 1966.
Burton, C. C.: The embryologic development and descent of the testes in relation to congenital hernia. Surg. Gynecol. Obstet. 107:294, 1958.
Cabot, H., and Nesbit, R. M.: Undescended testis. Arch. Surg. 22:850, 1931.
Campbell, H. E.: Incidence of malignant growth of undescended testicle: Critical statistical study. Arch. Surg. 44:353, 1942.
Campbell, H. E.: The incidence of malignant growth of the undescended testicle—A reply and re-evaluation. J. Urol. 81:663, 1959.
Campbell, M.: Undescended testicle and hypospadias. Am. J. Surg. 82:8, 1951.
Carroll, W. A.: Malignancy in cryptorchidism. J. Urol. 61:396, 1949.
Cherry, J. K.: Femoral hernia in children. Am. J. Surg. 106:99, 1963.
Clatworthy, H. W., Jr., and Thompson, A. G.: Incarcerated and strangulated inguinal hernia in infants: A preventable risk. J.A.M.A. 154:123, 1954.
Clatworthy, H. W., Gilbert, M., and Clement, A.: The inguinal hernia, hydrocele and undescended testicle. Problem in infants and children. Postgrad. Med. 22:122, 1957.
Clausen, E. G., Jake, R. J., and Brinkley, F. M.: Contralateral inguinal exploration of hernia in infants and children. Surgery 44:735, 1958.
Coles, J. S.: Operative cure of inguinal hernia in infancy and childhood. Am. J. Surg. 69:366, 1945.
Davison, C.: The surgical treatment of undescended testicle. Surg. Gynecol. Obstet. 12:283, 1911.
DeBoer, A.: Inguinal hernia in infants and children. Arch. Surg. 75:920, 1957.
Engberg, H.: Investigations of the endocrine functions of the testicle in cryptorchidism. Proc. R. Soc. Med. 42:652, 1949.
Engle, J.: Einige Bemerkungen über Langen verhältnisse der Baucheingeweide in Gesur Zustande. Wien Klin. Wochenschr. 39:705, 1857.
Ferguson, A. H.: Oblique inguinal hernia. J.A.M.A. 33:6, 1899.
Fischer, R., and Mumenthaler, A.: Is bilateral herniotomy indicated in unilateral hernia in infants and small children? Helv. Chir. Acta 24:346, 1957.
Fonkalsrud, E. W., deLorimier, A. A., and Clatworthy, H. W.: Femoral and direct inguinal hernias in infants and children. J.A.M.A. 192:597, 1965.
Fosburg, R. G., and Mahin, H. P.: Femoral hernia in children. Am. J. Surg. 109:470, 1965.
Gilbert, M., and Clatworthy, H. W. Jr.: Bilateral operations for inguinal hernia and hydrocele in infancy and childhood. Am. J. Surg. 97:255, 1959.

Gray, S. W., and Skandalakis, J. E.: *Embryology for Surgeons.* Philadelphia, W. B. Saunders Co., 1972.

Gross, R. E.: *The Surgery of Infancy and Childhood.* Philadelphia, W. B. Saunders Co., 1955.

Gross, R. E., and Jewett, T. C., Jr.: Surgical experiences from 1222 operations for undescended testes. J.A.M.A. *160*:634, 1956.

Halsted, W. S.: *Surgical Papers* (Vol. 1). Baltimore, Johns Hopkins Press, 1924.

Hamilton, J. B., and Mossman, H. W.: *Human Embryology* (4th ed.), London, Macmillan Press, Ltd., 1972.

Hand, J. R.: Undescended testes: Report of 153 cases with evaluation of clinical findings — Treatment and Results of follow-up to 33 years. Trans. Am. Assoc. Genitourin. Surg. *47*:9, 1955.

Hertzler, A. E.: Treatment of inguinal hernia in children. J.A.M.A. *61*:1879, 1913.

Herzfeld, G.: The radical cure of hernia in infants and children. Edinb. Med. J. *32*:281, 1925.

Hinman, F., Jr.: Optimum time for orchidopexy in cryptorchidism. Fertil. Steril. *6*:206, 1955.

Immordino, P. A.: Femoral hernia in infancy and childhood. J. Pediatr. Surg. *7*:40, 1972.

Ingall, J. R. F.: Femoral hernia in childhood. Br. J. Surg. *51*:438, 1964.

James, P. M.: The problem of hernia in infants and adolescents. Surg. Clin. North Am. *51*(6):1361, 1971.

Keeley, J. L.: Hernias and related problems in infants and children. Postgrad. Med. *53*:169, 1973.

Kieswetter, W. B.: Hernias — Inguinal and umbilical. Am. J. Surg. *101*:656, 1961.

Kieswetter, W. B., and Parenzan, L.: When should hernia in the infant be treated bilaterally? J.A.M.A. *171*:287, 1959.

Koontz, A. R.: *Hernia.* New York, Appleton-Century-Crofts, 1963.

Koop, C. E.: Inguinal herniorrhaphy in infants and children. Surg. Clin. North Am. *37*:1675, 1957.

LaRoque, G. P.: A modification of Bevan's operation for undescended testicle. Ann. Surg. *94*:314, 1931.

Lynn, H. B.: Hernia, hydrocele and undescended testicle. Am. J. Surg. *107*:486, 1964.

Lynn, H. B., and Johnson, W. W.: Inguinal herniorrhaphy in children. A critical analysis of 1,000 cases. Arch. Surg. *83*:573, 1961.

McLaughlin, C. W., Jr., and Coe, J. D.: Inguinal hernia in pediatric patients. Am. J. Surg. *99*:45, 1960.

McLaughlin, C. W., Jr., and Kleager, C.: The management of inguinal hernia in infancy and childhood. J. Dis. Child. *92*:266, 1956.

McVay, C. B.: Inguinal hernioplasty in infancy: The case against exploration of the contralateral side. In *Current Surgical Management,* Vol. III. Philadelphia, W. B. Saunders Co., 1965, pp. 482–485.

Martin, D. C.: The undescended testis: Evolving concepts in management. Urol. Digest *16*(11):17–31, 1977.

Mengel, W., Hienz, H. A., Sippe, W. G., II, and Hecker, W.: Studies on cryptorchidism: A comparison of histological findings in germative epithelium before and after the second year of life. J. Pediatr. Surg. *9*:445, 1974.

Mestel, A. L., Farber, M. G., and Chabon, I.: Femoral hernia in infancy and childhood. Arch. Surg. *79*:750, 1959.

Morgan, E. H., and Anson, B. J.: Anatomy of region of inguinal hernia. IV. The internal surfaces of the parietal layers. Q. Bull. Northwestern Univ. Med. Sch. *16*:20, 1942.

Mueller, C. B., and Rader, G.: Inguinal hernia in children. Arch. Surg. *73*:595, 1956.

Packard, G. B., and McLauthlin, C. H.: Treatment of inguinal hernia in infancy and childhood. Surg. Gynecol. Obstet. *97*:603, 1953.

Patten, B. M.: *Human Embryology* (3rd ed.). New York, The Blakiston Division of McGraw-Hill Book Co., 1968, p. 490.

Potts, W. J., Riker, W. L., and Lewis, J. E.: Treatment of inguinal hernia in infants and children. Ann. Surg. *132*:556, 1950.

Rajfer, J., and Walsh, P. C.: Hormonal regulation of testicular descent. J. Urol. *118*:985, 1977.

Ravitch, M. M., Snyder, W. H. Jr., and Welch, K. J.: *Pediatric Surgery.* Chicago, Year Book Med Publ, 1962, pp. 573–583.

Rea, C. E.: Histologic character of the undescended testis after puberty. Its significance with reference to the performance of orchidopexy. Arch. Surg. *44*:27, 1942.

Robinson, J. H., and Engle, E. T.: Some observations on the cryptorchid testis. J. Urol. *71*:726, 1954.

Rosenblatt, M. S.: Undescended testicle. Am. J. Surg. *69*:232, 1945.

Rothenberg, R. E., and Barnett, T.: Bilateral herniotomy in infants and children. Surgery *37*:947, 1955.

Rowe, M. I., and Clatworthy, H. W.: Incarcerated and strangulated hernias in children. A statistical study of high risk factors. Arch. Surg. *101*:136, 1970.

Russell, H. R.: The etiology and treatment of hernia in the young. Lancet *2*:1353, 1899.

Russell, H. R.: The inguinal hernia and operative procedure. Surg. Gynecol. Obstet. *41*:605, 1925.

Santulli, T. V., and Shaw, A.: Inguinal hernia: Infancy and childhood. J.A.M.A. *176*:110, 1961.

Scorer, C. G.: The incidence of incomplete descent of the testicle at birth. Arch. Dis. Child. *31*:198, 1956.

Scorer, C. G.: The anatomy of testicular descent, normal and incomplete. Br. J. Surg. *49*:357, 1962.

Scorer, C. G., and Farrington, G. H.: *Congenital Deformities of Testis and Epididymis.* New York, Appleton-Century-Crofts, 1971, pp. 58–74.

Smith, K. H.: Torsion of the spermatic cord. Br. J. Surg. *45*:280, 1957.

Snyder, W. H., Jr., and Greaney, E. M., Jr.: Inguinal hernia. In Benson, C. D., et al.: Undescended Testes, *Pediatric Surgery.* Chicago, Year Book Medical Publ., Inc., 1962, pp. 573–583, 1041–1064.

Sonneland, S. G.: Undescended testicle. Surg. Gynecol. Obstet. *40*:535, 1925.

Sparkman, R. S.: Bilateral exploration in inguinal hernia in juvenile patients. Surgery *51*:393, 1962.

Stewart, B. H.: Surgery of the scrotum and its contents. In Harrison, J. H., et al. (eds.): *Campbell's Urology,* Vol. 3 (4th ed.). Philadelphia. W. B. Saunders Co., 1979, pp. 2473–2498.

Swenson, O.: *Pediatric Surgery* (Vol. 1) (3rd ed.). New York, Appleton-Century-Crofts, 1969, pp. 559–579.

Torek, F.: Technic of orchidopexy. N.Y. J. Med. *90*:948, 1909.

Turner, P.: The radical cure of hernia in children. Proc. R. Soc. Med. *5*:133, 1912.

Wells, L. J.: Descent of the testes: Anatomical and hormonal considerations. Surgery *14*:436, 1943.

Woodburne, R. T.: *Essentials of Human Anatomy* (5th ed.) London, Oxford University Press, 1973, p. 377.

Zimmerman, L. M., and Anson, B. J.: *Anatomy and Surgery of Hernia.* Baltimore, Williams & Wilkins Co., 1967, p. 162.

## Supplemental Readings

Arey, L. B.: *Developmental Anatomy: A Textbook and Laboratory Manual of Embryology* (7th ed.). Philadelphia, W. B. Saunders Co., 1974.

Campbell, H. E.: The incidence of malignant growth of the undescended testicle: A reply and re-evaluation. J. Urol. *81*:663, 1959.

Culp, O. S.: Facts and fancies regarding anomalies of the male genitalia. J. Arkansas Med. Soc. *66*:429, 1970.

Davis, C. E., Jr.: Experiences with the surgical treatment of inguinal hernia in the child. Am. Surg. *135*:879, 1952.

Donovan, E. J., and Stanley-Brown, E. G.: Inguinal hernia in female infants and children. Surg. Gynecol. Obstet. *107*:663, 1958.

Estrin, J.: An improved technique of orchidopexy. Surg. Gynecol. Obstet. *116*:379, 1963.

Farrington, G. H.: Histologic observations in cryptorchidism: The congenital germinal-cell deficiency of the undescended testis. J. Pediatr. Surg. *4*:606, 1969.

Gans, S. L.: Sliding inguinal hernia in female infants. Arch. Surg. *79*:109, 1959.

Gilbert, J. B., and Hamilton, J. B.: Studies in malignant testes tumors — III. Incidence and nature of tumors in ectopic testes. Surg. Gynecol. Obstet. *71*:731, 1940.

Goldstein, I. R., and Potts, W. J.: Inguinal hernia in female infants and children. Ann. Surg. *148*:819, 1958.

Griscom, N. T., Cochran, W. C., Harris, G. B. C., Easterday, C. B. Umansky, I., and Frigoletto, F. D.: The processus vaginalis of the third trimester fetus with comments on inguinal hernia in childhood. Radiology *96*:107, 1970.

Hamilton, J. B., and Hubert, G.: Differential congenital hernias. Diagnosis of pseudocryptorchidism and true cryptorchidism. Endocrinology *21*:644, 1937.

Hartman, S. W., and Greaney, E. M., Jr.: Technique of orchidopexy. Surg. Gynecol. Obstet. *116*:629, 1963.

Healey, J. E.: *A Synopsis of Clinical Anatomy.* Philadelphia, W. B. Saunders Co., 1969.

Hollingshead, W. H.: *Textbook of Anatomy* (3rd ed.). New York, Harper & Row, 1974.

Hunter, R. H.: The etiology of congenital inguinal hernia and abnormally placed testes. Br. J. Surg. *14*:125, 1926.

Kieswetter, W. B.: Early surgical correction of inguinal hernia in infancy and childhood. Am. J. Dis. Child *96*:362, 1958.

Kieswetter, W. B.: Undescended testes. W. Va. Med. J. *52*:235, 1956.

Laufer, A., and Eyal, Z.: Contralateral inguinal exploration in child with unilateral hernia. Arch. Surg. *85*:521, 1962.

Lipschultz, L. I., et al.: Testicular function after orchidopexy for unilaterally undescended testis. N. Engl. J. Med. *295*:15, 1976.

Martin, D. C., and Menck, H. R.: The undescended testis: Management after puberty. J. Urol. *114*:77, 1975.

McVay, C. B.: Inguinal hernia in children (discussion). Arch. Surg. *73*:595, 1956.

Miller, A., and Seljelik, R.: Histopathologic classification and natural history of malignant testis tumors in Norway, 1959–1963. Cancer *28*:1054, 1971.

Minton, J. P., and Clatworthy, H. W., Jr.: Incidence of patency of the processus vaginalis: A study based on six hundred bilateral operations for inguinal hernia. Ohio Med. J. *57*:530, 1961.

Nyhus, L. M., and Harkins, H. N.: *Hernia.* Philadelphia, J. B. Lippincott Co., 1964, pp. 73–96.

Potts, W. J.: Should both inguinal canals be explored in a child with inguinal hernia? Med. Forum Mod. Med. *25*:36, 1959.

Schuster, S. R.: Recognition and management of inguinal hernia in infants and children. Q. Rev. Pediatr. *12*:201, 1957.

Snyder, W. H., Jr., and Chaffin, L.: Surgical management of undescended testes. J.A.M.A. *157*:129, 1955.

Walsh, P. C., et al.: Plasma androgen response to HCG stimulation in prepubertal boys with hypospadias and cryptorchidism. J. Clin. Endocrinol. Metab. *42*:52, 1976.

Wells, L. J.: Misconception of the gubernaculum testis. Surgery *22*:502, 1947.

White, J. J., Haller, J. A., and Dorst, J. P.: Congenital inguinal hernia and inguinal herniography. Surg. Clin. North Am. *50*(4):823, 1970.

Wyndham, N. R.: A morphological study of testicular descent. J. Anat. *77*:179, 1943.

Young, H. H.: Radical cure of hydrocele by excision of serous layer of sac. Surg. Gynecol. Obstet.

# 11

# Indirect Inguinal Hernia

*From the vantage point of 1933, it seems strange that progress was not more rapid (following Bassini's contributions). The obvious principle to be followed, complete sac extirpation and suture of the canal were not grasped at once, and even after they had been enunciated by Billroth, they were not followed even in his own clinic. Time was wasted on such frivolities as transplanting the sac (Kocher) or rolling it up to make a cork for the canal (Macewen).*

*E. Andrews (1935)*

## INTRODUCTION

This chapter will largely concern the indirect inguinal hernia as it appears in the adult. The preceding chapter dealt almost entirely with indirect inguinal hernia as it develops from the patent processus vaginalis; such hernias are repaired with a high degree of success by high ligation of the peritoneal sac after it has been carefully and thoroughly freed from the abdominal wall. Other types of indirect inguinal hernias will be considered in detail in Chapter 18, Sliding Inguinal and Femoral Hernias.

While it is true that most inguinal hernias are congenital in origin, it is becoming evident that not all indirect inguinal hernias are alike; and there is a variety of indirect inguinal hernia, appearing later in life, that is acquired in nature. Such indirect inguinal hernias may be compared to direct inguinal hernias in their pathogenesis. With increasing frequency, the congenital or saccular theory is being challenged as the sole explanation for groin hernias. Conner and Peacock (1973) speculated that factors other than a congenital sac accounted for some

indirect inguinal hernias that appear later in life—strongly suggesting that changes occurred in the supporting connnective tissue. Lichtenstein and Shore (1976) made similar observations regarding the adult variety of indirect inguinal hernias. The electromyographic findings recorded by Tobin and coworkers (1976) support the hypothesis that paralysis of inferior fibers of the transversus abdominis muscle occurred following appendectomy and may have contributed to the development of an inguinal hernia.

A diligent and thorough search of the medical literature on the subject of hernia indicated that worthwhile contributions have been made by many surgeons—some, performing in great institutions; others, laboring in small hospitals with extraordinary perception. At this point, we will consider matters of historic interest as they apply to indirect inguinal hernias.

## HISTORY

Marcy is recognized by some surgeons as an early contributor to the proper man-

155

agement of the internal abdominal ring in the repair of inguinal hernias. In 1871, he described a repair as follows: "The sac, unopened was pushed up with its contents into the abdominal cavity, and two stitches of catgut were taken through the walls of the ring." In 1881, he referred to a procedure in which he would "refresh the pillars of the ring or walls of the opening and close by sutures." In 1887, he again described his technique in which "stitches were placed at distances of about one-third of an inch to include both pillars of the ring" in order to close the ring securely.

There can be little doubt among scholars of hernia repair that the modern era of surgical treatment of hernia began with the work of Bassini. While it is true that other surgeons have made important observations and enduring contributions, it was Bassini who set a new standard of performance in hernia repair. As noted by Talbott in his biographic sketch (1970) of the surgeon, Bassini, besides completing his surgical education, continued postgraduate training under Billroth, Langenbeck, and Nussbaum and later occupied the chair of surgical pathology at Padua. Bassini recognized the significance of Lister's work and the need to control postoperative infection. He personally visited Lister and directly observed his monumental contributions toward the control of infection.

Before Bassini presented his experiences in 1887, Wood had reported a recurrence rate of 27 percent in 1886. In 1890, Bull reported a staggering recurrence rate of 36 percent, while Bassini, using an improved technique, reported a recurrence rate of 2.8 percent. Allowing for criticism on the grounds of inaccurate and short-term follow-up study of these cases, the results achieved by Bassini were still remarkable at that time in the development of the art of surgery for repair of inguinal hernias. I agree with Andrews (1935), Seelig and Chouke (1923), Pitzman (1921), Mahorner and Goss (1962), and Zimmerman and Anson (1967) that the modern operation for inguinal hernia begins with Bassini. He was the first to conceive and deliberately execute a planned procedure for repair of inguinal hernias.

Halsted was also a contemporary student of the problem of inguinal hernia repair and made a number of significant contributions concurrently with Bassini. Halsted, of course, worked completely independently; however, his contributions did in many ways parallel those of Bassini.

Bassini's indoctrination in the antiseptic method of surgery by Lister and his excellent knowledge in anatomy equipped him well for the repair of inguinal hernias. As described in 1887, Bassini's objective was to create a canal with two openings — i.e., the internal and external abdominal rings and two walls. The anterior wall was made up of the external oblique, while the posterior wall consisted of transversalis fascia (the vertical fascia of Cooper), the transversus abdominis, and the internal oblique. Bassini also had the courage and wisdom to open the peritoneal sac; in addition, he achieved high ligation of the sac. Most surgeons, prior to Bassini's time, were loath to open the peritoneal sac for fear of peritonitis; hence, they were content to ligate the sac with or without torsion. Such ligation was usually performed at the external inguinal abdominal ring. The opening of the peritoneal sac was a considerable advance. In addition, Bassini's use of silk to serve in place of various absorbable sutures was another noteworthy improvement in technique. Finally, he moved the spermatic cord laterally, closing the structures noted previously at the internal ring. Bassini's reported recurrence rate was 2.8 percent. Obviously, his reports were received with great enthusiasm, and Padua became a mecca for herniologists, in particular, and for surgeons, in general. Little wonder that Bassini's contributions were received so enthusiastically, for at long last one surgeon had devised a well-planned operative procedure for the correction of inguinal hernias — a problem that plagued mankind for centuries.

Following Bassini's report, initial reports from surgeons in other countries were equally encouraging. Judd (1911) reported a recurrence rate of 2.5 percent. Bull and Coley obtained more impressive results; their recurrence rate was only 0.8 percent prior to 1910, according to Andrews (1935).

However, as statistics on recurrence rates became more generally available, it soon became apparent that results were not as encouraging as earlier observers thought.

With indiscriminate and technically imperfect applications of the Bassini repair to both direct and indirect inguinal hernias, observation and long-term follow-up statistics led to the realization of the fact that the problem of groin hernias had not yet been conquered. The fact that excellent results had been obtained in infants and children was established early.

Taylor in 1920 found the recurrence rate to be 10.9 percent, while Erdman in 1923 reported an incidence of 7.5 percent. Such rates of recurrence were recognized as being too prevalent; a re-examination of anatomic knowledge and reassessment of surgical technique followed. Thoughtful surgeons were disturbed at results that were less than gratifying.

Following Bassini's report, other surgeons continued to study their results. The initial response was generally one of acceptance, but then came a period of re-evaluation. By 1924, Andrews cited several references that reported a recurrence rate ranging from 9 to nearly 11 percent following inguinal hernia repair. He acknowledged a very low recurrence rate in children; a figure of less than 1 percent was commonly reported. Upon recognition of the fact that the technique of hernia repair had not yet been perfected, interest in the subject became rekindled. Surgeons were aware that a hernia in an infant with a congenitally patent processus vaginalis was quite a different problem from a direct hernia in an adult or aged patient.

In 1924 Edmund Andrews, in a significant paper, stressed the importance of the endoabdominal (transversalis) fascia in hernia repair. He also pointed out that use of the internal oblique muscle in hernia repair was ill-conceived; thus, Andrews utilized only "white fascia" (aponeurosis) in his repairs. He deplored the use of red muscle (internal oblique) in hernia repair, noting that this maneuver would have an adverse effect on the sphincteric action at the internal ring. With clarity, Andrews illustrated his method of closure of the transversalis fascia at the internal ring.

Surgeons in divers places were frustrated at their results, and they looked at the matter of hernia repair critically. Connell of Oshkosh, Wisconsin, directed attention to the important technique of repair of the internal ring in 1908 and 1928. He recognized both the importance of the internal abdominal ring and the need for precise closure of the transversalis layer beneath the spermatic cord. His illustrations are clear and support the written description that, in fact, the transversalis fascial layer is closed snugly at the internal ring. Truly, "his was one voice in the wilderness," for the validity of his views was slowly accepted. The principle of separate closure of the transversus abdominis aponeurosis at the internal ring—i.e., the upper leaflet (transversus arch) is sutured accurately to the lower leaflet (iliopubic tract)—was slowly becoming established.

Pitzman in 1921 described what he called a fundamentally new technique for herniorrhaphy. He opposed suturing internal oblique and transversus abdominis muscles to Poupart's ligament, because this practice resulted in destruction of a certain amount of muscle tissue. His technique included high ligation of the peritoneal sac and suture of the transversalis aponeurosis and fascia down to the inguinal ligament. It was evident from the illustrations that in this method, the lower leaflet of transversalis fascia was included in the closure.

Being disenchanted with current methods of repair, Seelig and Chouke took one aspect of the problem to the laboratory in 1923. They concluded that normal muscle would not unite firmly with fascia or ligament. This concept was later disputed by Koontz (1956).

In 1925 Russell argued convincingly that those hernias of saccular origin could be cured by removal of the hernial sac. He insisted that oblique (indirect) inguinal hernias were always saccular and were never due to muscular weakness. He felt that high ligation of the sac was sufficient for repair of indirect inguinal hernias; this concept was unquestioned and widely accepted for years.

The origin and nature of hernia remained unsolved in 1923, when Sir Arthur Keith added a provocative concept through his identification of an "inguinal shutter." The internal oblique and transversus abdominis muscles approach the inguinal ligament upon contraction, thus, closing the inguinal gap. This fact is given as an additional reason for avoidance of suturing the internal oblique muscle to the inguinal ligament. According to Keith, the "shutter mechanism" should be preserved.

MacGregor in 1930 cautioned against transplantation of the internal oblique muscle since sutures placed through it would interfere with the valvelike closing action of this muscle.

Lytle contributed substantially toward a better appreciation of the importance of the internal abdominal ring, which he described at length in 1945. In 1970, he noted that a patent processus vaginalis was not the only cause of oblique hernia. Although removal of the sac with high ligation of the peritoneal ring was curative in infants, this procedure did not yield similar results in adults. Lytle spoke of the lateral and medial pillars of the internal abdominal ring. Both are derivatives of the transversus abdominis muscle. Closure of these structures is of importance in repair of indirect inguinal hernias seen in adults. Lytle pointed out that suture of the internal oblique muscle to the inguinal ligament was unsatisfactory and stressed the need for closure of the transversalis fascia.

Griffith in 1959 thoroughly reviewed the anatomy of the internal abdominal ring. He noted that the inguinal ligament and the internal oblique and transversus abdominal muscles do not enter into the defect at the internal ring, nor does the cremasteric muscle. Griffith emphasized that the actual defect exists in the transversus abdominis lamina with the peritoneal sac prolapsing through the defect. He felt that the cremaster muscle obstructed the view of the internal ring and that insufficient attention had been given to this important detail. Following excision of the cremaster and dissection and high ligation of the peritoneal sac, Griffith carefully closed the internal ring.

Madden and coworkers reviewed the pathologic anatomy and repair of inguinal hernias in 1971. These authors presented their views on the anatomy of the groin, and their respect for the transversus abdominis and its derivatives is clearly evident. The transversus abdominis layer is identified and precisely closed at the internal ring and through the remaining floor of Hesselbach's triangle.

The knowledge needed for proper repair

of indirect inguinal hernias in the adult evolved slowly. Clinical surgeons recognized that even though the Bassini repair had merit, it also had its limitations in certain situations. Through the efforts of Torek (1906), Connell (1908), Bates (1913), Pitzman (1921), Seelig (1923), and Andrews (1924), the need for accurate closure of the internal ring was recognized. The particularly important detail is accurate and snug closure of the transversus abdominis lamina at the internal ring. Triangulation of the transversalis fascia at the internal ring is a technical detail that contributes to achieving this end.

In England, Lytle in his article of 1945 noted that Colwell (1927), Ogilvie (1929), Turner (1933), Henry (1937) and Edwards (1943) all identified the need for closure of the internal abdominal ring.

Following Bassini's report, a number of procedures were advocated for repair of hernias. Surgeons were variously preoccupied with the hernial sac, the cord, with the "red muscle," the "shutter mechanism," the external oblique, the "conjoined tendon," and the transversalis fascia. Each enthusiast felt that he had the ultimate and simplest solution to the problem. Slowly, surgeons and anatomists began to identify the significant pathology of indirect inguinal hernias. They recognized fundamental differences between congenital and acquired hernias, as well as between direct and indirect inguinal hernias, and ultimately they perceived that all hernias protruded through the transversalis fascia. The anatomy of the groin underwent intense investigation, and important anatomic details were ferreted out by McVay and Anson. The pathology of congenital indirect inguinal hernias was finally understood. The existence of the patent processus vaginalis as a precedent to indirect inguinal hernias was appreciated. The fact that certain indirect inguinal hernias of adult onset are different from the simple congenital hernia is currently gaining recognition.

## OBSOLETE, OBSOLESCENT, AND CURRENT TECHNIQUES IN HERNIA REPAIR

To briefly note the current status of certain procedures once used in repair of hernias, I have listed certain techniques as obsolete, obsolescent, and current.

## Obsolete Techniques Once Advocated for Hernia Repair

Without going into discussion, the following techniques can now be considered obsolete in the repair of hernias:

Techniques that routinely sacrifice the testicle.

Techniques that ligate the peritoneal sac at the external ring.

Techniques that do not require opening the external oblique aponeurosis, especially in adults.

Techniques that require transplantation of the ligated stump of the peritoneal sac.

Techniques that use periosteal flaps or bone transplants.

Techniques that use muscle tissue as plastic repair.

Techniques that use cutis grafts and skin grafts.

## Obsolescent Techniques in Hernia Repair

A number of methods were once applied enthusiastically to hernia repair; however, with the passage of time, they have more or less fallen into disfavor. For example, fascia lata is almost completely replaced by synthetic materials that are universally available. Considered in this category are the following:

Techniques that utilize fascia lata.

Techniques that utilize fascial strips.

Techniques in which the cord is skeletonized.

Techniques that require division of the spermatic cord.

Use of catgut as the suture of strength in repair of hernias.

## Current Techniques Useful in Hernia Repair

A number of technical details have proved to be of great value in repair of groin hernias. These details have evolved slowly—largely through trial and error and repeated observations. They include the following:

Opening of the external oblique aponeurosis.

Dissection of the peritoneal sac to achieve freedom of peritoneum from the abdominal wall, permitting high ligation of the sac.

High ligation of the peritoneal sac.

Use of Hoguet maneuver in direct and femoral hernias.

Accurate identification and closure of the transversus abdominis lamina at the internal abdominal ring.

Triangulation of the transversus abdominis aponeurosis as a technical maneuver to permit precise and snug closure of internal ring.

Approximation of transversus abdominis arch to the iliopubic tract or femoral sheath (both are derivatives of the transversalis fascia).

Employment of the principle of multilayered closure.

Use of the relaxing incision.

Use of the transversus arch (not internal oblique muscle) in repair of the floor of Hesselbach's triangle.

Use of polypropylene (Marlex) mesh in appropriate cases, such as direct, recurrent inguinal or femoral hernias.

Use of Cooper's ligament in selected direct inguinal hernias, recurrent or femoral hernias.

Use of the preperitoneal approach in hernia repair.

## TECHNIQUE FOR REPAIR OF INDIRECT INGUINAL HERNIAS IN ADULTS

In my experience, I found that the simplest type of hernia to repair is the indirect inguinal hernia. This is particularly true when the hernia is of the congenital variety in a young individual; however, repair may not be difficult even when the hernia is quite large, and has been present for many years in an adult. Sliding hernias are not difficult to repair if important technical details are meticulously carried out (Chapter 18, Sliding Inguinal and Femoral Hernias). Certain principles are important and must be followed if success is to be achieved in nearly every instance. The description of the procedure that follows here will be directed largely toward the adult or elderly patient with an indirect inguinal hernia of moderate or large size. Fundamentally, the sac must be dissected free of the abdominal wall, high ligation of the preperitoneal sac achieved, and the floor of the inguinal canal must be repaired as needed.

Consideration must be given to the placement of the skin incision, since the patient's judgment of the surgeon's competency may be based on the surgeon's trademark, the healed incision. And, following the apprehension, trauma, and inconvenience associated with an operative procedure, the patient's evaluation of his operation may be more discriminating than usual. The skin incision is made approximately two centimeters above the inguinal ligament and parallel to Langer's lines (Fig. 11–1). It is good practice to mark the direction of the incision with the scalpel before actually incising the skin to assure correct placement of the incision. Smaller marks are made at right angles to the incision; these will serve as landmarks when the wound is being closed after the operation is completed. The dissection is carried out sharply and quickly through the fascial layers of Camper and Scarpa. Such an incision provides excellent exposure and heals with minimal scarring, if the subcutaneous tissue and fascial layers have been accurately approximated. If the

hernia is recurrent, then it is good practice to excise the old cicatrix when possible. Disfiguring postoperative scars suggest the possibility of an indifferent attitude on the part of the surgeon.

All blood vessels are clamped with fine forceps and tied with ligatures of fine silk. I have no strong opinions about the type of suture material used, provided that it has the necessary immediate strength and long-term holding power. The superficial external circumflex and the superficial epigastric and superficial external pudendal arteries and veins are frequently encountered and must be individually ligated. (Figure 2–2 in Chapter 2, page 19, shows the anatomy.) The incision is developed to the depth of the external oblique aponeurosis. I do not dissect off every vestige of areolar tissue at this point, since small vessels provide nourishment to this structure. The dissection is carried medially to the external ring so that the crura and the ring are easily recognizable. The ilioinguinal nerve can and should be identified at the external ring at this point. The dissection is carried inferiorly until the shelving border of the inguinal ligament is identified. Laterally, the dissection is carried out to a point just beyond the internal ring.

The external oblique fascia is opened at the level of the superior crus, care being taken to avoid injury to the ilioinguinal nerve (Fig. 11–2). The external oblique is dissected off the internal oblique to the degree dictated by the situation. For instance, if the patient is an infant, minimal dissection is indicated. On the other hand, in an aged adult with a large hernia and obvious weakness in the floor of Hesselbach's triangle, I elevate the superior leaflet of the external oblique as far upwardly and medially as possible, so that a relaxing incision can be made in the anterior sheath of the rectus muscle in selected cases. The iliohypogastric nerve becomes visible at this time and is easily safeguarded.

The inferior leaflet of the external oblique is dissected with a Küttner dissector until the shelving edge of Poupart's ligament is identified from the pubic tubercle to a point lateral to the internal or abdominal ring. An important technical point frequently overlooked at this stage of the

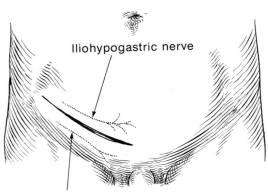

Iliohypogastric nerve

Ilioinguinal nerve

**Figure 11–1.** The skin incision is made approximately two centimeters above the inguinal ligament in a gentle curve following Langer's lines.

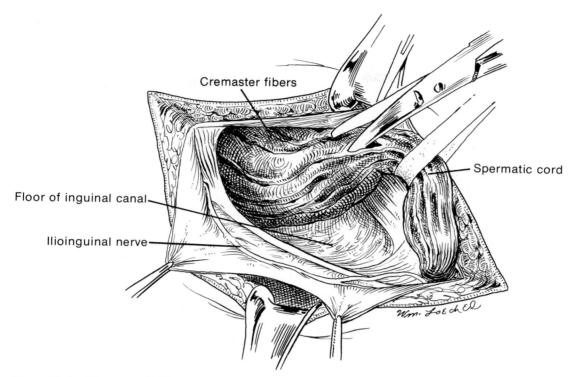

Cremaster fibers

Spermatic cord

Floor of inguinal canal

Ilioinguinal nerve

Wm. Loechel

**Figure 11–2.** The external oblique aponeurosis has been opened. The cord is freed from the inguinal floor. The freed ilioinguinal nerve is seen overlying the retracted lower leaflet of the external oblique aponeurosis. The cremaster muscle is being dissected free of the cord.

operation is the need for accurate demonstration of the reflected inguinal ligament. This applies to large hernias in adults and not to the congenital variety of hernia seen in an infant or child. Visualization of the reflected inguinal ligament makes mobilization of the complete cord together with the cremaster muscle a relatively simple matter. Traction on the cord should be minimal; and the cord structures, including the internal spermatic artery and the vas deferens should be protected from injury.

In large, long-standing indirect inguinal hernias in adults, the cremaster muscle is hypertrophied, and the cord with all its elements is often unwieldy and sausage-like. In such situations, I have found no harm, but several benefits, resulting from removal of at least a portion of the cremasteric muscle and fascia. The cremasteric muscle, however, should not be wantonly sacrificed, since it plays a role in maintaining the testicle in an acceptable position. Testicles deprived of all cremaster muscle may ride so low in the scrotum as

to be embarrassing or uncomfortable, or both. The ilioinguinal nerve is seen on the cord, dissected off, and preserved. The object is to remove only the thickened and troublesome cremasteric muscle from the internal ring to a point approximately two centimeters from the pubic tubercle. In this limited but important excision, it is not necessary to mobilize the testicle out of the scrotum unless other circumstances dictate the need for such a maneuver. It might be necessary to manage a coexistent hydrocele, or perform a biopsy if a suspicious lesion had been palpated on physical examination. If dissection of the cremaster is not carried out too far toward the scrotum, there is less danger of damaging the collateral circulation to the area. Any lipoma of the cord or preperitoneal protrusion of fat presenting at the internal ring is removed. A large lipoma of the cord significantly interferes with closure of the transversalis fascia, and removal is essential. These maneuvers are designed to reduce the mass of contents that could travel through the abdominal wall at the internal ring. Furthermore, the transversalis fascia is more accurately identified, and more precise closure of the internal ring is achieved. It is impossible to overemphasize the importance of this step in the repair of the indirect inguinal hernia, be it congenital or acquired. After the cremaster has been dissected off the cord, it is clamped proximally at the internal ring and distally near the pubic tubercle. Fine silk ligatures are used to ensure hemostasis. The external spermatic artery is easily identified and may be preserved, although its sacrifice has resulted in no problems in many patients. The genitofemoral nerve is also seen at this stage in the operation and preserved. No significant disturbances occur whenever the nerve is sacrificed, except for temporary anesthesia at the base of the scrotum.

The peritoneal sac is easily identified at the anterior, superior, and medial aspects of the spermatic cord (Fig. 11–3). The position is, of course, lateral to the deep inferior epigastric artery and vein. The upper portion of the sac is carefully incised, then meticulously explored. Intraoperative digital exploration should be carried out systematically to not only rule out the presence of a coexisting hernia, but also note any significant weakness in the abdominal wall that, when recognized, can be corrected so that actual herniation will not develop in the future. This detail is insufficiently emphasized in the literature on the subject of hernia repair. The index finger is first inserted through the opened sac. By sweeping the finger around the margins of the operative field from within, the deep inferior epigastric artery, the margin of the rectus sheath, Cooper's ligament, the region of the femoral ring, and the femoral artery are all identified. Any weakness is noted. Further digital exploration should be performed by palpating the area with the finger inserted between the peritoneum and the transversalis fascia. Using this technique, aponeuroticofascial weaknesses are further

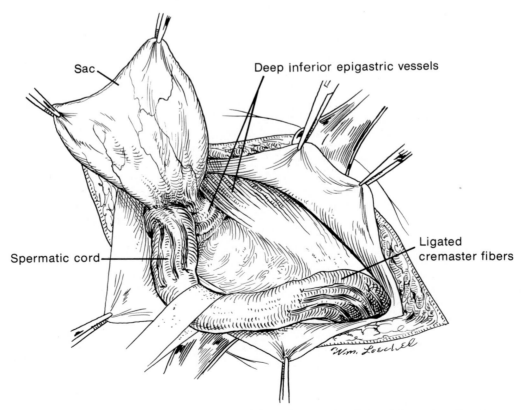

Sac

Deep inferior epigastric vessels

Spermatic cord

Ligated cremaster fibers

**Figure 11–3.** The peritoneal sac must be dissected free of the cord and the abdominal wall at the internal abdominal ring.

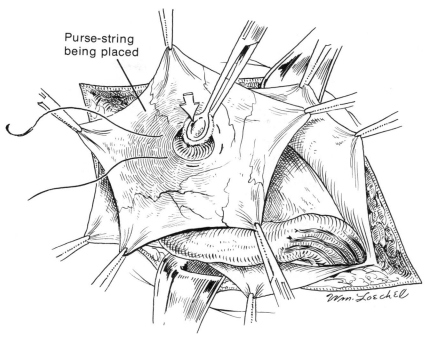

Purse-string
being placed

Wm. Loechel

**Figure 11–4.** The technical detail of high ligation of the sac is important in an orderly repair. The peritoneum must be freed of omentum, and adherent viscera must be detached. Appendices epiploicae or omentum must not be caught in the closure.

identified. The sac is completely freed of any adherent viscus as well as the abdominal wall, which permits high ligation of the peritoneal sac. Omentum and small intestine are most frequently adherent to indirect inguinal hernia sacs. A purse-string suture of heavy or number 2–0 silk or a nonabsorbable synthetic suture is used to achieve peritoneal closure (Fig. 11–4). The object is to achieve accurate closure of the peritoneum. Other methods of closure may be used with equal success. The suture is placed deep to any thickening in the peritoneal sac that might be present in long-standing hernial protrusions.

Repair is continued by closure of the transversalis fascia at the internal ring. At this point, the deep inferior epigastric artery is identified as it lies under the transversalis fascia. The transversalis fascia is grasped with a hemostat at this location. The maneuver, which I call triangulation of the transversalis fascia at the internal ring, is performed (Fig. 11–5). It is significant because accurate identification of both the internal ring and transversalis fascia is necessary, in this area of

critical importance, if repair is to be effective and safe. The second hemostat is placed on the transversalis fascia near the inguinal ligament at a point that is to become the newly fashioned internal ring. The third hemostat is placed on the transversalis fascia just above the cord. The internal oblique muscle is elevated with a small retractor, permitting identification of the superior leaflet of the transversalis fascia. The closure of the internal ring is now accomplished by bringing the transversalis fascia held in the two lateral hemostats together and suturing the fascia with medium or number 3–0 silk. For accuracy and safety, the suture nearest the cord is placed first. Since the cord and structures to be sutured are directly visualized, there is no possibility of including important cord structures in the line of suture. Usually three or four sutures of medium silk are sufficient to close the internal ring effectively. The aperture barely admits the tip of the index finger after closure and measures approximately one centimeter. Over a period of years, I have tended to close the ring more snugly. A hemostat may be placed into the

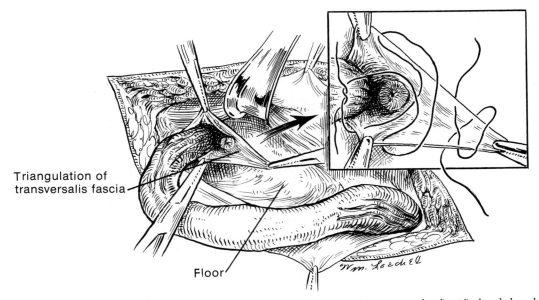

Triangulation of
transversalis fascia —

Floor

**Figure 11–5.** The components of the transversus abdominis lamina must be accurately identified and closed at the internal ring. Triangulation of the transversalis fascia (shown here) is a useful detail to help achieve accurate closure at the internal ring.

aperture and slightly opened to further test the accuracy of closure of the internal ring. Certainly, the aperture at the internal ring should not be so large as to admit the entire index finger. Obviously, the size of the deep ring should be tailored to the need of the individual patient, and the surgeon must retain the right to make a judgment as to the proper size.

Any weakness in the transversalis in the floor of Hesselbach's triangle is eliminated by the imbrication technique. When the indication for operation originally was the presence of an indirect inguinal hernia, a coexistent direct inguinal or a femoral hernia should not be overlooked.

Placement of the next row of sutures is not as simple as it might appear to be (Fig. 11–6). I would emphasize that it is not the internal oblique muscle that is sutured to the inguinal ligament. In fact, the internal oblique muscle is actually retracted out of the line of suture. Nor is it tendon, by strict definition, that is approximated to Poupart's ligament. The needle in its course through the abdominal lamina includes some musculoaponeurotic fibers derived from the internal oblique, the transversus abdominis, and the transversalis fascia above and the iliopubic tract and inguinal ligament below (Fig. 11–6). The integrity of the transversus abdominis lamina is

preserved with minimal tension upon the site of repair. Repair is achieved by approximating these layers with interrupted sutures of heavy or number 2–0 synthetic nonabsorbable sutures placed at intervals of one centimeter from the pubic tubercle to the internal ring. To reiterate, sutures are not placed into the internal oblique muscle, since preservation of the shutter mechanism would thereby be sacrificed.

A relaxing incision is made if the tension on the suture line is considered excessive. It is unnecessary to incise the rectus sheath when repairing a congenital indirect inguinal hernia.

One additional advantage of repairing hernias under local anesthesia is that the degree of tension on the repair may be accurately observed. Furthermore, the patient may be asked to cough, after repair, thus testing the adequacy of repair. If improperly placed or if inserted under undue tension, the suture may be seen to give way under the force of an explosive cough. Seeing the sudden failure of a suture for the first time is a most impressive experience for the young surgeon, and, as a result, the need for proper placement of sutures becomes painfully clear.

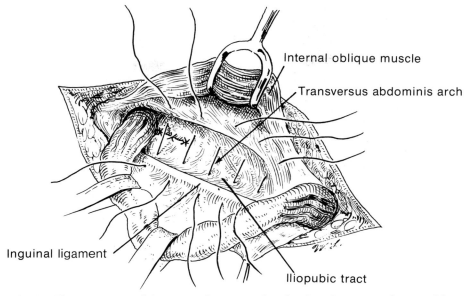

**Figure 11–6.** The transversus abdominis arch is sutured to the iliopubic tract and inguinal ligament.

The spermatic cord is placed under the fascia of the external oblique. Closure is achieved with imbricating sutures of medium or number 3–0 silk, or a synthetic nonabsorbable suture of comparable strength may be used (Fig. 11–7).

## TECHNIQUE OF CLOSURE OF SUBCUTANEOUS TISSUE AND SKIN

Significant improvements in modern wound closure techniques have resulted in greater comfort to the patient and a

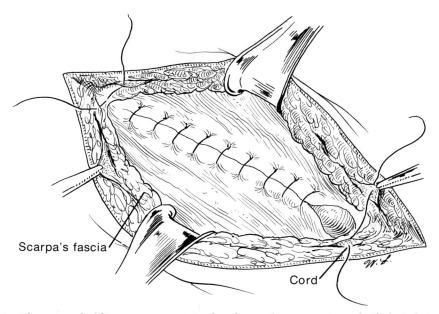

**Figure 11–7.** The external oblique aponeurosis is closed over the spermatic cord. Slight imbrication of this structure gives an excellent closure. Scarpa's fascia is then closed with interrupted sutures of number 3–0 plain catgut.

decrease in the incidence of "stitch abscesses." An article in a 1970 issue of the British Medical Journal briefly reviewed the subject of wound closure. The practice of wound approximation by strapping was practiced for many centuries. During the past half century, suture techniques using silk, nylon, or wire were popular and are still being used extensively. However, modern science has provided surgeons with small sterile strips of adhesive tape with excellent adhesive qualities and low allergenicity; this seemingly trivial advance in surgical materials has benefited both the patient and the surgeon.

### Tape Closure

The advantages of tape closure of the skin accrue to the patient, since the annoying pain incident to suture removal is avoided. The irritating experience of attempting suture removal with today's poorly designed and ineffective disposable suture removal sets is eliminated. According to Murray, Gilman, et al. in 1955 assessed the advantages of tape closure of wounds.

Rothnie and Taylor in 1963, as well as Bonnar and Low in 1968, used small adhesive tapes in approximating wounds in extremities with impaired circulation. Shepherd in 1966 used a similar method of closure in thoracic incisions, while Bonnar and Low used this type of material in gynecologic operations. Mary Shepherd

(1966), as a senior registrar in the Thoracic Surgical Unit of Harfield Hospital, used the sutureless technique for skin closure. Her technique is excellently illustrated. Conolly and associates in 1969 reported their extensive experience with adhesive tape wound closure. They found a reduced incidence of infection in contaminated wounds closed by this technique.

At the present time on my surgical service, nearly every herniorrhaphy incision, whether inguinal or umbilical, is closed with fine absorbable sutures for the subcutaneous fat and Scarpa's fascia and with small adhesive strips for approximation of the epidermis. For ten years, I have been using this technique with such increasing frequency that at the present time on my service, it is used for closure of nearly every incision employed in the repair of groin and umbilical hernias.

When tape closure of the wound is used, hemostasis must be meticulously carried out. Even small vessels with slight oozing are clamped with fine hemostats and ligated with number 4–0 sutures of silk or a comparable material. Dead space is eliminated by the approximation of subcutaneous fat and Scarpa's fascia with number 3–0 absorbable suture (Fig. 11–7). Synthetic absorbable sutures may be used for this purpose. The epidermal edges are brought together with placement of number 3–0 sutures at the subcuticular level (Fig. 11–8). These sutures may be of fine chromic catgut or synthetic absorbable material.

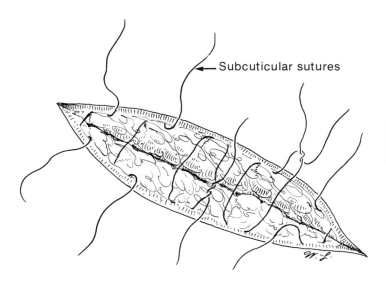

Subcuticular sutures

**Figure 11–8.** Subcuticular sutures of number 4-0 synthetic absorbable material bring the margins of the wound together.

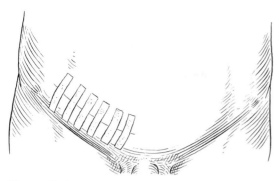

**Figure 11-9.** Small strips of adhesive nonallergic microporous paper are used to tape together the epidermal edges.

Prior to approximation of the epidermis, the skin is cleansed with saline. Care is taken to avoid running the saline over the skin and into the wound. The procedure of cleansing is repeated with an alcohol moistened sponge, and then compound tincture of benzoin is applied to the area. None of these solutions are permitted to enter the wound, which is protected with an appropriately held sponge. Finally, the small adhesive strips are placed so as to approximate the epidermis without overlapping or inversion (Fig. 11-9).

A bulky dressing is applied and allowed to remain in place for 48 hours. The patient may be safely discharged on or before the fourth postoperative day. With increasing frequency, patients are being discharged as early as the day of surgical repair, in which case, the patient is instructed to remove the small tapes in five to seven days after the operation. The appearance of the wound after such closure is testimony to the effectiveness of this type of closure.

Advantages of tape closure are numerous; I have had essentially the same experience with the method as reported by Conolly and coworkers (1969). The benefits of tape closure include the following:

1. Simple and rapid closure.
2. Excellent cosmetic result.
3. Elimination of needle tracts and "stitch abscesses."
4. Elimination of suture removal—the adhesive strips may remain in situ after the patient has been discharged from the hospital.

5. Elimination of intolerable pain in the case of suture removal in children.
6. Easy removal of strips by patient at home following warm tub bath.
7. Less postoperative incisional discomfort.

The argument that wounds approximated with adhesive strips show wide scars upon healing is not valid in my experience. However, the subcutaneous tissues and Scarpa's fascia are carefully approximated with number 3-0 plain catgut.

The use of strips of adhesive for wound closure is particularly appreciated by small children, who never understand that our kindness toward them is demonstrated by the pain we inflict whenever it is necessary to remove skin sutures with forceps and scissors. The results of such closure are cosmetically as good as, or better than, those resulting from skin suture techniques. Stitch abscesses and the small red crosshatchings often caused by skin sutures tied too tightly are not seen when adhesive strips are used for approximation of the epidermis.

### Problems Arising as a Result of Tape Closure

There are a few problems that may arise with tape closure. Failure of the tape to adhere means that the skin has not been properly cleansed or an oily substance has not been removed or a soapy film remains. The skin should be thoroughly cleansed with alcohol, and tincture of benzoin applied.

Of course, if a hematoma develops, the undue pressure may distract the wound edges; in such cases, evacuation of the hematoma and proper hemostasis are indicated.

Now and then, a small superficial blister will develop under the tape; this may be due to a sensitivity reaction, or it may arise from swelling of the wound. If the swelling is due to a seroma, evacuation under aseptic conditions will be helpful. The occurrence of an allergic response to small adhesive strips was rare in my experience. The advantages of tape closure of herniorrhaphy wounds far outweigh any minor problems that may occasionally arise.

## COMMENT ON THE TECHNIQUE OF REPAIR OF INDIRECT INGUINAL HERNIAS

The technique that I prefer for repair of indirect inguinal hernias in adults differs in several important details from Bassini's method; although the procedure is called a "Bassini repair," the differences are of fundamental importance and worthy of notice.

1. Bassini opened the floor of the inguinal canal from the internal ring to the pubic tubercle; this is unnecessary.
2. Bassini sutured the internal oblique, the transversus abdominis, and transversalis fascia to Poupart's ligament; this is not our practice.
3. In the method I describe, the cremaster muscle is excised only when it is thickened; this permits precise and snug closure of the transversalis fascia at the internal ring.
4. The transversus abdominis lamina above is sutured to iliopubic tract separately and accurately after performing a triangulation of this structure at the internal ring. All cord structures are directly visualized. In the repair, as I perform it, the integrity of the transversus abdominis lamina is preserved. Surgeons generally recognize the great importance of this technical detail.
5. The transversus arch is utilized to add strength to the floor of Hesselbach's triangle through its approximation to the iliopubic tract and inguinal ligament.
6. A relaxing incision is made in the anterior sheath of the rectus muscle to avoid excessive tension in selected cases. (The presence of a large hernia or coexisting direct inguinal hernia may require the use of such an incision.)
7. The internal oblique muscle is not sutured to the inguinal ligament.
8. I have become convinced that a hernia must be repaired long before the external oblique aponeurosis is reached. It is closed over or anterior to the cord in almost every instance.

It must be said that I make no claim of originality in the procedure just described for the repair of indirect inguinal hernias in adults. The principles employed have been advocated, to a varying degree, by a number of surgeons. Each detail has been accepted for continued implementation only after it has been utilized in hernia repair and found to be consistently effective. In the repair that I employ, extra consideration is given toward strengthening the floor of Hesselbach's triangle, since many of my patients are industrial workers who perform heavy work. Direct herniation is a constant threat to these individuals.

## CLINICAL STUDY

In an attempt to evaluate our clinical experiences with indirect inguinal hernias in older patients, a study was made using the available records of 548 patients operated upon at the Henry Ford Hospital between the years 1964 and 1968. A deliberate effort was made to secure records of older patients, since a report on congenital indirect inguinal hernias has been recorded in Chapter 10. It is felt that indirect inguinal hernias in adults represent, as previously stated, a somewhat different problem to the surgeon than do the congenital indirect hernias seen in infants and children.

### Incidence

The incidence of indirect inguinal hernias will vary considerably with the patient population studied. Harkins in a collected series (1952) found the incidence to be 56 percent. Glassow (1976) found that indirect inguinal hernias accounted for 60 percent of groin hernias among 13,108 herniorrhaphies. The incidence of indirect inguinal hernias among pediatric patients was found to be as high as 98 percent.

### Age

The age distribution shows that 437, or 80 percent, of the patients in this study were in the fifth decade of life, or older (Table 11–1).

## Table 11-1. AGE AND SEX INCIDENCE OF ADULTS WITH INDIRECT INGUINAL HERNIAS

| Age | Males | Females | Totals |
|---|---|---|---|
| 21 to 30 yrs | 22 | 3 | 25 |
| 31 to 40 yrs | 78 | 8 | 86 |
| 41 to 50 yrs | 101 | 9 | 110 |
| 51 to 60 yrs | 155 | 7 | 162 |
| 61 to 70 yrs | 109 | 12 | 121 |
| 71 to 80 yrs | 31 | 6 | 37 |
| 80 and up | 5 | 2 | 7 |
| *Totals* | 501 | 47 | 548 |

It is to be noted that 327, or 60 percent, of adult patients with indirect inguinal hernias were in the sixth decade of life, or older. This incidence of indirect inguinal hernias in older patients suggests to me that a type of indirect inguinal hernia in adults and aged patients has a pathologic basis somewhat different from that seen in infants and younger patients. Indirect inguinal hernias with an adult onset frequently present with a sac protruding through a large, patulous internal ring. One gains the impression that there is atrophy of tissues in the area of the abdominal ring. In this variety of indirect inguinal hernia, fatty infiltration, lipomas, and sliding components may be present in some combination.

As a result of this study, I am of the opinion that not all indirect inguinal hernias develop as a result of a patent processus vaginalis; some of them should properly be considered acquired rather than congenital or saccular. Pathologically, they resemble the direct inguinal hernia more closely than they do the congenital indirect variety. Of course, by definition they arise lateral to the deep inferior epigastric artery.

## Table 11-2. ANESTHESIA GIVEN TO 548 ADULT PATIENTS WITH INDIRECT INGUINAL HERNIAS

| Anesthesia | No. of Patients | Percent |
|---|---|---|
| Local | 299 | 54.6 |
| General | 128 | 23.4 |
| Spinal | 119 | 21.7 |
| Other | 2 | 0.3 |
| *Total* | 548 | 100.0 |

### Sex Distribution

The great preponderance of groin hernias in males is again confirmed. Five hundred and one individuals, or 91 percent, with indirect inguinal hernias were males; and only 47, or 9 percent, were females.

## Operative Treatment of 548 Adults with Indirect Inguinal Hernias

### Anesthesia

In this study, surgeons showed a preference for local anesthesia, but general and spinal anesthetics were given to significant numbers of patients (Table 11-2).

Although over 50 percent of the operations were performed under local anesthesia, some surgeons preferred general or spinal anesthesia. Spinal anesthesia had once been popular for hernia repair, but it is now used much less often. General anesthesia is advisable for those who refuse local anesthesia and for certain unstable individuals. It was necessary to resort to general anesthesia following an attempt at local anesthesia in one patient only. General anesthetic supplementation was necessary in one patient who had been given a spinal; these two cases are included in Table 11-1 as other forms of anesthesia. My own preference of anesthesia for the great majority of patients continues to be local anesthesia.

### Sutures

Silk was the preferred suture material in over 90 percent of the patients. Wire and synthetic nonabsorbable sutures were used in selected patients.

### Technique of Repair

Although there was some variation in details of repair, certain sound principles were followed consistently. Some operative notes were not sufficiently descriptive, so that data were undoubtedly left out. In spite of these shortcomings, I was able to determine consistency of method, even though a number of surgeons were involved in the repairs (Table 11-3).

Table 11–3.  **TECHNIQUE OF REPAIR
OF INDIRECT INGUINAL HERNIAS
IN 548 ADULTS**

| Technique of Repair | No. of Operations | Percent |
|---|---|---|
| Bassini | 353 | 61.8 |
| Halsted | 171 | 30 |
| Potts | 26 | 5 |
| Ferguson | 15 | 2 |
| McVay | 6 | 1 |
| Henry-Cheatle-Nyhus | 1 | 0.20 |
| *Total* | 571 | 100.0 |
| Bilateral simultaneous | 23 | 4.0 |
| Bilateral separate | 113 | 20.0 |

As was clear from the analysis of the 548 patients, surgeons at Henry Ford Hospital recognized that repair of an indirect inguinal hernia in adults as a rule required a different technique than was generally used in infants and children. For instance, the cremaster muscle was excised in 382 adults. A relaxing incision was considered advisable in 291 patients; this incision is almost never used in infants and neonates. The need for attention to the floor of Hesselbach's triangle is indicated by the fact that the master stitch was placed in 240 patients. A common denominator found in the repair of both infantile and adult indirect inguinal hernias is the insistence upon high ligation of the peritoneal sac. This important detail was attended to uniformly.

It might be well to comment upon the methods utilized in the repair of indirect inguinal hernias as applied to these cases.

### Bassini Repair

The Bassini repair was utilized in nearly 62 percent of the patients. I have described the method in detail earlier in this chapter. Although the repair we utilize is called a Bassini repair, it differs from the original operation as described by Bassini. (These differences were previously summarized in preceding pages.)

### Halsted Repair

The Halsted repair (see Chapter 13, Figs. 13–5 to 13–10) was utilized in 30

percent of the cases. Basically in this study the Halsted repair was performed much like the Bassini repair except that the spermatic cord was transplanted to a subcutaneous position—i.e., it lies upon the aponeurosis of the external oblique. Therefore, in this procedure the internal and external abdominal rings are superimposed; an undesirable consequence resulted from this practice and has been identified. If the transversus abdominis aponeurotico-fascial layer has not been snugly closed initially, the risk of an indirect recurrent inguinal hernia is significant.

The Potts' operation refers to the procedure popularized by Willis Potts of Chicago. In this method the important detail is careful dissection and high ligation of the peritoneal sac. Potts applied his procedure to infants and children. The method is suitable in patients with a patent processus vaginalis and an intact abdominal wall. It was used in only five percent of the adults. It is usually necessary to reconstruct the internal ring in adults by approximating the transversus abdominis lamina snugly about the cord.

### The Ferguson Operation

The Ferguson repair was utilized in only 2 percent of the adults. Ferguson was an outstanding and impressive surgeon who wrote a book, *Modern Operation For Hernia*, in 1907. He described an effective operation for indirect inguinal hernia, but his reason for the ultimate success of his procedure was wrong. First, his procedure was effective because he practiced high ligation of the sac. He did this "to restore the rotundity of the peritoneum." Second, he sutured the transversalis "nicely around the root of the cord." He did this to "obliterate a pathologic infundibuliform process and to make a new internal ring." With these two steps, Ferguson performed an effective repair for most indirect inguinal hernias. He then added an unnecessary step and stated:

The key to the radical cure of oblique inguinal hernia is to suture the internal oblique muscle and its tendon to the inner aspect of Poupart's ligament, as low down as possible without undue tension, after having ablated the sac and strengthened the internal ring with a few stitches above the root of the cord."

This was performed, cord in situ. Ferguson called his operation the "typic" or anatomic operation. He was especially critical of those who would mobilize the spermatic cord. The Ferguson repair, as originally described, is not at all popular among modern surgeons.

### McVay Repair

The McVay repair was infrequently used in the repair of indirect inguinal hernias in adults (only one percent of the cases in this series). The McVay repair is described in detail in Chapter 13 on direct inguinal hernia.

### Henry-Cheatle-Nyhus Repair

The Henry-Cheatle-Nyhus repair was utilized only once in this series of indirect inguinal hernias. The preperitoneal approach to the indirect inguinal hernia is one by which the defect can be clearly visualized and effectively repaired. The method, however, is not one that can be satisfactorily performed under local anesthesia. The Henry-Cheatle-Nyhus repair is presented in more detail in Chapter 15.

### Pathology of the Hernial Sac

The hernial sac must not be overlooked as a source of information that might identify coexistent pathology. Upon opening the peritoneum, the surgeon may observe ascitic or bloody fluid. Any excessive peritoneal fluid should be subjected to chemical and microscopic examination.

Digital examination through the opened peritoneal sac may result in the identification of a mass. The surgeon should recall

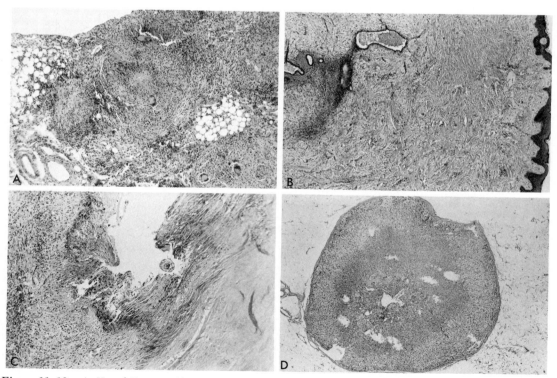

**Figure 11–10.** *A*, H and E stain of hernial sac removed at time of hernia repair. Note cellularity and presence of giant cells. Acid-fast bacteria were demonstrated on special studies. × 110.

*B*, Skin and hernial sac removed at time of umbilical herniorrhaphy. Endometrial glands and cellular infiltration were identified (H and E stain). × 45.

*C*, Echinococcosis cyst identified in inguinal hernial sac with removal during herniorrhaphy (H and E stain). × 110.

*D*, Adrenal rest identified by microscopic examination of hernial sac (H and E stain). × 45.

that the small bowel, omentum, sigmoid colon, appendix, ileocecal segment of the colon, bladder, Fallopian tubes, and ovary may be visualized or palpated, or both. On two occasions, I have seen carcinomatous implants in peritoneal sacs. Tuberculous peritonitis was diagnosed in another case (Fig. 11–10, A). I have seen a patient with endometriosis involving the peritoneal sac at the umbilicus (Fig. 11–10, B). Dr. B. M. Dahman, a House Officer, operated upon a patient with echinococcosis (Fig. 11–10, C). Adrenal rests are occasionally found in inguinal hernial sacs (Fig. 11–10, D).

Theoretically, derivatives from any organ within the peritoneal cavity may extend to involve a hernial sac by direct extension or metastasis. Because of the embryologic origin of the testicle in the lumbar area, splenic and adrenal tissue may be encountered in the inguinal region and hernial sac. Malignant cells can gravitate from the upper abdomen toward the pelvis—as occurs, for example, in carcinoma of the stomach. I am certain that if surgeons would be willing to report unusual cases in which diseases of the ab-

**Table 11–4.  SIGNIFICANT FINDINGS IN HERNIAL SACS AND GROIN HERNIAS**

| Author | Findings |
|---|---|
| Cullen (1916) | |
| Christopher (1927) | |
| Masson (1945) | |
| Dormandy (1956) | |
| Moore (1957) | ENDOMETRIOSIS |
| Scott (1960) | |
| Jimenez and Miles (1960) | |
| Serment et al. (1967) | |
| Toledo-Pereyra and Ward (1972) | |
| Ponka (This report, 1979) | |
| Lowenfels et al. (1969) | CARCINOMA |
| Sugerman (1960) | ECTOPIC |
| Disouza and Richard (1970) | PREGNANCY |
| Watson (1968) | |
| Sieber (1969) | SPLENIC TISSUE |
| Toledo-Pereyra and Ward (1972) | |
| MacLennan (1919) | |
| MacLennan (1922) | ADRENAL RESTS |
| Toledo-Pereyra and Ward (1972) | |
| Ponka (This report, 1979) | |
| Ponka (This report, 1979) | ECHINOCOCCOSIS |
| Ponka (This report, 1979) | TUBERCULOSIS |
| Ponka (This report, 1979) | MESOTHELIOMA |

**Table 11–5.  OTHER SIGNIFICANT FINDINGS IN 548 PATIENTS WITH INDIRECT INGUINAL HERNIAS**

| Finding | Number |
|---|---|
| LIPOMAS | 71 |
| HYDROCELES | 48 |
| SLIDING HERNIAS | 35 |
| Sigmoid | 19 |
| Iliocecal | 12 |
| Ovary and fallopian tube | 4 |
| INCARCERATION | 25 |
| Omentum | 13 |
| Small bowel | 9 |
| Appendices epiploacae | 3 |
| SPERMATOCELE | 2 |
| Total | 181 |

dominal cavity secondarily involve the peritoneal hernial sac, the list would be impressive. In Table 11–4, I noted some significant findings discovered in hernial sacs upon pathologic examination as reported by various surgeons. I have seen but one case in which the pathologist reported a mesothelioma in the hernial sac.

## Other Operative Findings Among 548 Patients with Indirect Inguinal Hernia

I am certain that significant operative findings are too often omitted from operative notes. The surgeon with experience is inclined to value the objective of brevity and, hence, may describe only what he considers essential details in his operative note.

It was remarkable that in this study (admittedly incomplete), 181 patients, or 33 percent, had accompanying significant pathology (Table 11–5).

### Lipomas

Fingerlike protrusions of adipose tissue along the path of the spermatic cord were encountered in 71, or 13 percent, of the patients studied. It is impossible to differentiate such lipomas from indirect inguinal hernias. Actually, they represent a variety of indirect inguinal herniation. Such lipomas enlarge the diameter of the cord; hence, an enlarged internal abdominal ring also is present. At other times, there is considerable adipose tissue at the internal ring, with the result that a large patulous opening is present.

Characteristically, the lipoma of the cord is found within the cremasteric sheath. Upon opening the cremaster, the digitlike circumscribed prolongation of adipose tissue can be easily identified and removed. The base of the lipoma should be ligated to avoid troublesome bleeding. A word of caution is in order at this point; in some patients, the spermatic cord is infiltrated with adult adipose tissue, and efforts at removal of such adipose tissue might compromise the circulation to and from the testicle. The veins of the pampiniform plexus are easily injured in such meddlesome dissection. It is essential to identify the transversus abdominis lamina at the internal ring, so that accurate and snug closure may be achieved. The internal ring in indirect inguinal hernias in adults, prior to repair, will often admit two or more fingers and must be reduced to approximately one centimeter in diameter.

## Hydroceles

Hydroceles were encountered in nearly 9 percent of patients studied. The testicle can easily be delivered during herniorrhaphy, and a hydrocelectomy performed. I have found that complete excision of the hydrocele sac is unnecessary and may result in swelling of the testicle. A generous portion of the endothelial sac is excised with good results.

## Sliding Hernias

Since the subject of sliding hernias is treated extensively in Chapter 18, it is worthwhile only to note again that sliding hernias occur on the left side more often than on the right. The sigmoid colon was present as the sliding component in 19 patients. The ileocecal segment was present in 12, and the fallopian tube and ovary were present in 4 patients. Thus, approximately 6 percent of this selected group of patients presented with sliding hernias. Approximately 9 percent of female patients had sliding hernias.

It is evident that the possibility of a sliding hernia is not remote when dealing with indirect inguinal hernias in adults.

## Incarceration and Strangulation

It is surprising that it was not necessary to resect small intestine in this series of 548 patients. Omentum was found incarcerated in the hernial sacs of 13 patients; and, in one instance, strangulated omentum was excised. It is of fundamental importance to clear the peritoneal sac of adherent omentum and small bowel prior to closure. In three patients, epiploic appendages were incarcerated in left indirect inguinal hernias. In one case, the epiploic appendage was excised because of strangulation. In dissection of fatty tissue at the internal abdominal ring, care must be exercised not to perform an inadvertent colotomy or to compromise the blood supply to the sigmoid colon.

The incidence of incarceration will vary with the patient population. When dealing with an indigent or neglected aged group of patients, the incidence of incarceration will be high. Zimmerman and Anson (1967) identified an incidence of strangulation of from 1.43 to 4.0 among patients with inguinal hernias from various sources. The rate of strangulation ranged from 6.45 to 32 percent among patients with femoral hernias; and in umbilical hernias, strangulation occurred in 1.95 to 17.2 percent of a comparable patient population. In our study of 488 patients with femoral hernias, 22, or 4.5 percent, required resection.

## Spermatoceles

In two patients benign lesions were excised that, upon pathologic examination, proved to be spermatoceles.

## Round Ligament in Indirect Inguinal Hernias

There were 47 female patients in this study; in 32, the operative note indicated that the round ligament was excised as a part of the operative procedure. There is a great advantage to excision of this structure, since the internal abdominal ring can then be closed completely. I have never seen ill effects from an excision of the round ligament, and I use this technique regularly when operating upon indirect inguinal hernias in adult females.

## The Appendix in Indirect Inguinal Hernias

Appendectomy was performed in three patients included in this study. In each case the appendix presented at the internal ring and was easily removed without complications. A word of caution is indicated here regarding appendectomy during herniorrhaphy. It is advisable to obtain the patient's permission for the procedure, lest the surgeon find himself in medicolegal entanglements. The subject of appendectomy and hernia repair will be considered in Chapter 24 on unusual hernias.

## Complications

Although complications following hernia repair have been declining in recent years, there is still room for improvement. The number of serious complications is quite small, but a great number of more or less trivial complications irritate both the patient and the surgeon. When one considers every systemic and local wound complication as well as various local and skin reactions, the total number is disconcertingly high. Since complications will be considered at length in Chapter 27, only those following repair of indirect inguinal hernias in adults will be summarized here (Table 11–6).

When reasonably accurate records of complications are kept, it can be seen that a systemic or local complication occurs in a significant number of patients. Some type of complication occurred in 26 percent of the patients. Wound complications occurred in 9 percent of the cases, and infections comprised nearly 3 percent of all complications; however, serious wound infections occurred in only 1 percent of the patients operated upon.

Some type of scrotal or testicular complication occurred in 6 percent of the patients. Testicular atrophy occurred in 0.55 percent of the patients; much more

**Table 11–6. POSTOPERATIVE COMPLICATIONS IN 548 ADULT PATIENTS WITH INDIRECT INGUINAL HERNIAS**

| *Wound Complications* | |
|---|---:|
| EARLY | 52 |
| Seroma | 22 |
| Hematoma | 9 |
| Minor wound infection | 8 |
| Wound abscess | 6 |
| Swelling and induration | 2 |
| Stitch abscess | 1 |
| Minor wound separation | 4 |
| LATE | 4 |
| Numbness | 3 |
| Keloid | 1 |
| | |
| *Skin Reactions* | 6 |
| Sensitivity to tape | 5 |
| Reaction to antiseptic | 1 |
| | |
| *Testicular* | 34 |
| Scrotal edema, swelling, induration, and ecchymosis | 20 |
| High riding testicle | 8 |
| Impotency | 3 |
| Atrophic testicle | 2 |
| Bilaterally atrophic testes | 1 |
| | |
| **Urinary Tract** | 11 |
| Urinary retention | 9 |
| Cystitis | 2 |
| | |
| *Pulmonary* | 11 |
| Bronchitis–pneumonitis | 3 |
| Atelectasis | 3 |
| Upper respiratory tract infection | 2 |
| Pulmonary infarcts (questionable) | 3 |
| | |
| *Thrombophlebitis* | 1 |
| | |
| *Complications Attributable to Spinal Anesthesia* | 3 |
| Headache | 1 |
| Backache | 2 |
| | |
| *Cardiovascular* | 4 |
| Vasovagal reaction | 1 |
| Congestive heart failure | 1 |
| Supraventricular tachycardia | 1 |
| Anginal attack | 1 |
| | |
| *Total* | 126 |

serious was the course of one patient with bilateral testicular atrophy.

A detailed discussion of complications will be found in Chapter 27.

## Deaths

There were no operative deaths in this group of 548 patients. It is to be expected that when dealing with adults and older

**Table 11–7.  LATE DEATHS IN 548 PATIENTS**

| Cause | Number |
|---|---|
| ARTERIOSCLEROSIS AND ARTERIOSCLEROTIC HEART DISEASE (Including myocardial infarction, coronary insufficiency, cerebral infarction, thrombosis, and hemorrhage) | 18 |
| CARDIAC FAILURE (Other causes) | 2 |
| CARCINOMA | 11 |
| Prostate | 3 |
| Stomach | 2 |
| Colon | 2 |
| Tonsil | 1 |
| Brain | 1 |
| Bladder | 1 |
| Larynx | 1 |
| CIRRHOSIS OF THE LIVER | 3 |
| GASTROINTESTINAL HEMORRHAGE | 2 |
| MISCELLANEOUS (Alcoholism, peritonitis, auto accident) | 3 |
| UNKNOWN | 2 |
| *Total* | 41 |

patients, deaths will occur from intercurrent diseases (Table 11–7). Thus, it can be seen that 7.5 percent of the patients died of intercurrent disease within 13 years of operative repair of their hernias. Arteriosclerosis and arteriosclerotic heart disease together with malignancies take the heaviest toll (Table 11–7).

*Recurrences*

We have seen in Chapter 10 that in infants and children with the congenital variety of indirect inguinal hernias, successful repair is to be expected. The recurrence rate in pediatric patients, and even older patients, with congenital indirect hernias was only 0.67 percent.

There were but five known recurrences among 548 patients having undergone repair of the adult type of indirect inguinal hernias, for a recurrence rate of less than 1 percent (0.91 percent). The recurrence rate would be somewhat higher if it were possible to conduct a long-term follow-up in which each patient would be individually examined. Only 37 percent of the patients were followed two years or longer.

Four of the five recurrences in this study were of the direct variety, arising within one to seven years from the time of repair. One was identified on physical examination, the patient being unaware of its presence. Neither infection nor hematoma was a factor in the recurrence.

I am left with the conclusion that execution of the repairs had been faulty and that sutures were placed too high on the internal oblique or "conjoined tendon." Tension at the suture site was therefore a significant factor in eventual recurrence of the direct hernias.

## SUMMARY

Indirect inguinal hernias in adults often present a clinical and pathologic picture that more closely resembles the one for direct inguinal hernias seen in adults rather than that for congenital indirect inguinal hernias seen in infants. Adult indirect inguinal hernias are more likely to be accompanied with lipomas of the cord, sliding components, and large patulous internal abdominal rings.

Closure of the peritoneum at the internal ring must command the attention and respect of the surgeon, for closure of the peritoneal sac may be more complicated than it is in infants. The internal abdominal ring must be freed of lipomas and sliding components. High ligation of the peritoneal sac and precise and snug closure of the transversus abdominis lamina are essential requirements to be met if repair is to be successful.

The floor of Hesselbach's triangle must not be disrupted in an overzealous attempt to correct a "weakness" in the floor. Sutures must not be placed too high into the internal oblique and transversus abdominis arch. In the larger hernias, judicious use of the relaxing incision is advisable.

NOTE:  References for Chapters 11 and 12 have been incorporated into one list, which can be found at the end of Chapter 12.

# 12

# Recurrent Indirect Inguinal Hernia

*It is frequently said that a surgeon's failures do not return
but look for a better surgeon.*

*Thieme, 1971*

## INTRODUCTION

Chapters 12, 14, and 16 will deal, respectively, with recurrent indirect, direct, and femoral hernias. Since the problem of recurrence following hernia repair is of enormous importance, I feel that each type of recurrence merits special consideration. By focusing attention on the specific defect seen and reflecting upon the pathophysiology, a better understanding of the problem will follow. It is hoped that this will lead to better results following repair of recurrent hernias. In most older texts, and even in the more current books, all the various types of recurrent hernias are simply lumped together under the general heading of "Recurrent Hernias"; however, I am convinced that each variety deserves special attention and thorough consideration.

## STATISTICS AND RECURRENT HERNIAS

The great discrepancy among recurrence rates following hernia repair reported by various authors is generally appreciated. Each study should be accepted on a basis of individual merit. For every case corrected surgically, long-term follow-up examinations by a competent surgeon are essential if a study is to have validity. Such studies are extremely difficult to accomplish for many reasons:

1. A significant number of patients move from one area to another and become lost to follow-up; this is especially true in industrial areas, such as Detroit, where there is a significant turnover of employees in industrial plants.

2. Too often when a patient has a recurrence, he is likely to report to another physician or hospital in the hope that a successful repair will be achieved. The occasional unhappy patient will absolutely refuse to respond to a letter of inquiry and reject an invitation to have a free examination.

3. In many studies, the follow-up period is of short duration. Although most hernias will recur within one year, some appear after 30 to 40 years.

4. Reports by patients submitted in letters or postal cards have a minimal value. Surgeons of experience know that a hernia might be present and undetected at one examination, only to appear after a period of activity. This can occur with indirect inguinal hernias, and direct inguinal hernias in obese

patients often must be palpated to be appreciated. Femoral hernias may be quite difficult to recognize. Statistics based upon reports from patients, without examination, must be accepted with reservations.

5. In order to compare one method of repair with another, similar patient populations must be subjected to the identical procedure. Repairing indirect inguinal hernias in infants is hardly comparable to repairing sliding indirect inguinal hernias in adult patients.

## Definition of Terms

Perhaps in no other area of surgical endeavor is there as much confusion as exists in regard to the "recurrent hernia." Surgical leaders in the field have not been able to agree upon a precise definition for the situation that is characterized by the reappearance of an old protrusion or the development of a new herniation following repair. Most surgical authors "throw up their scalpels in despair" and accept any protrusion in the groin as being a recurrence regardless of the initial defect; this attitude relieves the surgeon of the stress that accompanies critical thought on the subject.

In spite of the difficulty in arriving at an acceptable definition of recurrent hernias, some attempt must be made to improve the chaotic situation. The proper definition of any problem is the key to its eventual solution. We must thoroughly study hernias that reappear after repair.

Watson (1968) generously stated that any hernia occurring at the site of the initial operation should be classified as a recurrent hernia. Some authors feel that from a practical point of view, it matters little whether the recurrence is a reappearance of the initial problem, the development of a new iatrogenic hernia, or simply the result of a failure to recognize and repair the original hernia. They point out that the patient still faces the problem of having a hernia. Skinner and Duncan (1945) feel that any hernia recurring at the site of the previous inguinal hernia repair should be considered a recurrent inguinal hernia.

I feel that it is time to look at the matter more analytically than we have heretofore. Should a direct hernia that appears 40 to 50 years after the repair of an indirect inguinal hernia in an infant be called a recurrent hernia? Is the patient who is still hospitalized—recovering from a recent surgical attempt at repair of what proved to be an overlooked hernia—really suffering from a recurrent hernia? I have seen two instances in which patients with femoral hernias insist that the swelling in the groin had not been eliminated by a recent surgical procedure. In my judgment, this is a failure to identify the defect, and it should be so recognized. On more than one occasion, the patient, after having undergone repair of a direct inguinal hernia, appeared shortly thereafter with an indirect inguinal hernia in which the sac reached the scrotum. Should not these examples be more appropriately considered "overlooked hernias"?

What about the patient who identifies the time and event leading up to the reappearance of the hernia? I recall one patient who slipped while carrying a canoe on a camping expedition; and soon after that experience, pain and swelling appeared in the groin. Examination revealed a direct inguinal hernia—the same type that had been repaired four weeks earlier; this is an example of a direct recurrent inguinal hernia secondary to premature and excessive physical activity.

I have been impressed that 23 percent of patients with femoral hernias have had previous repairs of groin hernias. Should those be considered "recurrent hernias," or are they iatrogenically produced femoral hernias? It would be valuable information to know precisely what type of groin hernia repair preceded the appearance of the femoral hernia.

Even if surgeons cannot agree upon a precise definition of what constitutes a "recurrent hernia," I feel that a far more critical attitude is absolutely necessary if further progress is to be made toward resolving the problem.

Another extremely important aspect of the recurrent hernia problem is that far too often, the surgeon called upon to repair a recurrent groin hernia has operative notes containing vague, inaccurate, or even unavailable information as to how the original hernia was repaired. It is essential to know the original diagnosis and technique of repair. Unfortunately, operative notes too often fail to describe the method by which the original hernia was repaired. Designation of the method of repair by eponyms can at best provide only a general idea of how the repair was performed; important details frequently are not available. It would be most worthwhile if precise records of antecedent operative procedures were made available to the surgeon facing a recurrent hernia. Details describing the size and shape of the defect are usually lacking in most operative notes. Little descriptive information is included beyond noting that a direct, indirect, or femoral hernia is present. The size of the defect in the abdominal wall should be identified. The condition of the tissues should also be described. Thin attenuated tissues, in a patient with a large direct hernia and a chronic cough, are likely to remain in apposition poorly. Only when details are recorded accurately will worthwhile information be accumulated regarding the annoying problem of relapse following repair. Every attempt should be made to find out the original diagnosis and method of repair. It is hoped that the improvement in current operative notes will prove helpful. In order to encourage surgeons to examine the problem of recurrent hernias more critically, I suggest the simple classification shown in Table 12–1.

An *identical recurrence* is the appearance of a hernia of the same type as the one originally repaired. For example, if a direct inguinal hernia appears following a repair of the same type of hernia, we have an identical recurrence. It may develop within a short time and thus be considered an *early identical recurrence*, or it may be seen many years later and be considered a *late identical recurrence*. An early identical recurrence suggests failure to repair the hernia or poor choice of method of repair.

A *different recurrence* is the appearance of a type of hernia different from that initially repaired. For example, a different recurrence is when a direct hernia develops following the repair of an indirect inguinal hernia. Another example would be the appearance of a femoral hernia following the repair of a direct or indirect inguinal hernia. Again, the appearance of such a hernia may occur within a few weeks or after many years. These attempts at proper definition are not idle exercises. I am convinced that a direct inguinal hernia appearing 25 or 30 years following repair of an indirect inguinal hernia could hardly be called recurrence. The pathology of a direct hernia in such situations is similar to that seen in an ordinary direct inguinal hernia.

The appearance of a femoral hernia following repair of a groin hernia is a problem that is steadily attracting more attention. It is suspected that the type of original repair had something to do with the development of the new hernia. The question that arises is: "Do those repairs of groin hernias which utilize the inguinal ligament predispose the patient to development of femoral hernias?"

The overlooked hernia is not common, however, as long as it does occur, some discussion is warranted. The overlooked hernia may be the result of an improper preoperative or intraoperative diagnosis. The patient usually recognizes the problem in the immediate postoperative period and may indicate it by stating that the original swelling had not been eliminated. At other times, the protrusion is recognized by the patient in the somewhat later recovery period. I have repeatedly emphasized the need for a determined effort at correct clinical diagnosis; effort should also be directed at intraoperative diagnosis. Every patient should be considered a candidate for repair of direct, indirect, and femoral herniation, or of any combination thereof.

**Table 12–1.  CLASSIFICATION OF RECURRENT GROIN HERNIAS**

I. IDENTICAL RECURRENCE (Type identified)*
   A. Early
   B. Late

II. DIFFERENT RECURRENCE
   A. Early
   B. Late

III. OVERLOOKED HERNIA

IV. IATROGENIC HERNIA

*Each hernia should be identified as recurrent direct, indirect, or femoral, or combination thereof. The original operative note would be essential for any valid study of effectiveness of initial technique employed.

## Iatrogenic Hernia

More and more frequently, the possibility is being appreciated that when repairing one type of hernia, the surgeon creates another. For instance when performing an inguinal ligament repair (Bassini's or Halsted's), by placing sutures too high on the internal oblique, the surgeon may cause excessive tension on the repair site — resulting in femoral hernia.

The need for differentiation of types of recurrent hernias is stressed here because such an awareness leads to eventual elimination of the problem in many cases. The elimination of overlooked hernias depends upon proper identification of the hernia being repaired and has nothing to do with the technique of repair. Proper preoperative and intraoperative diagnosis will lead to corrective surgical treatment in most cases.

Some surgeons will argue that a patient considers a missed hernia to be a recurrence; this is, at least, a partial truth. The surgeon must be more critical of the tragic result caused by his failure to identify the defect correctly.

The statistics of Ryan (1953) on the matter of overlooked hernias are most instructive. With 154 indirect recurrent inguinal hernias, the surgeon failed to find the sac in 11 cases. With 124 direct recurrent inguinal hernias, one type of hernia was repaired, but another type was overlooked in 19 cases. Of 6 recurrent femoral hernias, there were 4 instances in which the femoral hernia was missed.

Martin and Stone (1962) noted a cause for recurrent herniation to be the failure to search for and identify a femoral hernia or an inguinal hernia of the other type during repair. They noted 12 instances in which hernias were overlooked.

Rydell (1963) studied the problem of recurrence among 65 patients with recurrent inguinal and femoral hernias. In 10 patients, the cause of recurrence was a missed indirect inguinal or femoral hernia.

The statistics in the preceding three references seem to support the view that some hernias "recur." But in fact, the hernias had never been repaired. Greater accuracy in preoperative and intraoperative diagnosis will significantly reduce the number of such "recurrences."

## Incidence

In spite of the fact that individual surgeons achieve and report very low recurrence rates following hernia repair. In the United States, the gross rate of recurrence for groin hernias approaches 10 percent — Thieme (1971) found the rate of recurrence to be 8.8 percent in Ann Arbor, Michigan; Quillinan (1969) found it to be 10 percent in Sacramento, California.

The low recurrence rate following repair of congenital indirect inguinal hernias in infants is generally recognized. Disposition of the hernial sac and appropriate attention to the transversalis fascia at the internal ring corrects this particular problem, and cures are reported in over 99 percent of infants operated upon. Nevertheless, even with this type of hernia, surgeons have reported some individuals with recurrent hernias 30 to 40 years after repair of a congenital hernia. The late-appearing hernia is usually direct in nature.

## THE ENIGMA OF THE RECURRENT INGUINAL HERNIA

Each variety — direct, indirect, and femoral — of recurrent hernia will be considered individually in Chapters 12, 14, and 16 respectively. At this point, however, it is worthwhile to identify the multitude of factors implicated in the causation of recurrence following groin hernia repair (Fig. 12–1). In this chapter, we will focus on the specific etiologic factors that, in combination, eventually result in recurrent indirect inguinal hernias. (Subsequent chapters will deal with recurrent direct and recurrent femoral hernias.)

I would like to state at this point, that I have not been able to identify infection and hematoma formation as being statistically significant factors in recurrence. Also, I have not found that sneezing, coughing, distension, straining, vomiting, and trauma are common factors in recurrences.

An improper diagnosis — both preoperative and operative — is an important factor in some recurrences. The surgeon who recognizes the enormous importance of technical factors and makes a proper choice of technique will be rewarded with excellent postoperative results.

# THE ENIGMA OF RECURRENT HERNIA

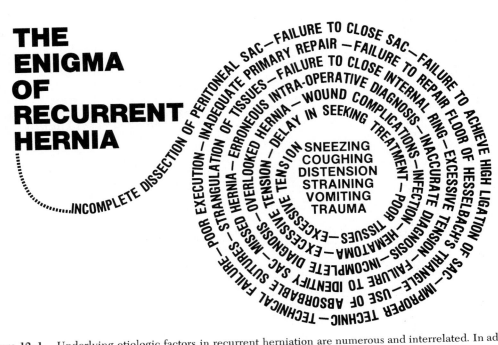

Figure 12–1.   Underlying etiologic factors in recurrent herniation are numerous and interrelated. In addition, exciting factors (such as coughing and straining) have a role that is less clear.

Martin and Stone in 1962 noted that in 123 recurrent hernias, the use of improper operative technique was noted as follows: by leaving too large an internal ring, or by not reducing the size of the cord in 72 of the cases (58.5 percent); by failing to recognize the sliding component in 16 cases; by failing to use a relaxing incision in conjunction with Cooper's ligament repair in 16 cases; by overlooking a coexistent hernia in 12 cases; and by performing an incomplete closure of the sac in 5 cases. In addition, the dissolution of absorbable sutures occurred in 2 cases. These authors have made significant observations. Through such an analytic approach, the hernia problem is solvable.

## Site of Recurrence

Once the (internal) ring itself is forced by the commencing recurrence of a hernial sac, it is doubtful if any repair medial to the ring, or on a plane superficial to it can effectively retard its progress.

*Lytle, 1945*

Obviously if we are speaking of indirect recurrent inguinal hernias, the protrusion will occur at the internal ring, lateral to the deep inferior epigastric vessels. The size of the ring in recurrent indirect inguinal hernias varies considerably, as does the length of the peritoneal sac. The presence of a long processus vaginalis, extending down to the testicle, suggests that the sac was overlooked. The presence of a lipoma at the internal ring indicates that too much tissue was permitted to egress through the aperture of the internal ring, thus leading to recurrence.

Closure of the internal ring becomes the critical issue. How large should the aperture be? What structures must be approximated? Etiologic factors in the genesis of recurrent indirect inguinal hernia will be considered later in this chapter.

Levy and coworkers (1951) found the incidence of recurrent herniation was higher after the Halsted repair method than after the Bassini repair method, regardless of the patient's age or the type of hernia. Levy and his colleagues observed that most of the recurrences were indirect; this was true even when the original hernia had been direct. They did not advocate routine use of the Halsted repair. Of the 141 recurrent hernias studied, approximately 50 percent were located at the internal ring; typically, the sac extended into the cord. Levy and his coworkers also found that one-half of the 1,282 recurrent hernias reported in the literature were located at the internal ring.

Of 300 recurrent groin hernia repairs in 284 patients, Postlethwait (1964) found that over 50 percent of the recurrences were indirect.

Martin and Stone in 1962 reported a recurrence rate of 3.8 percent in 2,751 primary inguinal herniorrhaphies. They noted that 77 percent of the recurrences were indirect, while only 16 percent were direct recurrences.

The low recurrence rate of hernia following repair in children is well known. Rydell (1963) reported no recurrences in 219 patients followed from 2 to 12 years. In 83 percent of these cases, the repair consisted of high ligation of the sac. In selected cases, the abdominal ring was repaired with a few sutures.

At other times, a sliding hernia forms a portion of the posterior-inferior portion of the sac. Here, failure to return the viscus to a position deep to the transversalis fascia contributes toward recurrence.

Thieme (1971) found that the internal ring was the site of recurrence in 48.6 percent of his cases.

It is difficult, indeed, to understand how a properly repaired indirect inguinal hernia can recur. It is the experience of knowledgeable surgeons that recurrent indirect inguinal hernias protrude through the supposedly repaired internal ring and that a newly developed sac then presents for a variable distance toward the external abdominal ring. The aponeurosis of the external oblique muscle forces the sac to follow the inguinal canal, if the initial operation was a Bassini repair or one of its modifications. This chain of events occurs even in cases where the peritoneal sac was identified and removed at the initial operation. Failure to achieve closure of the transversus abdominis lamina at the internal ring is the underlying deficiency. The presence, relatively soon after a primary operation, of a long, narrow peritoneal sac extending into the scrotum suggests that the sac was simply overlooked.

When the internal abdominal ring has not been sufficiently tightened, it is possi-

ble for the elastic peritoneum to undergo gradual stretching and enlarging. Once initiated, further enlargement occurs at the abdominal ring until the defect may measure 4 to 6 cm in diameter.

## High Ligation of the Peritoneal Sac

In indirect inguinal hernias, the hernial sac may have originated in infancy. In many infants, a patent processus vaginalis is directly responsible for the hernia (Chapter 10). Dissection of the peritoneal sac (freeing it from the abdominal wall) and high closure permit normal function of the internal oblique and transversus abdominis muscles at the internal ring.

In my opinion, the pathology of indirect inguinal hernias in adults is often different from that seen in infants. The indirect sac is acquired and develops in a manner that is similar to the appearance of direct inguinal hernias. In the type of indirect inguinal hernia under consideration here, the internal ring is large and patulous; often the area is infiltrated with adipose tissue, and the connective tissue is flimsy. Not infrequently, a sliding component is present. I feel that such hernias are acquired in nature (Chapter 18), similar to direct inguinal hernias in adults.

Opening of the peritoneal sac at the internal ring permits a careful examination for any possible combination of groin hernias. High ligation of the peritoneal sac is a fundamentally sound technical step in repair of indirect inguinal hernias in adults as well as in infants. It is interesting that very little is "sacred" insofar as hernia repair is concerned. Some individuals cite the relative weakness of the peritoneal membrane as a reason for ignoring it in hernia repair. Nevertheless, among surgeons of large experience, the details of complete dissection of the peritoneal sac from the abdominal wall and high ligation are considered to be extremely important. The fact that hernias may be repaired without closure of the peritoneal ring does not detract from the basic importance of this technical detail.

Prior to Bassini's time, hernial sacs were not opened for fear of peritonitis and death. The unopened sac was occluded by torsion. The contribution made by opening the peritoneal sac is fundamentally important, since it permitted accurate digital assessment of the condition of the inguinal area.

Russell (1925) advanced a strong opinion that oblique or indirect inguinal hernias are saccular in nature. He, therefore, advocated removal of the sac alone as a technique of repair. Prior to its ligation, the peritoneal sac must be freed circumferentially about the internal ring through the full thickness of the abdominal wall.

More recently, Griffith (1959) and Madden and coworkers (1971) called attention to important details concerning how high ligation is to be achieved. Griffith pointed out a significant detail where the peritoneum is freed from the transversus abdominis and transversalis fascia circumferentially above the internal ring. In the process of dissection, the belly of the internal oblique muscle is retracted upward; this cannot be done with sponge dissection, and sharp dissection is required. Medially the bladder is often recognizable, while inferiorly the vas deferens can be seen in the retroperitoneal position. After such meticulous dissection and careful ligation of the sac, the closed peritoneal stump will retract to a position deep to the transversalis fascia. These important details are by no means universally recognized or implemented in hernia repair.

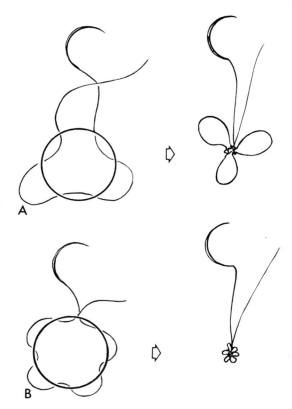

**Figure 12–2.** *A.* When large bites of the sac are taken, the purse-string does not securely close the defect, leaving open clefts through which recurrences may develop. *B.* Small superficial bites appose the peritoneum. (Reproduced from Postlethwait, R. W.: Recurrent inguinal hernias. Am. J. Surg. *107*:742, 1964 by permission of the author and the American Journal of Surgery.)

### Closure of Sac

A variety of factors enter into, or result in, ineffective closure of the peritoneal sac at the internal abdominal ring. Gross errors include the complete failure to identify the peritoneal sac; once identified, it is essential that the peritoneal sac be freed through the thickness of the abdominal wall to permit high ligation.

Proper placement of the suture at the internal ring means that the entire surface is occluded. Postlethwait (1964) has illustrated the importance of proper peritoneal closure (Fig. 12–2).

Omental adhesions or appendices epiploicae may interfere with precise peritoneal closure and must be detached.

Sliding components—including the ileocecal segment on the right, the sigmoid colon on the left, and the tube and ovary in females—must be properly managed. Technical details are illustrated in Chapter 18.

Martin and Stone (1962) noted indirect recurrent hernias within four months following surgery in two children under three years of age. There was improper management of the peritoneal sac and failure to achieve high ligation of the sac.

### OVERLOOKED HERNIA: CASE HISTORY

The failure to achieve high ligation of the peripheral sac resulted in a recurrent indirect inguinal hernia in this case history. The patient was a 62-year-old female, presenting with what the gynecologist diagnosed as a direct inguinal hernia. A Henry-Cheatle-Nyhus repair was carried out; well within a year, pain was consistently present in the groin. The patient stated that the pain was identical to that experienced preoperatively and that she felt a bulge. The patient underwent a second operation 16 months after her preperitoneal repair. At the second operation, a large indirect inguinal hernia was present. Using the inguinal approach, the indirect hernia was successfully repaired.

**Comment.** This case report points out the need for proper clinical evaluation as well as for accurate intraoperative examination. The large indirect inguinal hernia was never repaired. The same problem that appeared preoperatively persisted after her first repair; i.e., pain and swelling in the groin. Accurate diagnosis, dissection, and closure of the peritoneal sac, plus closure of the transversalis lamina, resulted in a cure.

## Excision of the Cremasteric Muscle

There is a difference of opinion as to the need for this step in the repair of every indirect inguinal hernia. Certainly in direct inguinal hernias, the cremaster muscle presents little interference to repair. In certain indirect inguinal hernias of long duration, however, the cremaster is thick and interferes with repair at the

internal ring. Nevertheless, it must be pointed out that the cremaster muscle is merely a continuation of the internal oblique muscle fibers and fascia over the cord. Thus, the muscle fibers largely occupy the anterior and inferior aspect of the cord (Fig. 12–3).

Excision of the cremaster muscle is hardly a recent development, and it should be noted that Bassini in 1899 removed cremasteric muscle. Of course, Halsted at first not only excised the cremaster but most of the cord structures as well. He abandoned his procedure of skeletonizing the cord, because hydroceles occurred postoperatively in about 30 percent of his patients.

Dr. L. S. Fallis of the Henry Ford Hospital taught this technical detail for over 30 years. In 1939 Dr. Fallis stated:

> However, when the surgeon decides to transplant the cord, the cremaster should be entirely cut away, since its presence interferes with accurate approximation of the structures at the medial margins of the canal.

Griffith in 1958 clearly illustrated his technique for excision of the cremaster; he emphasized the fact that accurate closure of the internal ring is greatly facilitated as a result of his technique. Griffith noted that Bassini in 1899 and Schillern in 1922 were others who had excised cremasteric

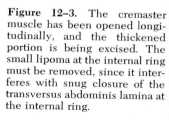

**Figure 12–3.** The cremaster muscle has been opened longitudinally, and the thickened portion is being excised. The small lipoma at the internal ring must be removed, since it interferes with snug closure of the transversus abdominis lamina at the internal ring.

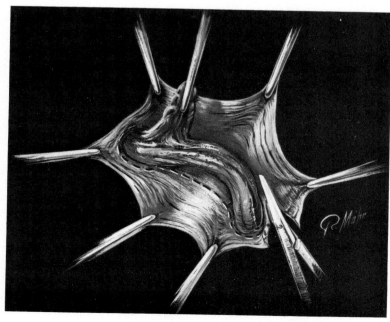

muscle in hernia repair. Bartlett in 1946 and Warren in 1949 also felt that excision of the cremaster facilitated repair of indirect inguinal hernias.

Not all surgeons look favorably upon excision of the cremasteric muscle. The postoperative result of this procedure is a testicle that rides in a distressingly low position in the scrotum, particularly in warm or hot weather. The cremaster muscle has, therefore, a function that is considered important by some patients and many surgeons.

It should be noted that in excising the cremaster, the external spermatic artery (which originates from the deep inferior epigastric artery) is usually sacrificed as well. The testicle derives its major blood supply from the internal spermatic artery, which arises from the abdominal aorta.

It can be concluded that excision of the cremaster facilitates repair of the larger indirect inguinal hernias. In such cases, the hypertrophic fibers interfere with clear identification of the transversalis fascia and, therefore, with accurate and snug closure of the internal ring. However, in cases in which the cremaster does not interfere with repair, I advise against its removal; this means that in direct and femoral hernias, the normal cremaster muscle is not disturbed. In indirect inguinal hernias, judgment should be exercised in deciding the fate of the cremaster muscle. When it presents no technical difficulties to repair, the cremaster is not resected.

### FAILURE TO EXCISE CREMASTER: CASE HISTORY

The patient was 53 years of age and had had two previous attempts at repair elsewhere. After each attempt, recurrence was prompt; the second hernia recurred 9 weeks postoperatively.

At the third operation, we found the cremaster to be markedly hypertrophied. A large peritoneal sac was identified at the internal ring. The cremasteric muscle was excised, and the peritoneal sac thoroughly dissected circumferentially at the internal abdominal ring. There was no direct or femoral hernia present. The peritoneum was closed with a purse-string suture of number 2-0 silk. The transversalis fascia was triangulated and carefully closed at the internal ring. In the repair of the internal abdominal ring, it is actually the transversus abdominis aponeurosis that is sutured to the iliopubic tract below. The integrity of the transversus abdominis lamina is preserved. Snug closure of the ring is essential. The procedure was completed as a Halsted repair, and nine years later the repair was still intact.

**Comment.** In this patient, failure to excise the hypertrophied cremasteric muscle made it impossible to achieve effective closure of the internal abdominal ring. The hernia recurred promptly after each of two previous attempts at repair. With excision of the cremaster, high ligation of the peritoneal sac, and accurate closure of the transversus abdominis lamina, repair was achieved.

### Spermatic Cord and its Relationship to Hernias

For centuries, the spermatic cord has plagued surgeons who deal with hernias. The pathway taken by indirect hernial sacs is well known. The need for identification and removal of the sac—and, similarly, the desirability of preservation of the vas deferens, the internal spermatic artery, and the pampiniform plexus along with the ilioinguinal nerve—is appreciated. Today's patients are far more concerned with preservation of testicular viability than were the patients of a quarter century ago.

The cremaster muscle is a continuation of internal oblique muscle fibers over the anterior and inferior portions of the cord. In an ordinary direct hernia, the cremaster is relatively small and presents no significant barrier to hernia repair. On the other hand, in long-standing indirect inguinal hernias the cremasteric muscle may become tremendously hypertrophied. The cord assumes a sausagelike proportion. In these situations, it is advisable to reduce the size of the cord, and the cremaster may be sacrificed completely or partially.

Halsted in 1892 originally excised some of the veins of the cord in his operation for cure of hernia. He believed that some of these veins were superfluous and, hence, excised all but one or two of them. The object was to reduce the incidence of recurrent hernias. However, by 1903 it was recognized that in about 10 percent of the patients in whom "skeletonization" of the cord was performed, atrophy of the testicles was a complication, As a result of this, the practice of "skeletonization" of the cord was abandoned. Nevertheless, the practice of excision of the cremasteric muscle, particularly in indirect hernias, remained.

The spermatic cord need not be sacrificed in order to achieve an effective repair of a hernia. All structures must be clearly identified and sutures placed under direct vision. Obviously, hemostasis must be complete.

The disposition of the spermatic cord in relationship to hernia repair will be discussed at length in Chapter 14.

## Closure of the Transversus Abdominis Lamina

This fundamental detail is respected and practiced by all surgeons who understand the genesis of indirect inguinal hernias. Furthermore, extraneous tissues and structures at the internal ring must be cautiously and completely removed or replaced deep to the reconstructed transversalis fascia.

As surgeons recognized that recurrences were all too prevalent following repair, explanations were sought. The anatomy of the internal ring received continuing scrutiny. The need for accurate identification of the transversalis fascia became apparent.

As an anatomist, Cooper recognized the importance of the transversalis fascia in 1803. Although Bassini actually repaired the inguinal floor from the pubic tubercle to the internal ring, he did not define the transversalis fascial layer at the internal ring as a distinct layer or structure. Bassini did include the endoabdominal fascia—i.e., transversalis fascia—in his repair, recognizing the importance of this detail. With the passage of time, the internal ring received increasing attention. Techniques that utilized the internal oblique muscle became suspect. Seelig and Chouke (1923) tried to show experimentally that muscle would not unite firmly to fascial or ligamentous structures. They urged fascia-to-fascia closure. Koontz (1926), however, could not confirm their observations. In the Ferguson technique,

the internal oblique muscle was sutured to Poupart's ligament over the spermatic cord, after high ligation of the hernial sac; this method has lost its popularity.

Not to be ignored is the "shutter mechanism" at the internal abdominal ring. Keith (1923) noted that as the internal oblique muscle contracts, the lower margin approximates the inguinal ligament—thus decreasing the size of the internal ring or the inguinal gap. This action may be seen when the patient is asked to cough or strain, while under local anesthesia. It is worthwhile to preserve the red muscle of the internal oblique during hernia repair by excluding it from the suture line. Lytle (1945) also supported the concept of a shutter mechanism in which the internal oblique and transversus abdominis layers participated as functional units. Griffith (1959) noted that as the arcuate fibers of the internal oblique muscle contract, they tend to approximate the inguinal ligament, resulting in a shutter action. The observations of Keith, Lytle, and Griffith should cause surgeons to consider the functional anatomy of the internal abdominal ring during hernia repair.

With a greater awareness of the functional anatomy of the internal ring, methods for identification and closure of the transversalis fascia emerged. White in 1906, Bates in 1913, Slattery in 1917, Pitzman in 1921, Connell in 1928, Lytle in 1945, and Griffith in 1958 all gave special attention to closure of the transversalis fascia at the internal ring. The illustrations of Griffith are especially clear.

Precise identification of the transversalis fascia and accurate and snug closure of the internal abdominal ring are now clearly established as essential technical details in successful repair of indirect inguinal hernias in adults (Fig. 11–5, p. 164). The most common error made in repair is attaching the transversus abdominis layer above to Poupart's ligament below. The inclusion of the transversalis fascia derivative, either the iliopubic tract or femoral sheath, is of fundamental importance. A more serious error is the use of internal oblique muscle in repair of the internal ring.

Martin and Stone (1962) reviewed records of 128 patients with 166 recurrent inguinal hernias. They noted that the internal ring was insufficiently tightened or the cord was insufficiently skeletonized in 72 of 123 patients in whom the technique was considered faulty. A sliding hernia was overlooked in 16, and a relaxing incision was omitted in 16. Martin and Stone recognized that another hernia had been overlooked, and incomplete sac closure was a factor in 5 recurrences. Their observations, I believe, are valid and indicate that in recurrent indirect inguinal hernias, improper surgical technique accounts for most failures.

## FAILURE TO CLOSE TRANSVERSUS ABDOMINIS LAMINA: CASE HISTORY

There is an abundance of literature dealing with congenital indirect inguinal hernias. In most cases, thorough dissection of the peritoneal sac and high ligation results in a successful repair. There is a need for individualization of treatment, even in congenital indirect inguinal hernias.

The patient was aged 13 years before repair of a congenital indirect inguinal hernia and correction of cryptorchidism were undertaken. At the operation, the patent processus vaginalis extending to the undescended testicle was found. Dissection of the cord and mobilization was such that the testicle could be placed into the upper scrotum. The surgeon achieved high ligation of the peritoneal sac, which was seen to retract upward. The external abdominal oblique aponeurosis was closed over the spermatic cord. Absolutely nothing was done to repair the internal ring, and its size was not even described in the operative note.

At the time of reoperation, an indirect recurrence of a moderate-sized hernia was found. The transversus abdominis lamina was closed snugly at the internal abdominal ring, and the repair was still intact seven years later.

**Comment.** This case illustrates the need for proper evaluation of each hernia as an individual problem. Although most congenital indirect inguinal hernias can be successfully repaired by thorough dissection of the peritoneal sac and high ligation thereof, some congenital hernias present excessively large internal abdominal rings, which must be repaired.

## FAILURE TO CLOSE TRANSVERSALIS LAMINA AT THE INTERNAL RING: CASE HISTORY

The patient was a 65-year-old male presenting with a large indirect inguinal hernia. The dissection of the peritoneal sac was adequate, but the closure of the internal ring was not. The transversalis fascia was not properly identified. Instead—to quote from the record—"The so-called conjoined tendon was brought down to the shelving portion of Poupart's ligament with a few interrupted heavy silk sutures." Clearly, the transversus abdominis lamina was never identified as such. A Bassini type of repair was completed, and the wound healed uneventfully.

Within five years, a large recurrent indirect inguinal hernia developed. The hernial sac had become enlarged and extended almost to the scrotum. The peritoneal sac was dissected free and high ligation performed. At the second operation, the transversus abdominis lamina was triangulated and closed accurately and snugly. The Bassini type of repair was completed, and the repair was sound 10 years later.

**Comment.** This case report clearly illustrates the need for accurate identification of the transversus abdominis arch above and the iliopubic tract below. These structures are derivatives of the transversus abdominis muscle and must be snugly closed about the cord. Once this had been accomplished, the repair remained sound in the patient 10 years later.

### Repair of the Floor of Hesselbach's Triangle

In spite of occasional arguments to the contrary, attention must be paid to the condition of the inguinal floor in aged patients with indirect inguinal hernias. There is no escaping the fact that even after adequate repair of the internal ring, direct hernias can appear in the floor of Hesselbach's triangle if this area is ignored.

The debate begins when any method of repair is offered as universally effective. Bassini in 1887 practiced high ligation and excision of the hernial sac. He strived to achieve a canal through the abdominal wall with two openings, one abdominal and the other subcutaneous. He visualized two walls: anteriorly, the external oblique aponeurosis, and posteriorly, a combination of three layers—the transversus abdominis, the internal oblique, and transversalis fascia (fascia verticalis Cooperi). For the first time, a relatively complete operative procedure was devised for repair of inguinal hernias. Halsted followed with his method, which was but a variant of the Bassini technique.

After the initial and great advances initiated by Bassini and Halsted, surgeons became increasingly critical of results obtained. Not all surgeons were able to duplicate the results reported by Bassini. Reassessment of the procedure came from many surgeons, and a variety of remedies were proposed. It was recognized that direct inguinal hernias tended to recur after repair by the Bassini technique. Appreciation of the anatomic differences between direct and indirect inguinal hernias followed.

Slowly it became obvious that a clearer understanding of anatomy of the abdominal wall was essential. The pathologic anatomy of groin hernias received greater attention. The need for precise technique was recognized.

Techniques for repair of the floor of Hesselbach's triangle remain controversial. Arguments center around the concepts of "normal anatomic relationships." Yet, it is clear that in a patient with a hernia, the anatomic structures are anything but normal. Some steps must be taken to correct the deficiencies. If the groin is intact (as it is in an infantile indirect inguinal hernia), then high ligation of the peritoneal sac will effect a cure. If, however, there is an additional defect in the inguinal floor (as often occurs in aged patients), then some rearrangement of tissues is necessary. The defect must be bridged through the shifting of available structures or through the use of implants. Techniques for repair of the floor of Hesselbach's triangle will be discussed at length in Chapter 13 on direct inguinal hernias. It is not enough that in the repair of hernias, reconstructive efforts are directed at the defect. Additionally, destructive or ineffective procedures must be omitted. For instance, suture of the internal oblique muscle itself to Poupart's ligament should be avoided. Suture of the

internal oblique muscle and aponeurosis, together with the transversus abdominis muscle and aponeurosis, to Poupart's ligament might be more destructive than constructive when achieved at the price of excessive tension at the suture line.

## CLINICAL STUDY

In an attempt to identify consistent occurrence of complications or errors in technique that might account for recurrence of indirect inguinal hernias, I studied available records of 101 patients who had undergone repair of indirect inguinal hernias during the years from 1962 to 1968 at Henry Ford Hospital. More records were not reviewed, since I felt that little or nothing would be gained by it. I am certain that the key to further progress in repair of hernias will depend upon far more accurate recording of diagnosis, accurate and detailed description of operative notes, and periodic postoperative evaluation by a physician. Lack of detailed information relevant to the preceding operation (or operations) is serious and a limiting factor when trying to gather information concerning effectiveness of any given method of repair.

### Age Distribution

It is noteworthy that recurrent indirect inguinal hernias are rarely seen in infants and children and infrequently seen in young adults. Only 11 hernias, or 11 percent, were seen in patients under 50 years of age (Table 12–2). In contrast, 89 percent of recurrent indirect inguinal her-

**Table 12–2. AGE OF PATIENTS WITH RECURRENT INDIRECT INGUINAL HERNIAS**

| Age | Number of Patients |
|---|---|
| 1 to 10 yrs | 0 |
| 11 to 20 yrs | 0 |
| 21 to 30 yrs | 4 |
| 31 to 40 yrs | 7 |
| 41 to 50 yrs | 16 |
| 51 to 60 yrs | 34 |
| 61 to 70 yrs | 30 |
| 71 to 79 yrs | 8 |
| 80 and Up | 2 |
| TOTAL | 101 |

nias were seen in patients aged 50 years or older. Fifty-two percent of the adult patients who presented initially with indirect inguinal hernias were in the sixth and seventh decades of life (see Chapter 11). In this chapter, 64 percent of the patients with recurrent indirect inguinal hernias were found to be in a comparable age group. The scarcity of recurrent hernias in infants, children, and young adults is testimony to the fact that either we are dealing with a simpler problem or we are repairing such hernias more effectively. I am satisfied with the explanation that hernias seen in adults and older patients cause more disruption of continuity of the abdominal wall and that the remaining tissues are often atrophic and fat-infiltrated.

### Sex

Not only do females develop indirect hernias less frequently than males, but they also experience fewer recurrences. Only 5 percent of patients with recurrent indirect inguinal hernias were females. Ninety-six of 101 patients with recurrent indirect inguinal hernias were males.

It is to be noted that 8.6 percent of 548 adult patients with indirect inguinal hernias were females (Chapter 11), but only 5 percent of recurrent indirect inguinal hernias were seen in females. Thus, it is at least suggested that repair of indirect inguinal hernias is somewhat more successful in females.

### Anesthesia

Local anesthesia was preferred in this group of adult patients (Table 12–3). Spinal anesthesia is being used less often in current practice than is noted in Table 12–3. General anesthesia is suitable for patients who wish to "go to sleep" and for surgeons who are not convinced of the effectiveness of local anesthesia.

## Technique of Repair

Interestingly, surgeons were essentially satisfied that two slightly different methods of repair were effective in the repair of recurrent indirect inguinal hernias (Table 12–4).

The technique of repair that is most often used in the repair of virginal indirect inguinal hernias is described in Chapter 11. The basic difference between the Bassini repair and the Halsted repair (as it is performed at Henry Ford Hospital) is in the position of the spermatic cord. In the Bassini repair, the cord lies upon the reconstructed floor, where the transversus abdominis arch has been sutured to the iliopubic tract and inguinal ligament below. In the Halsted procedure (as we perform it), the cord lies upon the aponeurosis of the external oblique aponeurosis. The spermatic cord is in a subcutaneous position, and the internal abdominal ring is superimposed upon the external abdominal ring. The Halsted technique was performed nearly twice as often (63 percent) as was the Bassini technique (33 percent) in the repair of 101 indirect recurrent inguinal hernias. This is surprising in view of the general objection of any technique that superimposes the external abdominal ring over the internal ring. The point must be made that closure of the peritoneal sac and repair of the internal ring are essential objectives to be

Table 12–3. ANESTHESIA FOR 101 ADULT PATIENTS WITH RECURRENT INDIRECT INGUINAL HERNIA

| Anesthesia | Number of Patients | Percent |
|---|---|---|
| Local | 61 | 60.4 |
| Spinal | 29 | 28.7 |
| General | 8 | 7.9 |
| Combination | 3 | 3.0 |

Table 12–4. METHOD OF REPAIR OF 101 INDIRECT RECURRENT INGUINAL HERNIAS

| Method | Number of Repairs | Percent |
|---|---|---|
| Halsted | 63 | 63 |
| Bassini | 34 | 33 |
| McVay | 4 | 4 |
| | 101 | 100 |
| Onlay tantalum | 6 | } 6.9 |
| Mesh implant Marlex | 1 | |

**Table 12–5.  DETAILS OF OPERATIVE
TECHNIQUE IN 101 RECURRENT
INGUINAL HERNIAS**

| Technical Detail | Number of Instances | Percent |
|---|---|---|
| High ligation of sac | 101 | 100 |
| Closure of transversalis fascia | 101 | 100 |
| Master stitch | 72 | 71.3 |
| Relaxing incision | 39 | 38.6 |
| Excision of cremaster | 31 | 30.7 |
| Repair sliding components | 14 | 13.9 |
|    Sigmoid      8 | | |
|    Iliocecal     4 | | |
|    Tube and ovary 2 | | |
| Excision of lipoma | 13 | 12.9 |
| Orchidectomy | 1 | 1.0 |

met if repair is to be sound (Table 12–5). The transversus abdominis lamina at the internal ring must be clearly identified and closed snugly in every case (Table 12–5).

Prosthetics were rarely used by most surgeons in the repair of recurrent indirect inguinal hernias. In fact, only one surgeon felt the need for prosthetic implants, and he accounted for the seven instances in which either tantalum or Marlex was used. In my opinion, the use of implants is rarely indicated in repair of indirect recurrent inguinal hernias. In the cases referred to here, the mesh was sutured to the inguinal ligament and to the aponeurosis of the internal oblique as an onlay graft.

## RECOMMENDED PRINCIPLES FOR REPAIR OF RECURRENT INDIRECT INGUINAL HERNIAS

The methods for repair of indirect inguinal hernias are detailed in Chapter 11. Fundamentally, the principles and methods discussed in that chapter apply to the problem of recurrent indirect inguinal hernias. Nevertheless, some special comments, which apply directly to recurrent indirect inguinal hernias, will be discussed here.

The previous cicatrix in the groin is excised or is utilized for the new incision if it permits adequate exposure. Occasionally, earlier incisions have been made at such a distance from the groin that a new incision is made approximately 2.5 centimeters above the inguinal ligament. Sharp dissection with scalpel is used to perform the dissection. Only fine silk ligatures are used to ligate blood vessels. As subcutaneous tissues are incised, the pampiniform plexus and vas deferens are cautiously approached and preserved. A clinical appraisal of the patient with recurrent hernia by the operating surgeon is most helpful in identifying the initial attempt as a Bassini or Halsted repair. At times, it is necessary to approach the deeper tissues from the medial or lateral extremes of the incision, since it is here that normal tissues may be found. If a Bassini repair was performed initially, then the cord structures will be found deep to the external oblique aponeurosis; and the dissection of the lower leaflet of the aponeurosis is continued until the shelving portion of Poupart's ligament is identified. Sharp dissection of the upper leaflet is continued until the sheath of the rectus abdominis is identified. The spermatic cord is identified by placing an umbilical cord tape or a soft rubber drain around it. In recurrent groin hernias the iliohypogastric and ilioinguinal nerves should always be kept in mind and preserved if at all possible; unfortunately, many times these nerves are absent during dissection as a result of previous surgery or are destroyed inadvertently in the process of a difficult dissection. The nerves too often are involved in cicatrix.

In recurrent indirect inguinal hernias, by definition, the sac finds its exit lateral to the deep inferior epigastric vessels. The sac and size of the internal abdominal ring will vary enormously. For instance, in one patient the indirect sac was quite large, yet was overlooked. The patient many years previously had undergone injection treatment for a groin hernia. The protrusion reappeared and, over a period of years, had enlarged. At operation, the tissue was organized into masses of cicatricial tissue with foreign body reaction. Much of this was excised, but the peritoneal sac was never identified. Postoperatively, the hernia promptly reappeared and re-operation was necessary. At the second operation the long indirect sac was identified and dissected free, and high ligation was carried out. The defect in the transversalis fascia was closed, and the repair completed with success.

Each recurrent indirect inguinal hernia deserves individual consideration. Is hypertrophied cremasteric muscle a deterrent to snug closure of the internal abdominal ring? If so, it is excised. Is a lipomatous mass protruding through the internal ring along the cord? If so, it is excised. Is a sliding inguinal hernia present and protruding through the internal abdominal ring, thus interfering with repair? If so, the sliding component is managed as described in Chapter 18.

Once the spermatic cord has been properly assessed and any abnormalities (such as hypertrophied cremasteric muscle, lipoma, and sliding components) identified, attention is directed toward high ligation of the peritoneal sac. Before the sac is dissected free, any incarcerated intestine is freed and any omental adhesions are detached. The peritoneal sac must be dissected free of the abdominal wall. Above, the internal oblique and transversus abdominis muscles are retracted upward and scissor dissection continued over the finger that has been placed in the peritoneal cavity for precise definition of the peritoneum. The dissection is continued about the perimeter of the sac, and inferiorly the vas deferens is freed from the peritoneum. At the inferior margin or portion of the ring, the vas deferens is in direct contact with the peritoneum except for the intervention of a minimal amount of connective tissue. Medially, the dissection is carried out until the adipose tissue overlying the bladder is identified. Care is taken in every case to achieve high ligation of the peritoneal sac, accomplished by placing and ligating a purse-string suture of number 2–0 silk (see Fig. 11–5, p. 164). Omentum must be excluded from the closed peritoneal ring. Identification of the deep inferior epigastric vessels is a worthwhile step in the repair; once they have been found, it is simple to locate the transversalis fascia, which overlies these vessels. Fine-pointed hemostats are applied to the transversus abdominis lamina at the medial margin of the transversalis fascia, and then to the inferior and superior leaflets of the fascia. The placement of three identifying hemostats is called *triangulation of the transversalis fascia at the internal ring* (see Fig. 11–5, p. 164). Traction on the medial clamp makes the transversalis fascia easily identifiable. The internal abdominal oblique muscle is re-

tracted upward, so that it is excluded from suture. The internal abdominal ring is then snugly closed with number 2–0 silk or with nonabsorbable synthetic suture. The first suture is placed nearest the cord under direct vision with the hemostats serving as guides. The repair is completed by placing sutures into the transversalis fascia where necessary. The size of the new internal ring must barely admit the tip of the index finger. If measured with a hemostat, the tip of the clamp should be inserted and opened for a width of approximately one centimeter. Obviously, the presence of a large cord will require a slightly larger aperture to avoid constriction at the site. It is noteworthy that, with the passage of time, I have steadily decreased the size of the internal abdominal ring.

The remainder of the repair may be completed as desired, but excessive tension must be avoided. The repair is usually completed by placing a row of interrupted number 2–0 synthetic nonabsorbable sutures between the transversus abdominis arch above and the iliopubic tract and inguinal ligament below (see Fig. 11–6, p. 165). In small indirect inguinal hernias, the relaxing incision is not necessary but should be used in those large defects requiring repair of the floor of Hesselbach's triangle. The spermatic cord is placed in subcutaneous position and wound closure completed as shown in Chapter 11.

Finally, the use of synthetic mesh in the repair of indirect inguinal hernias is seldom necessary. I find it rarely indicated, since most recurrent indirect inguinal hernias can be effectively repaired without prosthetics. Occasionally in patients who have had four or more recurrences, tissue destruction is great; and some reinforcement of the repair is justified. Here, suture of the Marlex mesh—as an onlay graft—to the inguinal ligament and transversalis fascia below and to the internal oblique aponeurosis above is a useful adjunct to repair. Sutures of number 2–0 silk or of synthetic nonabsorbable are placed at intervals of 2 centimeters about the defect and along the inguinal ligament. A small slit is made in the prostheses for passage of the cord.

The aponeurosis of the external oblique is usually closed over the spermatic cord.

Wound closure is identical to that described in Chapter 11 (Figs. 11–8 and 11–9, pp. 166 and 167.)

In the cases reviewed for this chapter, high ligation of the sac and precise closure of the transversus abdominis were accomplished in every case (Table 12–5). The cremaster was still present in 31 percent of the patients at time of repair of the recurrence, and excision was indicated. Sliding components and lipomas were present in over 26 percent of patients with recurrent indirect inguinal hernia (Table 12–5). This significant incidence of abnormalities at the internal ring suggests that some of them might have been overlooked.

The master stitch was placed in 72 patients, and a relaxing incision made in 39 patients. These technical details suggest that the surgeon felt there was a need for strengthening the floor of the inguinal canal and minimizing tension at the suture line (Table 12–5).

The details of technique, which have been described at length in Chapter 11 and in this chapter, are summarized in Table 12–5 for the sake of brevity.

## Causes for Failure, Resulting in Indirect Recurrent Inguinal Hernias

The complex and numerous interrelated factors that can result in recurrence of groin hernias have been summarized in Figure 12–1, which depicts this enigma-like problem.

After personally looking over an enormous number of patient's records, I feel that certain assumed causes for recurrence should be relegated to a position of less prominence. For instance, I have found that infection is an infrequent cause for recurrence. Hematomas are certainly uncommon etiologic factors in the genesis of recurrent hernias. Since most modern surgeons use nonabsorbable sutures, the factor of absorbability cannot be given great prominence as a cause for recurrence. Obesity does make repair technically more difficult, however, with the proper technique, hernias can be successfully repaired in patients who are overweight and their operative wounds will heal.

When all of the various causes and excuses are "tossed into the cauldron" of recurrent hernias, only technical factors and diagnostic errors retain their importance as significant etiologic factors. My opinion is that most indirect recurrent inguinal hernias are the result of a technical failure or an error in judgment as to choice of procedure. Most often, there is failure to achieve either high ligation of the peritoneal sac or snug closure of the transversus abdominis lamina at the internal ring or both.

In trying to determine the important cause (or causes) for recurrence among 101 patients with recurrent indirect inguinal hernias, operative notes were studied. Unfortunately, in several records it was difficult to ascertain which etiologic factor was the most important. In many cases, multiple factors were interpreted as contributing to the recurrence. For instance, in some instances the patient was left with a large internal abdominal ring, hypertrophied cremaster, and a sliding component. In others, the sac was considered as being unusually large or was even overlooked, as noted in Table 12–6.

As indicated in Table 12–6, most recurrent indirect inguinal hernias are the consequence of a technical error or failure. Failure to make a correct clinical or intraoperative diagnosis accounted for two "recurrent" indirect inguinal hernias.

It might be worthwhile to note that inadequate closure of the internal ring might be due to several causes. The surgeon might have simply left the internal ring too large after partial closure. Hypertrophied cremaster muscle, lipomas, and sliding components might have interfered with snug closure. In addition, a technical error might account for improper

**Table 12–6. ETIOLOGIC FACTORS IN 101 PATIENTS WITH RECURRENT INDIRECT INGUINAL HERNIAS***

| | |
|---|---|
| Failure to repair internal ring | 97 |
| Failure to achieve high ligation of sac | 58 |
| Failure to excise cremaster | 31 |
| Failure to manage sliding component | 14 |
| Failure to excise lipomas | 13 |
| Tissue atrophy (Marfan's syndrome 2) | 4 |
| Overlooked hernia | 2 |

*Total is more than number of patients because several factors were present in individual cases.

closure of the internal ring. It should be recalled that the transversus abdominis lamina is approximated at the internal ring and that suture of the internal oblique muscle to the inguinal ligament can be disastrous. This study supports the statement that a great number of patients will seek help elsewhere following the recurrence of a hernia. Only 17 of 101 patients had their initial repairs at Henry Ford Hospital. The type of original repair was not available in a majority of cases, but it was noted that the cord had been transplanted to a subcutaneous position in 18 of 45 patients for whom a description of the original operation was available. When the indirect inguinal hernia recurred after a Halsted repair, there regularly were other factors that had to be considered in the genesis of recurrences. Hypertrophied cremaster, lipomas, and sliding components were usually present in some combination.

Unfortunately in the great majority of cases, little was known of the variety of the original hernia or the type of repair; this important information should form a basis for any critical analysis of methods used in repair of hernias.

### Interval between Original Repair and Recurrence

The interval between the original repair and the recurrence of a hernia tells us something about the technique of repair. Two patients recognized the recurrent protrusion promptly; one was still in the hospital when he became aware of the hernia. In both cases, the hernia was simply overlooked. In eight patients, the recurrence was seen within six months, suggesting inadequate repair.

This study of 101 hernia repairs may be viewed with the legitimate criticism that it is small; nevertheless, useful information emerges. It is noteworthy that 57 percent of the recurrences were seen within five years of repair (Table 12–7). Recurrences appeared even after 25 years following hernia repair. The intervals, in years, were 26, 28, 30 (2 patients), 34, 40 (2 patients), 43, and 58; this listing is included here to emphasize the limitations of short-term follow-up studies.

### Number of Previous Repairs

In Table 12–8, I have summarized the number of previous repairs in 101 patients. It is remarkable that 101 patients with recurrent hernias required at least 224 attempts at repair before successful repairs were attained.

### Bilateral Repairs

The adverse effect of bilateral simultaneous repairs has often been alluded to in the literature. Sparkman (1962), in a study of 1944 patients with unilateral inguinal hernias, found that a hernia developed on the opposite side in 15.8 percent of the individuals.

In this study, 46 patients had both sides repaired at one time or another. Sixteen percent had bilateral simultaneous repairs. Bilateral simultaneous repair may be an explanation for recurrence of direct inguinal hernias (see Fig. 14–2, p. 218). The mechanism whereby tension is produced at the suture line is clearly illustrated. Since the pathology of indirect inguinal hernia in adults actually has some similarities to that of the direct hernia, the same attention must be given at surgery to

Table 12–7. INTERVALS BETWEEN REPAIR AND RECURRENCE IN 101 RECURRENT INDIRECT INGUINAL HERNIAS

| Interval | Number of Patients | Percent |
|---|---|---|
| 0 to 1 month | 2 | 1.98 |
| 2 to 6 months | 8 | 7.92 |
| 7 to 24 months | 16 | 15.84 |
| 2 to 5 years | 32 | 31.68 |
| 6 to 10 years | 12 | 11.88 |
| 11 to 15 years | 12 | 11.88 |
| 16 to 25 years | 9 | 8.91 |
| 25 years and up | 10 | 9.90 |

Table 12–8. NUMBER OF PREVIOUS REPAIRS IN 101 PATIENTS WITH RECURRENT INDIRECT INGUINAL HERNIAS

| Number of Patients | Previous Repairs |
|---|---|
| 1 | 4 |
| 2 | 3 |
| 14 | 2 |
| 84 | 1 |

minimize tension at the suture line. Relaxing incisions have an important role in this effort.

## Complications

Certain complications are seen more frequently following the repair of a recurrent hernia than following the original repair operation (Table 12–9). Wound complications and postoperative testicular problems are more common in recurrent hernias, as can be seen in a comparison between Table 11–6, p. 174, and Table 12–9.

## Late Deaths

Six of eight late deaths were due to arteriosclerosis and arteriosclerotic heart disease. One patient died of a pulmonary embolus, another of carcinoma of the colon. There were no operative deaths in this group of 101 patients with recurrent indirect inguinal hernias.

## Recurrences

There were two known recurrences in this study, for a rate of 1.98 percent. Sixty-four percent of the patients were followed two years or longer. Forty-four percent were followed six years or longer.

## SUMMARY

Among the most important factors in the genesis of indirect recurrent inguinal hernias are the following:

Failure to make an accurate preoperative diagnosis

Failure to locate the peritoneal sac

Incomplete dissection of the peritoneal sac

Low ligation of the sac—i.e., distal to the internal abdominal ring

Technical failures, such as

1. Failure to achieve high ligation of the peritoneal sac
2. Failure to close transversus abdominis lamina accurately at the internal ring
3. Failure to excise cremaster muscle (in selected cases)
4. Use of internal oblique muscle

**Table 12–9. POSTOPERATIVE COMPLICATIONS IN 101 PATIENTS WITH RECURRENT INDIRECT INGUINAL HERNIAS**

| Type of Complication | Number | Percent |
|---|---|---|
| WOUND | 16 | 15.84 |
| Hematoma | 4 | |
| Seroma | 4 | |
| Induration | 6 | |
| Infection | 2 | |
| TESTICULAR | 17 | 16.83 |
| Scrotal and testicular swelling | 15 | |
| Atrophic testicles | 2 | |
| URINARY RETENTION | 7 | 6.99 |
| Spinal anesthesia | 5 | |
| Local anesthesia | 1 | |
| General anesthesia | 1 | |
| PULMONARY | 3 | 2.97 |
| Lobar pneumonia | 1 | |
| Atelectasis | 2 | |
| GASTROINTESTINAL | 1 | 0.99 |
| Ileus | 1 | |
| THROMBOPHLEBITIS (treated with Heparin) | 1 | 0.99 |

instead of transversus abdominis aponeurosis

5. Failure to manage sliding components
6. Failure to excise lipomas
7. Strangulation of tissues by tying ligatures too tightly

Destructive sutures—placed lateral to spermatic cord into internal oblique and transversus abdominis muscles—that weaken the repair rather than support it.

Indirect inguinal hernias in adults can be repaired with a recurrence rate of less than one percent, provided that the surgeon is aware of the possible etiologic factors just described. Meticulous attention to detail is essential if uniform success is to be expected.

## REFERENCES*

Andrews, E.: A method of herniotomy utilizing only white fascia. Ann. Surg. 80:255, 1924.

Andrews, E.: A history of the development of the technique of herniotomy. Ann. Med. Hist. 7:451, 1935.

Bartlett, W., Jr. Observation on a concept of inguinal repair. Surg. Gynecol. Obstet. 83:55, 1946.

*Chapters 11 and 12 are included here in the References and Supplemental Readings.

Bassini, E.: Nuovo metodo per la cura radicale dell'erna inguinale. Atti Cong. Assoc. Med. Ital. 2:179, 1887.

Bassini, E.: Sopra 100 Casi di cura radicale dell'ernia operata. Archiv Atti Soc. Ital. Chir. 5:315, 1888.

Bassini, E.: Ueber Behandlung des Leistenbruches. Arch. Klin. Chir. 40:429, 1890.

Bates, U. C.: New operation for the cure of indirect inguinal hernia. J.A.M.A. 9:2032, 1913.

Bonnar, J., and Low, R. A.: Closure of surgical wounds of the lower abdomen by microporous tape. Lancet 1:1387, 1968.

Bull, W. T.: On the radical cure of hernia, with results of 134 operations. Trans. Am. Surg. 8:99, 1890.

Christopher, F.: Inguinal endometriosis. Ann. Surg. 86:918, 1927.

Connell, F. G.: Radical operation for the cure of oblique hernia. Surg. Gynecol. Obstet. 7:481, 1908.

Connell, F. G.: The repair of the internal ring in oblique hernia. J.A.M.A., 52:1087, 1909.

Connell, F. G.: Repair of internal ring in oblique inguinal hernia. Surg. Gynecol. Obstet. 46:113, 1928.

Conner, W. T., and Peacock, E.: Some studies on the etiology of inguinal hernia. Am. J. Surg. 126(6):732, 1973.

Conolly, W. B., Hunt, T. K., Zederfeldt, B., Cafferata, H. T., and Dunphy, J. E.: Clinical comparison of surgical wounds closed by suture and adhesive tapes. Am. J. Surg. 117:318, 1969.

Cooper, A. P.: *The Anatomy and Surgical Treatment of Abdominal Hernia.* (Volumes I and II). London, Longmans & Co., 1804 to 1807.

Cullen, T. S.: Adenomyoma of the round ligament and incarcerated omentum in an inguinal hernia together forming one tumor. Surg. Gynecol. Obstet. 22:258, 1916.

Dahman, B. M.: Personal communication.

Dormandy, T. L.: Inguinal endometriosis. Lancet 1:832, 1956.

D'Souza, C. R., and Richard, H. L.: Ectopic pregnancy in a hernial sac: A case report. Can. J. Surg. 13:166, 1970.

Erdman, S.: Inguinal hernia in the male. Ann. Surg. 77:171, 1923.

Fallis, L. S.: Personal communication.

Fallis, L. S.: The operative treatment of inguinal hernia. J. Med. Assoc. Georgia 28(8):316, 1939.

Ferguson, A. H.: *The Technic of Modern Operations for Hernia.* Cleveland, Ohio, Cleveland Press, 1907, pp. 280–288.

Glassow, F.: Inguinal hernia repair. Am. J. Surg. 131:306, 1976.

Griffith, C. A.: Inguinal hernia: An anatomic-surgical correlation. Surg. Clin. North Am. 39:531, 1959.

Halsted, W. S.: The radical cure of inguinal hernia in the male. Bull. Johns Hopkins Hosp. 4:17, 1893.

Halsted, W. S.: An additional note on the operation for inguinal hernia. Surgical paper by William Stewart Halsted. Johns Hopkins Press 1:306, 1924.

Halsted, W. S.: Excision of some of the veins of the cord in the operation for radical cure of hernia. Bull. Johns Hopkins Hosp. 3:76, 1892.

Halsted, W. S.: The cure of the more difficult as well as simpler inguinal ruptures. Bull. Johns Hopkins Hosp. 14:208, 1903.

Harkins, H. N.: Recent advances in the treatment of hernia. Ann. West. Med. Surg. 6:221, 1952.

Harkins, H. N., Moyer, C. A., Rhoads, J. E., and Allen, J. G.: *Surgery Principles and Practice* (2nd ed.). Philadelphia, J. B. Lippincott Co., 1957, p. 1026.

Jimenez, M., and Miles, R. M.: Inguinal endometriosis. Ann. Surg. 151:903, 1960.

Judd, E. S.: *Mayo Clinic Papers, 1904–1909.* Philadelphia, W. B. Saunders Co., 1911.

Keith, A.: On the origin and nature of hernia. Br. J. Surg. 11:455, 1923.

Koontz, A. R.: Views on choice of operation for inguinal hernia repair. Ann. Surg. 143:868, 1956.

Koontz, A. R.: Muscle and fascia suture with relation to hernia repair. Surg. Gynecol. Obstet. 42:222, 1926.

Levy, A. H., Wren, R. S., and Friedman, M. N.: Complications and recurrences following inguinal hernia repair. Ann. Surg. 133:533, 1951.

Lichtenstein, I. I., and Shore, J. M.: Exploding the myths of hernia repair. Am. J. Surg. 132:307, 1976.

Lowenfels, A. B., Rohman, M., Ahmed, N., and Lefkowitz, M.: Hernia sac cancer. Lancet 1:651, 1969.

Lucas-Championnière, J. L.: *Cure Radkale Des Hernies!* Avec une etude statistique de deux cent sacrante-quinze operations et cinquante figures intercalées dans le texte. Paris, Rueff, et Cie, 1892.

Lytle, W. J.: The internal inguinal ring. Br. J. Surg. 32:441, 1945.

Lytle, W. J.: A history of hernia. Med. Press 232:1, 1954.

Lytle, W. J.: The deep inguinal ring. Development, function and repair. Br. J. Surg. 57:531, 1970.

MacGregor, W. W.: Demonstration of true internal inguinal sphincter and its etiologic role in hernia. Surg. Gynecol. Obstet. 49:510, 1929.

MacGregor, W. W.: The fundamental operative treatment of inguinal hernia. Surg. Gynecol. Obstet. 50:438, 1930.

MacLennan, A.: On the presence of adrenal rests in the walls of hernial sacs. Surg. Gynecol. Obstet. 29:387, 1919.

MacLennan, A.: Radical cure of inguinal hernia in children with special reference to embryonic rests found associated with the sacs. Br. J. Surg. 9:445, 1922.

Madden, J. L., Saeed, H., and Agorogiannis, A.: The anatomy and repair of inguinal hernias. Surg. Clin. North Am. 51:1269, 1971.

Mahorner, H., and Goss, C. M.: Herniation following destruction of Poupart's and Cooper's ligaments. Ann. Surg. 155:741, 1962.

Martin, J. H., and Stone, H. H.: Recurrent inguinal hernia. Ann. Surg. 156:713, 1962.

Marcy, H. O.: The cure of hernia. J.A.M.A. 8:589, 1887.

Marcy, H. O.: The cure of hernia by the antiseptic use of animal ligature. Trans. Int. Med. Cong. 2:446, 1881.

Marcy, H. O.: A new use of carbolized catgut ligatures. Boston Med. Surg. J. 85:315, 1871.

McVay, C. B., and Anson, B. J.: A fundamental error in current methods of inguinal herniorrhaphy. Surg. Gynecol. Obstet. 74:746, 1942.

McVay, C. B.: *Hernia: The Pathologic Anatomy and The Anatomic Repair of the More Common Hernias.* Springfield, Ill., Charles C Thomas, 1954.

McVay, C. B., and Anson, B. J.: Aponeurotic and fascial continuities in abdomen, pelvis and thigh. Anat. Rec. 76:213, 1940.

Moore, W. R.: Inguinal endometriosis in bilateral hernia sacs associated with extensive pelvic endometriosis. Harp Hosp. Bull. 15(6):242, 1957.

Murray, P. J. B.: Closure of skin wounds with adhesive tape. Br. Med. J. 2:1030, 1963.

Pitzman, M.: A fundamentally new technique for inguinal herniotomy. Ann. Surg. 74:610, 1921.

Ponka, J. L., and Brush, B. E.: Sliding inguinal hernia in patients over 70 years of age. J. Am. Geriatr. Soc. 26(2):68, 1978.

Postlethwait, R. W.: Recurrent inguinal hernias. Am. J. Surg. 107:739, 1964.

Potts, W. J., Riker, W. L., and Lewis, J. E.: The treatment of inguinal hernia in infants and children. Ann. Surg. 132:566, 1950.

Quillinan, R.: Repair of recurrent inguinal hernia. Am. J. Surg. 118:593, 1969.

Rothnie, N. G., and Taylor, G. W.: Sutureless skin closure: A clinical trial. Br. Med. J. 2:1027, 1963.

Russell, R. H.: Inguinal hernia and operative procedure. Surg. Gynecol. Obstet. 41:605, 1925.

Ryan, E. A.: Recurrent hernias: An analysis of 369 consecutive cases of recurrent inguinal and femoral hernias. Surg. Gynecol. Obstet. 96:343, 1953.

Rydell, W. B.: Inguinal and femoral hernias. Arch. Surg. 87:493, 1963.

Schillern, P. G., Jr.: The choice of operation in inguinal hernia. Surg. Gynecol. Obstet. 34:230, 1922.

Scott, R. B.: External endometriosis: Mechanism of origin, theoretical and experimental. Clin. Obstet. Gynecol. 3:429, 1960.

Seelig, M. G., and Chouke, K. S.: A fundamental factor in the recurrence of inguinal hernias. Arch. Surg. 7:553, 1923.

Serment, H., Sudan, J. P., and Bossi, G.: A propos d'un cas d'endometriose du sac herniaire. Bull. Fed. Gynecol. Obstet. Franc. 19:199, 1967.

Shepherd, M. P.: Sutureless skin closure in a thoracic unit. Br. J. Surg. 53:445, 1966.

Sieber, W. K.: Splenotesticular cord (splenogonadal fusion) associated with inguinal hernia. J. Pediatr. Surg. 4:208, 1969.

Skinner, H. L., and Duncan, R. D.: Recurrent inguinal hernia. Ann. Surg. 122:68, 1945.

Slattery, R. V.: An operation for the radical cure of inguinal hernia. Lancet ii:455, 1917 (London).

Sparkman, R. S.: Bilateral exploration in inguinal hernia in juvenile patients. Surgery 51:393, 1962.

Sugerman, G. R.: Tubal pregnancy in a hernial sac: A case report. J. Newark Beth Israel Hosp. 12:160, 1961.

Talbott, J. H.: A Biographical History of Medicine. New York, Grune & Stratton, 1970, p. 1016.

Taylor, A. S.: The results of operations for inguinal hernia. Arch. Surg. 1:382, 1920.

Thieme, E. T.: Recurrent inguinal hernia. Arch. Surg. 103:238, 1971.

Tobin, G. R., Scott, C., and Peacock, E. E., Jr.: A neuromuscular basis for development of indirect inguinal hernia. Surgery 64:464, 1976.

Toledo-Pereyra, L. H.: The flora and fauna of hernial sacs! Minn. Med. 55:995, 1972.

Torek, F.: Combined operation for removal of appendix and cure of hernia. Ann. Surg. 43:665, 1906.

Warren, K. W.: Repair of inguinal hernia. Surg. Clin. North Am. 29:795, 1949.

Watson, L. F.: Hernia (3rd ed.). St. Louis, C. V. Mosby Co., pp. 281–297.

Watson, R. J.: Splenogonadal fusion. Surgery 63:853, 1968.

White, J. M.: Inguinal hernia. N.Y. Med. J. 84:71, 1906.

Wood, J.: Lectures on hernia and its radical cure. Br. Med. J. (Hunterian Lectures) 1:1185, 1233, and 1279; 1885 and 1886.

Zimmerman, L. M., and Anson, B. J.: Anatomy and Surgery of Hernia (2nd ed.). Baltimore, Williams & Wilkins Co., 1967, pp. 26 and 27.

## Supplemental Readings

Burton, C. C.: The evolution and classification of hernial operations. Surg. Gynecol. Obstet. 87:313, 1948.

Brandon, W. M. J.: Inguinal hernia—The sling operation. Br. J. Surg. 56:408, 1969.

Coley, F.: Three thousand consecutive herniotomies. Ann. Surg. 80:242, 1924.

Coley, W. B.: Review of radical cure of hernia during the last half century. Am. J. Surg. (Edit.) 31:397, 1936.

Doran, F. S. A.: Three methods of repairing the deep abdominal ring in men with primary indirect inguinal herniae. Br. J. Surg. 49:642, 1962.

Doran, F. S. A., and Lousdale, W. H.: Simple experimental method of evaluation for Bassini and allied types of herniorrhaphy. Br. J. Surg. 36:339, 1949.

Easton, E. R.: Incidence of femoral hernia following repair of inguinal hernia—Ectopic recurrence; Proposed operation of external and internal herniorrhaphy. J.A.M.A. 100:1741, 1933.

Edlich, R. F., and Kuphal, J. E.: Bioengineering analysis of sutureless wound closure. Int. Surg. 58:246, 1973.

Jelenko, C., Jelenko, J., Buxton, R. W., and Matthews, J. C.: The evolution of adhesive tape. Surg. Gynecol. Obstet. 126:1083, 1968.

Krieg, E. G. M.: Anatomy and physiology of the inguinal hernia in the presence of hernia. Ann. Surg. 137:41, 1953.

McNealy, R. W.: Are herniorrhaphies as successful as they should be? Lancet 59:262, 1939.

Ravitch, M. M., and Hitzrot, J. M., II: The Operations for Inguinal Hernia. St. Louis, C. V. Mosby Co., 1966.

Rice, C. D., and Steckler, J. H.: The repair of hernia with special application of the principles evolved by Bassini, McArthur and McVay. Surg. Gynecol. Obstet. 47:831, 1928.

Sampson, J. A.: Endometriosis of the sac of a right inguinal hernia associated with the pelvic peritoneal endometriosis and an endometrial cyst of the ovary. Am. J. Obstet. Gynecol. 12:459, 1926.

Schley, W. S.: Transposition of the rectus muscle and the utilization of the external oblique aponeurosis in the radical cure of inguinal hernia. Ann. Surg. 77:605, 1923.

Turner, P.: Inguinal Hernia. The Imperfectly Descended Testicle and Varicocele. Toronto, Canada, The Macmillan Company, Ltd., 1920.

# 13

# Direct Inguinal Hernia

*A direct inguinal hernia is such a totally different condition from the oblique type that it is unfortunate that the term "inguinal" seems to group them together.*

*Andrews and Bissell, 1935*

## INTRODUCTION

In this chapter we will consider the variety of hernias that protrude directly through the floor of Hesselbach's triangle. The defect (or defects) lies medial to the deep inferior epigastric vessels, above the inguinal ligament and lateral to the sheath of rectus abdominis muscle. By no means do all direct inguinal hernias present the same type or degree of abnormality.

## HISTORICAL BACKGROUND

For at least 16 centuries, direct inguinal hernias were not differentiated from the indirect variety. Zimmerman and Veith (1967) discovered the delightful work of Caspar Stromayr, who published his *Practica Copiosa* on July 4, 1559; however, the volume was to lie unappreciated in the city library of Lindau for 350 years. According to Zimmerman and Veith, the book was published in 1925 after the value of the work was recognized by Walter von Brunn. Stromayr recognized that the hernial sacs of some hernias follow the course of the cord. We recognize these as *indirect hernias*. Direct hernias, of course, do not follow the oblique path of the indirect sac.

Heister [according to Iason (1941)] de-scribed direct inguinal hernias in 1724. This knowledge, although interesting, had little practical value for nearly 175 years.

Hesselbach produced his anatomic observations in 1814, when he described the boundaries of his triangle (see Fig. 2–10, p. 28). Surgeons were unable to apply the anatomic knowledge prior to the discovery of asepsis and anesthesia. In the late nineteenth century—as the result of progress in both bacteriology and anesthesiology—surgeons were able to operate with minimal danger of infection and without pain. As a result of numerous efforts at an operative cure of hernia, surgeons began to recognize significant differences among the varieties of groin hernias.

## CLINICAL PATHOLOGIC CORRELATION AND CONSIDERATIONS

The direct inguinal hernia, for practical purposes, should be considered an acquired hernia; this is appropriate, since such hernias most often occur in an adult or elderly population. There is little to be gained by arguing that since the anatomic weaknesses or variations permitting ultimate direct herniation are present at birth, the resulting hernia should be considered congenital in origin.

Direct hernias characteristically appear in the adult or elderly patient. Andrews and Bissel in 1934 pointed out that in patients who ultimately develop direct hernias, there is a deficiency in the lower portions of the internal oblique muscle. Because of this deficiency, the transversus abdominis lamina in the posterior wall of the inguinal canal lacks the protection afforded by the internal oblique muscle. With atrophy of tissue due to aging or obesity and aggravated by increased intra-abdominal pressure, protrusion occurs through the weakest portion of the abdominal wall. Andrews and Bissell designated this area the *inguinal triangle*. Its upper boundary is the margin of the internal oblique; the lateral (or lower) boundary is the inguinal ligament, and the medial boundary is the sheath of the rectus abdominis muscle (Fig. 13–1). The enormous importance of the inguinal triangle, which is so difficult to repair when defective, has not been fully appreciated until recent years. Excessive tension at the suture line in repairing defects in this triangular area is most difficult to control.

Direct inguinal hernias protrude through the floor of Hesselbach's triangle, which is relatively weaker than the remaining abdominal wall. The force of protrusion is greater at this site than is the restraining capacity of the abdominal wall. Obesity has been recognized as a factor that results in increased intra-abdominal pressure. Fatty infiltration ap-

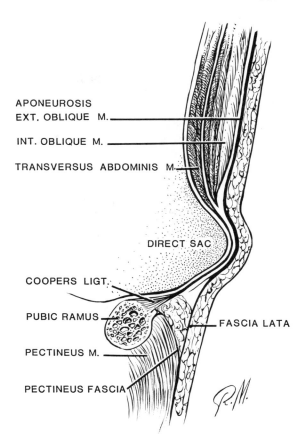

**Figure 13–2.** Sagittal view of the groin in a direct hernia, showing the large defect between the transversus arch and the inguinal ligament. (By permission of *Surgery, Gynecology and Obstetrics.* Modified from Andrews, E., and Bissell, A. D.: Direct hernia: A record of surgical failures. Surg. Gynecol. Obstet. 58:753, 1954.)

pears to decrease the holding strength of the abdominal wall layers.

Typically, the direct inguinal hernia develops slowly over a long period of time. The opening of the hernial sac is quite large when compared to the length of the sac, and as a result, direct hernias are easily reduced and rarely become incarcerated (Fig. 13–2). They do not, as a rule, descend into the scrotum; however, the largest hernias of this type may expand toward the upper scrotum.

## ANATOMIC CONSIDERATIONS

Every direct hernia, by definition, protrudes through the weakness in the abdominal wall in Hesselbach's triangle. Therefore, this triangle must be looked at

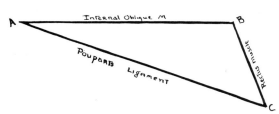

Fig. 6. The inguinal triangle. In order to obliterate this triangle surgically it is necessary to bring point *B* down to line *AC*. It is obvious that the entire pull of the rectus muscle is applied to prevent this. Such a closure can be made only by applying tension that augurs badly for the permanence of the result.

**Figure 13–1.** Andrews and Bissell's description of the inguinal triangle. (By permission of *Surgery, Gynecology and Obstetrics.* From Andrews, E., and Bissell, A. D.: Direct hernia: A record of surgical failures. Surg. Gynecol. Obstet. 58:753, 1954.)

in more detail, since the complexity of the problem will vary in relation to the precise site of protrusion. Although Hesselbach's triangle is the anatomic site of protrusion of direct inguinal hernias, it is the inguinal triangle of Andrews and Bissell that more clearly defines the site and character of the defect (see Fig. 13–1).

Practically, direct hernial sacs must exit first through a defect in the transversus abdominis lamina. After the external oblique has been opened and the spermatic cord identified, it is seen that the sac arises independently of the cord. The direct hernial sac is covered by an attenuated layer of fascia, which may be traced above to the transversus abdominis muscle and aponeurosis. Inferiorly, or toward the inguinal ligament, the transversalis fascia again becomes recognized as a structure of some substance. It runs in an identifiable, but thin, band just above Poupart's ligament toward the pubic tubercle and Cooper's ligament; this structure is variously designated as *iliopubic tract, Thomson's ligament,* and *bandelette iliopubienne.* Laterally, the deep inferior epigastric artery is an important anatomic landmark.

Andrews and Bissell (1934) have significantly pointed out that in direct inguinal hernias, the internal oblique and transversus abdominis muscles and their aponeuroses have a high insertion into the sheath of the rectus abdominis muscle. Upon contraction of these muscles, there is no defense mechanism against protrusion, since there is no significant tendency for the muscles to approximate Poupart's ligament. Thus, absence of sphincteric action at this site is a result of the musculo-aponeurotic deficiency.

## SITES OF PROTRUSION

There are essentially two portals of exit for direct inguinal hernias; both, of course, are situated medial to the deep inferior epigastric arteries.

First, the protrusion may occur through the middle fossa, which is situated between the folds of the deep inferior epigastric artery and the obliterated hypogastric artery.

Second, the protrusion may occur between the obliterated hypogastric artery

and the urachal fold. Practically, the medial boundary of a direct hernia of this type is actually the lateral portion of the tendon of the rectus abdominis muscle. The usual bulge due to a direct inguinal hernia is more or less diffuse and occupies a good portion of Hesselbach's triangle. The mouth, or opening, of the direct sac is usually quite large (see Fig. 13–2).

Perhaps the most difficult concept to teach resident physicians is that groin hernias must be viewed in three-dimensional perspective. The relationship of the transversus arch to Cooper's ligament and the inguinal ligament should be noted. How acute is the angle between the inguinal ligament and Cooper's ligament? How much tension is generated in the hernia being repaired by attaching the transversus arch to Cooper's ligament?

Occasionally, a diverticular type of sac presents medial to the deep inferior epigastric vessels; in such cases, the defect in the abdominal wall is small in diameter, but the sac is often four to six centimeters in length. This is the type of direct inguinal hernia often seen in females. Repair of such direct inguinal hernias is a much simpler problem than occurs when there is a large diffuse weakness in the floor of the inguinal canal.

## TECHNIQUES AVAILABLE FOR REPAIR

One area of hernia surgery that is always open to debate concerns techniques for repair of the posterior wall of the abdomen in the inguinal region. Here, *argumentum ex auctoritate* prevails. Those who would dissent with popularly held views are looked upon as surgical "heretics." Surgeons and anatomists speak convincingly of "normal" anatomic relationships in situations where, in fact, they do not exist. Who would argue that the patient with groin hernias has "normal" anatomic structures? The nearest semblance to a "normal" anatomic relationship of structures is seen in the patient with congenitally patent processus vaginalis. Even here, the long and open peritoneal sac is abnormal (although the abdominal laminae may be normal).

In the patient with direct inguinal hernia, the disposition of the internal oblique and transversus abdominis musculo-aponeurotic structures is such as to permit protrusion. In order to repair a direct inguinal hernia of some size, this defect in Hesselbach's triangle must be closed effectively and permanently. There are two obvious methods to achieve this goal. First, some shifting of structures of greater strength than those present in the defect is absolutely necessary if repair is to succeed. Second, a strong, well-tolerated, and durable prosthetic material could replace deficient tissue and add necessary strength. A combination of both principles constitutes an effective method of repair in selected cases.

Surgeons devised ingenious methods for disposition of the external oblique aponeurosis, other layers of the abdominal wall, and the cord and testicle.

A chaotic situation has been created as a result of innumerable operative techniques offered for repair of direct inguinal hernias. In order to identify common denominators, I have attempted to devise a simplified classification of the various techniques available for repair of such hernias. Minor variations in technical performance have too often served as justification for yet another eponymic designation of a recommended procedure. Sound principles are sometimes overlooked in the struggle to immortalize the name of proponents of assorted techniques that, too often, have little enduring value. The discussion that follows is an attempt to identify important broad differences in anatomic approach and to identify many, but by no means all, of the contributors who have left their "pen-prints" upon the rich history of surgical treatment of hernia. We will assume that technologically the modern era of herniology began with the work of Bassini and Halsted.

It is apparent from Table 13–1 that surgeons have been innovative in their approaches to the problem of hernia repair, in general. Proponents of the various techniques were enthusiastic in their recommendations, with the result that some of them enjoyed more than a fleeting popularity. Typical methods under each category will be described briefly, and an attempt will be made to identify the differences as well as the similarities between

**Table 13–1. MODERN TECHNIQUES FOR DIRECT INGUINAL HERNIA REPAIR**

I  *SINGLE-LAYERED CLOSURE*
 Halsted I (1890)
 Madden et al. (1971)
II  *MULTI-LAYERED CLOSURE*
 (Bassini-Halsted principle)
  Bassini (1887)
  Ferguson (1899)
  Andrews (1895)
  Halsted II (1903)°
  Fallis (1938)°
  Zimmerman (1938, 1952)
  Rienhoff (1940)°
  Tanner (1942)°
  Glassow (1943) Shouldice repair
  Griffith (1958)°
  Lichtenstein (1964, 1966)°
  Palumbo (1967)
  Smith (1977)°
III  *COOPER'S LIGAMENT REPAIR*
 (Lotheissen-McVay Principle)
  Narath (cited by Lotheissen, 1898)
  Lotheissen (1898)
  McVay (1942, 1958)
  (For more details and other contributions, see text and Fig. 15–3, p. 241.)
IV  *PREPERITONEAL APPROACH* (Closure of transversus abdominis lamina from within abdomen)
  Cheatle (1920)
  Henry (1936)
  Musgrove and McGready (1940)
  Mikkelson and Berne (1954)
  Nyhus et al. (1959)
  Condon (1960). See Nyhus, Condon, and Harkins (1960)
  Read (1976). Preperitoneal repair with prosthesis
  (For more historical facts, see Chapter 15.)
V  *REPAIR WITH PROSTHETIC MATERIALS*
  Koontz (1956)
  Usher (1960)
  (For more details, see Chapter 26.)

°Also added relaxing incision.

the various techniques in correcting the anatomic defect of direct inguinal herniations.

## Single-Layered Closure

The single-layered closure might be considered an oversimplification of the actual anatomic restructuring of the inguinal region—a method that is included in this group. Nevertheless, it is important to identify common denominators in the inexhaustible varieties of methods advocated for repair of hernias. Currently, few surgeons depend upon a single-layered closure for repair of the posterior abdominal wall.

In 1890 Halsted described a method of repair in which interrupted sutures of strong silk were passed so as to include everything between the skin and the peritoneum. In this procedure, the cord, reduced to the vas deferens and its vessels, was transplanted to the upper outer angle of the wound. Halsted closed the transversalis fascia, transversus abdominis muscle, and internal oblique and external oblique aponeurosis beneath the "skeletonized" cord with interrupted heavy silk sutures; this procedure was known as the "Halsted I repair." It was abandoned because of an unacceptably high incidence of postoperative testicular atrophy and hydroceles. Essentially, then, in his earliest procedure Halsted brought four layers of the abdominal wall to the inguinal ligament with a single row of heavy silk sutures. The cord was transplanted to its subcutaneous position in the process. The Halsted I procedure just described enjoyed only a brief period of usefulness and was never employed widely in this country or abroad.

Madden and his colleagues are among the few modern surgeons who depend essentially upon single-layered repair for correction of direct inguinal hernias after closure of the peritoneum. In 1971, he described his rationale for the technique he found effective. Madden sutures what he elects to designate as the medial segment of the transversus abdominis lamina to its lateral segment, known variously as the iliopubic tract, Thomson's ligament, and the femoral or deep crural arch. Madden's procedure is clearly illustrated in his published work (1971). Various terms are applied to objectives of repairs advocated by different surgeons. Madden calls his technique of repair anatomic because it restores the integrity of the transversus abdominis layer. In his procedure, Madden opened the tissue planes individually, then repaired them in reverse order.

## Multilayered Closure (The Bassini-Halsted II Principle)

The operations included in the multilayered closure group have been variously modified and have generated the most rhetoric. I have chosen the name "multilayered closure" for the technique in which the laminae of the abdominal wall are variously rearranged. This group includes a number of variants, and some of the better-known methods will be briefly described. In order to achieve some decrease in the total number of eponymic designations, I have included here several technical variants under the Bassini-Halsted II principle. By what authority do I feel justified in referring to this approach as the Bassini-Halsted II principle? Halsted himself recognized several features common to both the Bassini and Halsted repairs. In Chapter 11, I have described the modified Bassini operation as I perform it.

Since the efforts of Bassini and Halsted, most surgeons have chosen to repair defects in the inguinal area by approximating several layers of the abdominal wall. This category of procedures has attracted several variations (some of which are minor) in technique. Furthermore, the rationale for many repairs in which the inguinal ligament is used in reconstruction is challenged by some authorities, while others are equally convinced that the Cooper's ligament may be used with success. The arguments for both views must be presented in order to achieve a better understanding of the problem.

In 1895 E. Wyllys Andrews, an advocate of strict asepsis and careful hemostasis in his operative technique, described his method of imbrication of the external oblique aponeurosis over the spermatic cord. In his repair method, Andrews advised high ligation of the peritoneal sac. He sutured the "conjoined tendon" and transversalis fascia to Poupart's ligament, emphasizing that the ring should fit snugly about the spermatic cord. Thus far in describing Andrews' repair, we might be reviewing the technical details of a Bassini repair. Andrews observed that in some patients, the Bassini operation resulted in considerable tension at the suture line—i.e., following suture of "conjoined tendon" and internal oblique aponeurosis to Poupart's ligament. At this point, he recommended his method of imbrication. Andrews included external oblique aponeurosis, "conjoined tendon," and transversalis fascia in the posterior wall, then brought the lower leaflet of external oblique aponeurosis anterior to the spermatic cord. The repair might therefore be called the Bassini-Halsted-Andrews repair.

Ferguson described his method for hernia repair in 1899. I consider Ferguson's method to be obsolete for two reasons. First, leaving the spermatic cord undisturbed makes it impossible to assess the condition of the floor of Hesselbach's triangle. Second, the technique of suturing the internal oblique muscle over the cord and attaching it to the inguinal ligament is ill conceived. Muscle tissue is a poor structure to utilize for the purpose of reinforcement of the defective area. Excessive tension at the suture line of a repair precludes permanency of the reconstruction. Few surgeons today have the courage to resort to the Ferguson repair as a method of herniorrhaphy.

Most surgeons do agree on one anatomic defect in groin hernias—i.e., groin hernias must protrude through the transversus abdominis aponeurotico-fascial layer. Most surgeons also endorse the concept that this layer should be closed precisely. But discussing the way in which this closure is to be accomplished and the rationale for such closure provokes a debate that, at times, is charged more with emotion than with fact.

The greatest difference in opinion regarding effective repair of groin hernias concerns the use of the inguinal ligament as an anchoring structure. Following Bassini's reports and continuing for some time thereafter, there was no question as to the desirability of anchoring the abdominal laminae to Poupart's ligament, However, serious differences in opinion as to how groin hernias should be repaired began, in 1942, with the significant anatomic observations of McVay and Anson In that year, they recognized what was called a fundamental error in methods utilized by many surgeons. They pointed out the inguinal ligament was ill suited to serve as an anchoring structure for the layers of the abdominal wall. McVay and Anson emphasized that in fact, the margin of Poupart's ligament was normally free of attachments to the laminae of the abdominal wall. An instrument could easily be passed through an investing fascia between the inguinal ligament and the transversus abdominis aponeurosis. They further recognized that the latter structure actually has a firm attachment to Cooper's ligament. Thus, it would seem more appropriate to suture the transversus arch or the transversus aponeurosis to Cooper's ligament rather than to Poupart's ligament. In spite of the fact that many surgeons recognize these anatomic arrangements, there is a difference of opinion as to how hernias should be repaired.

Palumbo and colleagues described their modifications of the Bassini-Halsted repair in 1967. The method includes complete dissection of the peritoneal sac, followed by high ligation. The transversalis fascia is first closed, and then the internal oblique aponeurosis is sutured to the inguinal ligament with number 2–0 silk. In the process of repair, a new and snug internal ring is created. The external oblique aponeurosis is divided, so that its leaflets can be imbricated beneath the cord. In an extensive experience with this method, the authors report an overall recurrence rate of 1 percent.

Zimmerman, for example, recognized the validity of McVay's anatomic concepts but disagreed somewhat as to their application. According to Zimmerman, if the laxity of the inguinal ligament were an undesirable feature, its use in repair of inguinal hernias would first result in its upward displacement and then in femoral herniation. Such hernias do occur, but they are uncommon. Furthermore, it is well known that most recurrent groin hernias are of the direct or indirect variety. In a critique of the McVay repair, Zimmerman (1948) pointed out that identification of Cooper's ligament is technically more difficult and that there is greater danger in injury to the femoral vessels, particularly the femoral vein. Accessory obturator arteries may cause additional technical difficulties. Zimmerman, in another pertinent observation, noted that any operation in which a rigid, unyielding structure is used as an anchoring site must be wrong in conception. Excessive muscle pull exerted by the abdominal musculature must result in ischemic necrosis, with the sutures cutting through the tissue at the site of greatest tension.

Glassow (1976) has compared the experience of the Shouldice Hospital in

Toronto with that of Halverson and McVay in the repair of groin hernias. Surgeons at the Shouldice Hospital utilized the inguinal ligament in the repair, while Halverson and McVay utilized Cooper's ligament. Glassow, who found the Shouldice repair effective, utilizes the inguinal ligament in repair of inguinal hernias. As described by Glassow (1976), in the Shouldice repair the innermost of three musculoaponeurotic layers of the abdominal wall must be reconstructed. The strength of the floor of the inguinal canal is assessed by insertion of the finger deep to the transversalis fascia in the peritoneal space. The posterior wall is then divided according to the indications of each patient. Glassow considered the lower or lateral flap of transversalis fascia, which measures from 1 to 2 cm in width, vital to the success of the Shouldice repair; whereas McVay felt that the residual posterior wall was not suitable for repair. Glassow identified a flap of transversalis fascia that was "usually quite substantial and occasionally very strong." Thus, it is clear that a difference of opinion exists as to the quality of the residual transversalis abdominis layer in direct inguinal hernias. There is no disagreement with the view that the transversalis fascia is ultimately attached to Cooper's ligament.

In my opinion, it is essential to appreciate that Glassow recognized the importance of reconstituting the integrity of the transversalis fascial layer. He achieved repair of this layer by an overlapping technique with number 34 gauge monofilament stainless steel wire sutures. The transversalis fascia is carefully and snugly closed at the internal ring. In the completed repair, four lines of continuous nonabsorbable sutures are placed. Respect for the importance of the transversus abdominis lamina and for the ideal of multilayered closure without tension—accomplished with continuous nonabsorbable sutures of stainless steel wire—are desirable features of the Shouldice repair.

A variety of dispositions of the external oblique aponeurosis have been made by surgeons. E. Wyllys Andrews in 1895 showed a number of possible variations for closure of this structure. Poth as recently as 1971 described a method in which he used the rectus pyramidalis sheath.

It might be stated that in the proper management of the defect, what is done with the transversus abdominis aponeurotico-fascial lamina is far more important than what is done with the more superficial layers of the abdomen. The outer layers, including the external oblique aponeurosis, give direction to the path of the recurrence but cannot prevent relapses.

Other surgeons who have utilized variations of multilayered repair of the inguinal floor include Zimmerman, Fallis, Rienhoff, Tanner, and Smith.

Lichtenstein (1976) also challenged the concept that suture of the abdominal laminae to Cooper's ligament was the only desirable method for repair of direct inguinal hernias. He brought up the issue of excessive tension at the suture line that occurs when Cooper's ligament is utilized in repair. He noted that Poupart's ligament is actually nearer to the transversus abdominis arch than is Cooper's ligament. Furthermore, the distance between the transversus abdominis arch and Cooper's ligament increases significantly as the repair is carried laterally toward the femoral vein. I myself have found that tension is greatest at this site (see Fig. 14–8, p. 230). Again, the relaxing incision is essential to avoid undue tension at the suture line.

Doran (1955) emphasized the adverse effects of excessive tension at the suture line and pointed out that the result might be a recurrent hernia.

## Cooper's Ligament Repair (Lotheissen-McVay Principle)

The important fundamental anatomic observations of Anson and McVay have established the Cooper's ligament repair, or Lotheissen-McVay principle, as a sound technique for the repair of direct inguinal and femoral hernias.

Much earlier (1898), however, Lotheissen ingeniously utilized Cooper's ligament in the repair of a recurrent hernia in which the inguinal ligament had been destroyed in a previous attempt at repair.

He noted that Narath had performed a similar procedure.

Seelig and Tuholske in 1914 and Dickson in 1936 realized the desirable features of employing Cooper's ligament in repair of inguinal hernias, but McVay established the efficacy of the method. The qualities of Cooper's ligament that recommend its use as an anchoring structure include its accessibility and strength, as well as its direct attachment to bone. It is easily identified as a thick fibrous ridge along the iliopectineal eminence. Many surgeons have recognized the importance of the Lotheissen-McVay principle in hernia repair. Harkins noted that by 1949, at least forty publications had appeared on the subject, attesting to the significance of this method. He enthusiastically endorsed the principle of the McVay repair, and his illustrations in a 1949 issue of Surgical Clinics of North America (see Reference section) are recommended for the excellence of presentation.

## Preperitoneal Approach

The status of the preperitoneal approach in the repair of direct inguinal hernias is not completely clear at present. The method had been described by Cheatle in 1920 and was used by Henry for repair of femoral hernias in 1936. Larger experiences with the method were reported by Musgrove and McCready in 1949, Mikkelson and Berne in 1954, and Nyhus in 1959. Read in 1976 utilized the preperitoneal approach to place a prosthesis used in the repair of selected direct inguinal hernias. The subject of preperitoneal herniorrhaphy is presented in greater detail in Chapter 15.

## Hoguet Maneuver

The management of the peritoneal sac in indirect inguinal hernias is not a problem to most surgeons. It is generally accepted that dissection of the sacs and high ligation of the peritoneum are important steps in repair. In the case of a direct hernia, the sac may be ignored or inverted or dissected and ligated (after incising the transversalis fascia and peri-

toneum at the site of the herniation medial to the deep inferior epigastric vessels). The last technique, in my opinion, is dangerous, since injury to the bladder may occur.

Besides the alternatives just described, there is another technique—one that is, unfortunately, ignored by many surgeons. In 1920 Hoguet described his method for reducing the direct sac safely. He stated:

As mentioned before, an indirect sac can always be found in these cases (of direct hernia), although it may be very small. This sac is separated from the elements of the cord and opened. It has not been found necessary to divide the deep epigastric vessels, but by traction outwards on the indirect sac, all of the peritoneum of the direct sac may be pulled external to the vessels and the two sacs converted into one. By this proceeding, all possibility of injuring the bladder is eliminated, for as the peritoneum of the direct sac is pulled outwards under the epigastrics if the bladder folds are adherent to the under surface of the sac, they can be clearly seen. This redundant peritoneum of indirect and direct sac is then transfixed with a suture and cut away.

I have included Hoguet's description because of its clarity. Conversion of the direct sac into an indirect one is safe and simple. This maneuver permits digital exploration of the direct weakness and identification of a femoral hernia. It adds an important methodic dimension to the surgical treatment of groin hernias.

McClure and Fallis in 1939 recognized the value of the Hoguet maneuver and applied this principle to the reduction of peritoneal sacs due to femoral hernias. The maneuver of Hoguet is being increasingly recognized as a basic step in the repair of direct inguinal hernias. Harkins, Swenson, Burton, and Griffith are other surgeons who have seen the value of converting the direct sac into an indirect one. Fallis fully recognized the importance of the Hoguet maneuver, referring to it in 1938 and again in 1964. Lytle of Great Britain also called attention to this technique for conversion of the direct sac into an indirect one. More recently (1977), Qvist emphasized the usefulness of this method for managing the combination of simultaneous indirect-direct inguinal hernias.

### The Relaxing Incision

I consider the relaxing incision to be of such importance that Chapter 25 is devoted entirely to this subject. As can be seen in Table 13–1, the number of surgeons resorting to this important adjunct is increasing slowly, but definitely. The devastating effect of excessive tension on the line of repair is being more and more appreciated by surgeons. The relaxing incision is essential in repair of many direct inguinal hernias.

## TECHNICAL DETAILS OF REPAIR OF DIRECT INGUINAL HERNIAS

*Curative operations for hernia are now upon an entirely new basis, and form a highly perfected and specialized branch of the art.*

*E. Wyllys Andrews, 1895*

The direct inguinal hernia is frequently difficult to repair and should be considered on an individual basis. There are some direct hernias in which the defect in Hesselbach's triangle is quite small. The actual defect in the transversalis fascia in this area may measure only one to three centimeters. Such hernias are comparatively simple to repair. The difficulty arises in the repair of those direct hernias in which the entire floor is defective from the pubic tubercle to the internal ring. Furthermore, it is important to assess the magnitude of the weakness from the inguinal ligament to the arch formed by the internal oblique and transversus abdominis muscles above (Fig. 13–3). In years past, this structure was erroneously designated as the "conjoined tendon." It was found to be tendinous, albeit infrequently. Currently, it is called the transversus abdominis arch. In the repair of such hernias, it is essential that this attenuated area be strengthened. The hope that a large defect can be bridged successfully, consistently, and permanently by approximating available structures without any relaxing incision is ill founded. In the repair of direct hernias under local anesthesia, one of the serendipitous advantages is that the surgeon is able to see immediately the effect of his endeavors. Since the patient retains a great deal of his normal abdominal tonus as well as his reflexes, the repair may be tested by having the patient cough vigorously. In large direct inguinal hernias repaired without relaxing incisions in the anterior sheath of the rectus muscle, a single suture of number 2–0 silk will frequently give way under the strain of a single lusty cough. Since I have seen this occur with a single strand, I have resorted to the use of two strands of heavy silk or of synthetic nonabsorbable material for placing the master stitch in selected patients.

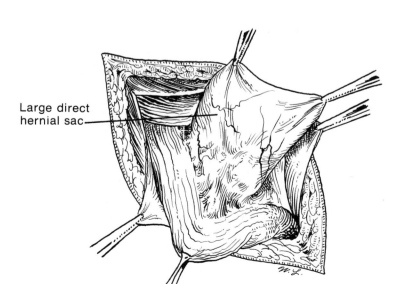

Large direct hernial sac

**Figure 13–3.** A large hernial sac protruding through the floor of Hesselbach's triangle.

There is no need to describe the skin incision or to proceed with any further detail of the procedure until the external oblique fascia has been opened, as was already described for indirect inguinal hernia repair (Figs. 11–1 and 11–2; pp. 160 and 161.

Access to the inguinal area is gained in the manner presented earlier. The large protrusion through the floor of Hesselbach's triangle is independent of the cord (Fig. 13–3).

The spermatic cord is elevated out of the floor of Hesselbach's triangle. Unless a combination of direct and indirect inguinal hernia exists, the cord is quite small. It is well known that in uncomplicated direct inguinal hernias, there is little or no hypertrophy of the cremaster muscle. For this reason, it is not necessary to excise the cremaster in every patient with an inguinal hernia. In fact, I seldom excise the cremaster muscle in patients with direct inguinal hernias.

The cremaster muscle is opened at the internal abdominal ring; the small tonguelike projection of peritoneum can be easily identified at the superior and medial margin. Placement of a loop retractor under the internal oblique muscle, along with gentle traction on the cord, makes identification easier.

I do not, as a rule, open the transversalis fascia medial to the deep inferior epigastric artery to achieve access to the peritoneal cavity, as there is danger to the bladder if this is done without due care. I have found it much safer to open the sac laterally to the deep inferior epigastric vessels. The area is carefully explored digitally for the presence of a femoral hernia, and the magnitude of the defect in the floor of Hesselbach's triangle is determined. Furthermore, with traction applied to the clamps placed about the sac, it is simple to convert the direct sac (and even a femoral sac) into an indirect sac as described by Hoguet

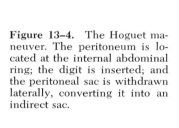

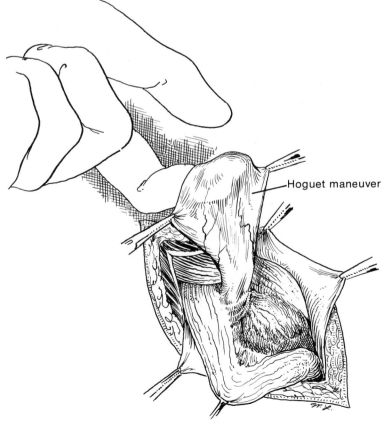

**Figure 13–4.** The Hoguet maneuver. The peritoneum is located at the internal abdominal ring; the digit is inserted; and the peritoneal sac is withdrawn laterally, converting it into an indirect sac.

Hoguet maneuver

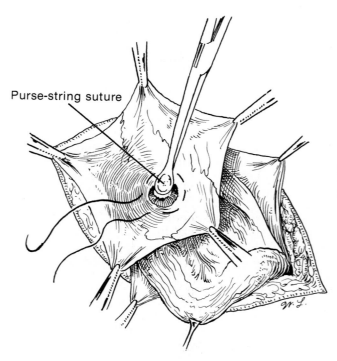

Purse-string suture

**Figure 13–5.** The peritoneal sac is closed with a purse-string suture of number 2–0 silk.

(Fig. 13–4). I wish to emphasize that the Hoguet maneuver reduces the peritoneal sac, regardless of its type. Some surgeons prefer to open the narrow, diverticular type of sac for inspection prior to ligation. The diffuse type of sac may be inverted, since there is little danger of incarceration of viscera.

A purse-string suture of heavy (or number 2) silk is placed to achieve peritoneal closure (Fig. 13–5). The ligated peritoneal sac withdraws to a position deep to the transversalis fascia (Fig. 13–6).

The transversalis fascia is triangulated at the internal ring and closed with sutures of number 3–0 silk. Accurate and separate closure of the transversalis fascia is just as important here as it is in the repair of indirect inguinal hernias, if recurrence as an indirect inguinal hernia is to be avoided (Fig. 13–7). Clear identification of structures and their precise approximation are mandatory if failures are

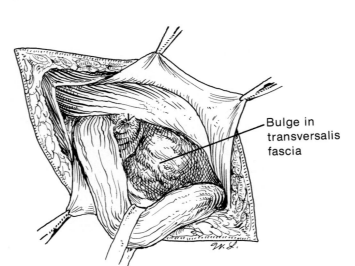

Bulge in transversalis fascia

**Figure 13–6.** After the Hoguet maneuver is performed, the bulge in the attenuated transversalis fascia must be eliminated.

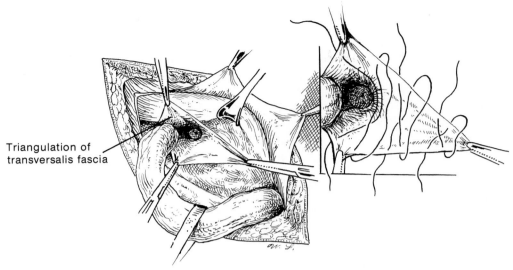

Triangulation of
transversalis fascia

**Figure 13–7.** The transversalis lamina at the internal ring is triangulated (for accurate identification) and closed snugly about the cord.

to be kept at an absolute minimum. Faulty, inaccurate closure of the transversalis fascia at the internal ring often accounts for indirect recurrent inguinal hernias after initial repair of direct inguinal hernia.

The next step in the repair may be subject to a difference in opinion as to its conduct and effectiveness. I have not found it necessary to excise the redundant and attenuated transversalis fascia.

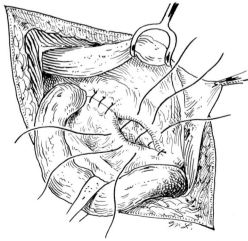

**Figure 13–8.** The attenuated transversalis fascia is imbricated, but it is the transversus arch—when sutured to either the inguinal ligament or Cooper's ligament—that provides strength in the repair.

Excision is acceptable if eventual closure is accurate. This structure is imbricated or inverted with sutures of number 3 or medium silk, placed at intervals of one centimeter from the pubic tubercle to the internal ring (Fig. 13–8). This imbrication is not to be misconstrued as the actual repair. I have no objection to the practice of excision of the attenuated transversalis fascia.

The external oblique aponeurosis is elevated, and the relaxing incision is made in the anterior sheath of the rectus muscle (Fig. 13–9). I make this incision as near the midline as possible, but in no circumstance would I carry this incision into the midline. Fortunately, it is not possible to reach the midline in most patients by elevating the external oblique aponeurosis. But should there be an instance in which there is failure of fusion of the external oblique, incision into the midline would result in a hernia. More significant is the fact that I have never seen a hernia develop as the consequence of a relaxing incision as we perform it. I would like to repeat that, in my opinion, the increasing use of the relaxing incision is the single greatest advance during the current quarter century toward the successful repair of hernias associated with large weaknesses in the floor of Hesselbach's triangle.

Accurate dissection and correct identification of structures in the medialmost

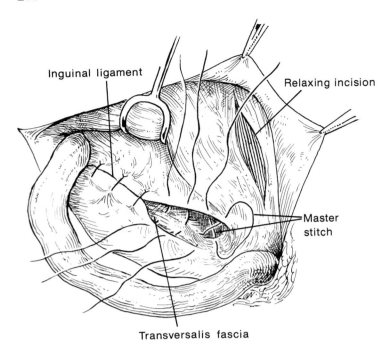

Inguinal ligament

Relaxing incision

Master stitch

Transversalis fascia

**Figure 13–9.** A relaxing incision is almost always needed to free the transversus arch from excessive tension. It is made obliquely in the anterior sheath of the rectus abdominis. Placement of the master stitch medially between the transversus abdominis arch, Cooper's ligament, Gimbernat's ligament, and the inguinal ligament occludes the medial aspect of Hesselbach's triangle. It is of paramount importance that the transversus arch is sutured to the iliopubic tract and inguinal ligament.

aspect of Hesselbach's triangle is of paramount importance at this point. I am referring to the medial projection of the inguinal ligament, the iliopubic tract, the medial portion of Cooper's ligament, and the projection of the internal oblique and transversus abdominis medially. This area is critical in the repair of the direct inguinal hernia and important in the repair of a femoral hernia.

As I have indicated, the variation in the magnitude of the weakness in the inguinal floor offers a choice in the technique of repair. In small direct inguinal hernias, I employ a method that is a variation of the Bassini repair. In the variation, placement of the medialmost suture (or "master stitch") includes Cooper's ligament, components of the internal oblique and transversus abdominis muscles, and Gimbernat's ligament (Fig. 13–9). In principle, this important stitch accomplishes attachment of the posterior abdominal wall to Cooper's ligament. Thus, the most powerful structures in the medial aspect of Hesselbach's triangle are shifted the shortest distance to strengthen the abdominal wall. Double strands of heavy (or number 2–0) silk or a synthetic nonabsorbable suture have been found effective and necessary in maintaining approximation of the structures just described. The remaining sutures are placed laterally and include fibers from the transversus abdominis and transversalis fascia, above, and the iliopubic tract and inguinal ligament, below.

During my years as a resident, I had been introduced to the Halsted I repair in which the external oblique was approximated under the spermatic cord. The theory was advanced that such a closure strengthened the floor of Hesselbach's triangle. The objection most commonly raised to such a closure was that the internal and external rings were superimposed upon each other, with resulting weakness at this point. According to those individuals who objected to this method of closure, indirect recurrences were more frequent at this site. In my opinion, it is the high ligation of the peritoneal sac as well as the accurate closure of the transversalis fascia at the internal ring that prevents indirect recurrences. In addition, I have found that it matters little what one does with the external oblique aponeurosis, provided that closure of the transversus abdominis layer is sound. Nevertheless, I have personally employed the Halsted I repair with less frequency in the past five years (Fig. 13–10).

The knowledgeable surgeon should have a number of techniques that he can

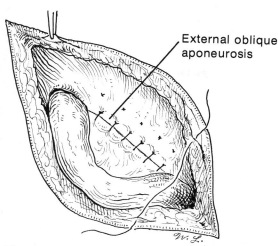

**Figure 13–10.**   The spermatic cord is replaced upon the imbricated aponeurosis of the external oblique.

execute skillfully, depending upon the needs of the situation at hand. Pioneer surgeons exemplified this quality on many occasions. In this context, the use of the Lotheissen-McVay repair of direct inguinal hernias is a case in point. When the weakness in the floor of Hesselbach's triangle is large, it may be sound to suture the internal oblique aponeurosis and transversus abdominis arch to Cooper's ligament. I first place the medialmost stitch (the master stitch) as already described. This suture consists of double strands of heavy silk or nonabsorbable suture, placed on a short stout needle. The use of such a needle is important, if breakage is to be avoided. Number 2–0 sutures are placed laterally, at intervals of approximately one centimeter, until the weakened floor is adequately repaired. It must be emphasized that two or three sutures placed indifferently will not effect a strong repair laterally near the femoral vein. If there is any doubt as to the proximity of the vein, then I dissect enough to properly visualize this structure. In the performance of the McVay repair, no less attention is given to the internal ring. The transversalis fascia had been closed, as previously described, using triangulation of the transversalis fascia. In addition, I suture the transversus abdominis and transversalis fascia to the inguinal ligament at the internal ring.

The need for the relaxing incision in the repair of the direct inguinal hernia by the McVay technique is an important detail, if excessive tension is to be avoided. The effects of tension upon the suture line are dramatically demonstrated when this repair is performed under local anesthesia, and the patient is permitted to cough.

The external oblique is approximated over the cord, which remains in the so-called Bassini position. As I have observed and participated in increasing numbers of hernia repairs, I am more convinced that the success or failure of a hernia repair is determined well before the external oblique is reached. In other words, what is done before the external oblique is reached is of far greater consequence than what is finally done with this structure.

The subcutaneous tissues are approximated with plain number 3–0 catgut. The epidermis is closed with adhesive strips.

## CLINICAL STUDY

This study was directed at patients with direct inguinal hernias but no other problems insofar as the groin area was concerned. Available records of patients operated on between 1950 and 1968 were reviewed. A total of 493 patients had 609 direct inguinal hernias repaired; 116 were repaired simultaneously. An additional 131 patients had the contralateral hernia repaired as a second, or separate procedure.

### Sex

There were 486 males and only seven females with direct inguinal hernias in this study. These statistics confirm the recognized fact that direct inguinal hernias are a rare event in females. The incidence of direct inguinal hernias in females was less than 1.5 percent of the total number of hernias; hence, 98.5 percent of direct inguinal hernias occurred in males.

The infrequent occurrence of direct inguinal hernias in females can be explained on an anatomic basis. The total muscle mass appears to have little to do with the capability of resistance to herniation. Rather, it is the stronger anatomic arrangement of the internal oblique and transversus abdominis in the female that is so effective in preventing herniation. The musculo-aponeurotic components of the internal oblique and transversus abdominis muscles connect much lower onto the rectus sheath and have a relatively wide attachment to the iliopectineal ligament.

### Age Distribution

Direct inguinal hernias are characteristically an affliction of adults and the elderly. Direct protrusions are rarely seen in infants and children. Of 609 hernias occurring in 493 patients, none had been seen in an infant or child under ten years of age (Table 13–2).

It can be seen that direct inguinal hernias occur in adults—in those whom the vicissitudes of life take their toll. Increasing abdominal pressure due to obesity, hard work, and intra-abdominal disease join together in various combinations to place increased pressure upon an abdominal wall that is undergoing some degree of atrophy incident to aging. Approximately 80 percent of the direct inguinal hernias occurred in patients in the fifth, sixth, and seventh decades of life. An additional 13 percent occurred in patients in the fourth decades of their lives.

### Anesthesia

Local anesthesia has been gaining in popularity, as reflected in Table 13–3. Nearly three-fourths of the operations were performed under local anesthesia. Local was combined with general anesthesia in four patients, and a similar number of patients with spinal anesthesia required such supplementation.

Chloroprocaine, as a one percent solution, was the most popular of local anesthetics used on this group of patients. Fifty cubic centimeters was the least amount of solution used, and one patient required 376 cubic centimeters of anesthetic solution. In over 70 percent of the patients, it was found that between 125 to 250 cubic

**Table 13–2. DIRECT INGUINAL HERNIA**

| Age | Number of Patients | Percent |
|---|---|---|
| 0 to 1 year | 0 | 0 |
| 11 to 20 years | 0 | 0 |
| 21 to 30 years | 22 | 4.46 |
| 31 to 40 years | 62 | 12.56 |
| 41 to 50 years | 160 | 32.45 |
| 51 to 60 years | 169 | 34.27 |
| 61 to 70 years | 68 | 13.79 |
| 71 to 80 years | 10 | 2.02 |
| 81 and up | 2 | 0.45 |
| TOTAL | 493 | 100.00 |

centimeters of one percent chloroprocaine provided excellent anesthesia. There were no major complications attributed to the local anesthetic.

### Suture Material

Silk continued to be the preferred suture material and was used in 591, or 97 percent, of the repairs. (Synthetic nonabsorbable sutures are slowly gaining in popularity.) Catgut was used in a single repair of a direct hernia in this study. Wire was used infrequently.

### Technique of Repair

There were some variations in method of repair used by the surgeons of Henry Ford Hospital, but fundamental requirements were generally met (Table 13–4).

The popularity of the Halsted repair at Henry Ford Hospital is attributed to Dr. Roy D. McClure, who received his surgical education under Dr. W. S. Halsted. Dr. Laurence Fallis continued the tradition

**Table 13–3. ANESTHESIA: 609 REPAIRS OF DIRECT INGUINAL HERNIAS**

| Type of Anesthesia | Number of Operations | Percent |
|---|---|---|
| Local | 443 | 72.74 |
| Spinal | 135 | 22.17 |
| General | 23 | 3.78 |
| Combinations | 8 | 1.31 |
|   Local and general = 4 | | |
|   Spinal and general = 4 | | |
| Total | 609 | 100.00 |

Table 13–4.  METHOD OF REPAIR:
609 REPAIRS OF DIRECT
INGUINAL HERNIAS

| Type of Repair | Number of Repairs | Percent |
|---|---|---|
| Halsted | 412 | 67.7 |
| Bassini | 150 | 24.6 |
| McVay | 44 | 7.2 |
| Henry-Cheatle-Nyhus | 3 | 0.5 |
| Total | 609 | 100.0 |

and made contributions of his own. The repair that carries the eponym "Halsted" is reproduced here because of its popularity (Figs. 13–4 to 13–10). Direct inguinal hernias were repaired by the Halsted method in 412, or 67.7 percent, of 609 operations in this study.

The Bassini repair was utilized in 150 patients, or 24.6 percent, of 609 repairs. The essential difference between the Halsted repair and the Bassini repair, as performed at our institution, is in the position of the cord. In the latter procedure, the spermatic cord lies under the aponeurosis of the external oblique.

The McVay repair is a sound approach to surgical correction of direct inguinal hernias. I was surprised that it was used in only 7 percent of 609 repairs. I am currently using the method with increasing frequency.

The preperitoneal approach was used in the repair of only three direct inguinal hernias. In each instance, the surgeon had entered the abdomen because of pelvic pathology.

## Details of Technique

Certain details of technique are carried out with uniform consistency. These are considered so important that they summarized here in Table 13–5.

High ligation of the peritoneal sac is considered an essential detail in the methodical approach to hernia repair. The peritoneum is initially identified at the internal ring, lateral to the deep inferior epigastric artery; and after complete evaluation of the inguinal triangle and the femoral ring, the Hoguet maneuver is performed. This approach, which minimizes the danger of inadvertent cystot-

omy, was performed in 88 percent of the repairs. The attentuated transversalis fascia was inverted without opening of the peritoneal sac in only 11 percent of the operations for direct inguinal hernias. The Hoguet maneuver was performed in 88 percent of the procedures when the peritoneum was initially identified at the internal ring. The value of the Hoguet maneuver is slowly being appreciated by increasing numbers of surgeons. Fallis recognized its importance in 1938, 18 years after it was described by Hoguet.

The relaxing incision has been recognized as an important adjunct to minimize tension at the suture line since 1892, when it was described by Wölfer. A vertical relaxing incision was made in the anterior sheath of the rectus abdominis muscle in 85 percent of the repairs. Such an incision is the simplest method to avoid excessive tension at the line of repair. Details of the relaxing incision are presented in Chapter 25.

Excision of the cremaster muscle had been common practice in the past; in 609 operations, it was excised in 79 percent of the repairs. There is no doubt in my mind that the indication for excision of the cremaster in patients with direct inguinal hernias is minimal, since it is not hypertrophied in uncomplicated direct herniations. Hence, it is currently my practice to leave the cremaster behind if it does not complicate the repair. Taking liberties with the cremaster jeopardizes the blood supply to the testicle and interferes with mobility and position of the testicle. In some patients, the testicle is suspended in an embarrassingly low position following excision of the muscle.

Table 13–5.  TECHNICAL DETAILS:
REPAIR OF 609 DIRECT
INGUINAL HERNIAS

| Technical Detail | Number | Percent |
|---|---|---|
| High Ligation of Sac | 540 | 88.6 |
| Hoguet Maneuver | 540 | 88.6 |
| Relaxing Incision | 516 | 84.6 |
| Excision of Cremaster | 479 | 78.6 |
| Master Stitch | 474 | 77.8 |
| Inversion Direct Sac | 69 | 11.3 |
| Use of Prosthetics | 15 | 2.4 |
| Excision Round Ligament | 6 | 0.9 |
| Bilateral Simultaneous Repair | 116 | 19.0 |

The master stitch is a most important technical detail in the repair of direct inguinal hernias. The suture, usually double strands of number 2–0 silk or synthetic nonabsorbable material, is placed between the medial portion of the transversus abdominis arch, Cooper's ligament, and a portion of Gimbernat's ligament. The suture is placed at the lowest margin of the transversus arch in order to minimize tension. This suture is placed as a figure-of-eight stitch and is inserted with a small "Mayo" needle; this needle is stout, since more fragile needles break too often during insertion into Cooper's ligament (Fig. 13–9). Basically, this suture would correspond to the first two sutures of an ordinary McVay repair. The master stitch was placed in 474, or 77.8 percent, of the repairs.

Prosthetic materials were used in only 15, or 2.4 percent, of the repairs. The reluctance of surgeons to bridge a defect in the groin with a strong, well-accepted material is difficult to understand. The defect in the inguinal triangle is occasionally of such magnitude that repair of the hernia without prosthetic support is doomed to failure, especially when so many direct inguinal hernias are bilateral defects (see Fig. 14–2, p. 218). Marlex mesh was the material used most often, and I currently favor its use.

The round ligament is usually excised in the repairing of groin hernias in females. Such an approach permits complete closure of the internal abdominal ring and facilitates repair. The defect that is present as a direct hernia in females is not at all difficult to repair.

Bilateral simultaneous repair was performed 116 times in this group of 493 patients; thus, in 24 percent of the patients, bilateral simultaneous repairs were accomplished. The arguments against such an approach will be presented in Chapter 14, which discusses direct recurrent inguinal hernias. I have performed bilateral simultaneous repairs for the following two reasons: first, a second procedure, with its attendant cost and disability, is avoided; and second, if proper attention is paid to technical details, the recurrence rate should be low. Methods that generate tension at the site of repair are avoided. Marlex mesh is used as a re-enforcing layer in some cases. The relaxing incision is extremely important in bilateral repairs.

In this regard, I should point out that an additional 131 patients had bilateral separate repairs. Thus, when adding 116 bilateral simultaneous repairs to 131 bilateral separate repairs, it is seen that approximately 50 per cent of patients with direct hernias will sooner or later have bilateral herniations. Whether the bilateral repair is done simultaneously or separately matters relatively little; the persistent problem of tension presents itself sooner or later and must be dealt with appropriately.

## Additional Procedures

A number of additional procedures may be performed on specific indication (Table 13–6). A total number of 67 additional procedures were performed during repair of direct inguinal hernias. Lipomas of the cord were considered to be of sufficient size to warrant excision in 36 patients. In 22 patients, hydrocelectomy was indicated. The bladder was found to be a sliding component in six patients. In each case the bladder was returned deep to the transversalis fascia into its retroperitoneal position, and then the McVay repair performed.

Incarceration of viscera is a rare occurrence in direct inguinal hernias. In one patient, omentum was adherent to a small-mouthed sac and, in another, a loop of small intestine was partially adherent to the peritoneal sac. Strangulation was not seen in any of the 493 patients, thus supporting the idea that direct inguinal hernias are rarely the site of visceral strangulation.

Table 13–6. ADDITIONAL PROCEDURES PERFORMED UPON 493 PATIENTS WITH DIRECT INGUINAL HERNIAS

| Procedure | Number | Percent |
|---|---|---|
| Excision Lipoma | 36 | 7.3 |
| Hydrocelectomy | 22 | 4.5 |
| Repair Sliding Hernia Bladder | 6 | 1.2 |
| Reduction Incarceration | 2 | 0.4 |
| Orchidectomy | 1 | 0.2 |

Orchidectomy was performed only once among 486 male patients in whom direct inguinal hernias were repaired. It is my opinion that testicles should not be wantonly sacrificed during hernia repair. The physiologic and psychologic effects of a functioning gonad are worth preserving (even at some inconvenience to the surgeon performing the repair).

### Late Deaths

A significant number of late deaths have occurred in a substantial group of cases, and this study confirms that fact (Table 13–7). As is true of the population in general, heart disease, malignancies and stroke were the leading causes of death in this study. Forty-seven, or 9.5 percent, of the patients died of intercurrent, unrelated diseases.

### Results

Direct inguinal hernias may be comparatively benign clinically, but they are far more difficult to repair than the congenital variety of indirect inguinal hernia. Even indirect inguinal hernias in adults can be repaired with uniform success. Direct inguinal hernias are difficult to repair because of the magnitude of the defect in the inguinal triangle. Approximation of the rectus abdominis sheath, the internal oblique, and the transversus arch to Poupart's ligament under excessive tension contributes to recurrences in some patients.

In 609 operations for direct inguinal hernia, there were 11 known recurrences, for a rate of 1.8 percent. Only 46 percent were followed for longer than one year. In this study, I could not confirm the opinion that bilateral simultaneous repairs result in a greater recurrence rate. It is seen that 116 patients had bilateral repairs of direct inguinal hernias, with four recurrences. Thus, recurrent hernias occurred in 3.44 percent of patients with bilateral repairs of direct inguinal hernias. Actually, 232 repairs were accomplished in 116 patients, for a recurrence rate of 1.72 percent among 232 repairs. Seven recurrences were seen in 377 patients with unilateral repairs, or in patients having the second repair as a procedure. Thus, the recurrence rate was 1.85 percent following repair of 377 unilateral repairs.

Meticulous attention to details must be paid during repair of direct inguinal hernias regardless of whether unilateral or bilateral repairs are being performed. Excessive tension must be avoided by use of the relaxing incision. The great reluctance to use prosthetic implants should be modified.

Bilateral simultaneous hernia repairs represent a great benefit to the patient by keeping pain and suffering to a minimum. The economic advantages due to a shortened hospital stay are obvious.

### SUMMARY

As recently as 1890, there was still doubt as to whether or not operative treatment of hernia was justified. Repairs consisted of ligation of the sac and, in some instances, closure of the pillars of the external oblique. The rate of relapse was reported

**Table 13–7. LATE DEATHS IN 493 PATIENTS FOLLOWING REPAIR OF DIRECT INGUINAL HERNIAS**

| | |
|---|---|
| *Arteriosclerotic cardiovascular disease* | 18 |
| Myocardial infarction 14 | |
| Congestive Heart failure 4 | |
| *Cerebrovascular disease* | 6 |
| Cerebrovascular accident 5 | |
| Aneurysm 1 | |
| *Malignancies* | 14 |
| Prostate 5 | |
| Colorectal 3 | |
| Stomach 3 | |
| Brain 2 | |
| Lymphoma 1 | |
| *Hypertensive cardiovascular disease* | 1 |
| *Miscellaneous* | 6 |
| Renal failure 2 | |
| Pneumonia 2 | |
| Pulmonary embolus 1 | |
| Septicemia 1 | |
| *Unknown* | 2 |
| Total deaths | 47 |

as varying from 27 to 42 percent within one year.

In 1890 Bassini advocated "slitting up the external oblique" from the external ring to a point approximately one inch beyond the internal ring. He advocated ligation of the sac at the internal ring and reconstruction of the inguinal canal. This was accomplished by suturing the internal oblique muscle to Poupart's ligament from the pelvic bone to the internal ring. The cord was placed under the external oblique layer. Bassini reported only seven recurrences in 262 operated patients, which represents a recurrence rate of less than 3 percent. In 1890 Halsted reported his procedure, which in several aspects was similar to the Bassini operation. He greatly reduced the size of the spermatic cord and transplanted it to a position external or superficial to the external oblique. The testicle was jeopardized frequently by the attempt at reduction of the size of the cord.

By 1903 Coley was able to report that in 917 operations by the Bassini technique for indirect inguinal hernia, there were only nine recurrences. He stated in 1936 that a permanent cure was to be expected in 95 percent of oblique inguinal hernias in adults.

It is evident that high ligation of the sac and repair of the internal ring were the basic requirements met for the successful repair of indirect inguinal hernias.

It soon became obvious that the direct inguinal hernia was more of a problem and that a simple Bassini repair failed to give the good results expected. Even as recently as 1924, recurrence rates of 16 percent were not uncommon. No one recognized the problem of direct inguinal hernia better than did Andrews and Bissell, who in 1934 pointed out that there was a deficiency of the internal oblique and transversus abdominis in the floor of the inguinal canal and described the inguinal triangle. They reported collected statistics in which the recurrence rate after repair of direct inguinal hernia varied from 41 percent to 32 percent during the years 1911 to 1933.

In 1938 Fallis reported that recurrence rates for direct inguinal hernia varied from 6 to 50 percent. He reported a recurrence rate of 11.6 percent in 154 operations for direct inguinal hernia. In his repair, he favored the use of a relaxing incision and transplantation of the cord to the subcutaneous position. It became clear that surgeons were able to repair indirect inguinal hernias reasonably successfully, but repair of the direct inguinal hernia was a more difficult problem. Various techniques were offered to strengthen the area of weakness in the floor of Hesselbach's triangle. Fascial flaps, fascial transplants, and fascial sutures were advanced. The results were still far from satisfactory. Why were the overall results so poor?

Zimmerman in 1940 stated that poor results after operation for hernia were in part due to a failure to differentiate adequately between direct and indirect inguinal hernias. He pointed out that in direct inguinal hernia, there is a deficiency in the lowermost fibers of the internal oblique muscle in the floor of Hesselbach's triangle and that the transversus aponeurosis is inadequate to withstand the increased intra-abdominal pressure. This confirmed the observations of Andrews and Bissell.

Further substantial progress in the treatment of hernia followed the anatomic studies of McVay and Anson. In 1941 McVay referred to an anatomic error in methods then being used in hernia repairs. He stated that the practice of suturing the various layers to the inguinal ligament was erroneous. The internal oblique and transversus abdominis muscles neither originate nor insert into Poupart's ligament. He advocated that the transversus abdominis, the transversalis fascia, and, if available, the internal oblique muscle be sutured to Cooper's ligament. This technique, according to McVay, more nearly restores the anatomic relationships to a normal state. It was McVay who provided the anatomic explanation for the success of the Lotheissen-McVay repair.

Properly performed, the Halsted procedure is an effective method of repair for most direct inguinal hernias. Attention must be paid to such details as precise closure of the transversus abdominis lamina at the internal ring, proper placement of nonabsorbable sutures, and use of the relaxing incision.

In my opinion, prosthetic materials should be used in selected direct inguinal hernias to bridge the gap between the transversus abdominis arch and Cooper's ligament or the inguinal ligament. The need to supply the strength of an implanted mesh without placing the burden of excessive tension upon the suture line is slowly but surely being recognized.

In my opinion, the next significant progress in effective repair will come when we learn to use the currently available, newer synthetic materials more appropriately and more frequently than we have in the past.

NOTE: References for Chapter 13 are included in the list of references at the end of Chapter 14.

# 14

# Recurrent Direct
# Inguinal Hernias

*I agree with those who feel that our statistics in this
operation (herniotomy) are materially better than our
results.*

*Pitzman, 1921*

## INTRODUCTION

Out of a voluminous literature on the
subject of hernia, it is possible to identify a
few papers of particular relevance to the
problem of direct inguinal hernias. The
first significant advances came about when
surgeons recognized the differences between direct and indirect inguinal hernias.

Currently, several surgeons are scrutinizing the structural and chemical content
of the supporting tissue in the groin. Tobin
and colleagues (1976) and Wagh and
coworkers (1971) have been interested in
tissue changes that might contribute
eventually to hernias of the groin. But in
the final analysis, it is the ability of the
abdominal wall to contain the viscera in a
normal relationship—even if exposed to
increasing intra-abdominal pressure—that
prevents herniation. Thus, any condition
that sufficiently increases pressure within
the peritoneal cavity can produce a hernia
at the weakest point; this area in aging
men is the *inguinal triangle.* To prevent
protrusion at this site, it is necessary to
devise some method of strengthening the
area. Two approaches are sufficient in this
regard; one, shifting of proximate strong
tissues to bridge the defect, and, two,

implanting a strong prosthetic material—a
procedure that, in my opinion, is not used
as often as it should be.

Regardless of which of the two procedures is employed, the avoidance of excessive tension is paramount in a successful repair. If tissues are shifted too far,
excessive tension and tissue necrosis can
lead to recurrence of the hernia.

## HISTORICAL BACKGROUND

E. Wyllys Andrews, in 1895, recognized
the consequences of suturing the internal
oblique muscle to the inguinal ligament.
His classic illustration (Fig. 14–1) vividly
depicts the tension that may result from
placing sutures too high on the transversus
arch. The same result occurs if we decide
to call the structure sutured to the inguinal
ligament the "conjoined tendon," or perhaps the internal oblique. I cannot understand how repair could be expected to be
uniformly successful if the internal oblique is shifted so far as to reach the
inguinal ligament.

The next substantial contribution came
from Andrews and Bissell in 1934, whose
contributions were of such fundamental
importance that I reproduced two of their

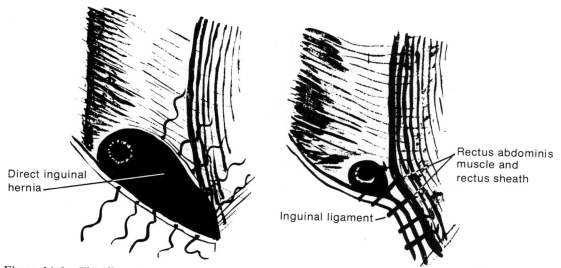

Direct inguinal hernia

Rectus abdominis muscle and rectus sheath

Inguinal ligament

**Figure 14–1.** This illustration was conceived by E. Wyllys Andrews in 1895. The artist's drawing dramatically illustrates the upward traction caused by placement of sutures high up on the internal oblique and the rectus sheath.

illustrations in Chapter 13. Figure 13–2 (see p. 197) shows a sagittal view of the width of the defect in Hesselbach's triangle that required repair. Whether the transversus arch (or any part of the abdominal wall in the area) or the "conjoined tendon" is sutured to Cooper's ligament or to the inguinal ligament, a certain amount of tension is inevitably created. Andrews and Bissell (1934) noted that in direct inguinal hernias, the lower fibers of the internal oblique were absent. I have observed that this muscle has a high insertion into the rectus sheath.

The second important observation advanced by Andrews and Bissell is that of the *inguinal triangle,* which is bounded medially by the rectus sheath, below by Poupart's ligament, and above by the internal oblique muscle. Figure 13–1 (see p. 197) calls attention both to the site of the underlying defect in direct hernias and, in a simple manner, to possible methods of repair and their consequences. Following repair of direct inguinal hernias, Andrews and Bissell cited recurrence rates reported by various authors during the years 1912 to 1932 as ranging from 6.4 to 32 percent.

Chronologically, the next noteworthy contribution came from McVay and Anson in 1942, when they identified a fundamental error in the methods of inguinal herniorrhaphy that were popular at the

time. McVay and Anson emphasized that the inguinal ligament was not the insertional site of the layers of the abdominal wall, and they identified Cooper's ligament as the attachment site of the posterior abdominal wall. These fundamentally important anatomic observations are of great value to the cognizant surgeon when he is facing complicated direct, recurrent direct and femoral hernias.

The relaxing incision must be mentioned at this point, since it is a means of decreasing tension at the line of suture. The evolution of the relaxing incision is described in detail in Chapter 25.

Besides the above contributions, I feel there must be a greater awareness among surgeons that direct inguinal hernias are, in fact, bilateral anatomic defects. Even if a direct inguinal hernia is seen as a unilateral defect, given sufficient time, a hernia will develop on the contralateral side in well over 50 percent of the patients.

In Figure 14–2, we present an illustration that clearly shows the magnitude of the problem in direct inguinal hernias (the arrows emphasize the lines of distracting forces). The rectus abdominis, internal oblique, and transversus abdominis muscles contribute toward tension developing in this region.

With full appreciation of the pathologic-

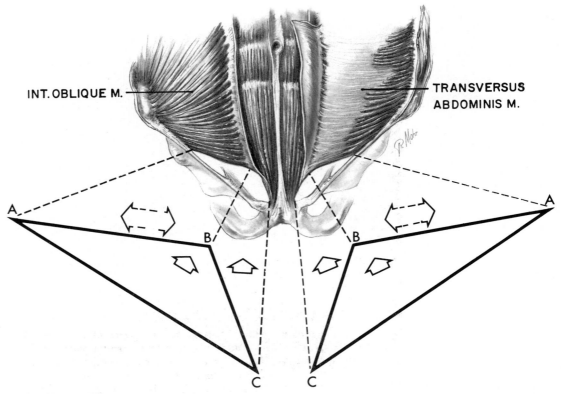

**INT. OBLIQUE M.**

**TRANSVERSUS ABDOMINIS M.**

**Figure 14–2.** In repairing bilateral inguinal hernias, it is important to recall the consequences of placement of sutures into the internal oblique and transversus arch. The arrows emphasize the lines of force exerted bilaterally by muscles in the area. Relaxing incisions and prosthetic materials are desirable adjunctive measures to combat excessive tension at the suture line.

anatomic problems facing the surgeon, successful repair is more likely to follow surgical efforts.

## INCIDENCE OF RECURRENT DIRECT INGUINAL HERNIAS

Historically, it has been recognized by surgeons that the recurrence rate following repair of direct inguinal hernias is unacceptably high. In 1912 Lameris (as cited by Andrews and Bissell, 1934) reported a recurrence rate of 28 percent following repair of direct inguinal hernias. Reported statistics vary widely, as can be seen in Table 14–1.

Stein and Casten in 1943 cited average recurrence rates of 10 to 15 percent for repair of direct inguinal hernias. In a review of the literature, they found that the recurrence rates following repair of direct inguinal hernias varied from 2.7 to 33.3 percent.

Rydell (1963) noted that recurrence rates varied with technique of repair. When a Cooper's ligament repair was employed for direct inguinal hernias, the recurrence rate was 3.6 percent; however, when other methods were used, the recurrence rate was 9.4 percent.

Recurrence rates two decades ago were higher than they are today; however, the number of relapses following hernia repair must be reduced even further. The commonly cited recurrence rate of 10 percent must be considered unacceptable; fortunately, many surgeons who have devoted special efforts to the problem are already demonstrating that better results are achievable.

Recurrence rates following preperitoneal repairs have been disturbingly high. Recurrence rates have been reported in

Table 14–1.  RECURRENCE RATE FOLLOWING REPAIR OF
DIRECT INGUINAL HERNIA

| Year | Author | Cases | Percent Recurred | Comment |
|------|--------|-------|------------------|---------|
| 1912 | Lameris Cited by Andrews and Bissell (1934) | — | 28 | Bassini Repair |
| 1920 | Taylor | 47 | 29 | |
| 1923 | Hoguet | 269 | 6.4 | |
| 1931 | Cattell | 51 | 7.8 | Fascial |
| 1936 | Fallis | 154 | 11.6 | |
| 1947 | Glenn | 220 | 8.1 | |
| 1964 | Palumbo et al. | 686 | 1.6 | Modified Bassini, Halsted and Andrews Repair |
| 1975 | Ross | 92 | 7.6 | |

the literature as follows: Dyson and Pierce (1965), 35 percent; Robertson (1966), 17 percent; Gregorie (1966), 14.8 percent; Lindholm et al. (1969), 12 percent; and Gaspar and Casberg (1971), 21 percent.

The preperitoneal approach to repair of indirect and femoral hernias gives excellent results, but direct inguinal hernias continue to recur in unacceptably high numbers following preperitoneal repair. In 1965 Dyson and Pierce identified a recurrence rate of 35 percent; and one year later, Robertson reported a recurrence rate of 17 percent following the preperitoneal approach to repair of direct inguinal hernias. Gregorie (1966) found a recurrence rate of 14.8 percent in a similar study. In 1969 Lindholm reported a recurrence rate of 12 percent, and in 1971 Gaspar and Casberg reported a disappointing recurrence rate of 21 percent following preperitoneal repair of direct inguinal hernias. As a result of such recurrence rates, the preperitoneal approach is hardly recommended as a method for repair of direct inguinal hernias.

### Time of Recurrence

Iason in 1941 estimated that 65 percent of recurrent hernias appeared within six months following repair, and 80 percent developed in the first year. He felt that only 6.5 percent appeared after two years.

As noted by Zimmerman in 1967, many surgeons believe that most recurrences are seen within six months postoperatively and that few recurrences occur after two years. He noted that relapses can occur many years postoperatively; thus, although a follow-up study of five years is adequate, he suggested that a study covering a ten-year period would be preferable.

Watson in 1948 stated that most surgeons quote a recurrence rate of 65 percent within six months and 95 percent within two years following repair. He reported in more detail on recurrence rates for 286 patients. Sixty-eight percent of the recurrent hernias analyzed by Watson occurred in the first six months following herniorrhaphy. Most significantly, 25 percent of the relapses occurred immediately. Failure to identify the hernia, selection of an ineffective procedure, poor operative technique, or a combination of these three factors must have accounted for most of the early recurrences.

Fallis (1937) studied two hundred operations and noted the time of postoperative recurrence as follows: the first six months, 22.5 percent; six months to one year, 15.5 percent; 12 to 24 months, 10 percent; two to five years, 19.5 percent; five to ten years,

14.5 percent; and 10 years and over, 18.5 percent.

Rydell (1963) reported 65 recurrent hernias (7.5 percent) among 871 adult patients. In 16 patients (24 percent), the recurrences were seen within 6 months; in 39 (60 percent), within 2 years; in 54 (82 percent), within 5 years; and in 11 (18 percent), from 5 to 10 years following repair.

In 1970 Halverson and McVay reviewed 1,211 inguinofemoral hernia repairs upon 1,088 patients. They cited that 62 percent of the recurrences appeared within 5 years; another 19 percent appeared within the next 5 years; and even 10 to 25 years after repair, an additional 19 percent of relapses were noted. Obviously, long-term follow-up examinations are needed if the data reported are to be reliable.

According to Qvist (1977), Edwards reported on 131 patients in whom 75 percent of the recurrences were indirect. In his study, 77 percent of the hernias reappeared within 18 months of the first repair.

As a result of this brief review of the literature, it is evident that most recurrences following hernia repair occur within 5 years; however, significant numbers of hernias appear as recurrences after as long a time as 10 to 25 years.

### Factors in Recurrence of Direct Inguinal Hernia

A search for some esoteric explanation for recurrence of direct hernias has proven to be fruitless. Although many contributing factors have been identified, a glance at Figure 12–1 (see p. 180) reveals the multiplicity of factors involved. There is no doubt that each of the etiologic factors plays a role of some importance in the genesis of recurrence. Such factors as hematoma formation and infection increase the likelihood of recurrence, but in all of my studies they played a role in only approximately two percent of the cases.

Patients with increased intra-abdominal pressure (such as occurs with excessive coughing, sneezing, or straining) pose a special threat to the line of repair of their hernias.

When all factors are considered critically, only two major causes for recurrence of direct inguinal hernias emerge. Excessive tension at the suture line is a most undesirable consequence to one's attempts at bridging the defect in the floor of the inguinal triangle. E. Wyllys Andrews (1895) recognized that suturing the internal oblique and rectus sheath to the inguinal ligament was likely to produce excessive tension; and he noted that even if primary union occurred, later movement of the abdomen and thigh resulted in separation (see Fig. 13–1, p. 197).

A second, more complicated factor contributing to recurrence is designated as poor technical execution. This factor includes problems such as the failure to place sutures into proper lamina. An important requirement is that the transversus abdominis lamina be closed. In this regard, it is not enough to use the attenuated stretched transversalis fascia. The transversus abdominis arch above must be sutured to the iliopubic tract below. The latter structure is usually available as an entity of some strength; however, if the repair is to gain its strength through the use of Cooper's ligament, then this structure must be identified from the pubic tubercle to the femoral vein. Interrupted sutures must be accurately placed between the transversus arch and Cooper's ligament, if a McVay repair has been selected.

In over one-half of the patients, a direct protrusion will occur on the contralateral side, sooner or later, if it is not already present at the time of repair. In any repair of direct inguinal hernias, it is advisable to consider the defect as being bilateral (see Fig. 14–2, p. 218).

Avoidance of tension when repairing a unilateral direct inguinal hernia is just as important as when dealing with bilateral simultaneous defects. The relaxing incision is a technical maneuver to combat excessive tension.

Use of absorbable sutures is to be avoided, since the loss of holding power is too rapid and fails to hold tissues in apposition long enough to permit proper healing.

Another problem related to the "poor technical execution" factor in recurrence is failure to use a prosthetic material in carefully selected cases. One may ask why synthetic mesh is not used in repair of certain direct virginal inguinal hernias when it proved to be so useful in repair of direct inguinal hernias that have recurred numerous times. Surgeons should overcome their reluctance to employ prosthetics in hernia repair. Of course, cases should be carefully selected for such implants.

In order to focus attention on the most important factors in the genesis of recurrent direct inguinal hernias, I may have been guilty of oversimplification. The surgeon who recognizes the devastating effects of excessive tension on repair of direct inguinal hernias and, then, carries out all important technical maneuvers with precision will enjoy a greater measure of success.

The role of experience in the successful repair of direct inguinal hernias is identified here in a separate section, but it applies to all hernias.

## THE IMPACT OF EXPERIENCE ON SURGICAL TREATMENT OF HERNIAS

For many years, young surgeons with minimal previous instruction were expected to repair most hernias. The procedure was considered to be "the house officer's operation." Too often the most inexperienced house officer was instructed by a colleague who was but one rung ahead on the ladder of surgical experience. On one occasion while visiting a medical center, I recall seeing two house officers spend four hours repairing bilateral inguinal hernias. Only later in the procedure did a more experienced surgeon add his knowledge of anatomy and surgical technique in order to complete the procedure.

I am convinced that hernias can be very complicated and may be misdiagnosed both preoperatively and intraoperatively. A knowledge of normal anatomy and pathology as it applies to hernia repair cannot be gained simply by graduating from a medical school or by completing one year of a rotating internship. Furthermore, instruction in repair of hernias must be planned well and provided by a surgeon of some experience. Delegation of major responsibility for repair of hernias to the youngest and most inexperienced member of the surgical team has contributed to the unacceptably high recurrence

rates reported by some authors. The next significant improvement in results following hernia repair will come when methods of instruction are improved. In this regard, I actively teach the importance of anatomy, proper diagnosis, and technical details as they apply to the hernia problem. The young surgeon must be assisted by a surgeon of some experience, if results are to improve.

In support of my opinion and to stress the importance of surgical experience in repair of groin hernias, I have recorded several direct quotations from various authors.

In referring to the rather poor results obtained in repair of hernia, Andrews noted in 1924 that we must face the fact "herniotomy is one of the operations most commonly done by the beginner in surgery."

Downes in 1920 recognized the circumstances that led to poor results following herniorrhaphy.

The explanation is that many surgeons have come to look upon the hernia operation as of almost minor importance, and to pass these patients along to young assistants or house surgeons without proper supervision, with the result that if the anatomy or the arrangement of the sac is unusual, the operation is likely to prove a failure.

Coley reviewed the status of the art and science of surgery as it related to herniorrhaphy in 1936—on the occasion of the fiftieth anniversary of Bassini's introduction of his method of repair.

There is no operation in surgery in which good results are more dependent on the skill and experience of the surgeon than is the operation for hernia. On the other hand, there has long been a tendency on the part of the general surgeon to regard herniorrhaphy as a comparatively minor operation, not worthy of his personal time and effort, but one that can be safely given to the house surgeon or assistant, men who have not been thoroughly instructed in the finer points of technique.

To the possibility that operations for repair are poorly done, Koontz in 1956 responded as follows:

I feel sure that is the case (poorly performed operations) in far too high a percentage of the total number of hernia operations performed in this country. One reason for this is that Chiefs of Service in a great many hospitals feel that the operation is of little importance and turn it over to junior members of their staff, giving them entirely too much leeway in their choice of the operation, and not properly supervising them in the actual operative technique employed.

Thieme stated the following in a paper in 1971 on recurrent inguinal hernia:

. . . Lacking a patient profile from which recurrence can be predicted, and so receive more individualized treatment, we are forced to conclude that surgical skill is the dominant factor in the success of repair of a recurrent hernia.

Skill in the art and science of surgery comes from experience gained through exposure to large numbers of patients. Anatomic details of the groin must be learned through cadaver dissection. Technical skill must be learned by performance; however, while experience is being acquired, the guidance and supervision of a mature surgeon is most desirable. Fortunately in this country a large number of capable surgeons are available to teach house officers who wish to learn that phase of surgical practice dealing with hernias.

## TYPE OF RECURRENCE OF DIRECT INGUINAL HERNIA

Surgeons repairing recurrent hernias should study the type of recurrence analytically, since only by identifying the type and magnitude of recurrence can the proper technique be selected for its correction. Although direct recurrent inguinal hernias occur in the floor of Hesselbach's triangle, differentiation of the type of recurrence is important. Not all direct recurrent inguinal hernias present as a large diffuse weakness in the inguinal floor. At least three common varieties of recurrent direct inguinal hernias can be identified, and I strongly suspect that their pathogenesis differs.

### A Classification of Recurrent Direct Inguinal Hernias

In order to further identify the type and magnitude of recurrent direct hernias, I propose a classification that identifies three varieties of recurrent protrusions.

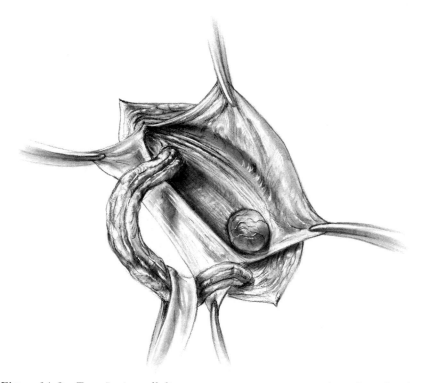

**Figure 14-3.**   Type I — A small direct recurrent protrusion near the pubic tubercle.

Admittedly, such a classification cannot identify all possible direct herniations; nevertheless, it calls attention to the fact that not all direct recurrent hernias are alike. The following varieties are easily recognized:

1. Type I — Small direct recurrence near the pubic tubercle.
2. Type II — Small direct protrusion through the floor of Hesselbach's triangle.
3. Type III — Large direct recurrent hernia in which most of the floor of the inguinal canal has been disrupted.

Type I would apply to the direct recurrent inguinal hernia in which a small protrusion occurs through a defect near the pubic tubercle (Fig. 14–3). It is quite possible that improper placement of the medial suture might be the cause for such a failure. The suture may have been placed too high upon the sheath of the rectus, resulting in excessive tension. The strength of the suture material is also at issue. Even though the recurrence is small, I feel the use of a relaxing incision is helpful. In Type I recurrent direct inguinal hernias, the lateral portion of the inguinal floor is strong.

Thieme (1971) found that 22.4 percent of the cases he studied occurred near the tubercle. Postlethwait (1971) found that 47 of 58 recurrent direct inguinal hernias oc-

curred near the tubercle. Skinner and Duncan (1945) also found that direct inguinal hernias commonly recurred near the pubic tubercle. In the cases I reviewed, the direct recurrence was small — appearing in the medial aspect of Hesselbach's triangle in 40.2 percent of 92 patients with recurrent direct inguinal hernias.

Type II direct recurrent inguinal hernias appear as comparatively small defects through the floor of Hesselbach's triangle (Fig. 14–4). The striking feature of these hernias is that the entire floor is strong, and a protrusion of preperitoneal fat finds its way through an isolated defect. Suture failure could produce such a defect; strangulation of tissue, caught in a suture that is tied too tightly, could produce the same result. In addition, if the suture were placed high up on the internal oblique (as in a Bassini or Halsted repair), it could cause distraction of tissues at the site. Of the 92 cases of direct inguinal hernias that I studied, 31.5 percent were of this variety.

Type III are the largest direct recurrent inguinal hernias. In this type, an extensive bulge occurs, occupying most of the floor of the inguinal canal (Figs. 14–5 and 14–6); this type of recurrence suggests poor technical performance, poor choice of procedure, or both. If sutures are placed high up on the transversus arch, or into the internal oblique, failure of this type is to

**Figure 14–4.** Type II — The recurrent defect protrudes through the floor of Hesselbach's triangle.

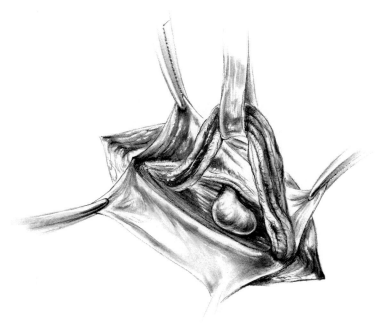

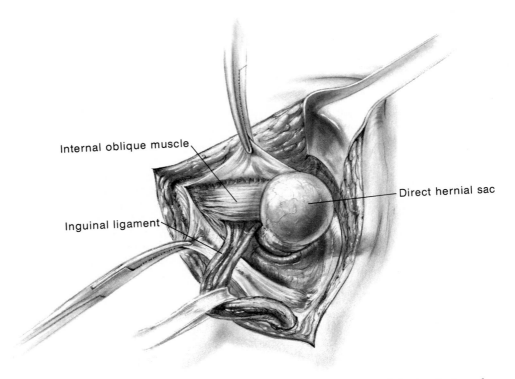

Figure 14-5. Type III—A large recurrent protrusion through the floor of the inguinal canal.

be expected. Failure to use a relaxing incision compounds the problem of tension. Tightly tied sutures, especially if placed at close intervals, can result in tissue necrosis at the line of suture. Should the patient have chronic pulmonary dis-

ease with coughing, the repair would be in future jeopardy. Thieme (1971) found such recurrences in 29 percent of his cases, while Postlethwait found that nearly one-half of his direct recurrent inguinal hernias were of the diffuse type. Of the 92 direct

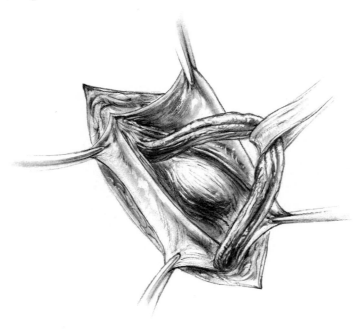

Figure 14-6. Type III—A variant of the direct recurrent inguinal hernia in which the entire floor of the inguinal canal is bulging.

inguinal hernias I studied, 28.3 percent were of the diffuse extensive type.

To my knowledge, this is the first attempt to establish a classification of direct recurrent inguinal hernias. I feel it is important to identify the type or types of recurrent herniations, and then to relate these observations to the type of original repair. This approach cannot but prove helpful in trying to resolve the problem.

## CAUSES FOR FAILURE — 92 PATIENTS WITH RECURRENT DIRECT INGUINAL HERNIAS

The causes for recurrent direct hernia are numerous, and often more than one reason can be cited for relapse of the hernia (Table 14–2). Although I found it extremely difficult to identify the specific cause or causes responsible for the recurrence of direct inguinal hernias, I am convinced nevertheless that excessive tension at the suture line is the single greatest cause for failure. The methods or techniques that may cause excessive tension at the suture line can be identified with some success.

## Excessive Tension as a Cause of Recurrence — Case in Point

The patient, a 44-year-old male, had undergone repair of a hernia, performed elsewhere, one year earlier. He was described as being well developed but with a left recurrent inguinal hernia.

At operation, the sac was disposed of properly; but the "conjoined tendon" was sutured to Cooper's ligament as the essential detail of repair. A relaxing incision was not made. Healing was acceptable; however, within two months, the patient had severe pain in the wound.

In seven months, the hernia was recognized as a recurrence. At the third operation, the recurrence was seen near the pubic tubercle. The hernia recurred as a direct at the site of greatest tension.

At this operation, a McVay repair was

Table 14–2.   **CAUSES FOR DIRECT RECURRENT HERNIAS IN 92 PATIENTS***

| | |
|---|---|
| *UNDUE TENSION UPON THE SUTURE LINE* | 80 |
|     Failure to use relaxing incision | |
|     Attachment of internal oblique to Cooper's ligament or the inguinal<br>      ligament under tension | |
|     Attachment of the transversus arch to Cooper's ligament or the inguinal<br>      ligament under tension | |
|     Attachment of sheath of the rectus to Cooper's ligament or the inguinal ligament | |
|     Bilateral simultaneous repairs | |
| *POOR TECHNICAL EXECUTION* | 64 |
|     Use of attenuated transversalis fascia for repair | |
|     Failure to identify Cooper's ligament and the transversus arch | |
|     Failure to use master stitch | |
|     Improper placement of sutures | |
|     Strangulation of tissues at suture line | |
|     Failure to achieve hemostasis | |
|     Postoperative wound infection | |
| *FAILURE TO PROVIDE NEEDED STRENGTH IN REPAIRS* | 13 |
|     Failure to use transversus abdominis arch | |
|     Failure to use a prosthesis | |
| *FAILURE TO IDENTIFY THE MAGNITUDE OF WEAKNESS* | 4 |
|     Overlooked hernia | |
| *MISCELLANEOUS* | 5 |
|     Wound infection | |
|     Severe chronic pulmonary disease | |
|     Atrophic tissues; aging; injection of sclerosing agents | |

*A total of 104 repairs were performed on 92 patients. The number of causes listed exceeds the number of patients because at times several etiologic factors entered into the recurrence in an individual patient.

performed and a relaxing incision added. The repair remained successful in a follow-up of eight years.

## Comment

The tension generated at the suture line in repair of direct inguinal hernias is enormous, particularly when sutures are placed into the rectus sheath or the so-called conjoined tendon. Whenever an attempt is made to shift the sheath and tendon of the rectus abdominis laterally to Cooper's ligament or the inguinal ligament, excessive tension results. Failure to add a relaxing incision can lead to failure of the repair.

In repair of such small direct hernias, it is essential initially to free the sac of the transversus abdominis lamina; then, the small defect must be closed with interrupted sutures.

Poor technical execution is also difficult to delineate, but certain errors can be recognized. For example, the transversalis fascia alone is not to be depended on if a sound repair is to be expected. If Cooper's ligament was not identified and if sutures were placed in the approximate vicinity of this important structure, the strength of the repair would be compromised. Use of the master stitch is a highly desirable technique for prevention of small medial direct recurrent inguinal hernias. Hematoma and wound infection were not identified as important causes for recurrence in the patients studied.

## TECHNICAL ERRORS AND POOR CHOICE OF TECHNIQUE—CASE IN POINT

Complicated surgical problems do not lend themselves well to statistical analysis. To illustrate the complexity of the recurrent hernia problem, the following report is presented:

The patient, 57 years of age, had had simultaneous bilateral inguinal hernia repairs performed elsewhere ten years earlier. The left inguinal hernia recurred within one year and was again repaired. Eight years later it recurred a second time, and a third repair was carried out. In the same year, a right recurrent hernia ap-

peared in the right groin. Within ten years the hernia on the left side reappeared for the fourth time and was repaired.

Finally, the patient was referred to Henry Ford Hospital for a fifth repair of the left recurrent direct inguinal hernia. The surgeon stated in his operative note that the transversalis fascia and rectus sheath were sutured to Cooper's ligament. Clearly, no relaxing incision was made, and the repair was performed under spinal anesthesia. The hernia recurred again on the left side in approximately ten months; thus, within one year after repair of a sixth recurrence, a femoral hernia appeared. The peritoneal sac was identified and dissected free, and high ligation performed. The surgeon again sutured transversalis fascia to Cooper's ligament under spinal anesthesia. A relaxing incision was considered to be unnecessary, and prosthetic materials were felt to be undesirable. Following this repair, the patient developed a severe wound infection; and upon healing, there appeared a larger recurrent direct and femoral hernia. Fourteen months later, the seventh repair was performed for what was described as a huge direct and femoral recurrent hernia. At this procedure, the sac was dissected free and high ligation performed. As a result of five previous operative procedures, the left testicle had become atrophic, and excision was advised at the seventh attempt at repair. At this procedure, Marlex mesh was implanted. It was attached to Cooper's ligament, the inguinal ligament, and the pubic tubercle. The mesh extended from the pubic tubercle to the region of the anterior superior iliac spine. It was anchored to the aponeurosis of the internal oblique above. The remains of the transversus abdominis arch had been sutured to Cooper's ligament, and the mesh attached over the repair. The internal abdominal ring had been closed earlier and separately to avoid recurrence as an indirect inguinal hernia; following this repair, the patient recovered and has remained without hernia for ten years.

## Comment

This case illustrates the serious nature of recurrence following hernia repair. Seven operative procedures were necessary to effect a cure. During the first five procedures, the blood supply to the testicle was compromised and orchidectomy was indicated. The serious nature of infection is seen after the sixth repair. Spinal anesthesia was used in three of the repairs at our institution. Such anesthesia provides excellent relaxation; this may cause the surgeon to overlook the need for a relaxing incision. Finally, after a number of reoperations, consideration should have been given to the use of mesh. It was not until the seventh repair that both a relaxation incision and mesh were employed with success. In the fifth and sixth repairs, it is felt that excessive tension contributed to the recurrence. The infection following the sixth repair was a devastating complication. The soundness of the McVay principle with the use of mesh was reaffirmed in the seventh repair.

Failure to provide needed strength in the repair can be identified in those cases where prosthetic implants resulted in successful repairs after a number of previous recurrences.

Failure to identify the magnitude of weakness or make a proper diagnosis occurred infrequently.

It is interesting that "poor tissues" were not mentioned as a cause for recurrence. Scar tissue is, of course, encountered as a problem in patients having repeated herniorrhaphies.

Concerning the problem of recurrent direct hernias, excessive tension and poor technical execution are two of the most important etiologic factors. Failure to provide adequate strength in the repair by avoiding the use of a prosthesis is another factor contributing toward recurrence in selected cases. Other factors are identifiable, but they are of secondary importance and occur infrequently.

## RECURRENT DIRECT INGUINAL HERNIA—COMPLICATED CLINICAL COURSE; NEED FOR SYNTHETIC MESH: CASE IN POINT

It is extremely difficult to identify the numerous factors that enter into the problem of recurrent groin hernias. The complexity of the problem is best explained by presenting the medical history of appropriate cases.

The patient was a 57-year-old male who had had an inguinal hernia repaired elsewhere. Four years later (at the age of 61 years), this obese male developed pain, redness, and swelling in the left groin. It was necessary to drain an abscess in the operative area. *Staphylococcus aureus* was the only organism recovered upon culture of the pus. One year later, the patient again underwent surgery for excision of an abdominal sinus. At the time of excision of the sinus tract, the surgeon noted a large defect in the floor of the inguinal canal with destruction of tissue and scarring. The area was permitted to heal; one year after excision of the sinus tract, the direct recurrent inguinal hernia was repaired with fascia lata. The inguinal ligament was utilized as an anchoring structure. The spermatic cord was transplanted to the subcutaneous position. Again, the patient recovered; however, one year later, a recurrence was discovered by an industrial plant physician.

I saw the patient and advised repair of a large direct–indirect recurrent inguinal hernia using Marlex mesh. Heavy cicatrix was present, and much of it was excised. The small indirect and large direct hernial sacs were converted into one sac utilizing the Hoguet maneuver. High ligation of the sac was performed; medially it was seen that a sliding hernia of the bladder was present. Transversalis fascia was identified at the internal ring and closed separately. It was necessary to repair the defect with Marlex mesh, which was sutured below to Cooper's ligament, the inguinal ligament, and the pubic tubercle. The repair was carried laterally beyond the internal ring. The upper portion of the mesh was attached to the internal oblique aponeurosis (Figs. 26–17 and 26–18, pp. 566–567). What was left of the transversus arch had been sutured earlier to Cooper's ligament. In effect, we depended on the McVay principle of using Cooper's ligament as an anchoring structure. With this effort, the patient made an uneventful recovery, and the repair was sound ten years later.

### Comment

This case illustrates the adverse effect of wound infection on tissues. The late appearance of infection in the posthernior-rhaphy period is noteworthy. The first repair of the recurrent hernia was poorly conceived because the inguinal ligament had been used as an anchoring structure on two previous occasions. Use of fascia lata was reasonable at the time because Marlex mesh was not yet available. Deep placement of the Marlex mesh one year later (after the second recurrence)—using Cooper's ligament, inguinal ligament, and pubic tubercle as anchoring sites—resulted in an intact groin after ten years' follow-up observation. The mesh was attached to the internal oblique aponeurosis above. Deep placement and wide anchoring of the mesh accounted for the good result.

## REPAIR OF RECURRENT DIRECT INGUINAL HERNIAS

The same technique for locating and identifying the aponeurosis of the external oblique is used in both direct and indirect recurrent inguinal hernias. Sharp scalpel dissection and effective hemostasis are extremely important.

After the external oblique aponeurosis has been opened, the type and extent of disruption of the transversus abdominis lamina should be evaluated.

As already described in the discussion on recurrent indirect inguinal hernias, the lower leaflet of the external oblique aponeurosis is dissected to the shelving edge of Poupart's ligament. At this point, the iliopubic tract may usually be identified. Sharp dissection is employed to free the superior leaflet, so that the internal oblique muscle and anterior sheath of the rectus is visualized. The cord must be identified and protected throughout the dissection. The attenuated transversalis should not be depended on by the surgeon.

I prefer to open the peritoneum at the internal ring (as described in Chapter 11 under the heading, Indirect Inguinal Hernia repair), although this is not always possible. Digital exploration must be thorough to identify a possible coexistent femoral hernia. The extent of the weakness is thoroughly evaluated. Furthermore, it is useful to explore the preperi-

toneal space and test the strength of remaining tissues. By opening the peritoneum laterally, the danger of bladder injury is minimal. If possible, a Hoguet maneuver is used to convert the direct peritoneal bulge into an indirect sac, at which point high ligation is carried out with a purse-string suture of number 2–0 nonabsorbable material.

The transversus abdominis aponeurosis is identified by elevating the internal oblique muscle upward with a small loop retractor. It should be recalled that in this area, the transversus abdominis lamina overlies the deep inferior epigastric artery. Inferiorly, the iliopubic tract or femoral sheath is available for completion of the repair of the internal abdominal ring. I always repair the internal abdominal ring independently of the repair of the direct inguinal hernia.

### Repair of Medial Recurrent Direct Inguinal Hernia (Type I)

A special note is necessary on the repair of a common and deceptive type of direct recurrent inguinal hernia—one that is comparatively small, usually painful to the patient upon activity, and difficult for the surgeon to repair successfully. The hernia under consideration is a small direct recurrent inguinal hernia that protrudes through the medial-most portion of Hesselbach's triangle, just lateral to the pubic tubercle. This hernia is often thumblike in size and configuration.

After the external oblique aponeurosis has been opened and the spermatic cord identified, the magnitude of the defect is evaluated. In the case under discussion, the internal ring had been securely closed, and the remaining portion of the floor of the inguinal canal well repaired. Thus, only this small medial defect remained to annoy both the patient and the surgeon. It is a more formidable task to repair this type of recurrent hernia than is generally appreciated. In such hernias, the sac must be dissected circumferentially, so that it may be properly closed. Such sacs need not always be opened, and they may well contain a portion of bladder wall. A purse-string suture placed at the base of the sac, inversion of the sac, and then ligation of

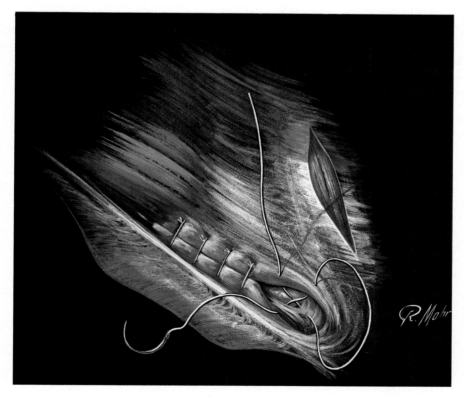

**Figure 14–7.** The two important technical details in repair of direct recurrent inguinal hernias include the master stitch and the relaxing incision. This artist's illustration shows details of placement of the master stitch.

the suture will dispose of the peritoneal sac; but the weakness in the transversalis lamina still remains. At this point, it is recommended that the Cooper's ligament be identified in its medial one-half or one-third. Using number 2–0 interrupted sutures of silk or synthetic nonabsorbable sutures, the transversus arch is sutured to Cooper's ligament (Fig. 14–7). Two or three such sutures may be necessary to close the defect. At this point, the surgeon may be mistakenly satisfied with his effort. One more important detail must not be overlooked. Even though the recurrent defect is small and the repair appears strong, a relaxing incision in the anterior sheath of the rectus abdominis is indicated. There is no better method for avoiding tension in this area where the forces of distraction are great upon coughing or straining. The fundamental principle in this repair is the proper reattachment of the abdominal wall to the iliopectineal ligament without tension.

## Repair of Small Recurrent Direct Inguinal Hernias (Type II)

There is a diverticular type of recurrent direct inguinal hernia in which the thin small sac protrudes through the floor of Hesselbach's triangle. The internal ring is intact, and the remaining portion of the inguinal floor is sound. In such cases, the dissection of the sac should be carried out through the thickness of the abdominal wall. Once it is clearly identified, it may be cautiously opened in order to avoid injury to the bladder. After the sac has been opened, careful digital exploration is performed to assure that the floor of the inguinal canal is otherwise intact. If so, the purse-string suture of number 2–0 silk is placed to achieve high ligation of the peritoneal sac. The defect in the transversus abdominis layer is then closed with interrupted sutures of number 2–0 silk or synthetic nonabsorbable sutures of comparable size. The remainder of the repair may be carried out as preferred by the surgeon. I have no great preference for the Bassini versus the Halsted repair at this point. Wound closure is completed as described in Chapter 11.

## Repair of Large Recurrent Direct Inguinal Hernias (Type III)

In this variety of direct recurrent inguinal hernia, the entire inguinal floor is disrupted. The defect occupies the area below the internal oblique muscle, above Poupart's ligament, and extends from the margin of the sheath of the rectus abdominis muscle to the deep inferior epigastric artery. Many of the hernias of this type have recurred repeatedly after a number of repairs. Some of them have had such complications as wound infections or hematomas. Atrophic testicles are seen with increasing frequency along with the re-recurrent hernias.

Again, the same principles of dissection as described in Chapter 12 are followed. The upper and lower leaflets of the exter-

nal oblique aponeurosis must be freed thoroughly. The inguinal ligament is identified below; the internal oblique aponeurosis is seen above. Often such recurrent hernias have been previously repaired by the Bassini or Halsted technique. The large recurrent direct hernia of this type presents as a diffuse bulge in the floor of Hesselbach's triangle. The internal ring is usually intact. The peritoneal cavity may be entered directly through the protruding sac; however, consideration and respect must be given to the bladder, which might form a portion of the sac of a sliding hernia. It becomes necessary to visualize the consequences of the contemplated repair. Excessive tension must be avoided.

The peritoneal sac is opened and carefully explored. The omentum and any adherent viscera are detached. The peritoneal sac may be closed with a purse-string suture or with interrupted sutures. Secure closure is essential. If a Lotheissen-McVay repair is planned, Cooper's ligament is identified from pubic tubercle to femoral vein (Fig. 14–8). It is surprising

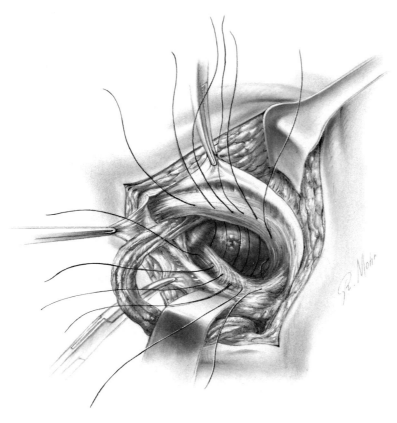

**Figure 14–8.** The hernial sac has been eliminated. Cooper's ligament is clearly identified, and sutures are placed between the transversus abdominis arch and Cooper's ligament. The lateral-most stitch (transition suture) includes transversus arch, femoral sheath, and Cooper's ligament.

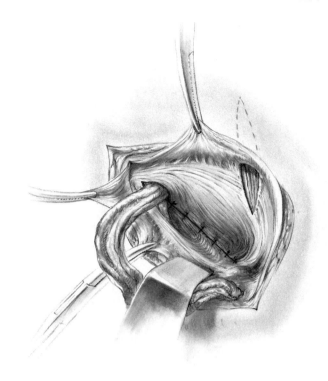

**Figure 14–9.** The Lotheissen-McVay repair for direct inguinal hernia has been completed. The transversus abdominis lamina at the internal ring must be precisely closed. Note the relaxing incision.

that Cooper's ligament is usually available and in good condition, because it had not been utilized in previous repairs. In a number of patients with recurrent direct inguinal hernias a Lotheissen-McVay repair together with a relaxing incision will result in a sound repair. This approach avoids the criticism directed toward the use of a foreign material in the repair of hernias (Fig. 14–9).

In hernias with repeated recurrences and attenuated tissues in the inguinal floor, I prefer to use a synthetic mesh as an implant. Number 2–0 synthetic sutures are placed into Cooper's ligament at intervals of less than one centimeter from the pubic tubercle to the femoral vein. The mesh will be anchored to Cooper's ligament via these sutures. The transversus abdominis arch is sutured separately to Cooper's ligament; next, the mesh is attached to Cooper's ligament. To accomplish this technical detail, the sutures that had earlier been placed through Cooper's ligament are first passed through the mesh at intervals of less than one centimeter and then tied. We now have, in effect, the Lotheissen-McVay repair, with additional support of a synthetic mesh that is an-

chored below to Cooper's ligament and above to the internal oblique aponeurosis. A relaxing incision is considered most important and is utilized almost without exception in these complicated cases. The mesh extends from the lateral margin of the rectus abdominis muscle to a point well beyond the internal abdominal ring. Thus, the entire inguinal floor is supported by a synthetic mesh (Figs. 26–17 and 26–18, pp. 566–567). The external oblique aponeurosis is then imbricated beneath the spermatic cord. Wound closure is completed as described in Chapter 11.

## Repair of Recurrent Direct Inguinal Hernias with Marlex Mesh and the Halsted Repair

The surgical approach to identification of recurrent direct inguinal hernias has been well described in preceding paragraphs.

Once the defect is identified, the decision is made as to whether or not a Hoguet maneuver is to be performed. If the internal abdominal ring is enlarged and the peritoneum is identifiable at this site, the peritoneum may be opened and the inguinal area carefully explored digitally. Careful examination is carried out to determine the strength of the floor of the inguinal canal and to rule out the presence of a femoral hernia. A Hoguet maneuver is performed, and the direct peritoneal sac is converted into an indirect sac. High ligation is carried out through placement of a purse-string suture, and then the transversalis fascia is accurately identified and snugly closed about the cord. A master stitch of number 2-0 silk or synthetic nonabsorbable material is placed between the transversus arch, Cooper's ligament, and a portion of Gimbernat's ligament; this suture must be accurately and deeply placed in order to occlude the medial portion of Hesselbach's triangle.

Repair of the inguinal floor is completed by suturing the transversus arch to the transversalis fascia and the inguinal ligament below. A relaxing incision is made in the anterior sheath of the rectus to minimize tension on the suture line.

A synthetic mesh is then attached to the inguinal ligament below and the internal oblique aponeurosis above. The mesh is implanted under tension, and wrinkling and reduplication of the mesh are both avoided. Number 2-0 sutures of synthetic nonabsorbable material are preferred.

The aponeurosis of the external oblique is closed under the spermatic cord as in the Halsted repair.

Wound closure is completed as described earlier in Chapter 11.

## CLINICAL STUDY

This study was directed at 92 patients who had undergone a total of 104 repairs for recurrent direct inguinal hernias during the years 1954 through 1968. The purpose of the study was to examine the problem of recurrent direct inguinal hernias critically. An effort was made to identify etiologic factors, types of recurrences, methods of repair and results. Of the original, or initial repairs, 74 were performed elsewhere and 18 were performed at Henry Ford Hospital; this confirms the observation that patients with recurrent hernias seek better results elsewhere.

Direct inguinal hernias are difficult to repair with success. In this study 8 pa-

**Table 14-3. AGE DISTRIBUTION — 92 PATIENTS WITH DIRECT RECURRENT INGUINAL HERNIAS**

| Age | Number of Patients |
|---|---|
| 1 to 10 yrs. | 0 |
| 11 to 20 yrs. | 0 |
| 21 to 30 yrs. | 2 |
| 31 to 40 yrs. | 5 |
| 41 to 50 yrs. | 22 |
| 51 to 60 yrs. | 29 |
| 61 to 70 yrs. | 26 |
| 71 to 80 yrs. | 7 |
| 81 and up | 1 |
| Total | 92 |

tients had 4 previous repairs; 9 patients had three previous repairs; 13 patients had 2 previous repairs; and 74 had 1 previous repair. Thus, 92 patients required a total of 243 attempts at repair. The economic consequences of recurrent herniation are staggering.

### Age

The age distribution is shown in Table 14-3. In general, it is the adult and aged patient who is likely to suffer from direct recurrent inguinal hernias.

Seventy-seven, or 84 percent, of the patients were in the fifth, sixth, and seventh decades of life. Infants, children, and young adults are rarely annoyed by such recurrences.

### Sex

Only three females, or 3.3 percent, had recurrent direct inguinal hernias. It was noted in Chapter 13 that in a study of direct inguinal hernias, the incidence of females was 1.5 percent. It is noteworthy that in general, repair of hernias in females is highly successful.

## Repair of Recurrent Direct Inguinal Hernias

### Anesthesia

Local anesthesia was employed in 58 procedures, or 55.8 percent, and spinal anesthesia was used in 40 procedures, or 38.5 percent. General anesthesia was se-

Table 14–4.  TYPE OF REPAIR – 104
OPERATIONS FOR RECURRENT
DIRECT INGUINAL HERNIAS

| Type of Repair | No. of Operations | Percent |
|---|---|---|
| HALSTED | 50 | 48 |
| McVAY | 37 | 36 |
| BASSINI | 17 | 16 |
| MESH USED° | 13 | 12.5 |

°Mesh was used in 13 patients to reinforce the three common types of repairs noted in this Table.

lected for six operations. The use of local anesthesia in recurrent inguinal hernias requires some adjustments in technique, since scarring limits diffusion of the anesthetic solution. The anesthetic agent must be injected repeatedly in small amounts as needed. Nevertheless, effective anesthesia can be achieved by local infiltration.

## Type of Repair

Traditionally, the Halsted method of repair, as described and illustrated in Chapter 13, has been popular at Henry Ford Hospital, particularly in the repair of direct inguinal hernias. The Bassini repair, as described in Chapter 11, has been used frequently in repair of indirect inguinal hernias. It is interesting that as we deal with direct recurrent inguinal hernias, the McVay repair becomes increasingly popular (Table 14–4).

## Technical Details in Repair

Among 104 repairs of recurrent direct inguinal hernias a number of technical details was considered important (Table 14–5).

It is unnecessary to repeat a discussion

Table 14–5.  TECHNICAL DETAILS IN
REPAIR OF 104 RECURRENT
DIRECT INGUINAL HERNIAS

| Maneuver | No. Times Used | Percent |
|---|---|---|
| Master stitch | 91 | 87.5 |
| Relaxing incision | 73 | 70.2 |
| Hoguet maneuver | 46 | 44.2 |
| Hernial sac inverted | 25 | 24.0 |
| Repair sliding hernia bladder | 5 | 4.8 |
| Use of prosthesis | 13 | 12.5 |

of the master stitch (Chapter 13), the relaxing incision (Chapter 25), or the Hoguet maneuver (Chapter 13) at this point, since these important details are amplified elsewhere as noted.

The direct hernial sac was inverted when the surgeon felt that nothing would be gained by further dissection. Usually, the bulge is oversewn by placing sutures between the transversus arch above to the iliopubic tract below. Regardless of the precise details, it is the transversus abdominis lamina that is closed over the protrusion. I would emphasize this technical maneuver is not designed to provide the actual strength to the repair. It is necessary to use the transversus abdominis arch in the actual repair. This structure is sutured to Cooper's ligament or to the inguinal ligament, depending on the method of repair selected.

Sliding hernias of the bladder were uncovered five times in 104 repairs of recurrent direct inguinal hernias. In each instance, the hernial mass was freed of the abdominal wall, inverted, the transversus abdominis lamina repaired and closure completed. There were no bladder injuries among 104 patients with direct inguinal hernias.

## Postoperative Complications

One patient should be considered as a postoperative death. The patient had been discharged from the hospital but died on the 27th postoperative day of a myocardial infarction.

There were two late deaths due to malignancy, and three others due to cardiovascular and cerebrovascular arteriosclerosis and its consequences.

Postoperative complications are summarized in Table 14–6. It can be seen that wound complications are common. These result from difficult dissection, which can be attributed to dense scarring in the area. There were no major wound infections. Some type of wound complication was seen in 14 percent of the repairs, but most of them were minor and caused no additional disability.

On the other hand, testicular complications were quite commonly seen. Five patients who presented with recurrent

Table 14–6.   POSTOPERATIVE COMPLICATIONS IN 92 PATIENTS
RECURRENT DIRECT INGUINAL HERNIA

| | | |
|---|---|---|
| *WOUND COMPLICATIONS* | | 16 |
| Early | | |
| Seroma | 6 | |
| Hematoma | 3 | |
| Minor wound infection | 1 | |
| Swelling and induration | 6 | |
| Late | | 5 |
| Numbness | 2 | |
| Pain | 3 | |
| *SKIN REACTIONS* | | 3 |
| Sensitivity to tape | 2 | |
| Reaction to antiseptic | 1 | |
| *TESTICULAR* | | 16 |
| Scrotal edema, swelling, induration and ecchymosis | 8 | |
| High-riding testicle | 2 | |
| Impotency | 3 | |
| Atrophic testicle | 3 | |
| *URINARY TRACT* | | 7 |
| Urinary retention | 5 | |
| Cystitis | 2 | |
| *PULMONARY* | | 5 |
| Bronchitis-pneumonitis | 1 | |
| Atelectasis | 2 | |
| Upper respiratory tract infection | 1 | |
| Pulmonary infarcts (questionable) | 1 | |
| *CARDIOVASCULAR* | | 1 |
| Myocardial infarct (fatal) | 1 | |

direct inguinal hernias had atrophic testes at the time they presented for repair. Two of these patients with atrophic testes had had four previous repairs; one patient had had three previous repairs, and one patient had had one side repaired, followed by unilateral testicular atrophy. The fifth patient had had previous hernia repairs elsewhere; one side was repaired 47 years earlier, and the other was operated 36 years before he appeared for his repair at Henry Ford Hospital. Both testes were atrophic. In this study, 5.4 percent of patients who presented for repair of direct recurrent inguinal hernias had atrophic testes.

Following hernia repair at Henry Ford Hospital, three additional patients developed testicular atrophy. The risk to the viability of the testicle increases significantly with increasing numbers of repairs for recurrence of hernias.

Urinary tract complications consisted of retention in five patients, four of whom had had spinal anesthesia. Only one of 58 patients having local anesthesia had difficulty voiding. Patients requiring repeated operations for hernia showed a significant increase in wound and testicular complications.

## Recurrence Rate

The recurrence rate following repair of this series of 92 patients was 6 out of 104 repairs. Fifty-two, or 56.5 percent of the patients were followed for three years or longer. Four of the six recurred as direct inguinal hernias, one as direct-indirect, and one as a femoral hernia. Four of the six patients had multiple recurrences, emphasizing that the recurrent direct inguinal hernia must be taken seriously.

As a result of this study, I have been less reluctant to employ mesh in repair of recurrent direct inguinal hernias. Reported recurrence rates following repair of recurrent inguinal hernias have varied from 33.1 percent, as reported by Thieme (1971) down to 3.1 percent as noted by Skinner and Duncan (1945). Fallis reported an incidence of recurrence of 13 percent, while Quillinan (1969) and Stein and Casten (1943) both recorded recurrence rates of 10 percent after attempts at repair of recurrent inguinal hernias.

In studying both direct and indirect recurrent inguinal hernias, I found that the recurrence rate following repair of indirect recurrent inguinal hernias was 1.98 percent; with direct recurrent inguinal hernias, the postoperative recurrence rate was nearly 6 percent.

## SUMMARY

Most direct recurrent inguinal hernias appear in three varieties: small hernias near the pubic tubercle, small to moderate diverticular hernias in the floor of Hesselbach's triangle, and large diffuse protrusions through the same area.

The small recurrent defect near the pubic tubercle may be due to improper placement of the medial-most suture. It may be placed too high on the rectus sheath or into the internal oblique. Excessive tension at the site of repair is the inevitable and undesirable result. Suture strength must be adequate, for the forces of distraction at this site are great. The knot must be securely tied, and a two-handed square knot with a minimum of four throws is mandatory to avoid slippage, or even untying of the knot. Finally, proper medial-most placement of the needle bearing the suture is not a simple matter; it must be placed into the medial extent of the transversus arch above and into Cooper's ligament below. The use of a small stout needle is advisable to avoid breakage.

Larger direct recurrent inguinal hernias may be due to several factors. Excessive tension will be generated if sutures are placed too high into the internal oblique and attached to the inguinal ligament. The result may be that sutures cut through the tissues or fracture. Again, improperly tied knots may fail to hold.

The relaxing incision is the simplest, easily available expedient to minimize tension.

Excessive tension at the suture line and faulty technical execution of any method of repair are the important factors leading to recurrence. In repairing recurrent direct inguinal hernias, it is essential to shift the transversus arch to an appropriate anchoring structure, or to use a prosthetic mesh. No matter what technique of repair the surgeon chooses, he must be acutely aware of the significant tension generated by shifting the abdominal wall to either Cooper's ligament or the inguinal ligament. The problem of tension is compounded by the propensity of direct hernias to exist as bilateral defects. It should be remembered that even when a unilateral direct hernia is repaired, the eventual appearance of a hernia on the opposite side is likely. The same forces of tension will come into play during repair of the second hernia, regardless of timing.

The known recurrence rate in this series is slightly over 6 percent, indicating that direct recurrent inguinal hernias are not easily repaired with success.

In my opinion surgeons are generally too reluctant to employ a prosthetic material in repair of direct inguinal hernias. It is entirely reasonable that an area of deficient holding strength be reinforced with a well-accepted strong implant.

## REFERENCES[*]

Andrews, E. Wyllys: Imbrication or lap joint method. A plastic operation for hernia. Med. Rec. 9:67, 1895.

Andrews, E., and Bissell, A. D.: Direct hernia: A record of surgical failures. Surg. Gynecol. Obstet. 58:753, 1934.

Andrews, E.: A method of herniotomy utilizing only white fascia. Am. Surg. 80:225, 1924.

Andrews, E.: The iliohypogastric nerve in relation to herniotomy. Ann. Surg. 83:79, 1926.

Bassini, E.: Nuovo metodo per la cura radicale dell' erna inguinale. Atti Cong Assoc. Med. Ital. di Chir. Z:179, 1887.

Bassini, E.: Uber die Behandlung des Leistenbruches. Arch. Klin. Chir. 40:429, 1890.

Burton, C. C.: Important considerations in the repair of direct hernia. In Nyhus, L. M., and Harkins, H. N.: Hernia. Philadelphia. J. B. Lippincott Co., pp. 186–192.

Cattell, R. B., and Anderson, C.: End results in the operative treatment of inguinal hernia. N. Engl. J. Med. 205:430, 1931.

Cheatle, G. L.: An operation for the radical cure of inguinal and femoral hernia. Br. Med. J. 2:68, 1920.

---

[*]Included here are the references for Chapters 13 and 14.

Coley, W. B. (ed.): Review of radical cure of hernia during the last half century. Am. J. Surg. *31*:397, 1936.

Coley, B. L.: Three thousand consecutive herniotomies. Ann. Surg. *80*:242, 1924.

Condon, R. E.: *In* Nyhus, L. M., and Harkins, H. N.: *Hernia*. Philadelphia, J. B. Lippincott Co., 1964, pp. 14–72.

Dickson, A. R.: Femoral hernia. Surg. Gynecol. Obstet. *63*:665, 1936.

Doran, F. S. A.: Inguinal herniorrhaphy. Lancet *2*:1307, 1955.

Downes, W. A.: Management of direct inguinal hernia. Arch. Surg. *1*:53, 1920.

Dyson, W. L., and Pierce, W. S.: Changing concepts of inguinal herniorrhaphy: Experience with preperitoneal approach. Arch. Surg. *91*:971, 1965.

Fallis, L. S.: Recurrent inguinal hernia. Ann. Surg. *106*:363, 1937.

Fallis, L.: Inguinal hernia. Ann. Surg. *104*:403, 1936.

Fallis, L. S.: Direct inguinal hernia. Ann. Surg. *107*:572, 1938.

Fallis, L. S.: The operative treatment of inguinal hernia. J. Med. Assoc. Ga. 28(8):316, 1939.

Fallis, L. S.: Halsted I repair of direct inguinal hernia. Important considerations in the repair of direct hernia. *In* Nyhus, L. M., and Harkins, H. N.: *Hernia*. Philadelphia, J. B. Lippincott Co, 1964, pp. 164–178.

Ferguson, A. H.: The Technic for Modern Operations for Hernia Cleveland Press, Chicago 1907, pp. 280–288.

Ferguson, A. H.: Oblique hernia. Typic operation for its radical cure. J.A.M.A. *33*:6, 1899.

Gaspar, M. R., and Casberg, M. A.: An appraisal of preperitoneal repair of inguinal hernia. Surg. Gynecol. Obstet. *132*:207, 1971.

Glassow, F.: Short stay surgery (Shouldice Technique) for repair of inguinal hernia. Ann. R. Coll. Surg. (Engl.) 58(2):133, 1976.

Glassow, F.: Femoral hernia following inguinal herniorrhaphy. Can. J. Surg. *13*:27, 1970.

Glassow, F.: Bilateral hernias in the female. Can. Med. Assoc. J. *101*:66, 1969.

Glenn, F.: The surgical treatment of 1545 herniae. Ann. Surg. *125*:72, 1947.

Gregorie, H. B., Jr.: Preperitoneal repair of groin hernias. J. S. C. Med. Assoc. 6:417, 1966.

Griffith, C. A.: Inguinal hernia. An anatomic-surgical correlation. Surg. Clin. North Am. *39*:531, 1959.

Halsted, W. S.: The radical cure of hernia. Bull. Johns Hopkins Hosp. *1*:112, 1890.

Halsted, W. S.: The cure of the more difficult as well as the simpler inguinal ruptures. Bull. Johns Hopkins Hosp. *14*:208, 1903.

Halverson, C. B., and McVay, C. B.: Inguinal and femoral hernioplasty. A 22 year study of the authors methods. Arch. Surg. *101*:127, 1970.

Harkins, H. N.: The repair of groin hernias. Progress in the past decade. Surg. Clin. North Am. 29:1457, 1949.

Harkins, H. N., and Schug, R. N.: Hernial repair using Cooper's ligament. Arch. Surg. 55:689, 1947.

Harkins, H., and Swenson, S. A.: A Cooper's ligament herniotomy. Surg. Clin. North Am. 23:1279, 1943.

Henry, A. K.: Operation for femoral hernia by midline extraperitoneal approach. Lancet *1*:531, 1936.

Hesselbach, F. K.: *Neuste Anatomisch Pathologische Untersuchungen über den Ursprung und das Fortschreiter der Leisten- und Schenkelbrüche.* Würzburg, Bäumgartner, 1814.

Hoguet, J. P.: Direct inguinal hernia. Ann. Surg. 72:671, 1920.

Hoguet, J. P.: Observations on 2468 hernia operations by one operator. Surg. Gynecol. Obstet. 37:71, 1923.

Iason, A. H.: *Hernia*. Philadelphia, Blakiston Co., 1941, pp. 105–107.

Koontz, A. R.: Inguinal hernias: Some causes of recurrence. Am. J. Surg. 82:474, 1951.

Koontz, A. R.: Views on the choice of operation for inguinal hernia repair. Ann. Surg. 143:868, 1956.

Lichtenstein, J. L.: Immediate ambulation and return to work following herniorrhaphy. Industr. Med. Surg. 35:754, 1966.

Lichtenstein, J. L.: Local anesthesia for hernioplasty. Calif. Med. 100:106, 1964.

Lindholm, A., Nilson, O., and Thomlin, B.: Inguinal and femoral hernias. Arch. Surg. 98:19, 1969.

Lotheissen, G.: Zur operation der Schenkelhernien. Zentralble. Chir. 25:548, 1898.

Lytle, W. J.: Inguinal hernia. *In* Rob, C., and Smith, R. (eds.): *Operative Surgery* (2nd ed.). London, Butterworth's, 1969, pp. 220–233.

Madden, J. L., Saeed, H., and Agorogiannis, A. B.: The anatomy and repair of inguinal hernias. Surg. Clin. North Am. *51*:1269, 1971.

Martin, J. D., Jr., and Stone, H. H.: Recurrent inguinal hernia. Ann. Surg. *156*:713, 1962.

McClure, R. D., and Fallis, L. S.: Femoral hernia. Report of 90 operations. Ann. Surg. *109*:987, 1939.

McVay, C. B., and Anson, B. J.: A fundamental error in current methods of inguinal herniorrhaphy. Surg. Gynecol. Obstet. 74:746, 1942.

McVay, C. B., and Anson, B. J.: Inguinal and femoral hernioplasty. Surg. Gynecol. Obstet. 88:473, 1949.

Mikkelson, W. P., and Berne, C. J.: Femoral hernioplasty suprapubic extraperitoneal (Cheatle-Henry) approach. Surgery 35:743, 1955.

Musgrove, J. E., and McCready, F. J.: The Henry approach to femoral hernia. Surgery 27:608, 1949.

Nyhus, L. A., Stevenson, J. K., Listerud, M. B., and Harkins, H. N.: Preperitoneal herniorrhaphy; a preliminary report in fifty patients. West. J. Surg. 67:48, 1959.

Nyhus, L. M., Condon, R. E., and Harkins, H. N.: Clinical experiences with preperitoneal hernial repair for all types of hernia of the groin. Am. J. Surg. 100:234, 1960.

Palumbo, L. T., Sharpe, W. S., Lulu, D. J., and Bloom, M. D.: Primary inguinal hernioplasty. Postgrad. Med. 42:505, 1967.

Palumbo, L. T., Sharpe, W. S., Shirley, W. G., and Benetti, A. F.: Primary direct inguinal hernioplasty. Am. J. Surg. 108:815, 1964.

Pitzman, M.: A fundamentally new technic for inguinal herniotomy. Ann. Surg. 74:610, 1921.

Postlethwait, R. W.: Causes of recurrence after inguinal herniorrhaphy. Surgery 69:772, 1971.

Poth, E. J.: Inguinal hernia repair using the rectus-pyramidalis sheath. Am. J. Surg. 122:699, 1971.

Quillinan, R.: Repair of recurrent inguinal hernia. Am. J. Surg. 118:593, 1969.

Qvist, G.: Saddlebag hernia. Br. J. Surg. 64:442, 1977.

Read, R. C.: Preperitoneal exposure of inguinal herniation. Am. J. Surg. *116*:653, 1968.

Read, R. R.: Preperitoneal, prosthetic inguinal herniorrhaphy without a relaxing incision. Am. J. Surg. *132*:749, 1976.

Rienhoff, W. F.: The use of the rectus fascia for closure of the lower or critical angle of the wound in the repair of inguinal hernia. Surgery 8:326, 1940.

Robertson, H. T.: Preperitoneal approach in the repair of inguinal hernias. Am. J. Surg. *112*:627, 1966.

Ross, A. P. J.: Incidence of inguinal hernia recurrence. Ann. Royal Coll. Surg. (Engl.) 57:326, 1975.

Rydell, W. E.: Inguinal and femoral hernias. Arch. Surg. 87:493, 1963.

Seelig, M. G., and Tuholske, L.: The inguinal route operation for femoral hernia with a supplementary note on Cooper's ligament. Surg. Gynecol. Obstet. *18*:55, 1914.

Skinner, H. L., and Duncan, R. D.: Recurrent inguinal hernia. Ann. Surg. *122*:68, 1945.

Smith, G. V.: *In* Hardy, J. D. (ed.): *Rhoads Textbook of Surgery: Principles and Practice* (5th ed.). Philadelphia, J. B. Lippincott Co., 1977, pp. 1323–1334.

Stein, H. E., and Casten, D.: Study of recurrences following inguinal hernioplasty. Surgery *14*:819, 1943.

Tanner, N. C.: A "slide" operation for inguinal and femoral hernia. Br. J. Surg. 29:285, 1942.

Taylor, A. S.: The results of operations for inguinal hernia. Arch. Surg. *1*:382, 1920.

Thieme, E. T.: Recurrent inguinal hernia. Arch. Surg. *103*:238, 1971.

Tobin, G. R., Scott, C., and Peacock, E. E., Jr.: A neuromuscular basis for development of indirect inguinal hernia. Surgery *111*(4):464, 1976.

Wagh, P. V., Leverich, A. F., Sun, C. H., White, H. J., and Read, R.: Direct inguinal herniation in men: A disease of collagen. J. Surg. Res. *17*:425, 1971.

Watson, L. F.: *Hernia* (3rd ed.). St. Louis, C. V. Mosby Co., 1938.

Wölfer, A.: *Zur Radikaloperation des Freien Leistenbruches.* Stuttgart, Beitr. Chir. (Festchr. Gewidmet Theodor Billroth), 1892, p. 552.

Zimmerman, L. M.: Recurrent inguinal hernia. Surg. Clin. North Am. *51*:1321, 1971.

Zimmerman, L. M., and Veith, I.: *Great Ideas in the History of Surgery* (2nd ed.). New York, Dover Publications, Inc., 1967.

Zimmerman, L. M.: The surgical treatment of direct inguinal hernia. Surg. Gynecol. Obstet. 66:192, 1938.

Zimmerman, L. M.: A critique of the McVay operation for inguinal hernia. Surg. Gynecol. Obstet. 87:621, 1948 (Editorial).

Zimmerman, L. M.: Essential problems in the surgical treatment of inguinal hernia. Surg. Gynecol. Obstet. 71:654, 1940.

Zimmerman, L. M.: Recent advances in surgery of inguinal hernia. Surg. Clin. North Am. *32*:135, 1952.

## Supplemental Readings*

Babcock, W. W.: The ideal in herniorrhaphy. Surg. Gynecol. Obstet. *45*:434, 1927.

Beekman, F., and Sullivan, J. E.: Analysis of immediate post-operative complications in 2000 cases of inguinal hernia. Surg. Gynecol. Obstet. *68*:1052, 1939.

Bloodgood, J. C.: Operation in 459 cases of hernia. Johns Hopkins Hosp. Rep. *7*:223, 1899.

Bull, W. T.: On the radical cure of hernia, with results of one hundred and thirty-four operations. Trans. Am. Surg. 8:99, 1890.

Chandler, S. B.: The anatomy of the inguinal (Hesselbach's) triangle. Ann. Surg. *124*:156, 1946.

Connell, F. G.: The repair of the internal ring in oblique inguinal hernia. J.A.M.A. *52*:1087, 1909.

Connell, F. G.: Repair of internal ring in oblique inguinal hernia. Surg. Gynecol. Obstet. *46*:113, 1928.

Jefferson, N. C., and Dailey, U. V.: Incisional hernia repaired with Tantalum guaze. Am. J. Surg. 75:575, 1948.

Komora, E. J.: Inguino-femoral anatomy; Aspects significant for inguinal herniorrhaphy. Am. J. Surg. *61*:380, 1943.

Krieg, E. G.: Anatomy and physiology of the inguinal region in the presence of hernia. Ann. Surg. *137*:41, 1953.

Mahorner, H., and Goss, C. M.: Herniation following destruction of Poupart's and Cooper's ligaments: A method of repair. Ann. Surg. *155*:741, 1962.

Ravitch, M. M., and Hitzrot, J. M., II: *The Operations for Hernia.* St. Louis, C. V. Mosby Co., 1960.

Schley, W.: Tranposition of the rectal muscle and the utilization of the external oblique aponeurosis in the radical cure of inguinal hernia. Ann. Surg. 77:605, 1923.

Garner, A. D.: Inguinal hernia. An analysis of 2643 operations. Am. J. Surg. 74:14, 1947.

Graivier, L., and Alfieri, A. L.: Bilateral Spigelian hernias in infancy. Am. J. Surg. *120*:817, 1970.

Longacre, A. B.: Follow-up of hernia repair. Surg. Gynecol. Obstet. *68*:238, 1939.

Myers, R. N., and Shearburn, E. W.: Recurrence rate of 2.6 percent following repair of 76 consecutive recurrent inguinal hernias.

Postlethwait, R. W.: Causes of recurrence after inguinal herniorrhaphy. Surgery 69:772, 1971.

Postlethwait, R. W.: Recurrent inguinal hernia. Am. J. Surg. *107*:739, 1964.

Ryan, E. A.: Recurrent hernias. Surg. Gynecol. Obstet. 96:343, 1953.

Usher, F. C.: The repair of incisional and inguinal hernias. Surg. Dig. (Apr.) 1971, pp. 7–14.

Weinstein, M., and Roberts, M.: Recurrent inguinal hernia: Follow-up study of 100 postoperative patients. Am. J. Surg. *129*:563, 1975.

*Chapters 13 and 14 included here.

# 15

# Femoral Hernia

The femoral hernia is the most deceptive of the three varieties of groin hernias. The small femoral hernia is easily overlooked in an obese patient; the incarcerated hernia of the Richter's type leads the diagnostician into making errors, while the apparently small anatomic defect lulls the unsuspecting surgeon into performing an operation that too often is only temporarily effective. Furthermore, femoral hernias are seen comparatively infrequently, with the result that recurrences are erroneously believed to be rare.

The need to define just what constitutes a femoral hernia might be questioned; yet in light of current knowledge, the modern surgeon must expand his understanding to include current practical anatomic knowledge.

## DEFINITION

A femoral hernia is one in which there is a protrusion of some abdominal or pelvic viscus, or preperitoneal fat, through the femoral ring and transversalis fascia into the crural region — through a lower small femoral hernial orifice. It must be emphasized that a dimple or depression at the femoral ring alone does not constitute a femoral hernia.

## ANATOMY

The anatomy and pathology of femoral hernias are better understood as the results of the contributions of McVay and

Anson (1942), Lytle (1957), and Nyhus and Condon (1960). McVay's contributions are valuable from an anatomic viewpoint, whereas Lytle called attention to the important details of the pathologic anatomy involved (Fig. 15–1).

The femoral canal has somewhat the shape of a cone or funnel. This concept is extremely important, since it includes not merely one but two orifices or rings. One of these — i.e., the femoral ring — serves as the inlet. The second, or smaller, opening, is the femoral hernial orifice, which is situated two or three centimeters inferiorly, or lower. It must be pointed out that the femoral hernia is recognizable as such after it passes through the femoral hernial orifice.

The femoral ring, measuring from one to three centimeters in diameter, is located at the iliopectineal line and most easily demonstrated by palpating the pelvic brim and Cooper's ligament through an abdominal or inguinal incision. A depression or dimple may be palpated at this site, but this alone does not necessarily constitute a hernia.

The anterior margin of the normal ring is the iliopubic tract, which is a derivative of the transversalis fascia as it contributes to the femoral sheath. The inguinal ligament in its medial portion has a free edge and can easily be elevated from the transversalis fascia and femoral sheath, as pointed out by Galludet (1931) and by McVay. The medial boundary of the femoral ring consists of the lateral attachment of the posterior inguinal wall onto the ligament of Cooper. Posteriorly, the margin of the

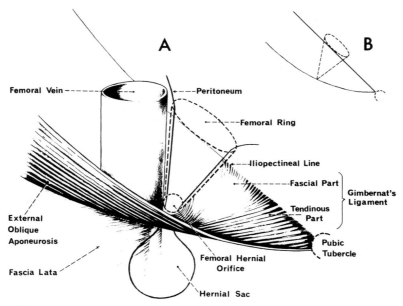

**Figure 15–1.** Lytle's concept of femoral hernia depicting the upper femoral ring and the lower femoral hernial orifice.

femoral ring is made up of the superior ramus of the pubis, Cooper's ligament, and pectineus fascia. The femoral vein comprises the lateral margin of the femoral ring. Actually, a connective tissue septum is present between the anterior and posterior portions of the femoral sheath. This structure is in close proximity to the vein.

The femoral canal, which is actually a potential canal, begins at the femoral ring and is normally present as a possible passageway for hernias. It is occupied by loose connective tissue, lymphatics, and lymph nodes of variable size and number. Here a single enlarged lymph node is known as the node of Cloquet in France, or as the node of Rosenmüller in Germany; both names are used in North America. The structures surrounding the femoral canal include the cribriform fascia anteriorly. The femoral vein and accompanying connective tissue are located laterally; the pectineus muscle and fascia lata, posteriorly.

Lytle's concept of a femoral hernial orifice, situated approximately two centimeters distal to the femoral ring, is a practical and useful one (see Fig. 15–1). It is at this point that a femoral hernia appears, continues downward and anteriorly, then presents at the fossa ovalis where the cribriform fascia is not of suffi-

cient strength to contain it. Fundamentally, the femoral hernia occurs because of a defect in the transversalis fascia. As Lytle has pointed out, many surgeons erroneously believe that the femoral ring is the site of constriction in femoral hernias. Actually, it is located further down—at the femoral hernial orifice, which is quite small, and usually measures approximately one centimeter in diameter. Lytle described the femoral hernia orifice in detail. The lateral edge is related to the femoral sheath. The lower portion of the lacunar ligament lies medially, the pectineal fascia posteriorly, and Hey's ligament anteriorly. The inguinal ligament lies in an anterior position, but it is situated above or cephalad to the femoral hernial orifice.

Any discussion of femoral hernia should include comment about rare forms of femoral herniation. The protrusion may occur in the prevascular location, or even farther laterally. I have seen a femoral hernia protrude into the thigh between the inguinal ligament and femoral vessels. This patient had previously undergone vascular surgical procedures on his femoral vessels.

Rhind (1971) reported a lateral femoral hernia bounded medially by the external iliac and inferior epigastric arteries, anteriorly by the inguinal ligament, and laterally and posteriorly by the iliacus muscle.

The anatomic variants of herniations into the thigh are more numerous than recognized; unfortunately, when they do occur, reports are too often lacking. Documentation of unusual femoral hernias would be worthwhile.

## ETIOLOGIC FACTORS

It has been difficult to establish definite causative factors leading to femoral hernia formation. Several theories have been advanced and ultimately rejected. For instance, few surgeons today will insist that femoral hernia is due to congenital abnormalities or the presence of a congenital sac. I will avoid complicating the matter unnecessarily by considering possible etiologic factors from two points of view—i.e, the congenital and the acquired theories of femoral hernia formation, both of which merit some discussion.

### The Congenital Theory

Historically, there was a period during which it was held that femoral hernias were due to congenital causes. Hamilton Russell in 1906 rejected the idea that the femoral hernia could be acquired, and he insisted that a developmental peritoneal diverticulum or sac in the femoral canal was required as a pre-existing condition. Murray in 1910 was of the same opinion. If one accepts the definition of the word *congenital* as "being present at or dating from birth," then the concept that femoral hernias are congenital becomes untenable. It is a rare event to see a femoral hernia in an infant or child, and even surgeons devoting their lives to surgery of infants and children rarely see femoral hernias.

Immordino (1972) found only 6 femoral hernias in 1600 groin hernias occurring in infants and children that were repaired at the New England Medical Center in Boston in a ten-year period. Three of the patients were four years of age or older, and three were two and one-half years of age or younger. It is noteworthy that four of these youngsters had undergone previous repairs of inguinal hernias.

At the Children's Hospital of Buffalo

(New York), Burke (1967) found femoral hernias in 16 children in a period of 28 years. Eight of his patients had undergone previous repair of inguinal hernias.

Significantly, there is no developmental event occurring in relation to the femoral canal comparable to the descent of the testicle from the posterior abdomen through the layers of the abdominal wall to its scrotal position.

Furthermore, if femoral hernias were congenital in origin, the preperitoneal sac or diverticulum should be demonstrable. Neither Keith nor McVay was able to demonstrate congenital peritoneal sacs.

I have never seen a congenital femoral hernial sac comparable to those seen often in indirect inguinal hernias in neonates, infants, and children.

### The Acquired Theory

In my experience, the age incidence strongly supports the concept that the femoral hernia is an acquired abnormality (Fig. 15–2). In reading the opinions of a

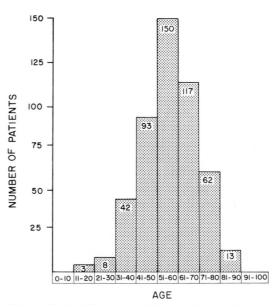

**Figure 15–2.** The age incidence of femoral hernia shows that such hernias are seen in large numbers in adults and aged patients.

number of contributors, I am impressed with the fact that some of them seek a single explanation for all femoral hernias. It is becoming obvious that several factors are operative in the causation of femoral hernias. Buckley, Koontz, Lytle, McVay and Monro, writing in Nyhus' book on hernia (1964), all favor the concept that the femoral hernia is an acquired defect.

Keith, in 1923, felt that increased intra-abdominal pressure caused protrusion or wedging of preperitoneal fat with femoral hernia formation. Buckley, also in 1923, stated that under the influence of increased intra-abdominal pressure, preperitoneal fat herniated under Poupart's ligament into the thigh, carrying with it a small peritoneal diverticulum. He then explained that once the protrusion passed the narrow neck, it is allowed to expand in the less-resistant tissues of the upper thigh. Buckley felt that the greater frequency of femoral hernia in women was due to the prolonged increase in intra-abdominal pressure incident to pregnancy.

McVay studied the anatomy of the inguinofemoral areas and concluded that the primary etiology of femoral hernia is the narrow attachment of the posterior abdominal wall to Cooper's ligament. As a result of the enlarged femoral ring, increased intra-abdominal pressure forces preperitoneal fat through the ring into the femoral canal, resulting in the formation of a femoral hernia.

Lytle in 1957 made an important observation when he suggested that the weakness lies in the femoral partition at the lower end of the femoral canal.

In the causation of femoral hernia, it appears that some anatomic abnormality exists, but oft-repeated and prolonged increase in intra-abdominal pressure is necessary as an exciting cause. A number of forces are capable of causing the increase in pressure, and pregnancy is merely one of these. Atrophy of tissue incident to aging may well be an additional factor. Increase in intra-abdominal pressure due to heavy work appears to be an important factor in the etiology of direct hernias; oddly, men who perform strenuous work and develop direct hernias do not present with femoral hernias in equal numbers.

## HISTORICAL CONSIDERATIONS

My comments will be directed toward those individuals who have contributed their anatomic observations and technical advances of enduring value to those dealing with the femoral hernia problem. Numerous instances of abdominal section for obstructed and strangulated hernias have been recorded, but the descriptions as to the technique of repair are entirely missing or so poorly described as to be

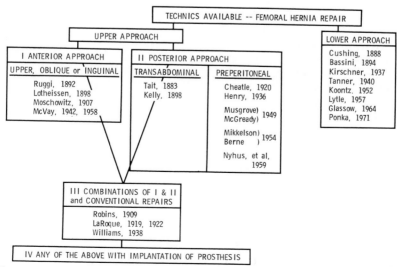

**Figure 15–3.** Various surgical techniques available for repair of femoral hernias as developed by a number of surgeons.

incomprehensible. I will avoid those reports in the literature dealing with isolated instances or operative procedures carried out mechanically, without appreciation of the anatomy involved. I hope to arrange the significant events in a simple but orderly and understandable manner (Fig. 15-3).

The preperitoneal or retroperitoneal approach to the repair of groin hernias has an interesting history. Lawson Tait in 1883 repaired a femoral hernia, which he discovered while operating for ovarian tumor through an abdominal incision. He attempted repair by closing the femoral ring.

Koontz (1963) pointed out that Kelly (the renowned gynecologist of Johns Hopkins Hospital of Baltimore during the Halsted era) would repair any coexisting femoral hernia when operating for gynecologic diseases. His method of repair, which was described in 1898, is worthy of note. He sutured Poupart's ligament to the "pubic portion of the fascia lata," utilizing the abdominal approach.

One of the best early descriptions of the preperitoneal repairs appeared in 1920 when Sir G. Lenthal Cheatle published a report consisting of 50 lines in the British Medical Journal and entitled, "An Operation for the Radical Cure of Inguinal and Femoral Hernia." His operation was performed through a rectus splitting incision. The rectus abdominis muscle was retracted: "the peritoneum is smoothed away by a dry swab from the parietes." He did not open the peritoneum "but the sac is ligatured at the peritoneal surface." After the peritoneal sac was ligated, it was allowed to slip back into the inguinal canal. Thus, he reasoned, it could not act as a guide for a recurrent hernia. He stated that the "muscle fibers and their sheaths are separately sutured." He added that there was nothing to stop the surgeon from occluding the internal ring at the same time.

Cheatle further stated that in one patient with a femoral hernia, the same procedure was used. He then described an addition to repair as follows: "I turned up a square inch of periosteum from the underlying pubes and attached it to the undersurface of Poupart's ligament and the outer margin of Gimbernat's ligament." No illustrations accompanied the article. Cheatle was unaware that other surgeons had used a comparable approach.

In a historically significant paper, Henry in 1936 described his operation, which he had performed only once at the Kasr-el-Aini Hospital in Cairo. He used a midline incision and the preperitoneal approach. Henry was familiar with this type of approach as a result of experience while operating for bilateral lesions of the pelvic ureter. As stated by Henry:

> The views obtained of the four relevant structures—Gimbernat's ligament, the hinder edge of Poupart's, the fascia covering the pectineus, the external iliac vein—was like that in a specimen prepared for demonstration.

He stated that this view convinced him that the femoral ring could easily be closed by "turning a flap of dense fascia covering the pectineus muscle and sewing it to the hinder edge of Poupart's ligament." The article by Henry is well illustrated and provides descriptions and illustrations that may be followed easily. He also refers to the anatomic features seen in inguinal hernias. Henry noted that the thickened transversalis could be easily identified; in addition, he had used the preperitoneal approach in the repair of direct inguinal hernias. The paper by Henry is an early and lucid presentation of the preperitoneal approach to repair of groin hernias; however, it was Cheatle who first used a flap of periosteum in the repair of a femoral hernia in 1920.

Musgrove and McCready used the Henry preperitoneal approach to femoral hernia repair in 1949.

Mikkelsen and Berne were interested in the procedure and in 1954 published a historically significant paper recording their experiences with the suprapubic extraperitoneal (Cheatle-Henry) approach to femoral hernioplasty in 113 patients. They have now operated on over 500 patients with remarkable results.

It is interesting to note in reviewing the literature on the preperitoneal approach for repair of groin hernias that urologists were the first to observe the anatomy involved and that easy access could be gained to the repair of groin hernias via the posterior approach. Henry as well as Riba and Mehn (1951), who also repaired hernias via the retroperitoneal route, were urologists.

The current popularity and interest in the preperitoneal approach to the repair of femoral hernias must be attributed to Nyhus and Condon and their coworkers. Until their publications appeared, the preperitoneal approach lay relatively dormant as a technique for repair of femoral hernias. In 1959 Nyhus, Stevenson, and Listerud published a preliminary report on the results of preperitoneal herniorrhaphy in fifty patients. Nyhus, Condon, and Harkins extended the technique for repair of all types of groin hernias in 1960. Nyhus and Condon are rightfully recognized as pioneers in the development of the preperitoneal approach to hernia repair because of their fundamental anatomic studies and the popularization of the procedure through their excellent illustrations and numerous publications.

The operative repair of groin hernias in which Cooper's ligament is utilized is known as the Lotheissen repair, the McVay repair, and Cooper's ligament repair. There is no doubt that the operation widely known today as the McVay repair was performed by Lotheissen in 1898. The procedure, as described by Lotheissen, will be discussed in detail in Chapter 19 on recurrent inguinofemoral hernia. In this publication, I will use both eponyms to refer to the Cooper's ligament repair. There are three very good reasons as to why, in my opinion, the procedure should be known as the McVay repair. First, McVay made basic and important contributions toward the proper understanding of the anatomy concerned with femoral hernias. Second, he pointed out the advantages of repairing the inguinal floor by suturing the transversus arch to Cooper's ligament. This repair precludes the egress of a femoral hernia. Third, he popularized the method through his teaching and the numerous publications dealing with the technique and results obtained.

Ruggi first sutured the inguinal ligament to Cooper's ligament in 1892, but Moschcowitz added repair of the inguinal floor by suturing the "internal oblique and transversalis" to the inguinal ligament over the cord or round ligament.

The lower approach to repair of femoral hernia was utilized by H. W. Cushing in 1888. He freed the peritoneal sac, then closed the femoral canal with a purse-string suture that included the falciform process, pectineus fascia, and Poupart's ligament.

Bassini performed a similar procedure in 1884, but his publication did not appear until 1894; by then he had accumulated 54 cases. Bassini ligated the peritoneal sac and excised the excess; Cushing used it to occlude the femoral canal. Bassini used interrupted sutures to approximate the falciform ligament or process to pectineus fascia, and additional sutures were placed between the inguinal ligament and pectineus fascia. Thus, the classical Bassini repair is a comparatively simple procedure.

## OPERATIVE TREATMENT— TECHNIQUES OF REPAIR

There are differences of opinion as to how femoral hernias should be repaired; each advocate has an anatomic basis for his recommended repair. McVay prefers repair of the posterior abdominal wall from a position above Poupart's ligament by suturing the transversus abdominis stratum (which includes the transversus abdominis muscle and transversalis fascia) to Cooper's ligament. Such a repair precludes the possibility of any viscus reaching the femoral canal. According to Lytle, the actual defect lies at the lower portion of the funnel or femoral canal at the femoral hernial orifice. Hence, he feels that an effective repair should restore the tissues of the femoral canal to normal by occluding the femoral hernial orifice. He accomplishes his objective from an approach below the inguinal ligament by placing a purse-string suture that approximates Gimbernat's ligament, pectineal fascia, fascia lata, and femoral sheath.

In my opinion, the well-informed surgeon has several techniques available to him for repair of femoral hernias. Each technique has its enthusiasts as well as its critics; therefore, it would be reasonable to conclude that femoral hernias can be successfully repaired by more than one method. The advantages and deficiencies of each method must be appreciated. The commonly used approaches are summarized in Figure 15–3 (see p. 241). The outline is specifically applicable to the treatment of femoral hernias.

## TECHNIQUE OF THE LOTHEISSEN-MCVAY REPAIR

The skin incision is made approximately two to three centimeters above and parallel to the inguinal ligament. The dissection is developed with a scalpel to the fascia of the external oblique. All blood vessels are clamped and ligated with number 4–0 silk. The external oblique aponeurosis is incised at the level of the superior crus, and the upper and lower leaflets are dissected free. After the upper, or medial, leaflet is elevated, the internal oblique muscle and aponeurosis and the anterior sheath of the rectus muscle are visualized.

The lower leaflet is dissected, so that the inguinal ligament is identified. The entire spermatic cord (or round ligament in the female) is elevated, and the floor of the inguinal canal is visualized. The area is inspected for indirect or direct hernias.

The cremaster muscle is divided to permit recognition of the peritoneal projection along the superior and medial aspect of the cord. The peritoneum is incised carefully and digital examination carried out to further identify weaknesses in the inguinofemoral area. I nearly always identify the peritoneal sac at the internal ring and enter the peritoneum at this point; the danger of injury to the bladder is greatly reduced.

The femoral hernial sac is withdrawn and converted into an indirect sac at the internal ring by the Hoguet maneuver. The peritoneal sac is closed with a purse-string suture of heavy or number 2–0 silk. High ligation of the peritoneal sac is essential. In large sacs, the excess peritoneum is excised.

If there is difficulty in reducing the femoral hernial sac, a combined approach may be used. Traction may be applied from above while pressure may be placed on the sac from below the inguinal ligament. Furthermore, the constriction may be released medially by incising Gimbernat's ligament.

The transversalis fascia is triangulated at the internal ring and closed separately with medium number 3–0 silk sutures. Precise closure of the transversalis fascia is of paramount importance if indirect recurrences are to be avoided (Fig. 15–4).

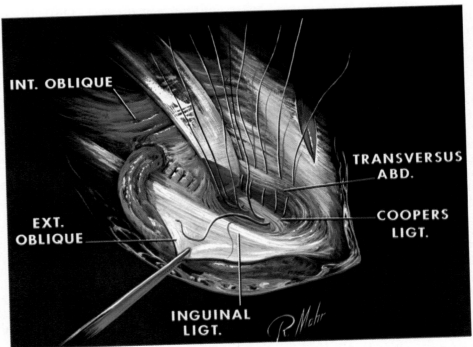

**Figure 15–4.** The artist's drawing of a Lotheissen-McVay repair in which the transversus abdominis arch is sutured to Cooper's ligament. The transversalis fascia is closed separately at the internal ring. (Reproduced by permission of publisher from Ponka, J. L., and Brush, B. E.: The problem of femoral hernia. Arch. Surg., *102*:420, 1971. Copyright 1971, American Medical Association.)

The transversalis fascia must now be opened or dissected off Cooper's ligament to permit accurate visualization of the dense, fibrous band of tissue, the iliopectineal ligament of Cooper. Any adipose tissue protruding through the femoral ring is removed. This dissection must then be carried laterally far enough to permit recognition of the femoral vein. The fact that Cooper's ligament must be clearly defined bears repetition. I have found that this dissection is often carried out incompletely and not far enough laterally. Furthermore, the femoral vein must be visualized if it is to be spared injury. The abnormal obturator artery must be looked for and avoided. I have seen three instances of troublesome bleeding following injury of blood vessels in this area. In one patient, the bleeding came from the femoral vein; in two others, severe bleeding followed injury to an abnormal obturator artery. Injury to the femoral vein should not occur if it is identified during dissection.

In recent years, I have come to appreciate the need for use of sutures of sufficient strength to hold the structures—namely, the transversus arch and Cooper's ligament—in apposition under conditions of unavoidable stress. Therefore, I have frequently used two strands of heavy number 2-0 silk or number 2-0 synthetic nonabsorbable sutures placed between these structures. A relaxing incision in the anterior sheath of the rectus is an important measure to decrease tension on the suture line.

Another word of caution is necessary. The approximation of the transversus abdominis aponeurosis or transversus arch must be carried far enough laterally to accomplish effective exclusion of the femoral ring so as to avoid recurrence of a hernia at this site. I have read operative notes in which only two sutures were used to approximate the transversus arch to Cooper's ligament. My recommendation is that a minimum of four sutures of heavy silk must be placed between these structures at intervals of approximately eight to ten millimeters between the transversus layer and Cooper's ligament if effective repair is to be achieved (Fig. 15–4). In tying these sutures, one must remember that approximation of the structures is de-

sirable and strangulation of the tissue must be avoided.

McVay has described a "transition suture," which is placed between the transversus layer, Cooper's ligament, and the medial portion of the femoral sheath.

I would add a note of caution that blind placement of sutures with a large needle (in the hope that Cooper's ligament has been included in the repair) is dangerous and inaccurate.

It is reassuring when performing the McVay repair under local anesthesia to have the patient give a lusty cough. The strength and effectiveness of the above repair can be visualized and, with a finger in the repaired area, palpated. Further sutures are unnecessary, but it bears repetition that the transversalis fascia must be closed precisely at the internal ring.

The aponeurosis of the external oblique is then closed after the cord or round ligament is replaced, and finally subcutaneous tissues and the skin are approximated.

The technique of wound closure is described and illustrated in detail in Chapter 11 on indirect inguinal hernia.

## UPPER APPROACH—MOSCHCOWITZ REPAIR

The Moschcowitz repair for femoral hernia has occupied a controversial position insofar as its usefulness in the repair of femoral hernia is concerned. The method is used less frequently in modern surgical practice. I will simply state that the procedure has a usefulness in very carefully selected patients. The anatomic position of the inguinal ligament in relation to the ligament of Cooper must be considered. If the angle between these structures is wide, then surgical approximation is likely to be temporary. If a great deal of tension is required to close the femoral ring by suturing Poupart's ligament to Cooper's ligament, then another technique should be considered. Although the Moschcowitz repair may be effective in selected patients, it is certainly not applicable to all patients with femoral hernia. Throckmorton in a discussion of the paper on femoral hernia by Ponka and Brush (1971) advocated the implantation of a prosthetic mesh over the femoral ring.

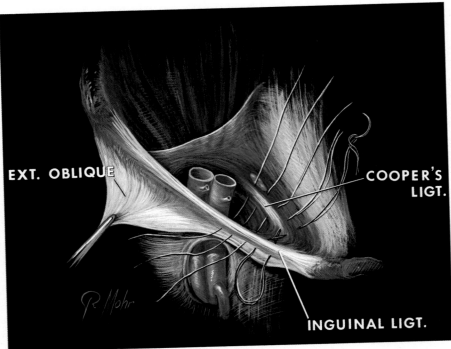

EXT. OBLIQUE

COOPER'S LIGT.

INGUINAL LIGT.

**Figure 15–5.** The Moschcowitz repair in which the inguinal ligament is sutured to Cooper's ligament.

I have used this technique and found it useful in certain recurrent femoral hernias as well.

The Moschcowitz method of repair is carried out through an incision made above and parallel to the inguinal ligament, much as it is performed for indirect or direct inguinal hernias (Fig. 15–5). Again, the incision is developed through the aponeurosis of the external oblique at the level of the superior crus. The upper and lower leaflets are dissected free, and the round ligament or spermatic cord is elevated from the floor of the inguinal canal. The ilioinguinal and iliohypogastric nerves are identified and preserved. The peritoneal prolongation is identified at the internal ring, and the peritoneum is opened. The peritoneal cavity is digitally explored. The Hoguet maneuver is performed, and thus the femoral sac is converted into an indirect sac. Moschcowitz converted the sac into a direct hernial sac. Fallis (while associated with McClure) applied the Hoguet maneuver to effect reduction of the femoral sac, converting it into an indirect sac. The peritoneal sac is closed with a purse-string suture of heavy silk. The transversalis fascia is triangu-

lated at the internal ring and closed separately with figure-of-eight sutures of heavy silk. The transversalis fascia is then opened in the floor of Hesselbach's triangle to permit visualization of Cooper's ligament. Any adipose tissue in the femoral ring is withdrawn upward, so that accurate apposition of the inguinal ligament with iliopubic tract and Cooper's ligament is possible. The sutures are first placed nearest the pubic tubercle, then are continued laterally in intervals until the femoral vein is reached (Fig. 15–5). Visualization of the femoral vein and Cooper's ligament must be clear. All required sutures are placed between these structures before any are tied. The sutures are tied from the medial aspect first, since it is where the tension is the least. Any modification of the technique just described is dictated by the needs of the individual patient.

I repair the floor by suturing the transversalis layer or transversus arch to the inguinal ligament and iliopubic tract beneath the cord.

The external oblique is closed over the cord with sutures of medium number 3–0 silk. Subcutaneous tissues are closed with number 3–0 plain catgut, and the skin is approximated with narrow strips of adhesive tape.

## LOWER APPROACH—THE BASSINI REPAIR

The designation of Bassini repair is often applied to numerous techniques performed through an incision below the inguinal ligament. The classical Bassini repair of a femoral hernia is one in which the femoral hernia sac is reached through an oblique or vertical incision in the upper thigh. The sac is dissected free, and a high ligation of the peritoneal sac is performed. Then the inguinal ligament and pectineal fascia and the fascia lata and pectineal fascia are approximated with interrupted sutures (Fig. 15–9).

The number of modifications of the Bassini technique is enormous. I shall describe two methods that have been found effective in selected cases. Some procedures carry individual eponyms simply as a result of employing a special type of suture.

## TECHNIQUE OF BASSINI-KIRSCHNER REPAIR OF FEMORAL HERNIA

The method of repair from below—the one that I prefer—is similar to an approach described by Kirschner. The oblique skin incision in the upper groin is developed through the subcutaneous fat and provides the patient with a more pleasing cosmetic result. All vessels are clamped and tied with number 4–0 fine silk. The fascia lata is incised transversely, and the peritoneal sac with preperitoneal fat is identified medial to the femoral vein and below the inguinal ligament. The sac is freed, then opened—with care being taken to avoid injury to the bladder. High ligation is performed, and then the excess sac is excised. It is remarkable how great a length of peritoneal sac may be obtained from this vantage point. The stump is permitted to withdraw into a position above the inguinal ligament, which it does easily (Fig. 15–6).

Next, the lowermost fibers of the external oblique and inguinal ligament are grasped with an Allis forceps and elevated upward. Such exposure permits visualization of the inferior aspect of the inguinal ligament, iliopubic tract, Cooper's ligament, and pectineus fascia. The femoral vein is easily identified and protected from this perspective. Sutures of heavy silk, number 2–0, are then placed between the inguinal ligament and iliopubic tract above and Cooper's ligament and pectineus fascia below in order to achieve closure of the upper femoral canal. A small, stout needle is essential here, since the maneuvers are carried out in close quarters. Care

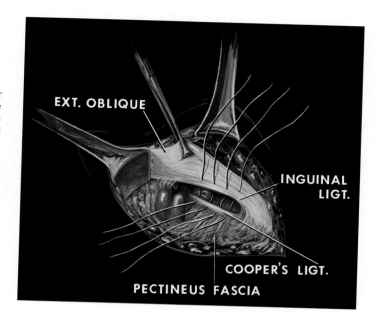

**Figure 15–6.** The Bassini-Kirschner repair of femoral hernia in which the inguinal ligament and transversalis fascia are sutured to Cooper's ligament and pectineal fascia through the inferior approach. (Reproduced by permission of publisher from Ponka, J. L., and Brush, B. E.: The problem of femoral hernia. Arch Surg., *102*:420, 1971. Copyright 1971, American Medical Association.)

EXT. OBLIQUE

INGUINAL LIGT.

COOPER'S LIGT.

PECTINEUS FASCIA

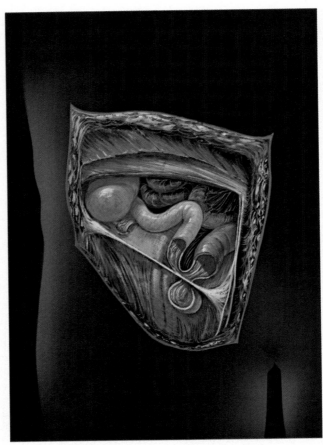

**Figure 15–7.** Artist's illustration of a Richter's hernia. The bowel lumen is partially occluded at the femoral ring. The proximal bowel is dilated while the distal intestine is more or less collapsed.

must be taken not to place sutures into the components of the spermatic cord. Subcutaneous tissues are approximated with fine number 3–0 plain catgut. Skin may be closed with Steri-strips or fine number 4–0 nylon sutures.

Dr. James Barron, formerly a member of the staff of Henry Ford Hospital, sutured the lowermost fibers of the inguinal ligament to the pectineus fascia. He then developed a flap of pectineus fascia, which was sutured to the lowermost extent of the external oblique.

The Bassini repair should not, in my judgment, be discarded. The peritoneal sac is dissected free and high ligation carried out. Then the falciform ligament or process is sutured to the pectineus fascia. Finally, additional interrupted sutures are placed between Poupart's ligament and the pectineus fascia (see Fig. 15–9). An

uncomplicated femoral hernia can be successfully repaired from below the inguinal ligament with minimal anesthesia and trauma to the patient. It is particularly applicable to women, since they rarely develop direct inguinal hernias. It has application in the repair of femoral hernias in men in whom other groin hernias have been successfully repaired. Furthermore, the procedure can be performed simply under local anesthesia. I agree with Koontz (1958), Monro (1964), Lytle (1957), Tanner (1942), and Glassow (1966) that the accurately diagnosed uncomplicated femoral hernia can be successfully repaired by any one of a number of modifications of a technique from a position below the inguinal ligament.

The Bassini repair has its disadvantages in that it does not provide access to the surgical correction of incarcerated and strangulated femoral hernias. It cannot be used as a method of repair of direct or indirect inguinal hernias when such combinations exist in the same patient.

## ABDOMINAL OR POSTERIOR APPROACH

If there is an area of confusion in regard to femoral hernia repair, it would most likely be found in the varied concepts of preperitoneal, properitoneal, or extraperitoneal and abdominal approaches to the repair of such hernias. The words preperitoneal, properitoneal, and extraperitoneal are synonymous and simply indicate that the peritoneal cavity has not been entered—the incision having been made through the abdominal paries at a distance from the groin. After dissection at the preperitoneal level, the peritoneal hernial sac is reduced and excised at the hernia site to permit repair of the hernia. After a selected incision has been made through the abdominal wall, the adipose tissue is easily separated from the abdominal wall and the inguinofemoral area is approached from its posterior aspect. Hence in an attempt to clarify this approach, it has also been called the "posterior approach" to femoral or inguinal hernia repair; this is in contrast to the classical or "anterior approach" whereby the incision is made anteriorly in the inguinal region.

On the other hand, in the abdominal approach to hernia repair the peritoneum is incised. The peritoneal defect at the inguinal or femoral ring is identified, and an incision must be made in the peritoneal sac in the region of the internal ring or the femoral ring. Transversalis fascia and its derivates, as well as Cooper's ligament, must be identified if hernias in the inguinofemoral area are to be repaired from this vantage point.

I have not discussed the procedure of Robins (1909), LaRoque (1919), and Williams (1938) in this section; although they made abdominal incisions in operative treatment of hernia, they used the conventional anterior approach in the repair of the abdominal wall defects.

The terms "posterior approach" should be applied to repairs carried out through dissection accomplished through exposure of the posterior abdominal wall from within the abdominal cavity. If the peritoneum has been incised, then the procedure cannot be called entirely retroperitoneal. On the other hand, if the dissection takes place with an intact peritoneal membrane, then the procedure is entirely preperitoneal, properitoneal, or retroperitoneal; and the repair is carried out through the posterior approach to the inguinofemoral region.

## TECHNIQUE OF REPAIR OF FEMORAL HERNIA THROUGH THE POSTERIOR APPROACH

As I have indicated, I have not used the preperitoneal approach regularly; however, it is recognized as an effective method for repair of femoral hernia by Musgrove and McCready (1949), Mikkelsen and Berne (1954), Nyhus, Condon, and Harkins (1960), McVay and Anson (1942), and Gaspar and Casberg (1971). Recurrence rates following the Cheatle-Henry-Nyhus repair of femoral hernias is variously reported as being between 0 and 2.5 percent. The technique of posterior repair for femoral hernias should be familiar to every abdominal surgeon. Detailed descriptions made available by Nyhus and Condon are recommended to the reader. I will briefly describe the techniques, which I have found to be useful and easily accomplished (see Fig. 15-8, A and B).

The posterior approach to repair of femoral hernia requires excellent relaxation. For this reason, either spinal or general anesthesia with curare are necessarily administered. This is one definite disadvantage of the posterior approach. Other techniques can be performed under local anesthesia. The incision used to gain access to the femoral region varies with the clinical situation. If the patient has some pelvic pathology in addition to a femoral hernia, a midline incision from the umbilicus to the symphysis pubis may be used. In an occasional patient, a transverse incision approximately midway between the anterior superior iliac spine and the pubic tubercle may be preferred. The length of the incision is influenced by the thickness of the abdomen. The incision is developed successively lateral to the rectus abdominis muscle through the external oblique aponeurosis, the internal oblique muscle, and the transversus ab-

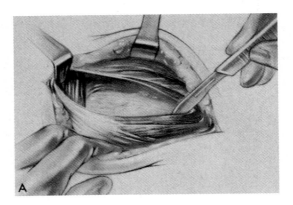

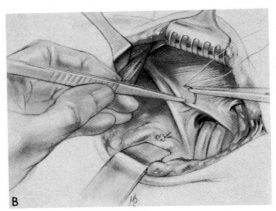
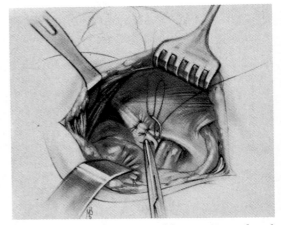

**Figure 15–8.**    Preperitoneal approach to repair of femoral, indirect, and direct inguinal hernia. (Reproduced by permission of J. B. Lippincott Company; from Nyhus, L. M., and Harkins, H. N.: *Hernia*. Philadelphia, J. B. Lippincott Co., 1964, pp. 271–306.)

*A,* The incision is made transversely approximately four centimeters above Poupart's ligament. The structures of the abdominal wall are incised down through the transversalis fascia permitting dissection at the preperitoneal level.

*B,* To repair a femoral hernia, the surgeon sutures the iliopubic tract to Cooper's ligament. Three sutures of number 2–0 synthetic nonabsorbable suture material will usually suffice and produce an excellent result.

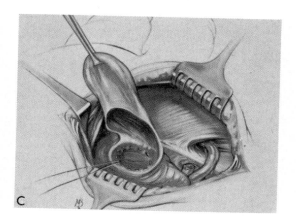
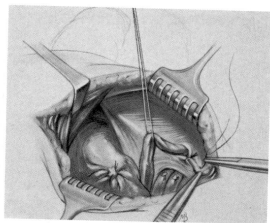
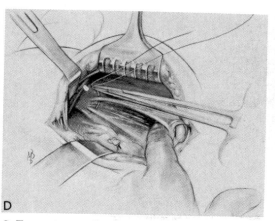
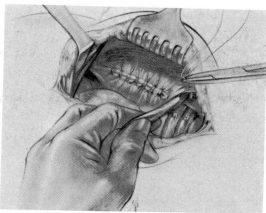

C, To repair an indirect hernia, the surgeon may free the peritoneal sac and perform high ligation, amputating the sac at the internal ring. The distal sac may be left in situ and the proximal peritoneal ring closed. The transversalis fascia derivatives are approximated with number 2–0 synthetic nonabsorbable sutures placed lateral to the cord, but in some patients sutures may be placed medially to the cord as well.

D, Repair of direct inguinal hernias is accomplished by approximating the transversus abdominis lamina above to the iliopubic tract below. In selected cases it may be necessary to approximate the transversalis fascial layer to Cooper's ligament. Excessive tension may be avoided by an appropriate relaxing incision. A similar approach may be utilized to repair indirect inguinal hernias that enlarge medially.

dominis muscle. The anterior sheath of the rectus muscle is divided, but the muscle itself is merely retracted to the side opposite of the repair. The transversalis fascia is incised tranversely, and the preperitoneal fat becomes visible. It is at this plane that the dissection is carried downward, exposing the area of Hesselbach's triangle posteriorly. The iliac vessels, Cooper's ligament, the femoral ring, and the internal ring are easily identified. The peritoneal sac and preperitoneal fat are withdrawn from the femoral ring and canal. At the preperitoneal plane, dissection may be easily carried out with either finger dissection or a small sponge held by an appropriate forceps. Cooper's ligament and the iliopubic tract (an analogue of the transversalis fascia) are clearly identified. The deep inferior epigastric artery may be ligated if it interferes with precise visualization of the structures just described.

The repair of the femoral defect usually requires three sutures of heavy or number 2–0 silk (or a comparable suture material). The sutures are accurately placed between Cooper's ligament and the iliopubic tract (see Fig. 15–8, B; p. 250). Incidentally, in the technique for repairing a right femoral hernia, the sutures are more easily placed with the surgeon's standing on the patient's left side.

The preperitoneal approach may be employed for repair of indirect inguinal hernias (see Fig. 15–8, C). The method is effective in repairing the defect at the internal ring where the transversus abdominis layers are comparatively easy to identify. Repair of direct inguinal hernias by the preperitoneal approach has had limited application because of high recurrence rates (see Fig. 15–8, D).

The excess of the peritoneal sac is excised; the peritoneum is closed, and the musculofascial layers of the abdominal wall are approximated with nonabsorbable sutures. I would emphasize the need for care in wound closure, since there is some danger of a postoperative or ventral hernia developing after repair. Although number 3–0 or number 4–0 chromic catgut may be used to close the peritoneum, heavier sutures should be used to approximate the aponeurotic layers. I use number 2–0 or heavy silk; in instances where I fear infection, monofilament wire or comparable synthetic sutures may be used. When-

ever the midline incision has been made it is repaired with heavy sutures, and the closure is further reinforced with heavy nylon retention sutures.

The preperitoneal approach to the repair of femoral hernias is useful and effective. The need for general or spinal anesthesia as well as relaxation is a relative drawback to more frequent use of the procedure. Another limiting factor is the need for an abdominal incision, which itself may become the site of a postoperative hernia. These disadvantages are offset by the excellent results obtained and the ease of repair. The posterior approach for repair of groin hernias is extremely useful to the surgeon who has performed abdominal section for some other pathologic process. Strangely, some surgeons who perform hernia repairs in significant numbers state with pride that they have never used the method—an attitude that defies my understanding.

## CLINICAL STUDY OF FEMORAL HERNIAS

Much of the data presented in this chapter was obtained from a review of 488 case histories of femoral hernias, selected at random from the medical records and treated at the Henry Ford Hospital since 1940. In a previous study Ponka and Brush (1971) found that the relative incidence of femoral hernias compared with that of other groin hernias was approximately 5 percent. In that report, they found that 10 percent of their patients had undergone previous surgical operations for femoral hernias at various institutions. Furthermore, 23 percent had operations for other groin hernias. Thus, 33 percent had previously undergone repair of some type of groin hernia. Such statistics should stimulate us into seeking explanations for results that are less than satisfactory. These statistics may be difficult to accept; however, Burton and Bauer (1958) found an incidence of 21.8 percent of recurrent hernias in their study. Furthermore, an additional 28.5 percent of their patients had undergone operations for inguinal hernias that later recurred as femoral hernias. McClure and Fallis, in a study made at Henry Ford Hospital in 1939, found that almost 23 percent had undergone operative procedures for inguinal hernia on the same side where the femoral hernia appeared. It is a reasonable assumption that from 1945 to 1970, surgeons have not greatly improved the lot of patients with groin hernias in general and femoral hernias in particular (Ponka and Brush, 1971).

I have come to realize that better results in treatment of femoral hernias will be forthcoming when the following criteria are appreciated and implemented:

1. Avoidance of diagnostic errors, both clinical and operative.
2. Recognition of the groin hernia as an inguinofemoral defect in which any combination of direct, indirect, and femoral hernia may be encountered in the same individual.
3. Understanding of the pathologic anatomy of the femoral hernia.
4. Utilization of sound principles and individualized application of any of a number of available effective techniques.

### Diagnostic Errors

Errors in diagnosis occur preoperatively and during the repair of inguinal hernias (Table 15–1). Prior to surgery (as I have noted in Chapter 3 on the diagnosis of hernia), the physician too often simply makes the diagnosis of inguinal hernia without any further evaluation. If an inexperienced surgeon then attempts repair without carefully exploring the area of the femoral ring digitally, the femoral hernia is overlooked.

In Table 15–1, I have summarized the erroneous clinical diagnoses recorded in 488 patients with proven femoral hernia; the list is one that the surgeon should always recall when considering the diagnostic possibilities. The importance of correctly identifying the defect instead of merely writing down the diagnosis of "inguinal hernia" cannot be overemphasized. Errors in diagnosis lead to errors in treatment, and it is a simple matter to overlook a femoral hernia at operation if it was not seriously considered in the differential diagnosis. I consider it an erroneous diagnosis if the clinician records "inguinal hernia" when, in fact, a femoral hernia was present.

**Table 15–1. ERRORS IN DIAGNOSIS OF FEMORAL HERNIA**

| | |
|---|---:|
| Inguinal hernia | 79 |
| Lymph node enlargement | 8 |
| Intestinal obstruction | 6 |
| Hydrocele | 4 |
| Saphenous varix | 4 |
| Lipoma | 3 |
| Fibroma, canal of Nuck | 2 |
| Lipoma, canal of Nuck | 2 |

Errors in the diagnosis of Richter's hernias are far too common (see Table 15–1). Nausea, vomiting, and abdominal pain should readily suggest the diagnosis of incomplete intestinal obstruction. The problems arising from a Richter's hernia (Fig. 15–7) are serious enough to warrant a detailed discussion in Chapter 23. The groin may be examined casually or not at all, and an incarcerated femoral hernia overlooked. Elderly patients may not always be aware of a protrusion, and in obese patients the small hernia may tax the diagnostic skill of even the most experienced clinician. At other times, patients will admit to having been aware of a swelling for as long as 25 years. The largest femoral hernia I ever saw had a loop of sigmoid colon in it (Fig. 15–10). At operation every groin must be examined for direct, indirect, and femoral hernias if errors are to be kept to a minimum.

### Age Distribution

Indirect inguinal hernias are often seen in neonates, infants, and children, whereas femoral hernias usually occur in adults and elderly individuals (see Fig. 15–2). Most femoral hernias occur in patients over 50 years of age. In fact, 70 percent of our patients were 50 years of age and older. Such evidence reinforces my opinion that femoral hernia is an acquired defect. Atrophy of tissue, weight loss, and a history of pregnancy are other etiologic factors to be considered.

Young patients seldom develop femoral hernias, and only 11 of the 488 patients were under 30 years of age. One remarkable woman, 19 years of age, had a femoral hernia after having borne four children.

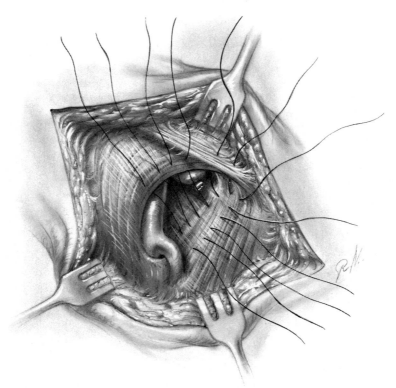

**Figure 15–9.**   In the Bassini repair of a femoral hernia, sutures are placed between the inguinal ligament and pectineal fascia as well as between the falciform process of the fascia lata and pectineal fascia.

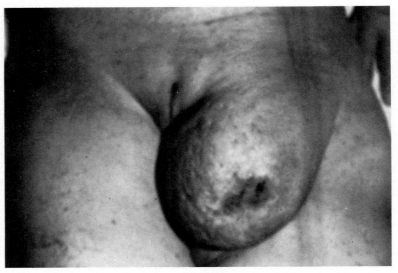

**Figure 15–10.**   This is a very large femoral hernia that contained sigmoid colon. Note ulceration of the skin.

## Sex Distribution

Glassow (1966) reviewed 1143 femoral hernia repairs and found the male/female ratio to be 5:3. Zimmerman and Anderson (1967) summarized the sex incidence of femoral hernias and found it to vary greatly. The ratios of male to female were variously reported as being 1:1.5 to 1:5. In many series the incidence of femoral hernia was two to three times greater in women than in men.

The statistics from this study of 488 patients must be interpreted with care, since the Henry Ford Hospital has the responsibility of treating large numbers of patients from industrial plants in Detroit, most of whom are men. There were 261 men and 227 women with femoral hernias in this study. One hundred and seventy-nine women had borne children. I have tried to substantiate the opinion that pregnancy predisposes to femoral hernia through stretching of the abdominal wall and increasing of intra-abdominal pressure; however, this is difficult to prove. On the other hand, women rarely develop direct hernias, and femoral hernias are far more common in women.

## Location of Hernia

An interesting observation has repeatedly been made insofar as the side of location of the femoral hernia is concerned. This study has shown that right-sided femoral hernias were encountered twice as frequently as those on the left; this observation is consistent with the findings of Burton (1958) and McClure and Fallis (1939). A satisfactory explanation for this great variation in location is not immediately apparent and will be further reflected on in the future.

## Bilateral Femoral Hernias

Femoral hernias were not often found to be bilateral in our experience. Somewhat less than 6 percent of 488 femoral hernias were found to be bilateral at the same examination. If one follows patients with femoral hernias for much longer periods of time, then this figure will increase. In some of our patients, the second femoral hernia appeared after 20 years. Bilateral, but separate, femoral hernias were found in nearly 13 percent of our patients. Mikkelsen and Berne (1954) reported the incidence of bilateralism to be as high as 20 percent.

## The Clinical Picture

The surgeon dealing with femoral hernias must be aware that the history given by the patient will vary enormously. I have summarized the varied clinical features seen in 488 patients with femoral hernias in Table 15–2. While it is true that many patients will complain of a nonreducible mass, certain elderly patients will present only with the clinical picture of intestinal obstruction. Cramping abdominal pain with vomiting and no abdominal distention may be due to a Richter's type of hernia. Since the incarceration and strangulation involve such a small portion of the bowel, only a most careful examination will reveal the presence of a groin mass. It is not uncommon for a patient with a Richter's hernia to be admitted with the incomplete diagnosis of intestinal obstruction (Fig. 15–11). The etiology of obstruction may be overlooked for a number of days—or until the embarrassing truth of a Richter's hernia is revealed in the bright lights of the operating room. Further details concerning the diagnosis of hernia are presented in Chapter 3.

Most patients will present with a mass in the groin, which appears after vigorous activity, coughing, or sneezing. In many patients the swelling recedes when the patient enjoys bed rest. The mass, by no means, always causes severe discomfort. Incarceration of omentum, ileum, and

### Table 15–2. CLINICAL FEATURES OF 488 PATIENTS WITH FEMORAL HERNIA

| | |
|---|---|
| Mass | |
|   painful, irreducible | 234 |
|   (swelling, lump, bulge, knot) | |
|   painless, irreducible | 139 |
|   painless, reducible | 54 |
|   painful, reducible | 45 |
| Pain alone | 16 |
| Obstructive symptoms | 46 |

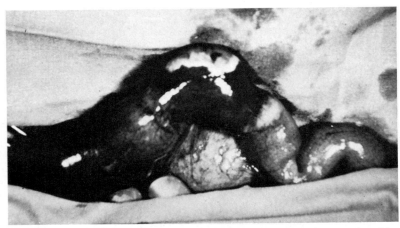

**Figure 15–11.**   Gangrenous intestine that was reduced from an incarcerated-strangulated hernia. The bowel at the apex was constricted in the unyielding femoral ring.

preperitoneal fat with compromise of blood supply will cause acute pain in most patients. Not all patients with obstructive symptoms will be found to have incarcerated intestine in the hernial sac at operation.

## Personal Observations on 488 Operations for Femoral Hernia

The observations recorded here have been made on 488 patients operated upon at Henry Ford Hospital since 1940 by various members of the Senior Staff and House Staff. Retrieving some of the older records was difficult but proved worthwhile, since changes in management and operative treatment became evident. For example, spinal anesthesia is currently being used less frequently. The McVay repair is being used with increasing frequency. In the 1940's there was often reluctance to operate upon patients over 60 years of age. Silk continues to be the suture material of choice. Patients are mobilized far more vigorously today. At the present time, they are being discharged in from two to five days; in the 1940's, ten days to two weeks was the length of hospitalization. Currently, infants and children are often operated on in the morning and discharged in the evening of the same day.

## Anesthesia

My personal choice of anesthesia in over 90 percent of the patients is local injection of an anesthetic solution (as described in Chapter 9). Bupivacaine as a 0.25 percent solution has been used most often. Local anesthesia has been found to be safe and effective. In the preoperative evaluation, arteriosclerotic, pulmonary, metabolic, and genitourinary tract diseases were found in a great many patients; in such patients, local anesthesia offers many advantages.

Several members of the staff prefer spinal or general anesthesia, but they also use local anesthesia in patients of advanced years or in those in poor physical condition.

Local anesthesia was used in 240, or in almost 50 percent of the patients; spinal anesthesia in 204, or approximately 42 percent; and general anesthesia was administered to 44 individuals, or 9 percent of the total of 488 patients. It is obvious that not all of the staff members favor the use of local anesthesia, which I find so satisfactory.

## Suture Material

I have been educated to use silk suture material, but other types of material are perfectly acceptable. There is only one condition that I would insist on—i.e., it must have the tensile strength to hold various structures in apposition. The peritoneum and transversalis fascia may be approximated with fine suture material; but when sutures are placed between the transversus arch and Cooper's ligament, heavy or number 2–0 silk must be the minimum strength. Silk was used in 428, or nearly 92 percent, of the 488 patients studied.

Catgut and wire were often used in cases of strangulated hernias where bowel was gangrenous. I always use catgut and wire when the risk of infection is great. Synthetic suture materials are being used with increasing frequency, a trend that I strongly support. These materials possess strength and durability.

## Hoguet Maneuver

This maneuver was described in 1929 when Hoguet used the technique to convert direct inguinal peritoneal hernial sacs into indirect sacs. The peritoneum is located at the superior and medial aspects of the cord where it is opened. The direct sac was converted into an indirect by lateral traction on the peritoneum. The same approach was applied to femoral hernias by McClure and Fallis in 1939. In this situation, the peritoneum is identified at the internal ring; after it is opened, the femoral sac is converted into an indirect sac. Complete reduction of the peritoneal sac is accomplished with minimal danger of injury to the bladder. The Hoguet maneuver was used in 137 of the 488 patients who were operated on.

## Relaxing Incision

The relaxing incision made in the anterior sheath of the rectus was utilized in 145 of the 488 patients undergoing femoral hernia repair. It is an important adjunct in the McVay repair if excessive tension is to be avoided. Details on the relaxing incision are presented in Chapter 25.

## Appendectomy

Appendectomy was performed in five patients in whom the appendix presented through the peritoneal sac. The appendectomy is easily performed when the cecum is redundant, and the appendix is readily delivered through the peritoneal ring. A determined effort is not made to perform an appendectomy if the appendix and cecum are difficult to deliver. There

were no complications incurred as a result of appendectomy in this small series.

Duari (1966) reported a case in which a Richter's hernia contained the appendix and the base of the cecum. Wakeley (1938) reported that the appendix is found in about one percent of all femoral hernias, a figure that I believe to be fairly accurate. Acute appendicitis along with femoral hernia is comparatively rare.

## Intestinal Strangulation and Deaths Associated with Femoral Hernias

It has long been recognized that femoral hernias are a notorious site for incarceration and strangulation of the intestine.

In 1939 McClure and Fallis found 21 incarcerations and strangulations among 90 patients with femoral hernias. Three of these patients died, for a mortality rate of 15.2 percent. Butters in 1948 found strangulation of intestine in 45 of 178 femoral hernias. Six patients died, for a mortality rate of 13.3 percent. Thomas, in 1967 at the Alfred Hospital in Melbourne, found that femoral hernias were associated with strangulation more frequently than all other hernias combined. Thomas found it necessary to resect gangrenous bowel in 34 of 100 patients. His mortality rate was an impressive 3 percent. Thomas cited several sources reporting mortality rates ranging from 6 to 23 percent following strangulated femoral henias.

Ponka and Brush (1971) found the incidence of strangulation-obstruction to be much lower in Henry Ford Hospital. Resection was necessary in only 2.3 percent of their patients.

## Incarceration—Strangulation

Femoral hernial sacs are surrounded by variable amounts of adipose tissue, but on occasion this adipose tissue undergoes compromise of its blood supply and may even become gangrenous. The peritoneal fat had undergone such changes in 38 patients. Omentum was found to be the abdominal viscus in 56 of the 488 patients operated on (Fig. 15–12).

Incarceration was the most common serious complication and occurred in 32 patients in whom the ileum was involved.

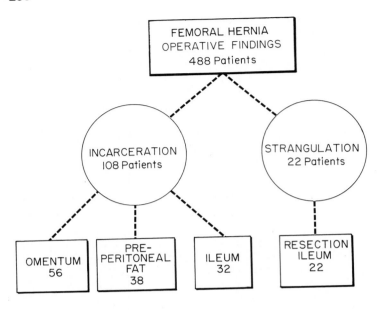

Figure 15–12.  Operative findings in 488 patients with femoral hernia.

Strangulation occurred in 22 patients requiring resection, for a resection rate of 4.5 percent among 488 patients.

Richter's hernia was present in ten patients, but not all of them required resection.

Bladder was present as a sliding component in 16 patients. The bladder was identified in large femoral hernias where it occupied the medial portion of the hernial sac. No bladder injuries occurred.

### Recurrences and Follow-up After Femoral Hernia Repair

The operations performed and the recurrences are summarized in Table 15–3.

The matter of recurrences will be discussed in detail in Chapter 16 on recurrent femoral hernias.

Although I have attempted to obtain an accurate follow-up study on my operations, even after a diligent effort the numbers of patients whom I could examine personally was disappointingly small. Numerous letters and phone calls were often nonproductive. After ten years postoperative, many patients had died—usually of arteriosclerosis, arteriosclerotic heart disease, and malignancy. The population of Detroit is certainly not a static one. Many had moved from the city without leaving a trace as to their new locations.

Only 221, or less than 50 percent, were followed six years or longer. Most disappointing was the fact that 135 patients were followed one year or less. Hence, no firm opinion can be offered as to our recurrence rate. Nevertheless, some useful information can be derived from this material, since all of our patients were subject to the same variables. I believe that some conclusions can be reached in considering the results of the various types of repairs. The overall recurrence rate for all types of repairs was approximately 6.7 percent.

It is seen that the McVay repair was most commonly performed. Furthermore, it was

Table 15–3.  OPERATIVE PROCEDURES AND RECURRENCES IN 488 PATIENTS WITH FEMORAL HERNIA

| Type of Repair | Operations | Recur. | Percent |
|---|---|---|---|
| McVay | 223 | 17 | 7.6 |
| Moschcowitz | 155 | 13 | 8.4 |
| Bassini | 102 | 3 | 3.0 |
| Preperitoneal | 8 | 0 | 0 |

selected as the procedure of choice when incarceration or strangulation was present (Table 15–3). It was also the procedure of choice when a combination of direct and femoral hernias was encountered. There were 17 recurrences in 223 McVay repairs, for a recurrence rate of 7.6 percent. It bears repeating that the McVay repair was selected for operative treatment of difficult and often complicated femoral hernias.

Patients on whom the Bassini repair was performed commonly had an easily recognized uncomplicated femoral hernia. Thus, it was selected as a procedure of choice for the most favorable types of femoral hernia. It was often employed in women and, at times, in men who previously had had inguinal hernias repaired successfully. In this highly selected group of 102 patients having the Bassini repair, there were three recurrences, for a recurrence rate of 3.0 percent.

Three statements should be made in regard to the Bassini repair. First, the procedure, properly used, is simple to perform and gives excellent results. Secondly, it is not utilized in complicated incarcerated and strangulated hernias or in those with multiple defects. Thirdly, the Bassini repair can be carried out easily under local anesthesia. I am in agreement with Lytle, Monro, Koontz and Glassow that the Bassini, or lower approach, should not be discarded because of its ease of performance and effectiveness in selected cases.

The Moschcowitz repair has been used with decreasing frequency in recent years, and there are a number of factors related to this decrease. McVay criticized the Moschcowitz technique, pointing out that because the inguinal ligament is relatively inflexible and Cooper's ligament is rigid, there is a great deal of tension created when these structures are approximated. This helps to explain the fact that the Moschcowitz technique yields the highest recurrence rate among the various techniques of repair. In a recent survey, I found 13 recurrences in 155 such operations, for a recurrence rate of 8.4 percent. Also, because of anatomic differences, the Moschcowitz technique has a limited applicability; in certain people the angle between the inguinal ligament and Cooper's ligament is so wide that when these two structures are approximated, enor-

mous tension develops. In light of the above facts, McVay's criticism of the Moschcowitz method must be taken seriously.

The preperitoneal or properitoneal approach, introduced by Cheatle (1920) and Henry (1963) and popularized by Nyhus and Condon (1960), was used in only eight patients with femoral hernia. I use this technique most often in cases where a femoral hernia is present along with other abdominal pathology. Repair is carried out with remarkable ease from the posterior vantage point. There is no doubt in my mind that it should be used more often than it is at present. There were no known recurrences recorded among our eight repairs.

## Complications

The frequency and magnitude of complications following hernia repair vary inversely with the knowledge and experience of the surgeon. Surgeons with a large experience in the field will have fewer problems and recurrences than will the neophyte. Nevertheless, complications do occur in the practice of all surgeons with a variable frequency. Some complications are unavoidable; others unpredictable — all of them annoying both to the patient and surgeon.

I am of the opinion that a summary of all noteworthy complications will be valuable, particularly to the young surgeon. He can become easily aware of what the complications might be and their relative frequency (Table 15–4).

Three hundred and eighty-four of 488 patients underwent operative repairs without complications, while 104 of them had one or more complications. Wound seromas were found to be the most common wound complications. Collections of serum are usually a minor problem, but they do worry the patient. These were aspirated under local anesthesia after careful aseptic measures were taken. Small seromas will often disappear in time without additional treatment.

Wound infection was a complication in 14 patients. Two distinct types of infection could be identified. Infections were seen most commonly in patients who had incarceration and strangulation of femoral

## Table 15-4.  COMPLICATIONS IN 488 PATIENTS OPERATED ON FOR FEMORAL HERNIA

| | |
|---|---:|
| 1. *Wound* | |
|    Seroma | 23 |
|    Infection (Major 11, Minor 3) | 14 |
|    Ecchymosis | 13 |
|    Hematoma | 8 |
|    Pain | 5 |
| 2. *Genitourinary* | |
|    Retention | 25 |
|    Infection | 14 |
|    Oliguria | 2 |
| 3. *Ileus* | 39 |
| 4. *Scrotal* | |
|    Swelling | 11 |
|    Hydrocele | 2 |
|    Atrophic testicles | 2 |
| 5. *Pulmonary* | |
|    Atelectasis | 11 |
|    Pneumonia | 3 |
| 6. *Skin* | |
|    Sensitivity to antiseptics | 3 |
|    Sensitivity to adhesives | 4 |
| 7. *Thrombophlebitis* | 7 |
| 8. *Spinal headaches* | 6 |
| 9. *Pulmonary emboli* | 3 |

hernias. The most common type of wound infection in femoral hernias is due to a mixture of gram-negative organisms. Among the organisms cultured from such wounds we found were: colibacilli, *Proteus*, staphylococci, and *Clostridium perfringens*. These organisms found their way into the wound through gangrenous bowel. When I repair hernias in which gangrenous bowel is encountered, I use single strands of wire and catgut suture. Silk should not be used if prolonged drainage and "spitting of silk" are to be avoided. Heavy braided silk is particularly troublesome in such cases.

The other type of recognizable infection occurs in clean operative wounds that become infected with staphylococci. The organisms in these cases come from the patient's skin or from the surgeon's hand through perforation of a glove. A number of other breaks in aseptic technique may occur in isolated instances.

Ecchymosis about the operated area is frightening to the patient, particularly if the penis becomes somewhat swollen and a dark purplish-blue color. Reassurance early in the postoperative period and hot tub baths later on in the period will restore the confidence of the patient that the problem is not a serious one.

Postoperative pain is considered a complication only when it remains a complaint after the wound is well healed and there is no apparent reason for its continuance. Tub baths, scrotal support, and analgesics will result in improvement in many patients.

**GENITOURINARY TRACT** complications occur with undesirable frequency. This is understandable when it is appreciated that 85 of 488 patients had recognized prostatism before their femoral hernias were repaired. Infection followed catheterization in 14 of 25 patients who had been unable to void. Oliguria and fluid and electrolyte imbalance occurred in two patients with strangulation obstruction who had been ill and vomiting for several days prior to treatment. Repair of the hernia after resection of the necrotic bowel plus fluid and electrolyte replacement resulted in eventual recovery of both patients.

Ileus was seen with surprising frequency. It occurred often in those patients who had nausea, vomiting and distention preoperatively. Patients with ileus postoperatively were found to have incarcerated omentum or intestine with regularity. Furthermore, most severe ileus followed resection of gangrenous bowel. I often insert the Miller-Abbott tube for intestinal decompression in such cases. In less severe ileus, the nasogastric tube functions effectively.

**SCROTAL SWELLING** occurs when there is excessive manipulation of the spermatic cord or when there is compromise of the blood supply to the testicle. In some instances, even minimal manipulation results in testicular swelling. Venous occlusion, for whatever reason, results in a large swollen testicle that is firm and tender to palpation. A scrotal hematoma may also cause swelling of the scrotum; in such cases there is less tenderness, and if the tension is not great, a normal testicle may be identified. Arterial occlusion of the internal and external spermatic arteries results in much less swelling, but tenderness is still present. Compromise of arterial supply results in testicular atrophy over a period of 6 to 12 months. The cause of arterial occlusion is not apparent in every case. Testicular atrophy occurred in 2 of 488 patients, while scrotal swelling was a problem for eleven others. Ice bags, scrotal suspensories, analgesics, and (later in the postoperative period) tub baths are considered to be the therapeutic endeavors for patients with scrotal swelling.

PULMONARY COMPLICATIONS included atelectasis in 11 patients and pneumonia in 3 seriously ill patients following resection of gangrenous small intestine. It is remarkable that pulmonary complications were not more of a problem, but early ambulation and the use of local anesthesia in poor-risk elderly patients contribute to these results.

SKIN REACTIONS to iodine and adhesive tape were uncommon. If care is taken to remove the iodine after its application in skin preparation, the reactions will be few indeed. The newer so-called nonallergenic paper and synthetic adhesive tapes provide an excellent means of holding the dressing in place. I find that the paper type of adhesive is very satisfactory.

THROMBOPHLEBITIS AND PULMONARY EMBOLISM were seen in only seven patients, with three having nonfatal pulmonary emboli. Local anesthesia followed by prompt ambulation is, in my opinion, the reason for such excellent results in many aged patients. Heparin was adequate therapy for patients with thromboembolic disease.

Pulmonary embolism is a continuing threat to elderly patients, but I am of the opinion that early ambulation is an effective measure towards its prevention. By early ambulation, I mean that the patient must be encouraged to walk immediately following surgical repair of the hernia. The most feeble patients often walk back to their rooms from the operating suite.

SPINAL HEADACHES were not a particularly common problem, but they are annoying when they do occur. Six patients of 204 having spinal anesthesia complained significantly of having headaches. Bed rest, hydration, and analgesics provided relief. Although I favor local anesthesia for hernia repair, I do not feel that the incidence of severity of headaches constitutes a strong argument against spinal anesthesia.

Only one patient insisted that he had difficulty walking after a spinal anesthetic. His recovery took two months and was eventually complete. No neurologic deficit could be demonstrated.

## Deaths

It is becoming apparent that the operation for femoral hernia, simple or incarcerated, can be done with little risk. Even elderly, acutely ill patients with compensated arteriosclerotic heart disease and degenerative diseases can be operated upon with an excellent prospect of survival. Of the 488 patients who were operated on there were only 3 hospital deaths.

One patient with an incarcerated femoral hernia had extensive carcinomatosis secondary to carcinoma of the parotid gland. This patient died of his malignancy on the third postoperative day and is considered an operative death.

The second patient had been on chemotherapy for carcinomatosis secondary to colonic carcinoma. This patient was in extremely poor condition and died on the fifth day following femoral hernia repair because of incarceration. She was also considered an operative death.

A third patient with severe arteriosclerosis died on the third postsurgical day, and at postmortem was found to have had a cerebrovascular accident.

Thus, the mortality in 488 patients was approximately 0.6 percent. The designation of the deaths recorded above as postoperative deaths required a great deal of self-discipline and generous interpretation of the term, "postoperative death."

Watson collected statistics on 700 patients operated on for nonstrangulated hernia in 1938 and found 9 deaths in all, for a mortality of 1.28 percent. The number of deaths in patients with strangulated hernias would be higher.

In 1938 McClure and Fallis of Henry Ford Hospital reported a mortality of 4.4 percent in 90 operations for femoral hernia. Two of the deaths were in patients aged 72 and 90 years. Burton in 1958 reported a mortality of 1.3 percent in 151 operations for femoral hernia. One of his patients died 25 days after repair of a presumed myocardial infarction.

The frightening mortality reported by several authors following incarceration and strangulation has been conveniently summarized by Zimmerman and Anderson (1967). They found the rates to vary from 3.5 to 32 percent after strangulation had occurred. The great advantage and safety of early operation are clearly evident when the various rates are compared.

Deaths following hernia repair should occur infrequently in modern surgical practice. A mortality of less than 0.5 percent for all operations for femoral hernia is not unreasonable when the procedures are performed under local anesthesia.

## SUMMARY

Femoral hernias demand the clinician's respect. The anatomic defect is small, but the potential consequences are lethal. Incarceration occurred in 32 of 488 patients and resection of gangrenous bowel was performed in 22, or 4.5 percent, of 488 patients. Furthermore, complications of incarceration and strangulation are serious because they usually occur in elderly patients with cardiac and pulmonary diseases.

Diagnosis of a small Richter's hernia requires a careful history and physical examination. Because the swelling is small, it may be easily overlooked.

There is a common misconception that repair of femoral hernias is a simple matter; the reason for this erroneous view is, to begin with, that femoral hernias are far less common than indirect and direct inguinal hernias.

A variety of methods are available for repair of femoral hernias. The Moschcowitz repair should be used in very carefully selected cases. Repairs from the subinguinal approach (including the Bassini and Bassini-Kirschner repairs) should be included in the surgeon's armamentarium, since the results are good in selected cases. The Lotheissen-McVay repair has been utilized in the most difficult cases, several of which had become incarcerated. In my current practice, the relaxing incision is used with greater frequency. Also, I am using prosthetic implants with regularity. A small sheet of synthetic mesh, properly implanted, provides great strength at the site of repair.

## REFERENCES

Bassini, E.: Neve Operations. Methode zur Radical Behandlung der Schenkel Hernie. Arch Kin. Chin., 47:1, 1894.

Bates, V. C.: New operation for the cure of indirect inguinal hernias. J.A.M.A. 60:232, 1913.

Buckley, J. P.: The etiology of the femoral hernial sac. Br. J. Surg. 12:60, 1924.

Burke, J.: Femoral hernia in childhood. Ann. Surg. 166:287, 1967.

Burton, C. C.: Current concepts of the anatomic clinical and reparative features of femoral hernia. Surgery 44:877, 1958.

Burton, C. T., and Bauer, R., Jr.: Femoral hernia: A review of 165 repairs. Ann. Surg. 148:913, 1958.

Cheatle, G. T.: An operation for the radical cure of inguinal and femoral hernia. Br. Med. J. 2:68, 1920.

Condon, R. E.: Cited in Nyhus, L. M., and Harkins, H. N.: Hernia. Philadelphia, J. B. Lippincott Co., 1964, pp. 14–62.

Cushing, H. W.: An improved method for the radical cure of femoral hernia. Bost M & S J, 119:546, 1888.

Duari, M.: Strangulated femoral hernia. A Richter's type containing caecum and base of appendix. Postgrad. Med. J. 76:726, 1966.

Galludet, B. B.: A Description of Planes of Fascia of the Human Body. New York, Columbia University Press, 1931.

Gaspar, M. R., and Casberg, M. A.: An appraisal of preperitoneal repair of inguinal hernia. Surg. Gynecol. Obstet. 132:307, 1971.

Glassow, F.: Femoral hernia: Review of 1,143 consecutive repairs. Ann. Surg. 163 (No. 2):227, 1966.

Henry, A. K.: Operation for femoral hernia by a midline, extraperitoneal approach, with a preliminary note on the use of this route for reducible inguinal hernia. Lancet 1:531, 1963.

Hoguet, J. P.: Direct inguinal hernia. Ann. Surg. 72:671, 1920.

Immordino, P. A.: Femoral hernia in infancy and childhood. J. Pediat. Surg. 7:60, 1972.

Keith, A.: On the origin and nature of hernia. Br. J. Surg. 11:455, 1923.

Kelly, H. A.: Femoral Hernia In Operative Gynecology, Vol. 2. New York, D. Appleton & Co., 1937, p. 4901.

Kirschner, W.: Allgemeine und Specielle: Chirugische Operationslehre; Die Operative Beseitigung der Bauchbruche. Berlin, Springer-Verlag, 1937, pp. 127–137.

Koontz, A. R.: Historical analysis of femoral hernia. Surgery 53(4):551, 1963.

Koontz, A. R.: Personal technique and results in femoral hernia repair: Report of 39 cases. Ann. Surg. 147:684, 1958.

LaRoque, G. Paul: The permanent cure of inguinal and femoral hernia. A modification of the standard operative procedures. Surg. Gynecol. Obstet. 29:507, 1919.

Lotheissen, G.: Zur radikal operation de Schenkelhernien. Zentralb. Chir. 25:548, 1898.

Lytle, W. J.: Femoral hernia. Ann. Roy. Coll. Surg. 21:244, 1957.

Mikkelsen, W. P., and Berne, C. J.: Femoral hernioplasty: Suprapubic extraperitoneal (Cheatle-Henry) approach. Surgery 35:743, 1954.

Monro, A.: Cited in Nyhus, L. M., and Harkins, H. N.: Hernia. Philadelphia, J. B. Lippincott Co., 1964, p. 199.

Moschcowitz, A. V.: Femoral hernia: A new operation for the radical cure. N.Y. State J. Med. 7:396, 1907.

Musgrove, J. E., and McCready, F. J.: The Henry approach to femoral hernia. Surgery 26:608, 1949.

McClure, R. D., and Fallis, L. S.: Femoral hernia:

Report of 90 operations. Ann. Surg. *109*:987, 1939.

McVay, C. B.: *Cited in* Nyhus, L. M., and Harkins, H. N.: *Hernia.* Philadelphia, J. B. Lippincott Co., 1964, pp. 215–230.

McVay, C. B., and Savage, L. E.: Etiology of femoral hernia. Ann. Surg. *154* (supplement 25):1961.

McVay, C. B., and Anson, B. J.: Methods of inguinal herniorrhaphy. Surg Gynecol. Obstet. *74*:746, 1942.

McVay, C. B., and Chapp, J. D.: Inguinal and femoral hernioplasty. The evaluation of a basic concept. Ann. Surg. *148*:499, 1958.

Murray, R. W.: Is the sac of a femoral hernia of congenital or acquired origin? Surgery *52*:688, 1910.

Nyhus, L. M., and Harkins, H. N.: *Hernia.* Philadelphia, J. B. Lippincott Co., 1964, pp. 271–306.

Nyhus, L. M., Condon, R. E., and Harkins, H. N.: Clinical experiences with preperitoneal hernial repair for all types of hernia of the groin: With particular reference to the importance of transversalis fascia analogues. Am. J. Surg. *100*:234, 1960.

Nyhus, L. M., Stevenson, L. R., Listerud, M. B., and Harkins, N. H.: Preperitoneal herniorrhaphy. A preliminary report on fifty patients. West. J. Surg. *67*:48, 1959.

Ponka, J. L., and Brush, B. E.: The problem of femoral hernia. Arch. Surg. *102*:417, 1971.

Ponka, J. L.: Incarcerated femoral hernia. Henry Ford Hospital Med. J. *15* (No. 3):203–214, 1967.

Rhind, F. R.: Lateral femoral hernia. J. Roy. Coll. Surg. *16*:299, 1971.

Riba, L. W., and Mehn, W. H.: Combined inguinal hernia repair and retropubic prostatectomy. Q. Bull. Northwestern U. Med. Sch. *25*:62, 1951.

Robins, A. C.: Rectus incision for reduction of strangulated hernia. With a report of a case of strangulated hernia in the sac of an undescended testicle. Old Dominion J. Med. Surg. *8*:324, 1909.

Ruggi, G.: Metodo operativo nuovo la cura radicale dell' ernia crurale. Bull. Scienze Med. di Bologna *7*(No. 3):223–228, 1892.

Russell, R. H.: Saccular theory of hernia and the radical cure. Lancet *2*:1197, 1906.

Tanner, N. C.: A slide operation for inguinal and and femoral hernia. Br. J. Surg. *29*:285, 1942.

Tait, Lawson: On the radical cure of exomphalos. Br. Med. J. *2*:1118, 1883.

Wakeley, C. P. G.: Hernia of the vermiform appendix. Lancet *2*:1282, 1938.

Watson, L. F.: *Hernia.* St. Louis, C. V. Mosby Co., 1938, pp. 292–326.

Williams, C.: The advantages of the abdominal approach to inguinal hernia. Ann. Surg. *107*:917, 1938.

Zimmerman, L. M., and Anderson, B. J.: *Anatomy and Surgery of Hernia.* Baltimore, Williams & Wilkins Co., 1967, pp. 228–261.

## Supplemental Readings

Andreason, A. T.: Twenty years experience with midline extraperitoneal approach to hernias of the inguinal and femoral regions. J. Int. Coll. Surg. *35*:713, 1961.

Blaisdell, F. W., Adams, D. R., Hall, A. D., and Gauder, P. J.: Preperitoneal hernia repair: Experience with 101 consecutive cases. Am. Surg. *30*:623, 1964.

Butters, A. G.: A review of femoral hernias with special reference to recurrence rate of low operation. Br. Med. J. *2*:743, 1948.

Chaitin, Horace: The Pfannenstiel incision for femoral hernia. Int. Surg. *51*(2):190, 1969.

Chevasse, T. F.: On a method of operating in strangulated hernia. Lancet *1*:865, 1882.

Fenwick, E. H.: Laparotomy as an aid to herniotomy. Lancet *2*:566, 1885.

Fischer, H.: Lotheissen's operation for femoral hernia. Ann. Surg. *69*:432, 1919.

Gaur, D. D.: Venous distention in strangulated femoral hernia. Lancet *1*:816, 1967.

Glassow, Frank: Femoral hernia following inguinal herniorrhaphy. Can. J. Surg. *13*:27, 1970.

Glassow, Frank: Recurrent inguinal and femoral hernia: 3000 cases. Can. J. Surg. *7*:284, 1964.

Glassow, Frank: Recurrent inguinal and femoral hernia. Br. Med. J. *1*:215, 1970.

Graffin, John M.: Incarcerated inflamed appendix in a femoral hernia sac. Am. J. Surg. *115*:364, 1968.

Halverson, K., and McVay, C. B.: Inguinal and femoral hernioplasty: A 22 year study of the authors' methods. Arch. Surg. *101*:127, 1970.

Hardy, John C., and Costin, J. R.: Femoral hernias: A 10 year review. J.A.O.A. *68*:696, 704–790, 1969.

Hull, H. E., and Ganey, J. B.: The Henry approach to femoral hernia. Ann. Surg. *137*:57, 1953.

Iason, A. H.: *Hernia.* Philadelphia, Blakiston Co., 1941, pp. 624–628.

Jennings, W. K., Anson, B. J., and Wright, R. R.: A new method of repair of indirect inguinal hernia considered in reference to parietal anatomy. Surg. Gynecol. Obstet. *74*:697, 1942.

Jones, Richard A.: Femoral hernia following inguinal hernioplasty. Am. Surg. *32*(10):724, 1966.

Keetley, C. B.: Thirteen cases of herniotomy for strangulated hernia. Br. Med. J. *2*:1195, 1883.

Koontz, A. R.: *Hernia.* New York, Appleton-Century-Crofts, 1963, pp. 90–105.

Lindholm, A., Nilsson, O., and Tholin, B.: Inguinal and femoral hernias. Results following 238 preperitoneal radical operations. Arch. Surg. *98*:19, 1969.

Lund, J., Hviot, V., and Kjeldsen-Andersen, J.: Inguinal and femoral hernioplasty. Five year follow-up of 284 cases of McVay repair. Acta Chir. Scand. *131*:72, 1966.

Mansfield, R. D.: A new approach to treatment of hernias of the groin. Am. J. Surg. *100*:462, 1960.

Meade, R. H.: The history of the abdominal approach to hernia repair. Surgery *57*:908, 1965.

McEvedy, P. G.: Femoral hernia. Ann. Roy. Coll. Surg. Engl. *7*:484, 1950.

McVay, C. B., and Anson, B. J.: Aponeurotic and fascial continuities in the abdomen, pelvis and thigh. Anat. Rec. *76*(2):213–231 (supplement), 1940.

Orr, T. G., Jr.: Richter's hernia. Surg. Gynecol. Obstet. *91*:705, 1950.

Palumbo, L. T., Sharpe, W. S., Gerndt, H. I., Magleetta, E. D., and Eidbo, W. B.: Primary inguinal hernioplasty. Our experience with 3,572 operations. Arch. Surg. *87*:949, 1963.

Robson, A. W. M.: Abdominal section for hernia. Practitioner *50*:417, 1893.

Souttar, H. S.: Surgical anatomy of femoral hernia. Br. Med. J. *1*:361–412, 1924.

Thomas, David: Strangulated femoral hernia. Med. J. Aust. *1*:258, 1967.

# 16

# Recurrent Femoral Hernias

Femoral hernias are the most treacherous of the groin hernias: they are not always easily recognized; they may be the site of incarceration and strangulation of the intestine; and they are more difficult to repair successfully. Femoral hernias are less commonly seen than are indirect and direct inguinal hernias; thus, surgeons are inclined to feel that efforts at repair of femoral hernias are more successful than they really are.

Serious attention must be given to the high recurrence rate of femoral hernias following antecedent repair of other groin hernias. It is recognized that an occasional femoral hernia might be overlooked at the time of repair of other groin hernias, but the inordinately high incidence of femoral hernias that appear subsequent to earlier herniorrhaphies cannot be ignored by surgeons who wish to improve their results. Femoral hernias are seen in from 15 to 45 percent of patients who have had prior repair of groin hernias (Table 16–1).

## FEMORAL HERNIA AFTER REPAIR OF INGUINAL HERNIAS

The matter of appearance of femoral hernias after repair of inguinal hernias has attracted attention of surgeons since 1933, when Easton called attention to the problem. Prior to that time, Taylor (1920) and later Iason (1941) had reported individual cases. Easton (1933) indicated that tension of abdominal wall might be transmitted to the inguinal ligament, with a resultant upward pull.

Jones in 1966 further called attention to the significant incidence of femoral hernias following repair of groin hernias in which the inguinal ligament was used as an anchoring structure. Several authors were aware of the same phenomenon.

In 1970 Glassow presented the experience at the Shouldice Hospital. He reported that 47 femoral hernias occurred following repair of indirect inguinal hernias and 57 appeared after repair of direct inguinal hernias.

Glassow analyzed the problem concerning the appearance of femoral hernias following repair of both direct and indirect inguinal hernias and concluded that such hernias may develop for the following reasons:

1. The femoral hernia might have been present at the initial operation, but it was overlooked.
2. A new hernia developed.
3. The femoral hernia was iatrogenically created.

One important point to consider is that excessive upward tension may disrupt the integrity of the femoral ring. Nearly all of the authors listed in Table 16–1 have recognized this possibility.

Furthermore, the forces of upward pull are greater when bilateral groin hernias are repaired. I have been impressed with the high incidence of bilateral repairs among patients who eventually developed recur-

Table 16–1.  INGUINAL HERNIA REPAIRS FOLLOWED BY FEMORAL HERNIAS*

| Year | Author | No. of Femoral Hernias Repaired | Prior Inguinal Herniorrhaphy | Percent |
|------|--------|---------------------------------|------------------------------|---------|
| 1939 | McClure and Fallis | 90 | 20 | 22 |
| 1948 | Fratkin | 20 | 9 | 45 |
| 1958 | Burton and Bauer | 165 | 46 | 28 |
| 1958 | Ludington | 62 | 26 | 35 |
| 1965 | Jones | 20 | 3 | 15 |
| 1966 | Glassow | 1143 | 255 | 23 |
| 1971 | Ponka and Brush | 216 | 49 | 23 |

*Initial data collected by Jones.

rent femoral hernias following repair of direct or indirect inguinal hernias.

Others who have recognized the possibility that use of the inguinal ligament in hernia repair might be counterproductive include Anson and McVay (1938) and McVay and Savage (1961).

## Recurrences Following Femoral Hernia Repair

Statistics referring to recurrences following repair of femoral hernias are not overabundant. The figures provided in Table 16–2 do not support the view that femoral hernias rarely recur following repair. I suspect that the reason for this situation is the low incidence of femoral hernias when compared to either direct or indirect inguinal hernias. More time must elapse before a substantial series of primary femoral hernias can be accumulated.

## ETIOLOGY OF RECURRENT FEMORAL HERNIAS: GENERAL DISCUSSION

The extremely high incidence of recurrent femoral hernias is an indication that the genesis of such hernias is not well understood. An attempt must be made to identify possible etiologic factors if the number of postoperative recurrences is to be decreased.

In discussing the reasons for failure, we must include the following: tension, poor choice of technical procedure or poor execution (or both), overlooked femoral hernia, wound hematoma, and wound infection. In a small percentage of recurrent femoral hernias, an etiologic factor cannot be easily identified. Consider the following example: can a femoral hernia that appeared 43 years after repair of an inguinal hernia be considered a "recurrent" hernia? In my judgment, the hernia in this case arose *de novo* and had nothing to do with the repair performed so many years previously. This example also emphasizes the need for effective record keeping. Some method must be devised so that surgeons can obtain records of antecedent operations. This unavailability of records, or incomplete operative reports, dealing with preceding repairs makes it exceedingly difficult to offer a valid study of the subject of recurrence of hernias. Greater accuracy in record keeping and general availability of such medical records to interested and responsible surgeons would be great steps forward in this field. Until such ideal circumstances are met, we must resort to a critical analysis of every bit of information available to us in order to improve results.

Table 16–2.  RECURRENCES FOLLOWING FEMORAL HERNIA REPAIR

| Year | Author | No. of Cases | Recurrence Rate (Percent) |
|------|--------|--------------|---------------------------|
| 1939 | McClure and Fallis | 54 | 9.7 |
| 1948 | Butters | 120 | 3.3 |
| 1966 | Glassow | 1143 | 0.2 to 6 |
| 1971 | Ponka and Brush | 216 | 6.5 |

## ETIOLOGY OF RECURRENT FEMORAL HERNIA (THE OVERLOOKED FEMORAL HERNIA)

There are numerous causes for recurrent femoral hernias. Perhaps more common a reality than generally appreciated is the overlooked femoral hernia. In my surgical lifetime, I myself am aware of four instances in which patients with recurrent femoral hernias noticed that the swelling in the groin—the problem for which the surgery was intended—was never corrected. The patient was aware of the recurrence while in the hospital or a few days thereafter, usually after the postoperative pain had subsided. Two of these patients were from the Henry Ford Hospital, and two came from other institutions. Undoubtedly, there are other such cases of overlooked hernias—the records forever lost in the complicated perplexity of inaccurate case reports, which are impounded and interred in the deep silent recesses of the Medical Records departments. Surgeons who have devoted a great deal of time to the hernia problem are aware that the overlooked femoral hernia occurs with uncomfortable frequency. I do not consider such hernias to be recurrences, since they were never repaired in the first place! Most authorities, however, tend to include overlooked hernias in the category of recurrences. In this discussion, I will do likewise—but with reservations as to the designation that such hernias are recurrent.

Femoral hernias are rather easily overlooked because of their small size; they are often well concealed in obese patients. The patient may be unable to give an accurate history of pain, since many of these patients are elderly. At other times, one defect may be overlooked when two are present. For example, when both indirect and femoral hernias are present simultaneously, the more obvious indirect may be repaired and the femoral hernia may be completely missed. Accurate diagnosis of defects in every patient is extremely important. Chapter 15 deals with diagnostic features of femoral hernias in more detail.

Femoral hernias may appear as protrusions after successful repair of indirect or direct inguinal hernias. It is not unusual for a femoral hernia to appear many years after a patient has undergone successful repair of an indirect inguinal hernia in infancy or childhood. It is extremely difficult to establish cause and effect in such cases because of the lack of accurate details concerning the original diagnosis and operative treatment. Femoral hernias that appear many years after the repair of direct or indirect inguinal hernias most likely develop de novo.

The continued popularity of the Bassini-Halsted repair of groin hernias inevitably leads the surgical statisticians to the inevitable conclusion that such repairs con-

### Table 16–3. FACTORS LEADING TO RECURRENT FEMORAL HERNIAS*

| Description | | No. of Patients |
|---|---|---|
| *Excessive Tension* | | 46 |
| Bilateral simultaneous repair | 23 | |
| Failure to use relaxing incision | 21 | |
| Sutures placed too high on internal oblique | 16 | |
| Increased intra-abdominal pressure | 4 | |
| (Ascites, cirrhosis, emphysema, abdominal carcinomatosis, and chronic cough) | | |
| *Technical Factors* | | 32 |
| Poor choice of procedure | 16 | |
| Failure to use prosthesis | 14 | |
| Inadequate repair | 2 | |
| *Overlooked Hernia* | | 3 |
| *Wound Infection* | | 3 |
| *Hematomas* | | 1 |
| *Etiologic Factors Not Easily Identified* | | 8 |
| *Iatrogenic Factors (Possible)* | | 16 |

*Number of factors exceeds that of patients (62) because several factors were operant simultaneously in individual patients.

stitute the great majority of operations to be later followed by recurrent femoral hernias. Once it has been theoretically established that groin hernias repaired by a technique utilizing Poupart's ligament predispose to femoral herniation, the search for an explanation can begin. It is reasonable to find fault with the original technique. One explanation is that suture of the internal oblique and transversus abdominis musculoaponeurotic plate to Poupart's ligament results in tension, pulling the latter structure upward and disrupting the normal femoral ring. Another explanation is that tension on the transversalis fascia, or iliopubic tract, opens up the femoral ring.

## ETIOLOGIC FACTORS IN RECURRENT FEMORAL HERNIAS

Often, the causes for recurrence of femoral hernias are numerous, evident, and interrelated; at other times, they are difficult to identify (Table 16–3). Individual case reports will help to explain the problem of recurrence.

### Excessive Tension

Excessive tension at the repair site could be recognized as a factor in a large number of the 62 cases studied. Bilateral hernia repairs had been performed initially in slightly over one-third of the patients. In nearly one-third, the relaxing incision was omitted. In 16 patients, the operative note stated that sutures were placed into the internal oblique or "conjoined tendon."

### Recurrent Femoral Hernias—Multiple Causative Factors: Case in Point (Bilateral Repair)

The numerous and complex interrelated factors leading to recurrent herniation is well illustrated in the following case report.

The patient was an active female, 55 years of age, who had undergone two previous repairs on each side performed elsewhere within a period of two years. Reappearance of the hernias was prompt

following bilateral operations on one occasion. The patient appeared for the third repairs at Henry Ford Hospital. At this time, simultaneous Moschcowitz repairs were performed on the right and left groins.

Two months later, the patient returned with complaints of discomfort and swelling; at this time, a recurrent right direct inguinal hernia was diagnosed—making this the third recurrence.

At the time of the fourth repair, the surgeon described a massive direct recurrence in which the sac contained the tube and ovary. These structures were removed, and high ligation of the peritoneal sac achieved. The surgeon wisely elected to perform a Lotheissen-McVay repair. The patient recovered nicely but developed a seroma, which required aspiration.

Four months following earlier Moschcowitz repairs, the patient developed a left femoral recurrent hernia, thus making the fourth recurrence. The surgeon elected to employ Marlex mesh in the repair, anchoring it to Cooper's ligament below and the internal oblique aponeurosis above.

### *Comment*

Bilateral simultaneous repairs were performed upon this patient on two previous occasions without benefit of relaxing incision or reinforcing mesh. Prompt recurrence was strong evidence of poor choice of procedure and execution.

Failure to use mesh after the second and third repairs, I believe, is bad practice. Tissue strength is compromised when excessive scarring is present.

The choice of the Lotheissen-McVay repair was a good one, since both direct and femoral hernias can thereby be eliminated.

Any patient with numerous recurrences requires special attention, and the use of mesh should be entertained. Tension at the site of repair must be strictly avoided.

### Technical Factors

Technical factors, including poor choice of procedure and poor execution of the procedure, are difficult to identify in some cases. The choice of a Moschcowitz repair after a previous failure of such a repair was considered a poor choice of procedure.

Another example of poor choice of procedure was recognized when a McVay repair failed to hold only to be repeated without a relaxing incision. The result was a reappearance of the hernia as a femoral and direct inguinal hernia.

An inadequate repair was recognized when the repair was not carried far enough laterally toward the femoral vein.

## Recurrent Femoral Hernia — Inadequate Repair: Case in Point

The patient was a female, 41 years of age, who presented with a left direct and femoral hernia. The surgeon identified a small femoral hernia. He then stated: "The femoral defect, though small, was rather superficial and easily closed with a single heavy figure-of-eight master stitch." The procedure was completed as an inguinal ligament repair in which the transversus arch was sutured to Poupart's ligament. Soon after the repair the swelling was again recognized below the left inguinal ligament.

### Comment

In this case, the surgeon recognized the femoral defect but failed to repair it adequately, resulting in a promptly "recurrent" hernia. Actually, it was never repaired. Sutures should have been placed laterally between the transversus arch and Cooper's ligament, so as to occlude the femoral ring to a point near the femoral vein. Instead of the single figure-of-eight suture, a minimum of four to six sutures should have been inserted. These should be of number 2–0 silk or synthetic nonabsorbable material. A Lotheissen-McVay, Moschcowitz, or Bassini-Kirschner repair would have been a good choice of method.

Immediate recurrence after repair indicates the possibility of an overlooked hernia or a technically inadequate operative procedure.

Failure to use mesh was considered to be faulty technique, but it is also question-

able surgical judgment. Tantalum or Marlex mesh was implanted successfully in 13 patients in my study with failure in only one patient. The mesh was improperly anchored and failed to prevent recurrence of a femoral hernia. In my practice, I often use Marlex mesh when dealing with hernias that have recurred a number of times.

## Other Factors

In some instances, identification of the overlooked femoral hernia is made by the patient, who recognizes it as the same defect for which repair was initiated. In other instances, the surgeon identifies a defect at the femoral ring, then fails to carry the repair laterally far enough resulting in a prompt recurrence.

We will not elaborate here on the deleterious effects of infection and hematoma on the healing of an operative wound; they are not common factors in the etiology of recurrent femoral hernias.

In 8 of 62 patients, I could not easily identify the etiologic factors that might have resulted in recurrent femoral hernias.

In 16 patients, it was suspected that iatrogenic factors were operative in causing recurrent femoral hernias. In these, the inguinal ligament was used as the anchoring site of the abdominal wall, and tension was considered to be excessive.

This retrospective analysis undoubtedly has its limitations, but there is no doubt in my mind that recurrent femoral hernias are caused by a number of factors. Tension, poor choice of procedure, and faulty execution of a groin technique are important factors in recurrences.

One detail bears emphasis: although anatomists and surgeons agree that the defect to be repaired in femoral hernias is small, relatively rigid structures are utilized in attempts to repair such hernias. Cooper's ligament has no flexibility or elasticity whatsoever, and the inguinal ligament is tautly drawn between the anterior superior iliac spine and the pubic tubercle. Thus, in attempting to occlude the femoral ring by approximating these two structures, considerable tension is the undesirable consequence.

## RECURRENT FEMORAL HERNIA—CLINICAL STUDY

It is most difficult to accumulate a substantial number of records of patients with recurrent femoral hernias. My series is quite small, consisting of 66 recurrent femoral hernias repaired among 62 patients. Four patients had bilateral recurrent femoral hernias. The records of these patients were gathered from our files beginning in the year 1945 up to and including 1974. Only by studying specific types of recurrences in detail can we expect further improvement in our results.

### Age and Sex

In a study recorded in Chapter 15 of 488 femoral hernias, I found the incidence to be 53.5 percent in males and 46.5 percent in females. In this study of recurrent femoral hernias, 22 (or 35.5 percent) recurred in females and 40 (or 64.5 percent) recurred in males. It would appear that repair of femoral hernias is somewhat more successful in females; this is consistent with the fact that the female abdominal wall is anatomically so constructed that it is better able to withstand the stresses to which it is exposed.

### Age Distribution

Femoral hernias are rarely seen in infants and children and infrequently seen in young adults. The same observation applies to recurrent femoral hernias (Table 16–4). Interestingly, femoral hernias tend to occur in older patients: 71 percent in this

**Table 16–4. AGE DISTRIBUTION: RECURRENT FEMORAL HERNIAS—62 PATIENTS**

| Age | Number | Percent |
|---|---|---|
| 1 to 10 | 0 | 0 |
| 11 to 20 | 0 | 0 |
| 21 to 30 | 2 | 3.2 |
| 31 to 40 | 4 | 6.5 |
| 41 to 50 | 12 | 19.4 |
| 51 to 60 | 17 | 27.4 |
| 61 to 70 | 21 | 33.8 |
| 71 to 80 | 4 | 6.5 |
| 81 and over | 2 | 3.2 |

**Table 16–5. NUMBER OF PREVIOUS REPAIRS—62 PATIENTS WITH RECURRENT FEMORAL HERNIAS**

| No. Previous Repairs | No. of Patients | Percent |
|---|---|---|
| 1 | 36 | 58. |
| 2 | 14 | 22.6 |
| 3 | 5 | 8.1 |
| 4 | 4 | 6.5 |
| 5 | 2 | 3.2 |
| 6 | 1 | 1.6 |
| Total | 62 | 100.0 |

study occurred in patients 50 years of age and older.

### Number of Previous Repairs

Even in this small series of 62 patients, it is evident that repair of femoral hernias is too often followed by recurrence (Table 16–5). It can be seen from Table 16–5 that 26 patients required a total of 75 repairs. In all, 62 patients required 105 repairs. The need for better surgical management of femoral hernias is clearly evident.

## Operative Management

### Anesthesia

Local anesthesia was preferred for most of the patients requiring repair of femoral hernias. Local anesthesia was used for 63.6 percent; spinal anesthesia for 27.3 percent; and general anesthesia was selected for only 9.1 percent of the repairs.

### Technique of Repair

Sixty-two patients underwent a total of 66 repairs of recurrent femoral hernias; four patients had bilateral simultaneous repairs. The methods chosen for repair have been described in detail in Chapter 15.

### Utilization of the Lotheissen-McVay Repair

The Lotheissen-McVay repair was the preferred method of repair, being used in 45.5 percent of the repairs (Table 16–6).

Table 16–6.  **REPAIR OF 66 RECURRENT FEMORAL HERNIAS — METHOD OF REPAIR**

| Method | No. Repairs | Percent |
|---|---|---|
| Lotheissen-McVay | 30 | 45.5 |
| Moschcowitz | 18 | 27.3 |
| Bassini-Kirschner | 12 | 18.2 |
| Bassini | 4 | 6.0 |
| Henry-Cheatle-Nyhus | 2 | 3.0 |
| Total | 66 | 100.00 |

The need to approach the recurrent femoral hernia from an approach above the inguinal ligament is clear. By this route it is possible to identify either recurrent direct inguinal hernias or recurrent indirect inguinal hernias, or both. Rarely, direct, indirect, and femoral hernial sacs are present simultaneously. Thus, if combinations of defects are suspected, the inguinal approach is indispensable.

The Lotheissen-McVay repair has steadily gained in popularity as a method for repair of recurrent femoral hernias in our practice (see Fig. 14–8, p. 230).

In this approach the dissection is carried out from a vantage point above the inguinal ligament. If a groin incision is present from earlier surgical repair, the cicatrix makes dissection difficult. Sharp dissection offers many advantages; once mastered, it makes dissection of the area much less traumatic. The skin incision is made in such a manner as to excise the previously healed incision. If the earlier incision had healed with only a thin line, the new incision may be made through it to the aponeurosis of the external oblique. In the process of developing the incision, the cord structures must be constantly looked for and protected. The veins of the pampiniform plexus and the vas deferens are identified by direct vision. Usually the spermatic cord is found under the external oblique aponeurosis. A small rubber tape or gauze sling may be used to isolate the cord and facilitate its manipulation.

The transversalis fascia (or the remains of it), is incised obliquely, and Cooper's ligament is identified with sharp and blunt dissection. The femoral hernial sac is identified at this point. Dissection of the globular mass below the inguinal ligament is completed, and the protrusion may be freed through circumferential dissection about it. At times, a small incision may be required in Gimbernat's ligament. I prefer to identify the peritoneum at the internal ring and perform a Hoguet maneuver if this is reasonable. On the other hand, if the internal ring has been previously well repaired, the peritoneum may be opened medially to the deep inferior epigastric vessels, similar to the technique used when a direct hernial sac is opened. Care is exercised to avoid injury to the bladder. Again, the femoral peritoneal sac is reduced at this time, forming what amounts to a direct peritoneal sac. The bladder may comprise a sliding portion of the sac. High ligation of the peritoneal sac is performed, and then reconstruction is begun. The transversus abdominis arch (or the remains of it) is sutured to Cooper's ligament with interrupted sutures of number 2–0 silk or of nonabsorbable synthetic sutures. Repair is carried out by careful placement of sutures approximately one centimeter apart from the pubic tubercle medially to the proximity of the femoral vein laterally (see Fig. 14–8, p. 230, and Fig. 15–4, p. 244). Two or three such sutures are not enough; six or eight sutures might be too many and might interfere with the blood supply to an area already in jeopardy. Some judgment is necessary. Laterally, a suture is placed between the transversus arch, the femoral sheath, and the ligament of Cooper to prevent herniation at this site. The need for a relaxing incision in this situation is great and, in my opinion, indispensable to sound repair. The internal ring must be individually evaluated; if it admits more than the tip of the digit, the transversalis fascia must be identified separately and closed. It might be worthwhile to again state that the transversalis fascia above is sutured to its counterpart below, which is the iliopubic tract or femoral sheath and not the inguinal ligament.

Closure of the skin and subcutaneous tissues is accomplished as shown in Chapter 11, Figures 11–7 and 11–8, pp. 165 and 166.

### Utilization of the Moschcowitz Repair

In the 1940's and 1950's the Moschcowitz repair was frequently employed in repair of femoral hernias, but the method is used infrequently today.

The Moschcowitz method of repair of femoral hernias has a comparatively limited place in the repair of virginal femoral hernias and should be of rare use in the repair of recurrent femoral hernias. The Moschcowitz repair can be utilized in selected femoral hernias when the angle between the inguinal ligament and Cooper's ligament is not too great. If tension is excessive upon approximation of these two structures, then the method should be abandoned. I was surprised that the Moschcowitz repair was used in 18, or 27 percent, of the operations for recurrent femoral hernias.

Experience teaches us that recurrent femoral hernias must not be taken lightly. Although the defect is not large, permanent closure is the goal of surgery. The Moschcowitz repair is rarely used for repair of recurrent femoral hernias in my practice because of unacceptably high recurrence rates. The method is illustrated in Chapter 15, Figure 15–5, page 246.

### Utilization of the Bassini-Kirschner Repair

The Bassini-Kirschner repair, performed via the inferior approach as described in Chapter 15, has gained in popularity on my service (Fig. 15–6, p. 247). It has proven a useful method in repair of selected patients with recurrent femoral hernias. The recurrent femoral hernia should be approached as an individual problem. The recommendation that all femoral hernias must be repaired in the same manner is ill conceived. For instance, when the surgeon is facing the problem of a recurrent femoral hernia, certain information should influence his approach. In a female who has had an inguinal hernia repaired previously, it is most likely that an indirect inguinal hernia was the initial defect. Direct hernias are rare in females (see Table 7–2, p. 84). Hence, when a femoral hernia appears following successful repair of a groin hernia in a female, full attention can be directed to the defect at hand. Recurrent femoral hernias appearing in males who have had successful repair of groin hernias may also be approached from below with far less danger to the spermatic cord.

Approach of a recurrent femoral hernia through the inferior approach has much to recommend it. Dissection through an area free of dense cicatricial tissue is more simply accomplished. The procedure may be carried out under local anesthesia through a transverse or an oblique skin incision below Poupart's ligament. Then the incision is developed through the subcutaneous fat. The globular hernial sac is seen with incision of the attenuated fascia. It is dissected free of surrounding tissue, so that the pectineus fascia is seen posteriorly. Laterally, the femoral vein is identified; above and anteriorly, the external oblique aponeurosis and the inguinal ligament may be identified. The sac and contents are dissected circumferentially until the entire sac is free. This means that Cooper's ligament can be demonstrated posteriorly and superiorly. With elevation of the external oblique aponeurosis after application of an Allis clamp, it is possible to visualize the inguinal ligament. From this vantage point, the transversalis fascia is also encountered. The peritoneal sac is completely freed and ligated with a purse-string suture of number 2–0 silk. The excess sac is amputated, and the stump retracted to a point above Cooper's ligament. It is now a simple matter to suture the inguinal ligament and transversalis fascia to Cooper's ligament, after the method described as the Bassini-Kirschner repair (see Fig. 15–6, p. 247). Three or four sutures of number 2–0 silk or synthetic nonabsorbable sutures will result in a strong repair in most cases. If desired, however, a small flap of pectineus fascia may be liberated and turned upward over the repair and sutured to the external oblique aponeurosis. Closure of the subcutaneous tissue and skin completes the operation. This operation inflicts a minimum of surgical trauma upon the patient and may be performed upon seriously ill patients with a high degree of safety. The Bassini-Kirschner repair was used in 12, or 18.2 percent, of the repairs.

The classical Bassini repair is simple and safe to perform and is an optional method for consideration. Interrupted sutures of number 2–0 silk are placed between inguinal ligament, pectineal fascia, and the falciform process and fascia lata (Fig. 15–9, p. 254). The method is used infrequently in repair of recurrent femoral hernias; it was used in only 4 of 66 repairs in this study.

## Utilization of Prosthetic Implants

The need for some method of increasing the structural strength in the groin is slowly being recognized by increasing numbers of surgeons. The concept of shifting of a portion of the abdominal wall to bridge a gap in the groin has been exercised almost to the point of exhaustion. Surgeons persist in attempts to suture the inguinal ligament, or the transversus arch, to Cooper's ligament—too often, with failure. The transversus abdominis arch was approximated to Cooper's ligament, with a number of failures. It is noteworthy that in our cases, an implant was not utilized until a number of recurrences with conventional methods were recorded.

In 66 repairs of recurrent femoral hernias, mesh was used in nearly 22 percent. Tantalum mesh was used in the 1950's, but currently Marlex mesh is used exclusively.

Two methods of fixation of the prosthetic material are utilized. In one method the mesh is attached to Cooper's ligament and the inguinal ligament, thus completely obliterating the femoral ring. In the other method, the mesh is attached to Cooper's ligament inferiorly, then attached to the aponeurosis of the internal oblique muscle above. The mesh is tailored to fit an area from the pubic tubercle to the region of the anterior superior iliac spine, where it is attached to the inguinal ligament as well. Number 2–0 synthetic nonabsorbable material is used almost exclusively for this purpose. Placement of sutures inferiorly is done under direct visualization from the pubic tubercle to the femoral vein. Attachment above is to the transversus arch and aponeurosis of the internal oblique muscle.

## Utilization of the Henry-Cheatle-Nyhus Repair

The Henry-Cheatle-Nyhus preperitoneal approach was used in 2 of 66 recurrent femoral hernias (see Fig. 15–8, B; p. 250). The method is technically sound but does not lend itself for performance under local anesthesia. Nevertheless, it should be utilized in selected patients who have undergone a number of attempts at previous repair.

### Inguinofemoral Recurrent Hernias

Large recurrent simultaneous direct and femoral hernias occur frequently enough to warrant an individual chapter. Such hernias are largely iatrogenic in nature and present a real challenge to the surgeon. Inguinofemoral recurrent hernias are described in detail, along with surgical management, in Chapter 19.

### Postoperative Complications

In one patient, wound infection occurred as a postoperative complication; a culture study revealed staphylococci. In two patients, hematomas were troublesome and required drainage. Four patients developed seromas. These individuals had multiple previous repairs, and two of them had prosthetic implants (Marlex mesh, in one; Tantalum, in the other). Three patients had ecchymosis in the operative area, all of which resolved uneventfully. Five patients developed testicular swelling, and two eventually had atrophic testes. Both of these individuals had undergone two previous herniorrhaphies.

Three patients developed postoperative urinary retention, and one had a troublesome urinary tract infection.

Two patients developed atelectasis, and one additional patient required treatment of pneumonitis.

One individual required treatment of thrombophlebitis.

There were no fatalities among 62 patients undergoing repair of recurrent femoral hernias.

### Recurrences

It was necessary to review records of patients dating back to 1945 in order to locate those with recurrent femoral hernias. Only 15 of the 66 recurrent femoral hernias had been initially repaired at Henry Ford Hospital. Only 30 of 62 patients were followed 5 years or longer. It was impossible to draw any conclusion as to which method might be superior to others. It was seen that failures followed every method used. Furthermore, I gained the impression that it is care as well as judgment in performance of the individual operation that has much to do with success and is most difficult to evaluate.

Even though the Moschcowitz repair was used in 18 patients, two such repairs were followed by recurrences. One recurrence was seen after a McVay repair. Subsequently, this hernia was successfully repaired with mesh attached to Cooper's ligament. The fourth recurrence followed a Bassini repair of a recurrent femoral hernia. Thus, the recurrence rate for 66 repairs was 6 percent; this recurrence rate is similar to that seen after repair of direct recurrent inguinal hernias.

Insofar as prevention of recurrences, Halverson and McVay (1970), in discussing the problem, suggested that recurrence rates would possibly have been lower had they used a synthetic mesh (such as Marlex) in cases where strength of the repair was in doubt.

Unfortunately, despite every effort at correct preoperative and operative diagnosis and meticulous surgical technique, the surgeon may find that an occasional hernia will recur, and the result will defy explanation.

## SUMMARY

A *recurrent femoral hernia* should involve, strictly speaking, the reappearance of a femoral hernia following prior repair of a hernia of the same variety. Yet the practicing surgeon too frequently encounters a femoral hernia that appears after earlier repair of either a direct inguinal hernia or an indirect inguinal hernia, or both. Surgeons must be aware of the possibility of creating a femoral hernia while repairing an inguinal one.

In the genesis of recurrent femoral hernias, the most important factor is excessive tension created by the repair. Bilateral repairs, failure to use relaxing incisions, and placement of sutures too high onto the internal oblique, or the rectus sheath, are all counterproductive measures.

There is need for an individual approach to the patient with recurrent femoral hernia. For example, in the female the floor of the inguinal canal is of such strength that a direct inguinal hernia is a rare finding; hence, it is meddlesome to disrupt the floor of Hesselbach's triangle as a routine practice. On the other hand, if an elderly male has an enlarged external abdominal ring, a bulge in the inguinal floor, and a femoral hernia, it would be essential to approach the defects through an incision above the inguinal ligament. Such an approach permits thorough intraoperative evaluation together with an effective method of repair. In patients with incarceration of intestine and suspected strangulation, the transinguinal approach is recommended. Each patient with a recurrent femoral hernia requires careful clinical evaluation prior to selection of a method of repair.

Careful attention to detail is essential in performance of any method of repair selected for a given patient. No method will yield superior results if poorly performed.

There is slowly mounting evidence that prosthetic implants should be used more frequently in the repair of recurrent hernias and in bilateral repairs.

The recurrence rate of 6 percent indicates that the problem of recurrent femoral hernia is not yet solved.

## REFERENCES

Anson, B. J., Reimann, A. E., and Sigart, L. L.: The anatomy of hernial regions. II–Femoral hernia. Surg. Gynecol. Obstet. 89:752, 1949.

Anson, B. J., and McVay, C. B.: Anatomy of inguinal and hypogastric regions of abdominal wall. Anat. Rec. 70:211, 1938.

Burton, C. C., and Bauer, A. R., Jr.: Femoral hernia: Review of 165 repairs. Ann. Surg. 148:913, 1958.

Burton, C.: Current concepts of the anatomic, clinical and reparative features of femoral hernia. Surgery 44:877, 1958.

Cheatle, G. L.: An operation for the radical cure of inguinal and femoral hernia. Br. Med. J. 2:68, 1920.

Condon, R. E.: The anatomy of the inguinal region in its relationship to groin hernias. In Nyhus, L. M., and Harkins, N. H. (eds.): Hernia. Philadelphia, J. B. Lippincott Co., 1964, pp. 14–62.

Dunphy, J. E.: The diagnosis and surgical management of strangulated femoral hernia. J.A.M.A. 114:394, 1940.

Easton, E. R.: Incidence of femoral hernia following repair of inguinal hernia-ectopic recurrence; Proposed operation of external and internal herniorrhaphy. J.A.M.A. 100:1741, 1933.

Fratkin, L. B.: Femoral hernia following inguinal herniorrhaphy. Can. Med. Ass. J. 58:365, 1948.

Glassow, F.: Femoral hernia following inguinal herniorrhaphy. Can. J. Surg. 13:27, 1970.

Glassow, F.: Femoral hernia: Review of 1143 consecutive repairs. Ann. Surg., *163*:227, 1966.

Henry, A. K.: Operation for femoral hernia by a midline extra-peritoneal approach; With a preliminary note on the use of this route for reducible inguinal hernia. Lancet *1*:531, 1936.

Halverson, K., and McVay, C. B.: Inguinal and femoral hernioplasty. Arch. Surg. *101*:127, 1970.

Iason, A. H.: *Hernia*. Philadelphia, Blakiston Co., 1941.

Jones, R. A.: Femoral hernia following inguinal hernioplasty. Am. Surg. *32*:725, 1966.

Lotheissen, G.: Zur radikal Operation der Schenkel hernien. Zentralbl. Chir. *25*:548, 1898.

Ludington, L. G.: Femoral hernia and its management with particular reference to its occurrence following inguinal herniorrhaphy. Ann. Surg. *148*:823, 1958.

McClure, R. D., and Fallis, L. S.: Femoral hernia; Report of 90 operations. Ann. Surg. *109*:987, 1939.

McVay, C. B., and Savage, L. E.: Etiology of femoral hernia. Ann. Surg. *154*:25, 1961.

McVay, C. B., and Anson, B. J.: A fundamental error in current methods of inguinal herniorrhaphy. Surg. Gynecol. Obstet. *74*:746, 1942.

Mahorner, H., and Goss, C. B.: Herniation following destruction of Poupart's and Cooper's ligaments: A method of repair. Ann. Surg. *155*:741, 1962.

Mikkelsen, W. P., and Berne, C. J.: Femoral hernioplasty: Suprapubic extraperitoneal (Henry-Cheatle) approach. Surgery *35*:743, 1954.

Moschcowitz, A. V.: New operation for radical cure of femoral hernia. J.A.M.A. *48*:899, 1907.

Nyhus, L. M.: The preperitoneal approach and iliopubic tract repair of all groin hernias. *In* Nyhus, L. M., and Harkins, N. H. (eds.): *Hernia*. Philadelphia, J. B. Lippincott Co., 1964, pp. 271–306.

Ponka, J. L.: Incarcerated femoral hernia. HFH Med. J. *15*(3):203, 1967.

Read, R. R.: Pre-extraperitoneal approach to inguinofemoral herniorrhaphy. Am. J. Surg. *114*:672, 1967.

Taylor, A. S.: The results of operations for inguinal hernia. Arch. Surg. *1*:382, 1920.

# 17

# Combined Direct-Indirect and Femoral Hernias; Recurrent Multilocular Inguinal Hernias

## INTRODUCTION

In examining several books on the subject of hernia, I found it most interesting that the problem of multilocular hernias was given little consideration. I am certain that the authors were fully aware of the problem; however, I felt a more prominent treatment of the subject was warranted because of the frequency with which combinations of hernias occur. Also, a more accurate clinical and intraoperative diagnosis would result from recognition of this frequency.

Why give so much attention to something that is generally known? In my opinion, to be forewarned is to be prepared. Certainly, every surgeon prefers to enter the operating arena with a well-planned course of action rather than an extemporaneous one. To reiterate, it is certain that a correct diagnosis is more likely to be made when the clinician entertains the possibility that more than one hernia exists; in addition, the surgeon who is alert to this possibility is less likely to overlook the presence of a second hernia.

Classifications of groin hernias that recognize only three varieties of hernias—i.e.,

direct, indirect, and femoral—must be considered incomplete. An additional designation must be added for combinations of direct, indirect, and femoral hernias. Actually, combined herniations are encountered more frequently than are femoral hernias.

I find the term "multilocular" to be an especially good one for this condition. The diagnosis might be recorded as multilocular, direct-indirect, or direct and femoral hernia. In such hernias, more than one protrusion is present in the groin simultaneously.

The fact that indirect and direct inguinal hernias are common types of groin hernias is well appreciated. The incidence of femoral hernias is approximately 5 percent of all hernias. Zimmerman and Anson (1967) accumulated 100,114 hernias in a collected review; of these, 81.4 percent were listed as inguinal and 5.3 percent as femoral. However, this large series did not include a breakdown into direct, indirect, and multilocular inguinal hernias. In my study, I found the incidence of combinations of inguinal hernias to be 7.6 percent of groin hernias in males and 3.1 percent in females.

## INCIDENCE OF COMBINED DIRECT-INDIRECT AND FEMORAL HERNIAS

Most physicians, and many surgeons, have a tendency to accept direct, indirect, and femoral hernias as the types of protrusions commonly encountered in the lower abdomen and groin. Although some combination of direct-indirect and femoral hernias is more common than the femoral hernia alone, this fact is not reflected in the literature dealing with the subject of hernia.

Hoguet's significant contribution in 1920 provided a substantial step toward proper identification of combinations of defects in the groin. He noted that when a direct hernia is present, a definite sac or a peritoneal protrusion, varying in size, could be identified at the internal ring. Another of his contributions—the Hoguet maneuver—is described in detail in Chapter 13 on direct hernia.

Watson in the third edition of his book, *Hernia* (1948), made a short statement on the matter of double, or "saddlebag," hernias. He pointed out that when one is operating for direct inguinal hernias, the indirect component can be overlooked unless the sac is opened at the internal ring. I feel that identification of the peritoneum lateral to the deep inferior epigastric artery is of fundamental importance, since from this point of entry digital examination for direct and femoral hernias is easily performed. Watson's suggestion of asking the patient to cough, if the herniorrhaphy is being performed under local anesthesia, aids in identifying the type and extent of the weakness.

Any valid statistical study regarding the relative incidence of direct, indirect, femoral, or combined types of hernias should reflect the age and sex of the group being studied. For instance, any study of hernias in infancy and childhood will reveal the great preponderance of indirect inguinal hernias in this group, and a study of direct inguinal hernias will disclose a high incidence in males. As the age of the patient population being studied increases, so does the incidence of direct inguinal hernias, as well as that of the combined forms of hernias.

Grace and Johnson (1937) studied hernias in patients over 50 years of age. If we consider the 710 indirect inguinal hernias, 286 direct inguinal hernias, and 119 combined types of groin hernias in their study, we find the incidence to be 63.7 percent, 25.6 percent and 10.7 percent respectively. Therefore, the need for emphasizing the significant incidence of multilocular inguinal hernias in adults is clear.

In a more recent study of personal cases, Ljungdahl (1973) found the incidence of femoral hernias to be 3.6 percent, while the incidence of combined herniations (which included direct, indirect, and femoral) was 4.1 percent.

Lichtenstein (1970) studied 627 consecutive herniorrhaphies and found the incidence of various types of hernias to be as follows: indirect, 33 percent; direct, 32 percent; direct-indirect, 8 percent; and femoral, 2.6 percent. Of 91 recurrent cases studied, the following were found: direct, 55 percent; indirect, 31 percent; direct-indirect, 10 percent; and femorals, only 1 percent. Direct-indirect hernias were more commonly encountered than were femoral hernias, yet such combinations have merited little attention in the past.

Palumbo and Sharpe (1971) found the incidence of direct-indirect, or "saddlebag," hernias to be 16 percent.

Among 745 patients, Dodd (1970) found the incidence of "pantaloon" hernias to be 29 percent. But Glassow (1976), in a much larger experience with 13,108 cases, found the incidence to be 6 percent.

Rowe and Skandalakis (1973) described an unusual patient with bilateral hernias as follows: direct, indirect, femoral, and supravesical hernias. Such multiple hernias are rare; however, the possibility of some combinations of defects should at least be considered.

The significant incidence of multilocular inguinal hernias should alert the surgeon to the possible presence of such combined defects in every adult and aged patient with groin hernias.

### Direct–Indirect Inguinal Hernias

By definition, one cannot escape the obvious fact that a direct–indirect inguinal hernia has two protrusions: one, medial to the deep inferior epigastric vessels; and the other, lateral to them.

Combinations of direct and indirect inguinal hernias are seen most commonly in men of advancing years. Thus, the indirect component of the combination of hernias is likely to be due to the same pathophysiologic mechanism that applies to direct inguinal hernias. Both components, in my opinion, are acquired herniations.

The direct-indirect inguinal hernia has been variously designated as a "pantaloon," "saddlebag," and dual, or double, hernia. The terms "saddlebag" and "pantaloon" are most often applied simply because they are so descriptive. In addition, the term multilocular is also applicable to such hernias.

Watson (1948) recognized that there could be several reasons for recurrence following repair of multilocular hernias. For example, one sac of a combination of sacs might be overlooked; or, in the presence of an obvious indirect sac, a subtle direct one might be easily overlooked. The presence of a small femoral hernia could also be difficult to demonstrate. One must insert the examining finger searchingly into the peritoneal cavity. Each potential hernia site must be given individual attention. I prefer the approach in which the peritoneal cavity is entered at the internal abdominal ring and, from this portal of entry, a methodical digital exploration is carried out. Not only are direct inguinal hernias considered in this approach, but the femoral ring is digitally examined as well. This approach, which is advocated by Hoguet, is described in detail in Chapter 13 on direct inguinal hernias.

It is usually the direct component of direct-indirect hernias that receives the attention of the surgeon. Commonly, the defect in the floor of the inguinal canal is diffuse and wide-mouthed, and is readily recognized once the cord is lifted out of the inguinal canal. This obvious hernia may divert the surgeon's attention from a defect at the internal ring. Any enlargement of the internal ring should not go unnoticed. The cremaster sheath should be opened at the internal ring, and the small indirect peritoneal sac can then be identified. It is at that site that I prefer to enter the peritoneal cavity, regardless of the type of hernia present.

## Direct-Indirect-Femoral Hernias

Such combinations as direct, indirect, and femoral herniations are not common.

But, they do exist, and unless the surgeon is aware of the possibility he may overlook one or two of the components while directing his attention to the most obvious of the protrusions. In such cases, variations in size of the component protrusion is great. For example, the direct inguinal hernia might be prominent, while the indirect and femoral herniations might be quite small. Unless the internal ring is examined and the peritoneum identified at that site, a small indirect inguinal hernia might be easily overlooked. If the direct sac is simply inverted and oversewn with imbricating sutures, the femoral ring may totally escape exploration; and, thus, a femoral hernial component might be overlooked. It is conceivable that some of the femoral hernias appearing after repair of indirect or direct inguinal hernias might initially have existed as small defects. Femoral hernias are notoriously easy to overlook.

## Direct-Femoral

Such combinations as direct-femoral hernias are especially treacherous if the surgeon does not elect to open the peritoneum. The protrusion through the floor of the inguinal canal may lead the surgeon to the erroneous conclusion that only a direct hernia is present, since the smaller femoral hernia can easily be overlooked. Also, it is possible that some of the femoral hernias attributed to inguinal ligament repairs are actually small femoral hernias, which were missed at the time of initial repair. Digital exploration of the groin, with attention to the region of the femoral ring, will help identify any combination of defects.

## Indirect-Femoral

Although the indirect-femoral hernia is an unusual combination, the fact remains that it does exist. The indirect peritoneal sac is usually easily identified at the internal abdominal ring, but the femoral component may be comparatively small.

I recall reviewing more than one record in which the surgeon felt justified in describing an "enlarged femoral dimple," which eventually culminated in a recurrent femoral hernia. The femoral defect may be small and easily missed.

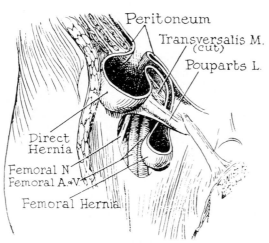

**Figure 17–1.** Unusual bilocular hernia as recognized by Zimmerman. Reproduced with permission of publisher from Zimmerman, L. M., and Anson, B. J.: *Anatomy and Surgery of Hernia* (2nd ed.). Baltimore, Williams & Wilkins Co., 1967.

## Unusual Groin Hernias

Increasingly, unusual hernias are appearing about the groin as a result of vascular surgical procedures upon the femoral vessels. Some are inguinofemoral in type (as described in Chapter 19). Others protrude through the prevascular space between the inguinal ligament and the femoral artery. Occasionally, a protrusion is seen lateral to the femoral vessels.

Zimmerman and Anson (1967) described a rare bilocular interparietal inguinofemoral hernia. They recognized two cases where a direct protrusion was accompanied with a protrusion into the femoral canal (Fig. 17–1).

A variety of protrusions is possible in and about the inguinal area, but these are quite rare. (There is a brief discussion concerning this matter in Chapter 24 on unusual hernias.)

## TECHNIQUE FOR REPAIR OF COMBINATION RECURRENT DIRECT–INDIRECT INGUINAL HERNIAS

Obviously, in repairing recurrent combined direct–indirect inguinal hernias, one must deal with both components; nevertheless, I have seen recurrences due to inadequate repair of either type of hernia.

The technique of repair that is useful in the uncomplicated case is taken from an actual patient's record, as follows: The patient was a 60-year-old male who had had cryptorchidism as an infant. Two bilateral simultaneous repairs, which had been performed elsewhere, were followed by prompt recurrence. The hernias had been present since the age of 13. As the hernias enlarged and became more troublesome, the patient began wearing a truss. At the age of 55, the patient developed congestive heart failure, which responded to therapy; however, the hernias again became troublesome. The patient wished to have the hernias repaired under local anesthesia. We felt that epinephrine should not be used with this patient and injected 1 percent Nesacaine as described by Ponka (1963).

The skin was properly prepared with iodine and alcohol, and anesthesia was achieved; then the previous cicatrix on the left side was excised. The bleeding points were individually ligated with fine silk sutures after the vessels were grasped by fine-pointed hemostats. Sharp scalpel dissection was used throughout. The aponeurosis of the external oblique was identified, and it was observed that the last repair had been a Bassini repair. The external oblique was incised in the region of the superior crus, and the upper and lower leaves of the external oblique aponeurosis were dissected free utilizing sharp dissection. The spermatic cord was found to be markedly thickened; it was freed from the inguinal floor, and a cord tape was applied for ease of identification. The hypertrophied cremaster muscle was present and excised between clamps, and the stumps ligated. The peritoneum was identified at the internal abdominal ring and opened on its superior aspect. Examination revealed a complete congenital scrotal hernia in which the sigmoid colon constituted the posterior wall. The peritoneal sac was dissected free of the cord; a Hoguet maneuver was performed, reducing the lemon-sized direct hernia. Then the peritoneum was incised medially and laterally to the sliding component (see Fig. 22–18, p. 000). The medial and lateral peritoneal leaflets were approximated, and the peritoneal sac was closed with a purse-string suture of number 2–0 silk.

The transversalis fascia–transversus abdominis aponeurosis layer was identified, triangulated, and closed with figure-of-eight sutures of number 3–0 silk. A generous relaxing incision was made in the anterior sheath of the rectus abdominis. The redundant, attenuated transversalis fascia was imbricated. Cooper's ligament was clearly identified, and sutures of number 2–0 silk were placed between the transversus arch and Cooper's ligament. As the femoral vein was approached, a suture was placed between the transversus arch, the femoral sheath, and the iliopubic tract. The patient was asked to cough vigorously, and it was seen that a strong repair had been achieved. The aponeurosis of the external oblique was imbricated beneath the cord, and the wound was closed with interrupted sutures of number 3–0 nylon.

The skin was prepared for repair of the right side, and new sets of drapes and instruments were utilized. Local anesthesia was used without incident. Sharp dissection was again utilized: the aponeurosis of the external oblique was opened, and the spermatic cord was isolated. Here a smaller indirect sac was identified, but a rather large direct hernia was also present. A Hoguet maneuver was performed, with the result that a large peritoneal sac was produced. High ligation was achieved with a purse-string suture of heavy silk. The transversus abdominis lamina was identified and closed with heavy silk sutures. A large relaxing incision was again performed. The attenuated transversalis fascia was imbricated. A McVay repair was performed much as described for the left-sided hernia. The aponeurosis of the external oblique was imbricated beneath the cord. The wound was closed with three interrupted sutures of number 3–0 nylon.

The causes for recurrence of these hernias are numerous. The patient had two bilateral repairs in early childhood with prompt recurrence. The failure to excise the cremaster, to achieve high ligation of the peritoneal sac, to deal properly with a sliding hernia, to repair the floor of Hesselbach's triangle, and to use a relaxing incision all contributed to the recurrences.

Utilization of the McVay repair, with special attention to separate closure of the transversus abdominis, contributed to a satisfactory postoperative result with which the patient was still happy seven years after repair.

## DIRECT-INDIRECT-FEMORAL HERNIAS—CLINICAL STUDY

In the past, the matter of multilocular hernias received very little attention. The reason became apparent to me when I tried to retrieve records of patients with combinations of groin defects. Most records were indexed under the designation of indirect, direct, or femoral hernias. It was extremely difficult to identify records of patients with simultaneous direct, indirect, and femoral defects (Fig. 17–2). Nevertheless, I was able to collect records of 93 patients seen during the years from 1960 to 1968 who had multilocular hernias.

Regrettably, the follow-up study of patients in this series was of comparatively short duration. Only 67 percent, or 63 patients, were followed from 3 to 15 years. In spite of such limitations, however, I felt that the study of such combined hernias was helpful in gaining a better appreciation of the total hernia problem.

It is noteworthy that seven (7.5 percent) of the patients expired of causes unrelated to their operations. Five succumbed to arteriosclerotic heart disease, and two died of malignancies.

### Sex Incidence

Combined types of direct-indirect and femoral hernias are uncommon in females. This observation again supports the fact that the abdominal wall in females is better able to withstand the pressures to which it is exposed. Only 7.5 percent of multilocular hernias occurred in females

Table 17–1.  AGE INCIDENCE:
93 PATIENTS WITH COMBINED
DIRECT-INDIRECT AND
FEMORAL HERNIAS

| Age | Number of Patients | Percent |
|---|---|---|
| 1 to 10 years | 0 | 0 |
| 11 to 20 years | 0 | 0 |
| 21 to 30 years | 1 | 1.1 |
| 31 to 40 years | 6 | 6.5 |
| 41 to 50 years | 14 | 15.1 |
| 51 to 60 years | 27 | 29.0 |
| 61 to 70 years | 29 | 31.1 |
| 71 to 80 years | 14 | 15.1 |
| over 80 years | 2 | 2.2 |
| Total | 93 | 100.00 |

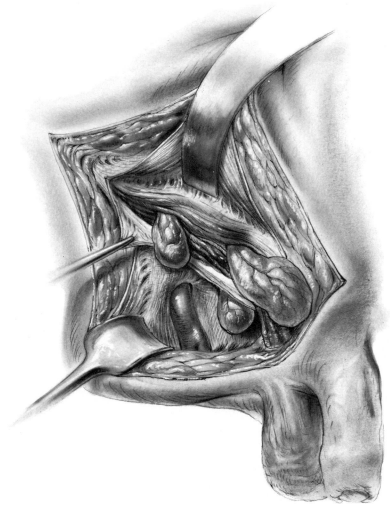

**Figure 17–2.**   A recurrent hernia with direct, indirect, and femoral hernial components. Such hernias are best repaired by the Lotheissen-McVay technique (see Fig. 14–8, p. 230).

(or, conversely, 92.5 percent occurred in males).

### Age Incidence

The age incidence of combined direct-indirect and femoral hernias is most interesting (Table 17–1). Seventy-seven percent of patients with multilocular inguinal hernias were in the fifth decade of life or older. Such evidence suggests that changes in tissues occurring with advancing years have something to do with the protrusions at numerous sites. Not one multilocular hernia occurred in patients in the first two decades of life, and only one was seen in a patient in the third decade of life.

## Types of Multilocular Hernias Seen

Before initiating this study, I had some idea that combined direct-indirect, or pantaloon, hernias were the most common of the multilocular hernias. This study provides some information as to the relative frequency of the various types (Table 17–2).

Table 17–2 clearly emphasizes the need for proper preoperative and intraoperative evaluation of every patient with groin hernias. Although the direct-indirect variety of multilocular herniation constituted 75 percent of the cases operated upon, other combinations occur with sufficient frequency to warrant concern on part of the surgeon.

Another significant observation in this study is that when a multilocular hernia is present on one side, there is great likelihood that a hernia of some type is present on the contralateral side. Slightly over 40 percent of the patients had either bilateral simultaneous hernias or bilateral separate hernias repaired. The exact type of hernia on the opposite side was difficult to determine, since many of the repair operations were performed elsewhere.

## Anesthesia

It was not surprising that local anesthesia was preferred for most of the older patients in this series. Local anesthesia was used for 72, or 77 percent, of the patients operated on; spinal anesthesia was used in 14, or 15 percent, of the patients; general anesthesia was used for just 3 patients; and one individual required that the local anesthesia be supplemented with general anesthesia.

One patient, age 73 years, had a repair attempt of an inguinal hernia performed elsewhere under general anesthesia. The operation was discontinued because he developed a cardiac arrest. He was later operated on under local anesthesia with success.

## Type of Repair

Several different approaches were used to correct the various combinations of direct, indirect and femoral hernias. The surgeons selected those procedures which they felt would correct the defects, as they

### Table 17–2. TYPES OF MULTILOCULAR INGUINAL HERNIAS REPAIRED IN 93 PATIENTS

| Type of Hernia | Number of Operations | Percent |
|---|---|---|
| Direct-Indirect | 79 | 75.2 |
| Direct-Femoral | 11 | 10.5 |
| Indirect-Femoral | 8 | 7.6 |
| Direct-Indirect-Femoral | 7 | 6.7 |
| Total | 105° | |

°Note: Twelve patients had bilateral combinations; hence, there are more operations than patients.

were encountered in individual patient (Table 17–3).

### The Halsted Repair

The Halsted repair was selected for the repair of almost half of the combined hernias. The peritoneal sac was invariably identified at the internal adbominal ring, and a Hoguet maneuver performed. In this procedure, the transversus abdominis lamina is separately closed at the internal ring following triangulation (see Fig. 13–4, p. 205).

The relaxing incision is considered to be of great importance in the repair of hernias with combined defects. The anterior sheath of the rectus was incised in 72 of 105 operations, or nearly 70 percent.

The attenuated transversalis fascia may be excised or imbricated over this bulge in the floor of Hesselbach's triangle. At this point, the transversus arch is sutured to the iliopubic tract and inguinal ligament with interrupted sutures of number 2–0 nonabsorbable material. The medial-most suture in the repair is the master stitch (see Fig. 14–7, p. 229). In the Halsted repair, the spermatic cord was placed in the subcutaneous position.

### The McVay Repair

It is interesting that the frequency with which the McVay repair is used varies with the type of hernia. For example, this technique is not popular in repair of indirect inguinal hernias. In such cases, the McVay repair was used in one percent of operations (see Chapter 11). The technique was considered more desirable as a method of repairing direct inguinal hernias, and it was used in 7 percent of direct inguinal hernias (see Chapter 13).

In hernias with combined loculations, the McVay repair was employed in 25, or nearly 24 percent, of the operations.

### Table 17–3. TYPE OF HERNIA REPAIR: 105 MULTILOCULAR HERNIAS

| Type of Repair | Number of Operations | Percent |
|---|---|---|
| Halsted | 50 | 47.6 |
| McVay | 25 | 23.8 |
| Bassini | 23 | 21.9 |
| Moschcowitz | 7 | 6.7 |

In the McVay repair the peritoneal sac is identified at the internal abdominal ring, and thorough exploration of the inguinal floor and femoral ring performed. Again, the Hoguet maneuver is used to convert the direct or femoral peritoneal sac into an indirect sac. The sac is closed with a purse-string suture of heavy silk. The transversus abdominis layer is closed with the technique noted for the Halsted repair. The attenuated transversalis fascia may be excised or imbricated. The important detail here is that it is the strong transversus abdominis arch that must be used in the actual repair. Cooper's ligament must be visualized from the pubic tubercle to the femoral vein laterally. Interrupted sutures are placed between the transversus arch and Cooper's ligament. These are not ligated until all sutures are placed under direct vision. They are tied in order, beginning with the medial-most suture. The suture material should be number 2–0 nonabsorbable material or comparable wire sutures. Once all the sutures have been placed, the need for a relaxing incision becomes evident; and it is used with great regularity. In my opinion, it should only be omitted in the exceptional case.

In the McVay repair, particular attention must be paid to the lateral extent of the repair, or that nearest the internal abdominal ring. The transition suture is placed between the transversus arch, Cooper's ligament, and the femoral sheath.

Although the Halsted repair is effective as a method of repair of direct and indirect inguinal hernias, it is not designed to repair the femoral defect. The McVay repair, properly performed, will remedy direct, indirect, and femoral hernias as well.

### The Bassini Repair

The Bassini repair was utilized as the method of repair in 23, or 22 percent, of 105 patients with combined types of hernias. The method was performed as illustrated in Chapter 11. It is applicable to patients with combined indirect and direct inguinal hernias.

### The Moschcowitz Repair

The Moschcowitz repair was utilized to obliterate the femoral ring in the presence of a femoral hernia. In the group of cases included in this study, an additional direct or indirect inguinal hernia was present along with the femoral hernia. Hence, the Moschcowitz repair was accompanied by a Bassini or Halsted repair in order to repair the internal abdominal ring and the floor of Hesselbach's triangle. The Moschcowitz repair was utilized in 7, or 6.7 percent, of 105 patients with multilocular hernias.

The McVay repair was used quite frequently as shown in Table 17–3. Obviously, such a repair has the capability of correcting the direct, indirect, and femoral defects as well. The Bassini and Halsted types of repair are applicable to direct and indirect combinations only. The Moschcowitz repair alone can eliminate the femoral defect, but some additional procedure is necessary to repair the defect in the floor of the inguinal canal. Furthermore, indirect hernias can only be prevented if the internal ring is closed snugly.

In the repair of four hernias with multiple defects, the surgeons utilized Marlex mesh, suturing it to Cooper's ligament below and the aponeurosis of the internal oblique above (see Chapter 26).

### Technical Details of Operative Procedures

In the repair of 105 direct–indirect inguinal hernias, a number of technical details, which facilitated or augmented the repairs, were carried out. These details of repair have been described in Chapters 11, 12, and 13; hence, it will be unnecessary to review them here. Nevertheless, it is useful to summarize the important technical maneuvers. The frequency of their use is shown in Table 17–4. The Hoguet maneuver was used consistently to convert the direct (and, in some cases, the femoral) hernial sac into an indirect sac. High ligation of the sac is considered to be important (Fig. 17–3). Excision of the cremaster was a fairly routine procedure during repair of hernias with combined loculations. The master stitch was also considered important as indicated by its use in nearly 70 percent of the repairs. The need to minimize tension at the suture line was recognized by the surgeons; a relaxing incision was used in approximately 70 percent of the repairs. As can be seen in Table 17–4, other adjunctive procedures were infrequently utilized.

Table 17–4. **TECHNICAL DETAILS EMPLOYED IN REPAIR OF 105 COMBINED HERNIA DEFECTS**

| Technical Detail | Number of Times Used | Percent |
|---|---|---|
| Hoguet Maneuver | 91 | 86.7 |
| Excision Cremaster | 75 | 71.4 |
| Master Stitch | 73 | 69.5 |
| Relaxing Incision | 72 | 68.6 |
| Excision Lipoma of Cord | 8 | 7.6 |
| Repair Sliding Hernia | 6 | 5.7 |
|   Sigmoid  4 | | |
|   Bladder  2 | | |
| Hydrocelectomy | 2 | 1.9 |
| Use of Prosthesis | 4 | 3.8 |
| Orchidectomy | 1 | 0.9 |

Sliding hernias were identified in 5.7 percent of the operations. The surgeon cannot afford to overlook the possibility of a sliding component in the repair of any hernia in the adult, especially in those of advanced years.

Most combined hernias can be repaired successfully without prosthetic materials.

Prosthetics were employed in only 3.8 percent of 105 operations.

## Complications

The types of complications seen are similar to those encountered with other groin hernias. These will be summarized in Table 17–5. There were no major wound infections, but two minor superficial infections required treatment.

Two patients suffered postoperative atrophy of their testicles. Another patient had an atrophic testicle secondary to mumps many years prior to repair of the hernia. The remaining complications are self-explanatory and will be discussed in detail in Chapter 28 on postoperative complications.

## Recurrences

There were 5 recurrences in 105 operations, for a recurrence rate of 4.8 percent.

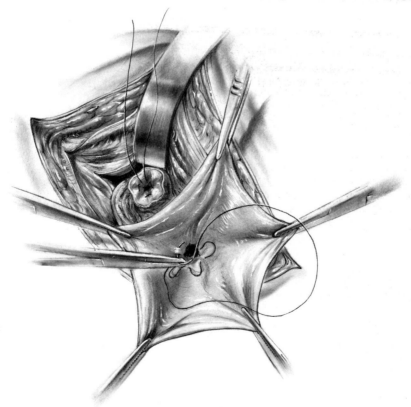

**Figure 17–3.** The Hoguet maneuver is useful in reducing multilocular hernial sacs. In this case, however, the direct and femoral peritoneal sacs were reduced through an opening of the direct peritoneal sac.

**Table 17–5. POSTOPERATIVE COMPLICATIONS IN 93 PATIENTS WITH COMBINED DIRECT, INDIRECT AND FEMORAL HERNIAS**

| Wound Complications | | 7 |
|---|---|---|
| *Early* | | |
| Seroma | 2 | |
| Hematoma | 2 | |
| Superficial wound infection | 2 | |
| Ecchymosis | 1 | 4 |
| *Late* | | |
| Pain | 2 | |
| Numbness | 2 | 10 |
| Testicular | | |
| Scrotal swelling and edema, ecchymosis, induration | 6 | |
| High-riding testicle | 1 | |
| Painful testicle | 1 | |
| Atrophic testicle | 2 | 10 |
| Urinary Tract | | |
| Urinary retention | 8 | |
| Urinary tract infection | 2 | 2 |
| Anesthetic | | |
| Post-spinal headache | 1 | |
| Hypotensive episode | 1 | |

This is a significant incidence of postoperative recurrences, indicating a need for improvement.

In two of the five patients, the recurrences were immediate. The reason for failure was obvious in one case. The patient had a direct and femoral hernia, both being recognized. Then, in the operative note, the surgeon described placement of two sutures between the transversus abdominis arch and Cooper's ligament. The repair was obviously not carried far enough laterally to exclude the femoral ring, and a femoral recurrence was the result. In the second case, prompt recurrence followed a bilateral simultaneous repair that had been performed for direct-indirect hernias; no relaxing incision had been made. The recurrence was of the direct type. The adverse effect of tension on the suture line was a factor in the reappearance of the direct hernia.

The third patient underwent bilateral Bassini repairs for direct–indirect inguinal hernias. A direct inguinal hernia recurred two years later and was successfully repaired by utilization of the McVay technique with a relaxing incision. Excessive tension was probably a factor in this recurrence.

The fourth recurrence was of the femoral type in a patient who had undergone repair of a direct and femoral hernia two years earlier. Utilization of the Moschcowitz repair for the femoral component was probably due to an error in surgical judgment. A McVay repair was later successful.

The fifth patient is of special interest. Marlex mesh was sutured over the femoral ring during the repair of a direct and femoral hernia. This repair failed, and the direct hernia recurred. In this case, a larger portion of mesh should have been used; attachment to Cooper's ligament and to the aponeurosis of the internal oblique would have resulted in a strong repair.

## RECURRENT DIRECT-INDIRECT AND FEMORAL HERNIAS

Combinations of groin hernias recur far more frequently than most surgeons recognize. Femoral hernias, whether virginal or recurrent, attract more attention than is directed at various combinations of recurrent inguinal and femoral hernias.

Dodd (1970) presented a case report in which a patient had a recurrent hernia with three inguinal sacs: one was indirect; the second was direct; and the third protruded through the transversalis aponeurosis near the pubic tubercle. He found that in the repair of inguinal hernias since 1962, only 4 of 122 repairs in his practice had three sacs, for an incidence of 3.3 percent. In these cases, the sacs were direct-indirect and femoral. Dodd noted that the incidence of multilocular hernias is rarely mentioned in the literature. He pointed out the need for thorough intraoperative exploration to avoid overlooking an occult hernia.

In an attempt to investigate those hernias which occurred in various combinations, I isolated records of 70 patients who had recurrent hernias with two or three types of combined simultaneous defects. These patients had been seen at Henry Ford Hospital during the years 1960 through 1968.

### Sex Incidence

The sex incidence of simultaneous combined hernias was found to be consistent with the general observation made in previous chapters; that is, groin hernias occur far more frequently in males than in fe-

**Table 17–6. AGE INCIDENCE IN 70 PATIENTS WITH RECURRENT DIRECT-INDIRECT-FEMORAL HERNIAS**

| Age | Number of Patients |
|---|---|
| 0 to 10 years | 1 (age 4 years) |
| 11 to 20 years | 0 |
| 21 to 30 years | 1 |
| 31 to 40 years | 1 |
| 41 to 50 years | 11 |
| 51 to 60 years | 17 |
| 61 to 70 years | 24 |
| 71 to 80 years | 14 |
| 81 years and older | 1 |
| Total | 70 |

**Table 17–7. TYPES OF RECURRENCES IN 70 PATIENTS WITH MULTILOCULAR HERNIAS**

| Type of Recurrence | Number of Patients | Percent |
|---|---|---|
| Direct-Indirect | 46 | 59.0 |
| Direct-Femoral | 13 | 16.7 |
| Indirect-Femoral | 8 | 10.2 |
| Inguinofemoral | 6 | 7.7 |
| Direct-Indirect-Femoral | 5 | 6.4 |
| Total | 78 | 100.0 |

males. Nearly 93 percent of recurrent direct-indirect and femoral hernias occurred in males.

### Age Incidence

Patients with recurrent direct-indirect and femoral hernias have a similar age distribution to those with primary multilocular hernias (Table 17–6). This group of patients tends to be older than individuals who have indirect inguinal hernias alone. The differences in ages of patients can be appreciated by comparing Table 17–6 with Table 11–1 on page 169.

One unusual patient, a 4-year-old infant, had a recurrent direct–indirect inguinal hernia following earlier repair of an indirect inguinal hernia. In my opinion, this reflects the meddlesome nature of those surgeons who insist on repairing the inguinal floor, even in children.

### Types of Recurrent Multilocular Hernias

It is interesting to consider the various anatomic forms of recurrent multilocular hernias (Table 17–7). The appearance of a variety of hernia that is referred to as the inguinofemoral type of recurrence in Table 17–7 is of fundamental significance. This variety is definitely iatrogenic in origin. A hernia of this variety is only seen after an earlier attempt at repair of a groin hernia. It emphasizes the destructive nature of certain techniques of repair. The protrusion in a recurrent inguinofemoral hernia is one that presents simultaneously as both a direct and a femoral hernia. In this hernia, the inguinal ligament has been destroyed as a result of either surgical

misadventure or excessive tension placed upon it through faulty suture technique. The insistence on suturing the internal oblique and rectus sheath to the inguinal ligament or to Cooper's ligament under excessive tension ends in failure more often than we fully appreciate.

If Table 17–2, page 281, is compared with Table 17–7, page 285, it can be seen that other virginal types of combined hernias compare favorably with the various kinds of recurrent multilocular hernias.

### Number of Previous Repairs

Patients with recurrent combined direct-indirect and femoral hernias too often require a number of repairs before success is attained (Table 17–8). It can be seen in Table 17–8 that 19 patients required a third repair, while 7 individuals required a fourth operative procedure. In all, 70 patients required a total of 193 operative attempts at repair before the defects were largely eliminated. The need for careful attention to surgical details is evident

**Table 17–8. NUMBER OF REPAIRS AMONG 70 PATIENTS WITH RECURRENT COMBINED DIRECT-INDIRECT AND FEMORAL HERNIAS**

| Number of Repairs | Number of Patients |
|---|---|
| 1 | 41 |
| 2 | 19 |
| 3 | 7 |
| 4 | 1 |
| 5 | 1 |
| 6 | 1 |
| Total | 70 |

when it is realized that most patients with multilocular hernias will require at least two attempts at repair, and many will require a third operation.

As a result of numerous operative procedures, the testicle became atrophic in five individuals.

## Factors Leading to Recurrence of Multilocular Hernias

*The most direct effect in the prevention of recurrences which the surgeon can exert, however, is in the conduct of the operation.*

Postlethwait, 1964

I must accept the criticism that the preceding study of causative factors in genesis of recurrent hernias has the limitation inherent in retrospective analysis. Nevertheless, attempts at determining causes for recurrent hernias are infrequently made and seldom recorded. I reviewed the individual clinical records of 70 patients and scrutinized the operative notes for any useful information they might yield.

In individual cases, numerous factors contributed to recurrence. For example, an individual patient might present with a sliding hernia and an enlarged internal abdominal ring. In addition, the floor of the inguinal canal might have been weakened by the placement of sutures high into the internal oblique, resulting in excessive tension at the repair site.

Excessive tension may result when the rectus sheath is approximated to either inguinal or Cooper's ligaments. Omission of a relaxing incision aggravates the situation, and further tension is added by performing bilateral repairs, either separately or simultaneously.

In spite of the limitations of incomplete records, I feel that this attempt at identifying causes for recurrence of groin hernias will prove useful (Table 17–9).

The striking incidence of bilaterality in 70 patients with multilocular hernia commands attention. Thirty patients had initial bilateral simultaneous repairs and, in addition, 19 had bilateral separate repairs. Thus, 49 of 70 patients, or 70 percent, had bilateral repairs of groin hernias. It is becoming clear that the undesirable effect of bilateral repairs is the creation of excessive tension at the suture line. Any method

**Table 17–9. FACTORS CONTRIBUTING TO RECURRENCE OF MULTILOCULAR HERNIAS IN 70 PATIENTS**

| | |
|---|---|
| *Undue Tension at the Suture Line* | 53 |
| Sutures placed high on the internal oblique. | |
| Sutures placed into the rectus sheath. | |
| Failure to use the relaxation incision. | |
| Bilateral simultaneous repairs. | |
| Bilateral separate repairs. | |
| *Poor Technical Execution* | 38 |
| Failure to close the internal ring adequately. | |
| Failure to achieve high ligation of the sac. | |
| Failure to excise the cremaster muscle. | |
| Failure to excise lipomas of the cord. | |
| Failure to manage sliding component properly. | |
| Failure to occlude the femoral ring. | |
| Failure to use the master stitch. | |
| *Failure to Provide Needed Strength in Repairs* | 18 |
| Failure to repair floor of inguinal canal. | |
| Meddlesome attempt to repair the floor of the inguinal canal. | |
| Failure to use a synthetic mesh. | |
| Destructive effect of inguinal ligament repairs. | |
| *Overlooked Hernia* | 3 |
| *Hematoma and Infection* | 1 |
| *Attenuated Tissues* | 4 |
| *Miscellaneous* (Obesity, severe cough, emphysema, and bronchitis) | 15 |

to be employed in correction of such defects must minimize the forces of distraction (Fig. 14–2). The failure to provide needed strength in initial repairs of multilocular hernias becomes apparent when it is appreciated that mesh was utilized in nearly 30 percent of the second and third repairs with success.

Such factors as hematomas, infection, and attenuated tissues do not enter into the genesis of recurrent multilocular hernias in a significant number of instances.

I am forced to conclude that excessive tension at the line of suture, poor technical execution of the selected procedure, and failure to provide needed strength in the repair account for most of the failures in repair of multilocular hernias. More frequent use of synthetic mesh is desirable in repair of bilateral multilocular hernias.

## Operative Treatment of Recurrent Direct-Indirect-Femoral Hernias

Operative repair under local anesthesia was performed in 50 patients, or in slightly over 71 percent. Spinal anesthesia was preferred for 13 patients, or in slightly under 20 percent of the repairs.

Subtle changes in operative approach

Table 17–10. TYPE OF REPAIR: 78
RECURRENT MULTILOCULAR HERNIAS*

| Type of Repair | Number of Operations | Percent |
|---|---|---|
| Halsted (5 with mesh) | 43 | 55.1 |
| McVay (14 with mesh) | 25 | 32.1 |
| Bassini (2 with mesh) | 4 | 5.1 |
| Moschcowitz (4 with mesh) | 6 | 7.7 |
| Total | 78 | 100.0 |

*Prosthetic implant was used in 25 or 32.1 percent of the repairs.

Table 17–11. TECHNICAL DETAILS
EMPLOYED IN REPAIR OF 78
RECURRENT DIRECT-INDIRECT-
FEMORAL HERNIAS

| Technical Detail | Number of Times Used | Percent |
|---|---|---|
| Hoguet Maneuver | 53 | 67.9 |
| Excision Cremaster | 27 | 34.6 |
| Master Stitch | 62 | 79.5 |
| Relaxing Incision | 38 | 48.7 |
| Excision Lipoma of Cord | 10 | 12.8 |
| Repair Sliding Hernia | 13 | 16.6 |
| Sigmoid  8 | | |
| Cecum  2 | | |
| Bladder  3 | | |
| Use of Prosthetics | 25 | 32.0 |

are seen in techniques selected for repair of recurrent multilocular hernias (Table 17–10).

Two obvious departures from our customary approach to repair of groin hernias are noted in Table 17–10. First, there is a slight increase in use of the Lotheissen-McVay repair. Second, prosthetics were used in 32 percent of repair of recurrent multilocular hernias. Both of these modifications in surgical repair indicate recognition of the undesirable effect of conventional repairs—i.e., excessive tension on the line of repair. Furthermore, the limited usefulness of the inguinal ligament in repair of complicated multilocular hernias is being recognized more clearly in current practice.

Currently, Marlex mesh is the material which I prefer for implantation; it is utilized in nearly every patient in whom it appears that some implanted material is desirable to strengthen the repair without increasing tension at the suture line.

### Technical Details of Operative Procedures

A number of important technical details must be carried out if repair of recurrent multilocular groin hernias is to be successful. These details have been amply described and illustrated in Chapters 10 through Chapter 16 (Table 17–11).

In over one-third of the repairs, hypertrophied cremaster interfered with proper closure of the internal ring. Lipomas also interfered with snug closure of the internal abdominal ring. Furthermore, sliding com-

ponents (consisting of sigmoid, cecum, and bladder) required attention before repair of the internal ring could be achieved. Thus, in nearly one-third of the procedures, it was necessary to deal with sliding components of various types.

The master stitch was utilized in nearly 80 percent of the repairs in order to provide strength at the medial angle of the repair. This detail is important to prevent recurrence at the medial-most portion of the repair.

Because of the use of synthetic mesh implants in over 30 percent of repairs of multilocular hernias, the relaxing incision was used less frequently than is our custom. The mesh is implanted in such a manner as to absorb some of the tension at the repair site.

### Complications

The number of complications in this series of 78 repairs appears to be inordinately high. Yet when one considers that 70 patients had undergone a total of 193 operative procedures, the reasons for these complications become apparent (Table 17–12).

The danger to the testicular blood supply increases with the number of repairs; in this series, our repairs accounted for postoperative atrophy in three individuals. Each individual had repeated procedures prior to the last repair. Also, it can be recalled that six patients already had testicular atrophy when they appeared for yet another repair.

The other complications in Table 17–12

**Table 17–12. COMPLICATIONS FOLLOWING REPAIR OF 78 RECURRENT MULTILOCULAR HERNIAS**

| | | |
|---|---|---|
| *Wound Complications* | | 9 |
| Hematomas | 3 | |
| Seromas | 2 | |
| Infection | 1 | |
| Ecchymosis | 3 | |
| *Scrotal and Testicular Complications* | | 8 |
| Testicular atrophy | 3 | |
| Testicular swelling | 2 | |
| Testicular pain | 1 | |
| Scrotal swelling | 2 | |
| *Urinary Tract Complications* | | 3 |
| Urinary retention | 2 | |
| Urinary tract infection | 1 | |
| *Pulmonary Complications* | | 3 |
| Atelectasis | 2 | |
| Pneumonitis | 1 | |
| *Phlebothrombosis* | | 2 |

will be considered in Chapter 28 on post-operative complications.

## Recurrences

I can report only two recurrences in 78 repairs of recurrent multilocular hernia for a recurrence rate of 2.6 percent. Only 58 percent of the patients were followed longer than three years. The reason for this favorable recurrence rate is elusive, but I suspect that the use of synthetic mesh to repair the defects contributes to the good results in these complicated cases. In addition, a senior surgeon usually plays an active role in repair of unusual hernias.

## SUMMARY

Combined hernias with indirect, direct, and femoral components can be repaired successfully, provided that the significance of each defect is recognized and that the appropriate technical procedure is utilized in repair. In this study, the recurrence rate of 4.8 percent is probably too low; however, it clearly establishes the fact that hernias with combined loculations recur with greater frequency than do indirect inguinal hernias (with a recurrence rate of 0.91 percent).

When combinations of groin hernias were being repaired, it was found that the indirect component was repaired with uniform success and that recurrences appeared as direct and femoral hernias.

Armed with such knowledge, the surgeon should pay particular attention to the floor of Hesselbach's triangle and to the femoral ring. With greater utilization of the McVay repair for correction of direct and femoral defects, better results can be anticipated.

Recurrent multilocular hernias are more frequent than is generally recognized. Besides the frequent association of bilateral simultaneous repairs, the improper use of the inguinal ligament as an anchoring structure predisposes to such recurrences.

In selected cases, the use of a prosthetic implant will strengthen the area while minimizing tension.

## REFERENCES

Dodd, H.: Inguinal herniae in older patients: Why do they recur? Br. J. Clin. Prac. 22:5, 1968.
Dodd, H.: Recurrent inguinal hernia with three sacs. Br. Med. J. 1:173, 1970.
Glassow, F.: Short-stay surgery (Shouldice technique) for repair of inguinal hernia. Ann. R. Coll. Surg. Engl. 58:133, 1976.
Grace, R. V., and Johnson, V. S.: Results of herniotomy in patients more than 50 years of age. Ann. Surg. 106:347, 1937.
Hoguet, J. P.: Direct inguinal hernia. Ann. Surg. 72:671, 1920.
Lichenstein, I. L.: *Hernia Repair Without Disability.* St. Louis, C. V. Mosby Co., 1970.
Ljungdahl, I.: Inguinal and femoral hernia. An investigation of 502 own operated cases. Acta Chir. Scand. (Supplement) 439:1–81, 1973.
Palumbo, L. T., and Sharpe, W. S.: Primary inguinal hernioplasty in the adult. Surg. Clin. North Am. 51:1293, 1971.
Ponka, J. L.: Seven steps to local anesthesia for repair of inguino-femoral hernia. Surg. Gynecol. Obstet. 117:115, 1963.
Postlethwait, R. W.: Recurrent inguinal hernia. Am. J. Surg. 107:739, 1964.
Rowe, J. S., and Skandalakis, J. E.: Multiple bilateral inguinal hernias. Am. Surg. 39:269, 1973.
Watson, L. F.: *Hernia* (3rd ed.). St. Louis, C. V. Mosby Co., 1948.
Zimmerman, L. M., and Anson, B. J.: *Anatomy and Surgery of Hernia* (2nd ed.). Baltimore, Williams & Wilkins Co., 1967, p. 20.

## Supplemental Readings

Cowell, E.: Recurrent inguinal hernia. Br. Med. J. 2:330, 1946.
Fallis, L. S.: Direct inguinal hernia. Ann. Surg. 107: 572, 1938.
Qvist, G.: Saddlebag hernia. Br. J. Surg. 64:442, 444, 1977.
Rains, A. J. H., and Ritchie, H. D. (eds.): *Bailey and Loves Short Practice of Surgery* (16th ed.). London, Lewis, p. 1070.
Skinner, H. L., and Duncan, R. D.: Recurrent inguinal hernia. Ann. Surg. 122:68(Supplemental), 1945.

# 18

# Sliding Inguinal and Femoral Hernias

## DEFINITION

A completely satisfactory definition of a sliding hernia is not as simple a matter as it might seem. A generally acceptable definition for a sliding hernia is that it is one in which a viscus constitutes a portion of the hernial sac wall, such as in sliding hernias of the cecum and sigmoid colon. This definition, however, is inapplicable when we discuss the extrasaccular or extraperitoneal variety of hernia in which the viscus is actually outside the peritoneal sac but does pass through the internal abdominal ring. On other occasions, the viscus (e.g., a portion of the bladder) may appear in a sac in the retroperitoneal position as, for instance, in a large direct hernia.

It is important to remember that the mere presence of some abdominal organ in a hernial sac does not necessarily indicate a sliding hernia. Adhesions between the intestine or omentum and the peritoneal sac also do not meet the requirements of such a hernia.

A sliding hernia is one in which an abdominal viscus, with its peritoneal and retroperitoneal attachments, has abandoned its normal anatomic position in the peritoneal cavity and has found its way through one of the potential orifices of the abdominal cavity. In this new, abnormal location, the viscus may be intraperitoneal or extraperitoneal. It often constitutes a portion of the hernial sac wall when it remains completely or partially in continuity with the peritoneal cavity. Some-times the abdominal organ remains completely in its extraperitoneal position as, for instance, in a sliding hernia of the bladder.

## HISTORICAL CONSIDERATIONS

Knowledge of the sliding type of hernia has been gained slowly indeed. Publications dealing with hernia in general are abundant, but those specifically considering sliding hernias are comparatively few in number. Articles dealing with the subject have appeared sporadically. As recently as 1942, Burton stated, "The most serious, the rarest, and the most difficult herniae to repair are the sliding herniae of the large bowel."

The following notes of historical interest have largely been selected from the work of Treves (1887), Carnett (1909), Walton (1913), Burton (1942), and Williams (1947). The chapter on sliding hernias, by Moretz, in Nyhus' and Harkins' book, *Hernia*, has also been drawn upon. An excellent review of the subject of inguinal hernias in children, written by Snyder and Greaney, can be found in *Pediatric Surgery*, by Benson and associates.

Galen apparently recognized the sliding hernia as early as the second century A.D. Burton acknowledges Rousselus in 1559, Geiger in 1631, and Spigelius in 1645 as early contributors to the knowledge of sliding hernias.

Treves discussed the problem at length,

in "Hernia of the cecum." In this article, he stated that the cecum had been found in the umbilical, inguinal, and femoral regions. He referred to a case, recorded by Arnaud in 1732, in which the hernia had been present for 20 years; it had a circumference of 27 inches and extended to midthigh. The hernial sac contained ileum, cecum, and colon. Surgical intervention became necessary because of obstructive symptoms. At operation, gangrenous areas were found in the intestine. Treves quoted Arnaud as saying: "I employed one hour and a quarter in dividing the adhesions and bridles which connected the colon to the hernial sac." Uncertain as to the best method of management, he finally decided upon resection of the ileocolic segment. The patient made a good recovery but was left with a permanent fecal fistula. There is some danger in speculation, but in my judgment, Arnaud had encountered a complicated sliding inguinal hernia.

Percival Pott in 1783 described the sliding hernia in his treatise on the subject. In 1809 Scarpa stated that as the sliding hernia, consisting of the colon, cecum, and appendix, descended through the internal ring into the scrotum, the natural peritoneal attachments were drawn downward as well. Pelletan in 1810 and Cloquet in 1819 held similar views. Hesselbach in 1816 also recognized this special type of hernia.

Lawrence in 1838 presented what I consider to be the first detailed account of a sacless cecal sliding hernia. The cecum was inadvertently entered during the operative procedure, and fecal matter escaped. Thirty-six hours later, fecal discharges were seen in the wound. The patient died, and the postmortem examination confirmed Lawrence's observations. Treves challenged the concept of a sacless cecal hernia on an anatomic basis by pointing out that the cecum is normally covered with peritoneum.

Liston in 1838 and Sir Astley Cooper in 1839 made further observations on the nature of sliding hernia.

Banks in 1887 made a classic observation when he said, "I may here remark in passing that of all the forms of hernia with which I am acquainted, those in which what may be called a landslip of cecum takes place present the greatest obstacles to return of the bowel, and involve the greatest risk to the patient."

Morris in 1895 recognized sliding hernias of the sigmoid and cecum and was a pioneer in surgery for sliding hernia. His method of liberating the sliding component from the cord and returning the viscus to the peritoneal cavity was an important, original contribution. He incised the peritoneum on either side of the sliding viscus, thus permitting its return to the peritoneal cavity, and he reperitonealized the bowel with the peritoneal leaflets derived from the sac. Carnett stated that van Heuversyn, Morris, Gouilliard, Raffin, Tuffier, Weir, and Singley all fashioned peritoneal flaps in order to surround the gut entirely with peritoneum. Few, if any, surgeons today attempt reperitonealization of the bowel.

In my opinion, modern understanding of the various types of sliding hernias began with the work of Carnett. In a classic article in 1909, he classified cecal hernias as either simple or gliding. The gliding hernias were further subdivided into intrasaccular, extrasaccular (or parasaccular), and sacless. In the simple variety of hernia, the cecum lies free in the sac. In the gliding, or sliding, types of cecal hernia, there is some degree of attachment posteriorly. In the extrasaccular, or parasaccular, hernias, the cecum is not contained within the sac but lies on the posteroexternal surface. In the sacless variety, the cecum passes through the internal ring, free of a sac and minus its own serous covering. This type of sliding hernia must be extremely rare.

Hotchkiss described his method of managing large sliding hernias of the sigmoid in 1909. He freed the sac from the full extent of the cord and reconstructed the mesentery of the sigmoid.

Kirchner in 1911 reported his technique for repair of sliding hernias in which he invested the sliding portion of the bowel with peritoneal flaps derived from the hernial sac. He created medial and lateral leaflets of peritoneum by incising the peritoneum on each side of the viscus. This enabled him to reduce the viscus into the peritoneal cavity. Closure of the peritoneal ring was the next step, followed by secure closure of the internal ring. His method of repair was fundamentally sound, in my opinion.

In 1913 Walton of London, an assistant surgeon to the Dreadnaught Hospital, wrote on the subject of extrasaccular hernia. He studied the problem carefully and presented his technique for repair, which included reperitonealization of the cecum. His approach was unduly complicated; it is not popular today.

Walton developed a classification of hernias based on the one suggested by Carnett. It includes three subgroups: simple hernia, extrasaccular hernia, and sacless hernia. Reference was also made to Stoney's observation that in cases of sliding hernia, the iliac colon was more frequently the sliding component.

Prior to Walton's efforts, hernia of the bladder received very little attention. Albucasis in the twelfth century and Guy de Chauliac in 1363 referred to the problem of hernia of the bladder. Walton gave credit to Cloquet in 1819 and to Lockwood in 1889 for early descriptions of hernias in which the bladder was the sliding component. Eccles in 1902 was the first to describe three varieties of sliding hernia of the bladder. In certain large groin hernias, the bladder may be covered with peritoneum. At other times, the bladder forms only a portion of the sac wall, and it may be partially covered with peritoneum. The bladder rarely descends into the hernia entirely free of peritoneum. Eccles recognized that the bladder may find its way into a femoral hernial sac as well.

Erdmann in 1908 was of the opinion that the bladder more commonly prolapsed into femoral hernias than into the inguinal variety. The bladder will be found on the medial portion of the sac wall. The distended bladder may look deceptively like a hernial sac.

Watson in his book on hernia did much to clarify the problem of sliding hernia of the bladder. He fully appreciated the various possible anatomic locations in which the bladder, as a sliding component, could be found. His illustrations of the pathologic anatomy are excellent.

It is clear that by 1913 hernias of the right colon, cecum, appendix, sigmoid colon, and bladder were well recognized. Furthermore, it was understood that unless the surgeon was aware of the pathology at hand, the various viscera could be easily injured—with complications and increased morbidity, at best, or disaster and death to the patient if a technical error went unrecognized.

Commencing in 1919, La Roque was an enthusiastic advocate of the muscle-splitting incision above the internal ring for all inguinal hernias. He continued his interest in this technique and refined it further in 1924. Five years later, he applied the principle of the secondary muscle-splitting incision to sliding hernias. Watson, Moschcowitz, Graham, Williams, Brown, and Koontz were among the surgeons employing secondary incisions for the repair of sliding hernias.

In 1920 Criley described his experience with seven sliding hernias of the bowel and two involving the bladder. His article, like that of Treves, is significant in that he reviews and relates the genesis of sliding hernias to embryologic development.

Prior to the year 1923, I could find no specific reference to sliding hernias in children. David then described sliding hernias of the cecum and appendix in three young patients. He considered embryologic factors, such as the rotation of the cecum and ascending colon and the descent of the testicles, in the genesis of sliding hernias in children.

Moschcowitz in 1925 stated that the quality of the literature on sliding hernia was good, bad, or indifferent. He also alluded to the difficulty involved in making the proper diagnosis. In a given case, the surgeon may fail to think of the possibility of a sliding hernia, or the differential diagnostic features may be so elusive that the diagnosis cannot be established with absolute certainty. He referred to two well-known mistakes made by operating surgeons with considerable experience, as follows:

1. Designating a hernia to be sliding when it is merely a simple hernia in which a loop of intestine is adherent to the sac.
2. Hemorrhage caused by attempting to dissect the viscus (colon or bladder) from its blood supply.

He should have emphasized the third hazard, namely, accidental entry into the bowel or bladder.

Moschcowitz felt that two mechanisms

were responsible for the resultant sliding hernia: (1) a pulling mechanism, and (2) a pushing mechanism. He proposed that a McBurney type of counter-incision be made to facilitate repair and permit reversal of the mechanisms that allowed the hernia to occur in the first place.

In 1930 Bevan described his experiences with sliding hernias of the ascending colon and cecum, sigmoid colon, and bladder. His illustrations showing the blood supply to the colon in sliding hernias are excellent. He describes his method of repair; although rather complicated, it does not require an additional abdominal incision. His method of repair was effective because he replaced the sliding component deep to the transversalis fascia.

In 1935 Graham noted that there was a lack of unanimity of opinion as to the proper operative procedure that should be used in the repair of sliding hernias. He reviewed the genesis of sliding hernia, as cited in Moschcowitz's work. Graham recommended the use of a paramedian incision through which the sliding viscus could be returned to the peritoneal cavity and advised the classic Bassini repair for correcting the defect in the abdominal wall.

Mackid in 1936 also advised using a secondary rectus incision as an adjunct for repair of sliding hernias of the sigmoid. Strangely enough, he stated that he had never seen a sliding hernia on the right side that involved the cecum.

Zimmerman and Laufman presented their sound views in regard to the pathology and treatment of sliding hernias in 1942. They were of the opinion, which I share, that disposition of the sac and treatment of the hernia were unduly complicated. They point out that the sac, with its contained intestinal floor, is easily dissected from the cord in the same way as is commonly done for other hernias, with the dissection carried down through the abdominal ring. This permits return of the viscus into the abdominal cavity deep to the transversalis fascia. Closure of the transversalis fascia is absolutely necessary. Zimmerman and Laufman do not advocate opening the sac for direct hernias in which the sliding viscus is the bladder. Repair of the transversalis fascia and re-enforcement

of the inguinal floor, however, are necessary.

In a review of sliding hernias in 1942, Burton advocated the use of the Hoguet maneuver, in which the peritoneal sac is opened at the internal ring. Any direct redundant peritoneal sac is converted into an indirect sac. He credited Morris, van Heuversyn, and Gouilliard with employing similar techniques in the management of the hernial sac in sliding hernias. The sac was incised on either side of the viscus; next, the peritoneal leaflets were sutured posteriorly, thereby covering the bare area. The margins, or leaflets, of the peritoneum were then closed together with the pertioneal sac after the contents were returned to the peritoneal cavity. Finally, excess peritoneal sac was excised.

Williams in 1947 advocated the use of the La Roque approach for the repair of sliding inguinal hernias. The advantages cited by Williams include:

1. Dissection from above insures a better view of the blood supply to the colon; it is easier and safer.
2. Excess peritoneum is removed.
3. A new mesocolon is constructed.
4. Unusual conditions of the sac can be readily recognized and corrected.
5. The colon may be fixed to the abdominal wall.
6. The muscle-splitting incision above the internal ring gives better access to the sac than does the rectus incision.

Brown in 1943 advocated making a muscle-splitting incision above the internal ring in order to avoid injury to the nerve supply. His method is essentially that advocated by La Roque. In 1952 Koontz also recommended the La Roque approach for the repair of difficult sliding hernias of the large bowel.

Sensenig and Nichols in 1955 found it possible to repair sliding hernias without a concomitant abdominal incision. In 53 patients, followed up for at least 2 years, there were 4 definite recurrences.

In 1956 Ryan of Toronto presented a study containing detailed statistical analysis of 313 consecutive indirect sliding inguinal hernias. He concluded that an additional abdominal incision was never mandatory and that indirect sliding hernias could be repaired with a recurrence rate of less than one percent. He did not feel it was necessary to resect the hernial sac if it was freed from the cord and abdominal wall and placed deep to the transversalis fascia. This is a most important principle, which I strongly endorse.

Ryan observed the increased incidence of sliding hernias with age; most of these hernias were not of congenital origin. He emphasized the relationship of obesity to sliding hernias and noted that such hernias were often large and long-standing, with a lax abdominal ring. He observed that the sacless sliding hernia was rare. In his experience, early ambulation had a beneficial effect on the patient.

Ryan and his colleague, E. E. Shouldice, pointed out the need for early recognition of sliding hernias. They advised separation of the herniating mass from the transversalis fascia at the internal ring. According to Ryan and Shouldice, the spermatic cord must be separated from the hernial sac and its contents. The excess of the sac could be removed, but this was not considered an essential step. Closure of the transversalis fascia over the replaced protruding mass was a most important detail. Repair of the floor of the inguinal canal was described as being a routine procedure. A counterincision, or muscle-splitting incision, was considered unnecessary. Other surgeons who have repaired sliding hernias without counterabdominal incisions are Bevan, Burton, Kirchner, Laufman, Maingot, Ponka, and Zimmerman.

Roberto in 1953 reported an unusual hernia in an infant, five weeks old, in which the uterus, adnexa, and bladder formed a portion of the sac wall.

Since 1957 there has been a great awareness of the problem of sliding hernias in infants. Wiley and Chavez described their experiences with 52 infant females with inguinal hernias. Sixteen of the 52 patients had adnexa in the hernial sac. In 10 cases, the hernial sac consisted of the right tube and ovary. One hernial sac contained both tubes, ovary, and uterus. In their operative technique, Wiley and Chavez split the sac on either side of the mesosalpinx in order to return the sliding component to the peritoneal cavity and permit closure of the peritoneum.

De Boer observed in his practice that all inguinal hernias in infants and children were indirect. In his study (1957), all but one of the female children with incarceration were found to have ovaries in the hernial sac.

Goldstein and Potts in 1958 reported their views on the management of sliding inguinal hernias. They had treated 42 infants with hernias in which the tube or the ovary, or both, made up a portion of the sac. In two of these infants, the sacs contained the uterus, tubes, and ovary. In eight more patients, both tube and ovary were incarcerated in the sac.

A method for disposing of the sliding component was described by Goldstein and Potts. The technique consists of identifying the sac, opening it, and incising the peritoneum on each side of the adnexa, parallel to the vessels, in such a manner as to avoid compromise of the blood supply. The viscus is returned to the peritoneal cavity, and high ligation of the sac is then achieved. This method is simple, sound in principle, and effective in correcting the defect.

Gans in 1959 presented his experience with sliding inguinal hernias in female infants. He found that the 19 sliding inguinal hernias he encountered represented 28 percent of all hernias in female infants in his series. His method of repair is quite similar to that of Goldstein and Potts, whom he credits with putting the subject of sliding hernia in the female infant in the proper perspective.

In 1959 I reported specifically on the method that I prefer for the repair of large bilateral sliding hernias, the incidence of which is low, indeed. Ryan found only 8 instances of bilateral sliding hernias in 7000 inguinal hernias. Barrow found 1 in 1000 men of military age, while Burton only found 2 bilateral sliding hernias in 2614 operations.

Allen and Condon found inguinal protrusions, or bladder ears, in 9 percent of the urographic studies made of 406 infants under 1 year of age. This 1961 study demonstrates the position of the bladder at the internal ring. In some instances, the bladder may descend down the inguinal canal. Another important observation was that, as the infant grows into adulthood, the bladder assumes its normal protected position. The bladder ears fill when the bladder is filled to a certain capacity. With further filling, the bladder becomes more globular, and these physiologic diverticula disappear. A distended bladder then is in danger of injury.

Shaw and Santulli illustrated and described their method of management of sliding hernias of the urinary bladder in infants in 1967. They accurately described the sliding bladder component as occupying the medial portion of the sac wall. The bladder may appear in a paraperitoneal or intraperitoneal position. They pointed out that the fat about the infantile bladder in this area may be difficult to recognize. Bladder injuries occurred in 2 infants over a 14 year period during which 2378 infants had been operated upon.

Shaw and Santulli used the technique of repair, which was advocated by Goldstein and Potts and described by Gans, for the repair of 32 sliding hernias. The procedure was performed without complication or visceral injury.

Important observations on the management of sliding hernias, as viewed in historical perspective, include the following:

1. Early recognition of a sliding hernia is important if technical errors are to be avoided. Injury to the bowel or bladder is a possibility, unless the surgeon is alert to the abnormality at hand.
2. Sliding hernias of the cecum, ascending colon, and sigmoid colon are indirect and usually acquired. These hernias commonly occur in older men.
3. Direct sliding hernias, often found in elderly men, contain bladder.
4. Indirect sliding hernias in infant females may contain the fallopian tubes, the ovaries, and even the uterus. The adnexa are more commonly seen in such hernias.
5. Infant males should be suspected of having bladder in the vicinity of the internal abdominal ring, particularly if the bladder is enlarged.
6. Most sliding hernias are indirect. Direct sliding hernias contain bladder, femoral sliding hernias also contain the bladder and, in the female, the adnexa.

7. Early separation of the hernial sac and its contents from the cord is an important operative detail.
8. The peritoneal sac should be freed well into the internal ring. High ligation of the peritoneal sac remains a fundamental requirement for effective repair. The peritoneal sac should be opened at its anterior-superior aspect.
9. By incising the peritoneum medially and laterally to the sliding viscus—the adnexa in the female infant or the bowel in the adult—it is possible to return the sliding viscus to the peritoneal cavity. High ligation of the sac is then accomplished.
10. Counterincisions, either of the McBurney type (La Roque) or secondary abdominal incision (Graham), have been used by renowned surgeons, but the necessity for making such incisions is debatable.
11. The sliding component must be replaced into a position deep to the transversalis fascia or into the peritoneal cavity. Snug closure of the transversalis fascia at the internal ring is absolutely necessary for successful repair.
12. Repair of the floor of Hesselbach's triangle is important in direct sliding hernias. The McVay repair may be used for these hernias or for femoral hernias.
13. The repair of indirect sliding inguinal hernias in infants requires freeing the sac from the cord (or round ligament), incising the peritoneum medially and laterally to the viscus, and replacing the sliding component into the peritoneal cavity, followed by high ligation of the peritoneal sac.

## A NEW CLASSIFICATION OF SLIDING HERNIAS

The current method of classifying sliding hernias is less than complete, for it does not incorporate the total pathologic and anatomic picture. The current classification is based on the relationship of the viscus to the peritoneum and mesentery. Sliding hernias may be of the indirect, direct, or femoral variety. They are most often acquired; although congenital sliding

### Table 18–1. A NEW CLASSIFICATION OF SLIDING HERNIA

| Type of Sliding Component | Variety of Hernia | Viscus | Relative Frequency |
|---|---|---|---|
| **VISCEROPARIETAL**<br>The sliding viscus and attached parietal peritoneum form an intimate portion of the sac wall. The cecum, ileum, and sigmoid colon are the most common examples of this type. | INDIRECT INGUINAL | Sigmoid colon<br>Cecum or appendix, or both<br>Cecum, ileum, appendix<br>Right colon, cecum, ileum<br>Fallopian tube and ovary<br>Bladder<br>Uterus | Common<br>Common<br>Infrequent<br>Uncommon<br>Uncommon<br>Uncommon<br>Rare |
| **VISCEROPARIETAL** | DIRECT | Bladder | Uncommon |
| **VISCEROMESENTERIC**<br>The viscus and its mesentery are found in the hernial sac, but the mesentery actually makes up the sliding portion of the sac wall. The appendix with its mesentery and the fallopian tube and ovary are good examples of this type of hernia. | INDIRECT INGUINAL | Sigmoid colon<br>Appendix<br>Cecum or ileum, or both<br>Fallopian tube and ovary | Common<br>Uncommon<br>Uncommon<br>Uncommon |
| **EXTRAPERITONEAL**<br>In this type, the peritoneal sac is smooth and intact. The viscus, such as the cecum or bladder, remains in the retroperitoneal position in close proximity to the peritoneal sac. | DIRECT | Bladder<br>The bladder is found in the medial portion of the sac. | Uncommon |
| **EXTRAPERITONEAL** | FEMORAL | Bladder | Uncommon |
| **EXTRAPERITONEAL** | INDIRECT | Cecum<br>Appendix<br>Bladder | Rare<br>Rare<br>Rare |

hernias occur more frequently than was formerly believed.

Most texts on the subject deal with sliding hernias of the cecum and sigmoid colon. They refer briefly to sliding hernias of the bladder and rarely discuss sliding hernias containing the fallopian tube, ovary, and uterus. I have formulated a new classification, which I hope will bring the various types of sliding hernias to the attention of surgeons. This classification is simple and practical and presents the problem of sliding hernias in a broader perspective (Table 18–1).

### Simple Hernia

In the simple hernia, the peritoneum forms a complete sac that protrudes through the abdominal wall (Fig. 18–1). If the hernia contains the omentum or a viscus, the hernial sac completely surrounds the contents. Adhesions between the omentum or viscus and the sac do not alter

the fundamental nature of a simple hernia. Figures 18–2 to 18–6 are diagrammatic representations of sliding hernias viewed from behind, or from the posterior aspect. These illustrations present important anatomic details from a practical point of view

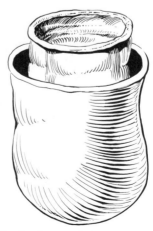

**Figure 18–1.** In the simple hernia illustrated here, the peritoneum forms a complete sac.

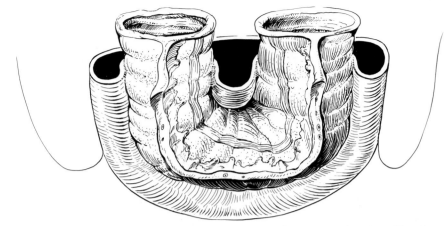

**Figure 18–2.** The visceroparietal type of sliding hernia, as seen from a posterior view. The sigmoid colon and its mesentery form an intimate portion of the posterior portion of the sac.

for the surgeon, since he is interested in the blood supply to the sliding viscera involved in sliding hernias. Figure 18–1 illustrates the simple hernia in its elementary form.

## Visceroparietal Hernia

This is the most common type of sliding hernia, in my experience. In the visceroparietal type of sliding hernia, the viscus and parietal peritoneum constitute the posterior aspect of the sac wall (Fig. 18–2). The sigmoid colon is also frequently found to be a component of the sac wall. These hernias, usually long-standing, have been

slowly enlarging. Eventually, the use of a truss fails to control the protrusion. The sliding hernia in which the ileocecal segment forms a portion of the sac wall is a good example of the visceroparietal type (Fig. 18–3). It should be recalled that the ileocecal sliding hernia is viewed from the back.

## Visceromesenteric Hernia

The viscus and its mesentery are found in the hernial sac. However, in this variety, the mesentery forms an integral part of the posterior wall of the hernial sac. If the mesentery is divided near the viscus, such

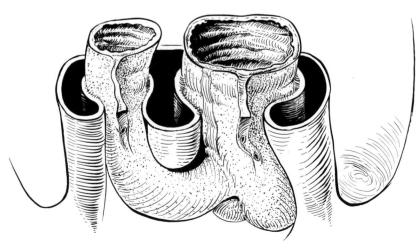

**Figure 18–3.** The ileocecal segment, as viewed from behind, forms a portion of the sac wall of a right indirect sliding inguinal hernia.

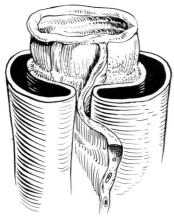

**Figure 18-4.** In the visceromesenteric sliding inguinal hernia, the mesentery of the viscus forms a portion of the sac wall.

as the appendix or right colon, there is danger of compromising the blood supply to that part. In other examples of this type, the fallopian tube, the ovary, and in certain instances, the sigmoid colon may form a portion of the hernial sac (Fig. 18–4).

### Extraperitoneal Slider

In the extraperitoneal slider, the viscus protrudes through the defect in the abdominal wall but lies outside the sac (Fig. 18–5). The viscus, free of peritoneum, is located in the extraperitoneal position. The cecum (rarely) or the bladder (more

frequently) may be found in such sliding hernias. This particular variety of sliding hernia is extremely rare, in my experience, but is included here for the sake of completeness.

Combinations of these types of sliding hernias are possible but not at all common (Fig. 18–6). For instance, a sliding hernia of the sigmoid may simultaneously present with features of the visceroparietal and visceromesenteric varieties.

The bladder is not often found in hernias, but the surgeon should be aware of this possible occurrence. In Figure 18–7, the appearance of the bladder in an indirect (*right*) and a direct (*left*) hernia is illustrated simply. It is possible for a diverticulum of the bladder to be covered by peritoneum in these locations; also, the bladder may be extraperitoneal.

Even less frequently, the bladder may find its way into a femoral hernial sac. The location of the bladder may be in the retroperitoneal or extraperitoneal position (Fig. 18–8). It should be pointed out that, rarely, the bladder may be found in a femoral hernial sac, surrounded by peritoneum (Fig. 18–9).

### DEVELOPMENTAL AND ANATOMIC CONSIDERATIONS

Certain developmental events are of importance to the surgeon. It should be recalled that in the fetus the intestinal tract

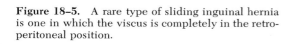

**Figure 18-5.** A rare type of sliding inguinal hernia is one in which the viscus is completely in the retroperitoneal position.

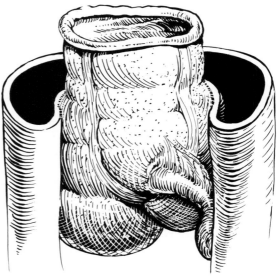

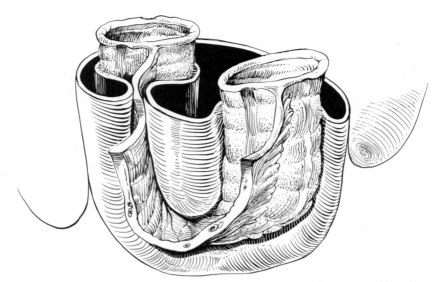

**Figure 18–6.**   Combinations of visceroparietal and visceromesenteric sliding inguinal hernias are seen occasionally. In this illustration, the sigmoid colon and its mesentery form a portion of the sac wall.

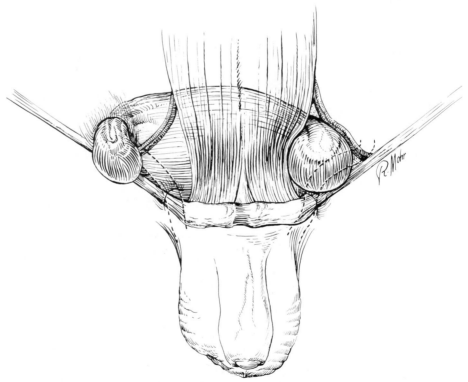

**Figure 18–7.**   A composite illustration to show the appearance of an indirect (*right*) and a direct (*left*) sliding inguinal hernia. The position of the spermatic cord is shown by the broken line.

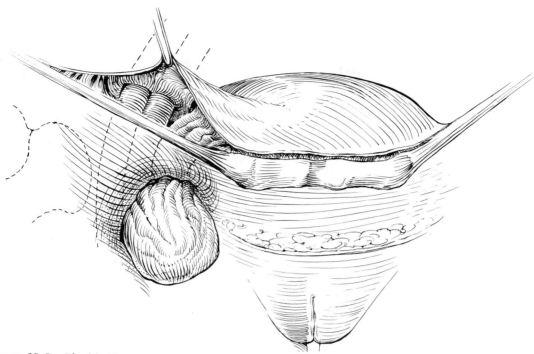

**Figure 18–8.** The bladder may appear in a femoral hernial sac in the extraperitoneal position, as shown in this illustration.

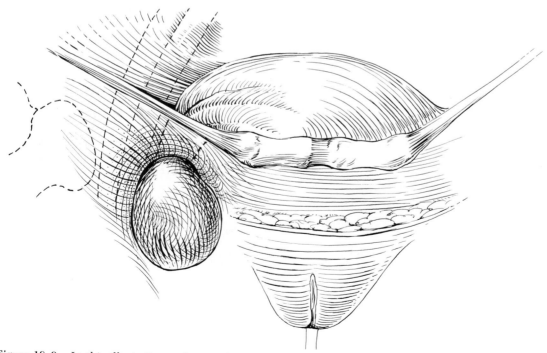

**Figure 18–9.** In this illustration, a diverticular protrusion of the bladder has found its way into a femoral hernia. Note that the bladder is covered with peritoneum, in this instance.

is a straight tube. Differential growth rates and changes due to intestinal rotation account for differences in size and ultimate location of the individual structures.

The cecum is that portion of the colon lying below a line, passing above the ileocecal valve. It is normally covered with peritoneum, has no mesentery, and lies freely in the peritoneal cavity. After the colon has returned to the abdominal cavity, it is suspended by a mesentery. The cecum is situated originally in the subhepatic area in the right upper quadrant. As growth of the colon continues, the cecum reaches the iliac fossa in the right lower abdominal quadrant, where it is ordinarily found. However, the cecum may be found farther down into the pelvis, or it may remain in the right upper quadrant. Ordinarily, the cecum is an intraperitoneal viscus, but there are instances in which dorsal fixation of the cecum to the posterior abdominal wall has

occurred. This type of anatomic situation provides the conditions that are favorable for the occurrence of a cecal sliding hernia.

As stated previously, the ascending colon is suspended by a mesentery early in embryologic development. However, as it comes to lie against the parietal peritoneum, a fusion fascia is formed. Thus the blood supply comes from the medial aspect. During surgery, an incision can be made into the peritoneum at the lateral margin of the bowel without danger. Furthermore, using blunt dissection at the level of the fusion fascia, the ascending colon and cecum can be rotated well toward the midline. These anatomic facts, when recognized and appreciated, permit safe mobilization of the ileocecal colonic segment in dealing with a large sliding hernia (Fig. 18–10).

The sigmoid colon commences at the iliac crest and joins the rectum at the third

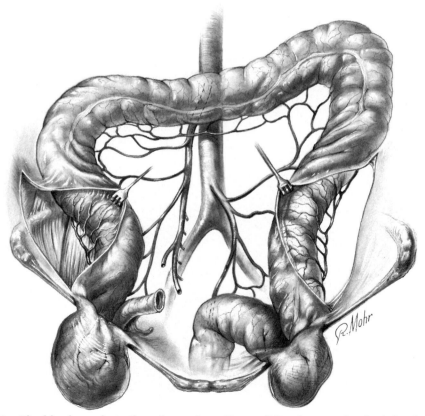

**Figure 18–10.** The blood supply to the colon as it applies to sliding hernias. On the left side, the inferior mesenteric artery, by means of its sigmoid branches, supplies the portion of colon found in a sliding hernia. On the right side, the ileocolic artery and ileal branches are of major concern.

sacral vertebra. The iliac portion, lying in the iliac fossa, is without a mesentery. The pelvic portion of the sigmoid colon commences at the pelvic brim and is suspended by a mesentery of variable length. The blood supply to the sigmoid colon is provided by the inferior mesenteric artery and its sigmoid arterial branches. Mobilization of the sigmoid colon may be safely performed when the peritoneum is raised laterally and the dissection is continued medially at the level of the fusion fascia. Mobilization of the sigmoid colon can be done safely, provided that sound anatomic principles are employed.

The urinary bladder finds its way into hernias in infants who have certain congenital disorders and in elderly men who develop direct inguinal hernias. The bladder wall is normally thick and easily recognized because of its muscular trabeculations; however, when greatly distended, it may resemble a serous sac.

In the infant the bladder is found rather high up in the pelvis, with the result that the base may be quite near the internal rings. As the infant grows, the pelvis is enlarged and the bladder assumes its position as a pelvic organ.

When distended, the bladder may reach up to the umbilicus and extend laterally to the inguinal rings. It is retroperitoneal when viewed from the peritoneal cavity, but laterally, anteriorly, and inferiorly it is extraperitoneal. Owing to enlargement or herniation, the bladder may find its way through the internal abdominal ring and remain extraperitoneal. Congenital factors, such as abnormalities in muscular development or a patent processus vaginalis, create favorable circumstances for the development of a hernia in which the bladder is a component. In my experience, the urinary bladder appears most often in large direct hernias, but it is also seen in femoral hernias. The bladder may also be identified medially in the largest indirect hernias when the floor of Hesselbach's triangle is weak and the defect almost reaches the margin of the rectus abdominis muscle.

In the female infant, the canal of Nuck may remain patent. This compares with the patent processus vaginalis in the male. The ovaries in their developmental descent move through a shorter distance than do the testes. In the male, the testes descend beneath the peritoneum in close relation to the abdominal wall. In the female, the ovaries and the uterus stretch the peritoneum and are suspended by a structure resembling a mesentery. It is a combination of factors (e.g., a patent canal of Nuck and unusual mobility of the adnexa and uterus) that leads to sliding hernias in female infants.

## THE INGUINAL APPROACH FOR THE REPAIR OF SLIDING HERNIAS

There are two schools of thought as to the proper management of sliding hernias. One group of surgeons (La Roque, Moschcowitz, Williams, and others) advocates a counterincision into the abdominal wall. Some surgeons add a McBurney incision above the internal ring, while others prefer vertical incisions that are paramedian or even midline. There is no unanimity of opinion as to how or where this counterincision should be placed.

The second method is one in which the repair is accomplished through the groin incision that is necessarily made in every patient undergoing groin hernia repairs. I prefer to complete the operation through the inguinal incision. Zimmerman and Laufman, Burton, Ryan and Shouldice of Toronto, and Maingot are other surgeons who consider the secondary abdominal incision unnecessary.

Safe and effective repair of a sliding hernia properly begins with recognition of the problem at hand. An accurate diagnosis is necessary at the earliest moment if complications or even disaster are to be avoided. A long-standing hernia in an elderly, obese male should arouse the surgeon's suspicion that he might be dealing with a sliding hernia. If it is difficult to maintain the hernia in a reduced state, then the likelihood of its being sliding is increased. The incidence of sliding hernias in female infants is greater than had heretofore been suspected. The presence of a tube, an ovary, and even the uterus in the hernial sac of female infants should be recognized early in the operative procedure. The surgeon's awareness that a portion of the bladder may find its way into a hernial sac of the

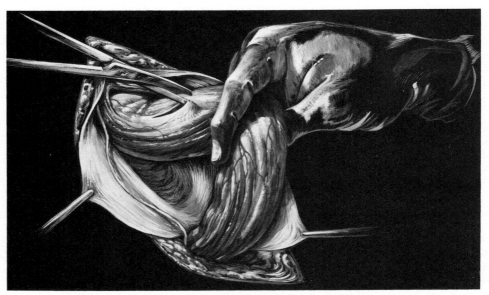

**Figure 18–11.** The external oblique muscle has been incised. The enormous thickening of the spermatic cord, along with hypertrophied cremaster muscle, is commonly seen in long-standing sliding hernias.

infant will result in less injuries to this structure.

The same type of skin incision is used as is described under indirect inguinal hernia (see Fig. 11–1, p. 160). The incision is quickly carried through the subcutaneous fat and the external oblique fascia. In large sliding hernias, the spermatic cord is markedly enlarged as a result of hypertrophy of the cremaster muscle. The enlarged, thickened cord, along with its contents, is impressive (Fig. 18–11).

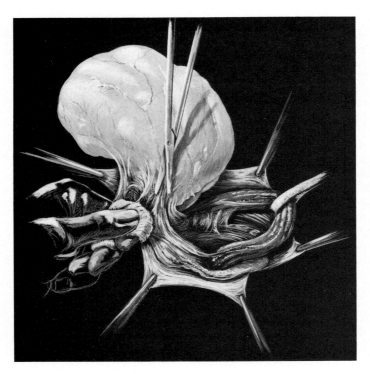

**Figure 18–12.** The cremaster muscle has been excised. The enormous hernial sac with the sliding viscus is being separated from the spermatic cord.

The ilioinguinal nerve is freed from the cord and preserved. The cremaster muscle is excised between hemostats and the stumps ligated with fine silk. Small sliding hernias, particularly of the sigmoid colon, may present problems if the surgeon is not constantly aware that the posterior-inferior portion of the sac wall may actually be composed of the sigmoid itself. The hernial sac is usually large and thick, and the viscus may be recognizable upon palpation.

In my opinion, it is best to separate the sac from the cord before it is opened. This procedure has been practiced for 15 years, with excellent results (Fig. 18–12).

There is no firm anatomic attachment of the sliding hernial sac and its contents to the cord. The areolar tissue may be easily and safely divided under direct vision. The freeing of the sac must be complete and well beyond the internal ring. In this connection it should be recalled that mobilization of the sliding hernia is comparable to mobilization of the right or left colon in preparation for resection. It must be possible to return the sliding viscus to the abdominal cavity deep to the transversalis fascia. The same principles apply when one is dealing with a sliding hernia involving the right colon, the cecum, the appendix, or the sigmoid colon on the left side. Large sliding hernias can be managed as easily as smaller ones, provided that mobilization of the sliding component has been carried out at the proper plane.

The anterior portion of the sac is then carefully opened near the internal abdominal ring. Only the peritoneum is incised, lest a viscus be injured. The area is examined digitally in order to evaluate the magnitude of the problem. The femoral area and the floor of Hesselbach's triangle are tested. Dissection of the peritoneum is carried out with the index finger in the sac. The sac must be freed completely about the internal ring so that high ligation is possible (Figs. 18–13 and 18–14).

In order to free the sliding component, the peritoneum is incised medially and laterally to the viscus. The incision is carried to a depth beyond the internal abdominal ring (Fig. 18–15). This permits return of the viscus with its blood supply into the peritoneal or abdominal cavity, where it properly belongs. No attempt is made to reperitonealize the posterior aspect of the viscus. This method has never, in my experience, created any immediate or delayed complications.

The medial and lateral leaflets of peritoneum are approximated with a heavy silk

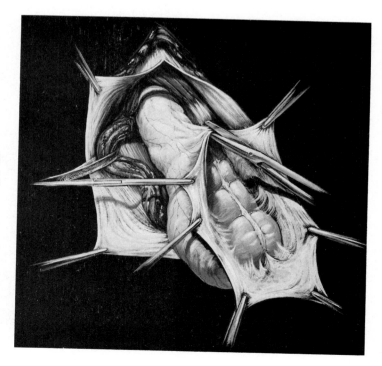

**Figure 18–13.** The hernial sac is being opened on its superior aspect. Only the superior portion of the sac is opened initially.

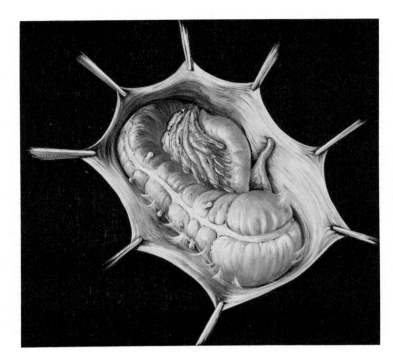

**Figure 18–14.** Cecum, appendix, and terminal ileum make up the posterior portion of the hernial sac in this huge ileocecal sliding hernia.

**Figure 18–15.** The incision is made in the peritoneum medially and to the sliding viscus laterally.

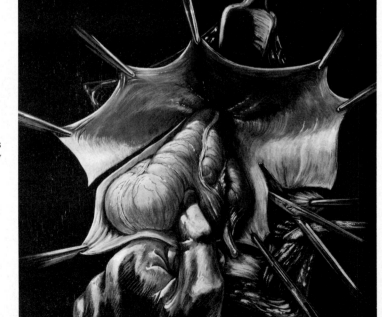

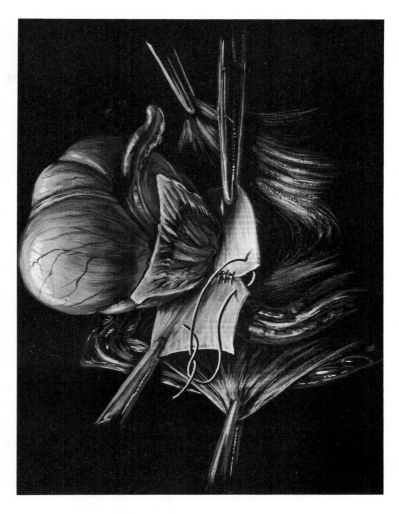

**Figure 18–16.** Medial and lateral leaflets of peritoneum are being approximated, forming a complete peritoneal ring.

suture (Fig. 18–16). Complete closure of the peritoneum is accomplished with a pursestring suture of heavy silk (Fig. 18–17).

In a direct or femoral hernia, the peritoneal sac is opened at the internal ring. The direct or femoral peritoneal sac is converted safely into an indirect sac, using the maneuver of Hoguet (Fig. 18–18). Again, I feel that digital exploration of the area is necessary if the proper operative procedure is to be performed. By opening the peritoneum laterally, there is no danger of injury to the bladder. In a direct hernia, opening the peritoneum in the floor of Hesselbach's triangle can be dangerous, particularly if the bladder is distended at the time. If the viscus in the sliding hernia is retroperitoneal, such as the bladder, it must be returned to its position deep to the

transversalis fascia. Any extrasaccular or extraperitoneal hernia is similarly managed. The important detail to remember is that the viscus must be returned to its position deep to the transversalis fascia after being separated from the cord.

The transversalis fascia is then triangulated at the internal ring for proper identification and accurate closure (Fig. 18–19). The first suture of medium silk is placed nearest the cord, since the transversalis fascia and the cord at its point of exit from the abdomen can be best visualized at this time. The internal ring is reduced to approximately one cm in size. It barely admits the tip of the index finger. If the ring is large enough to admit the entire finger, it is too large, in my judgment.

In a few patients, I have been able to

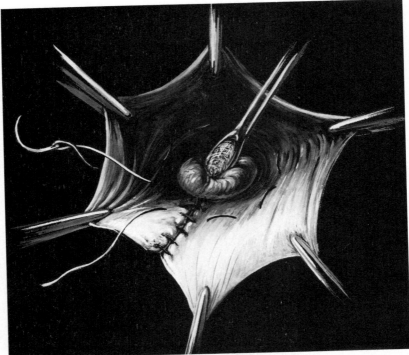

**Figure 18–17.** A pursestring suture of heavy silk has been employed to achieve high ligation of the peritoneal sac.

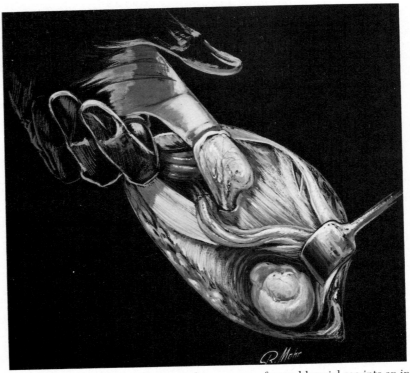

**Figure 18–18.** The Hoguet maneuver is being used to convert a femoral hernial sac into an indirect sac. The same procedure may be employed to reduce a direct hernial sac, which is converted into an indirect hernial sac.

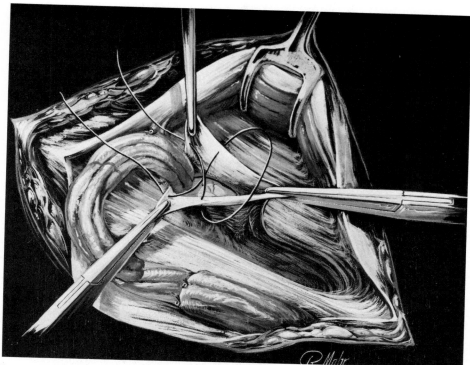

**Figure 18–19.** Accurate and firm closure of the internal ring is easily accomplished by triangulation of the transversalis fascia at the internal ring. The suture nearest the cord is placed first, since exposure is optimal at this stage of the procedure.

close the transversalis fascia and internal ring more effectively by placing one or two sutures of medium silk lateral to the cord. In these instances, the internal ring was usually large, and medial closure alone was felt to be inadequate. These sutures should not be placed deeply, lest the shutter mechanism of the musculature be disrupted.

If the operation is being performed under local anesthesia and the patient is asked to cough at this point in the repair, the effectiveness of the repair can easily be demonstrated.

A relaxing incision is added if the defect is large and if there is an accompanying weakness in the floor of the inguinal canal. Excessive tension on the suture line must be avoided.

In the surgical procedure for indirect inguinal sliding hernias, I close the inguinal floor by suturing the transversus abdominis and transversalis fascia to the iliopubic tract and inguinal ligament in order to strengthen the floor of Hesselbach's

triangle. I have not found it necessary to use the McVay repair in the ordinary, uncomplicated, indirect sliding inguinal hernia.

## REPAIR OF SIGMOID SLIDING HERNIAS

The repair of sliding hernias of the sigmoid colon follows the same principles as those previously described for ileocecal sliding hernias. The cord is large, owing to the hypertrophy of the cremaster muscle. The hernial sac is again freed from the cord after excision of the hypertrophied cremaster. The large hernial sac containing the sigmoid colon is freed from the cord (Fig. 18–20).The peritoneal sac is then carefully opened in its superior aspect in order to avoid injury to the sigmoid colon (Fig. 18–21). The peritoneum is incised medially and laterally to the sigmoid colon (Fig. 18–22), and the leaflets are approximated (see Fig. 18–17).

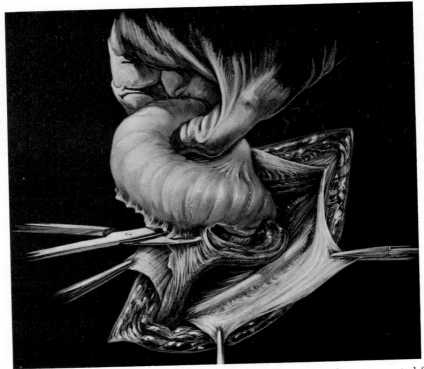

**Figure 18–20.**  An intact hernial sac, containing a sigmoid sliding hernia, is being separated from the cord.

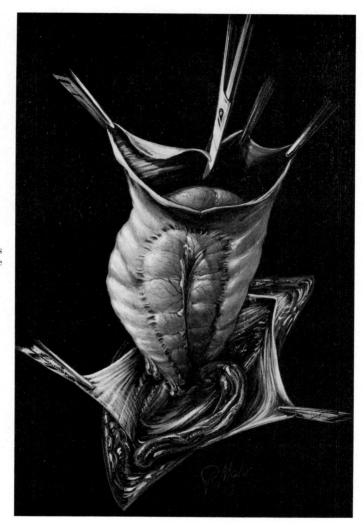

**Figure 18–21.** The freed hernial sac is being opened in its superior aspect. The cremaster muscle has been excised.

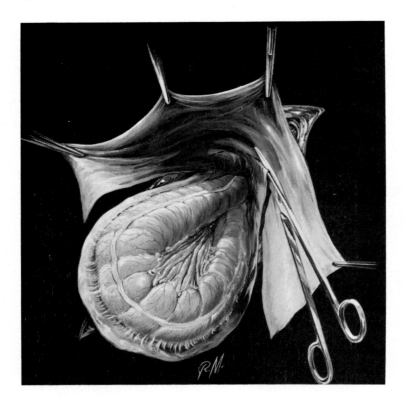

**Figure 18–22.** The peritoneal sac is incised medially and laterally well down into the abdomen in order to free the sliding viscus and to permit high ligation of the sac.

The repair is completed by closure of the transversalis fascia and by subsequent repair of the inguinal floor.

In the repair of the direct sliding inguinal hernia, the bladder must be returned to its proper anatomic position deep to the transversalis fascia. Excessive dissection about the bladder is meddlesome surgical practice and frequently results in dysuria postoperatively. The McVay technique is effective in the repair of large direct inguinal hernias and femoral sliding hernias.

When the bladder finds its way into a femoral hernial sac as a sliding component, it occupies the anterior-medial aspect of the sac. The sac and its contents must be freed so that they may be returned to their normal position in the abdominal cavity, deep to the transversalis fascia. The sac in a sliding hernia of the bladder is managed somewhat differently from that in a sliding hernia of the cecum or the sigmoid colon. The peritoneum is not separated from the bladder medially. The peritoneal sac is freed both superiorly and laterally. Excessive dissection of the peritoneum over the bladder is avoided. After the peritoneal sac has been properly

ligated, the repair of the femoral hernia is completed.

The principles referred to in the repair of direct sliding inguinal hernia are also used in the repair of sliding hernia in female infants. The indirect sac is freed at the internal ring, then opened and inspected carefully. The fallopian tube, the ovary, and even the uterus have been found in such hernial sacs. The peritoneum is incised medially and laterally to the sliding viscus or viscera (Fig. 18–23, A). Bleeding is controlled by careful hemostasis. The sliding components are returned to the abdominal cavity (Fig. 18–23, B). Then the peritoneal ring, free of any interfering viscera, is accurately closed with a pursestring suture of silk (Fig. 18–23, C). The transversalis fascia must be carefully repaired if recurrence is to be avoided. The floor of Hesselbach's triangle need not be disturbed. I have yet to see a direct inguinal hernia in a female infant.

In repairing sliding hernias of the bladder, it may be necessary to resort to the McVay technique in order to strengthen the floor of Hesselbach's triangle. These usually occur as direct hernias but occa-

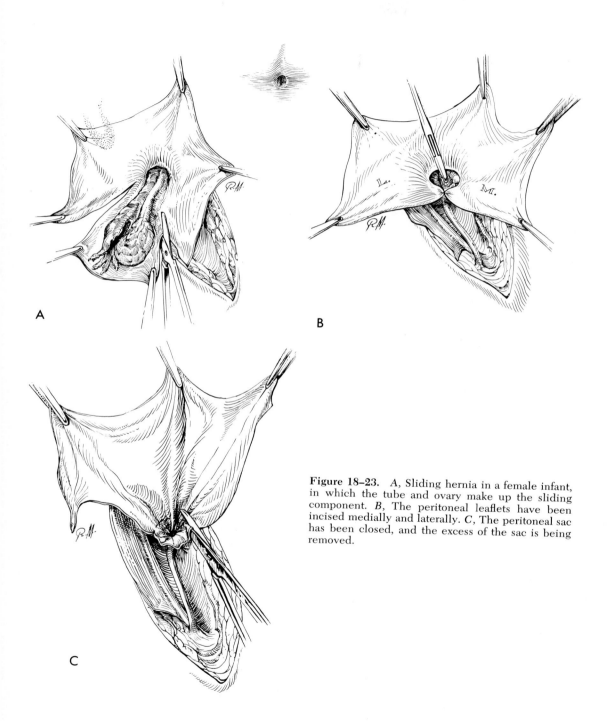

**Figure 18–23.** *A*, Sliding hernia in a female infant, in which the tube and ovary make up the sliding component. *B*, The peritoneal leaflets have been incised medially and laterally. *C*, The peritoneal sac has been closed, and the excess of the sac is being removed.

sionally appear as femoral hernias. Large indirect hernias of a long-standing nature may contain a portion of the bladder medially. Although I frequently used the Halsted repair in the past, I rarely use it today. If the cord is placed subcutaneously in a thin individual, some discomfort may ensue. If the preceding details have been properly carried out, the sliding hernia is repaired before the external oblique aponeurosis has been reached. The fate of the external oblique aponeurosis at this point in the procedure is a minor consideration, in my opinion. In current operative procedure, the spermatic cord is placed in a position under the external oblique aponeurosis. Closure of the subcutaneous tissues and skin is accomplished in the same manner as is used for indirect inguinal hernia (see Figs. 11–8 and 11–9, pp. 166–167).

## REPORT ON 350 SLIDING INGUINAL HERNIAS: A SUMMARY

During the years 1942 to 1968, surgeons of the Henry Ford Hospital operated on 350 sliding inguinal hernias. These cases had been indexed as sliding hernias in the medical records department. Additional sliding hernia cases were discovered after careful study of operative notes. The observations made and the experience gained from this exposure will be summarized. The late Dr. Henry N. Harkins and Dr. L. S. Fallis, former Chairman of the Department of Surgery, are two of the well-known surgeons who operated on some of the earlier patients.

### Sex and Age Distribution

The age incidence in this study is noteworthy. Although Henry Ford Hospital is located in an industrial center and mainly treats adult patients, it has always had an active pediatric department. The relative infrequency of sliding hernias occurring in infants and children is striking. Only 7 of the 350 patients with hernias were under the age of 7 years. Male infants, though often subject to congenital hernias and associated anomalies of the testes, rarely present with sliding hernias. Only one of the seven infants was a male;

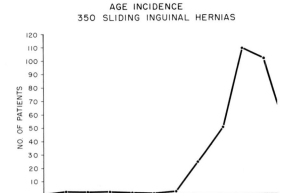

**Figure 18–24.** Age incidence: 350 sliding inguinal hernias.

he was found to have an indirect sliding hernia of the cecum and appendix when he was eight months old. The other youngsters were the only females among 350 patients with sliding hernias.

A breakdown of the patients into incidence by decades is worthy of some discussion. Figure 18–24 shows clearly that sliding hernias are found most often in elderly patients. Of the total 350 patients, 220 were between the ages of 51 and 70 years. These statistics, in my opinion, lend strong support to the concept that sliding inguinal hernias in the adult are acquired.

### Clinical Features

Patients with sliding hernias often refuse surgical treatment for many years, depending upon trusses for relief. Finally, these appliances fail, and surgical correction is mandatory. The patient may describe the swelling in the groin as having enlarged over many years. Nineteen patients had hernias for 25 to 50 years. The truss failed to maintain reduction in 13 of these individuals.

One hundred and sixty-two patients were operated upon less than four years after onset of their hernias. This may be explained by the fact that 168 of the total 350 patients were industrial workers or were covered by workmen's compensation; therefore, they sought medical care early for whatever disability they had.

Heavy work was performed by 156 of the

**Table 18–2. DURATION OF SLIDING HERNIAS**

| Duration | No. of Patients | No. Wearing Trusses |
|---|---|---|
| 25 years and longer | 19 | 13 |
| 15 to 24 years | 20 | 4 |
| 10 to 14 years | 30 | 3 |
| 5 to 9 years | 34 | 0 |
| 0 to 4 years | 162 | 0 |
| Undetermined | 48 | 0 |
| "Many" years | 37 | 7 |

350 patients with sliding hernias. Again, it should be noted that these patients were from an industrial area.

Table 18–2 summarizes the lengths of time that the various age groups sustained hernias before seeking surgical correction. Several elderly patients could not recall with any accuracy when their hernias were first observed, but undoubtedly, they were present for many years. Trusses failed to help seven out of 37 individuals in this group.

Sliding hernias often appear large when presented to the surgeon; nevertheless, they are reducible almost without exception. However, even after reduction, they will promptly protrude unless pressure

**Table 18–3. CLINICAL DIAGNOSTIC IMPRESSIONS OF 350 PATIENTS WITH SLIDING HERNIAS**

| Type of Hernia | No. of Patients |
|---|---|
| INDIRECT SLIDING INGUINAL HERNIA | 14 |
| INDIRECT INGUINAL HERNIA | 199 |
|     Indirect inguinal | 132 |
|     Bilateral indirect | 28 |
|     Indirect scrotal | 21 |
|     Scrotal | 7 |
|     Incarcerated | 7 |
|     Recurrent indirect | 4 |
| INGUINAL HERNIA (Not further described) | 88 |
|     Inguinal | 48 |
|     Recurrent inguinal | 20 |
|     Bilateral inguinal | 20 |
| DIRECT INGUINAL HERNIA | 43 |
|     Direct inguinal | 32 |
|     Direct recurrent | 2 |
|     Bilateral direct | 9 |
| DIRECT-INDIRECT INGUINAL HERNIA | 6 |

over them is continued. Only seven patients of the total 350 presented with incarcerated sliding hernias.

## Preoperative Diagnosis

The attitude that sliding hernias cannot be diagnosed preoperatively is deplorable, in my opinion. It creates an unreceptive state of mind in the diagnostician, thereby eliminating any possibility of making the proper diagnosis. It is my conviction that a determined effort to make the correct diagnosis in every patient will eventually lead to the successful recognition of sliding hernias in an acceptable number of instances. Furthermore, by merely suspecting the possibility of a sliding hernia, the surgeon may well avoid injury to the colon or bladder. Diagnosis of hernia is treated more completely in Chapter 3. Every elderly obese patient with a long-standing hernia that is reducible but reappears easily should at least be suspected of having a sliding hernia. In the larger sliding hernias, the examiner will be impressed with the feeling that some viscus forms an intimate part of the sac. It is true that there are no pathognomonic signs for sliding hernia; yet the correct diagnostic impression can be made with surprising frequency. Table 18–3 summarizes the clinical diagnostic impression in the patients studied. In only 14 patients was the possible presence of a sliding hernia considered in the differential diagnosis. The clinical impression of sliding hernia was infrequently recorded.

In only 14 patients, the correct diagnosis was suspected and entered into the record. In 199 cases, the presence of an indirect inguinal hernia was appreciated, but in some of them there was no attempt at differential diagnosis. For instance, in seven patients, the diagnosis was a noncommittal "incarcerated" hernia; in seven others, "scrotal hernia" was the impression. A further effort at making a correct diagnosis would often have been productive. In 88 patients, the diagnosis offered was a comfortable one of "inguinal hernia" with no further description. In 43 patients, the diagnosis was direct inguinal hernia, whereas only 17 actually had such a hernia. Twenty-three patients were erroneously diagnosed as having direct hernias, when, in fact, they had sliding hernias. These errors arose from deficiencies in two main areas: first, in failing to describe in sufficient detail the findings in physical examination of patients with inguinal hernia and, second, in failing to differentiate direct from indirect sliding inguinal hernias. A determined effort by the physician to make the proper diagnosis will result in a higher incidence of correct diagnoses.

### Anesthesia

In the early years of this study, spinal anesthesia was by far the most popular. However, because of the problems of headaches and backaches following spinal anesthesia, I began to resort more and more to the use of local anesthesia. One-hundred and eighty-two sliding inguinal hernias were repaired under local anesthesia; 141 were repaired under spinal anesthesia; and 27 were repaired under general anesthesia.

Infants, children, and young adults are often given general anesthesia. Neurotic patients are not candidates for either local or spinal anesthesia. Finally, a small number of patients simply want to be "put to sleep." For such patients, general anesthesia is recommended if they are suitable candidates otherwise.

## Operative Findings

Table 18–4 summarizes the important findings in this series of sliding inguinal hernias. The small indirect inguinal sliding hernia is the type most commonly seen in our practice. In this variety, the sigmoid colon is found to constitute the inferior portion of the hernial sac near the cord. These hernias are often associated with large abdominal rings. In obese individuals, the area is infiltrated with fat. The larger indirect sliding hernia may contain the cecum and contiguous structures or a large loop of sigmoid colon. Hernias of the bladder are most often direct but may be femoral. We have seen the medial portion of the bladder in huge indirect inguinal hernias. Sliding hernias are uncommonly seen in small boys but are somewhat more frequently seen in female infants. In these cases, the tube, ovary, and even uterus may be seen in the hernial sac.

### Suture Material

Our preference in suture material was silk. Since Dr. Roy D. McClure—first Surgeon-in-Chief of the Henry Ford Hospital—had been Dr. William S. Halsted's house officer, it is not surprising that he brought the "silk technique" with him to Detroit. Silk was the suture material of choice used in 334 out of the total 350 patients. Catgut alone and catgut with wire were used in 12 patients. Synthetic sutures

**Table 18–4. OPERATIVE FINDINGS IN 350 PATIENTS WITH SLIDING HERNIAS**

| Type of Hernia | No. of Patients |
|---|---|
| LEFT INDIRECT INGUINAL HERNIA | 260 |
| Large | 57 |
| Moderate | 72 |
| Small | 131 |
| RIGHT INDIRECT SLIDING INGUINAL HERNIA | 64 |
| Large | 30 |
|   Ascending colon, cecum, ileum, and appendix | 3 |
|   Ascending colon, cecum, appendix | 2 |
|   Cecum and appendix | 10 |
|   Cecum and ileum | 9 |
|   Cecum | 6 |
| Moderate | 15 |
|   Ascending colon and cecum | 1 |
|   Cecum and appendix | 9 |
|   Cecum | 5 |
| Small | 19 |
|   Cecum | 14 |
|   Appendix | 5 |
| DIRECT SLIDING HERNIA OF BLADDER | 17 |
| Bilateral | 4 |
| Right | 8 |
| Left | 5 |
| FEMORAL SLIDING HERNIA OF BLADDER | 4 |
| INDIRECT SLIDING HERNIA IN FEMALE INFANT | 5 |
| Left indirect sliding hernia (Tube and ovary) | 3 |
| Right indirect sliding hernia (Tube and ovary) | 2 |
| Total | 350 |

**Table 18–5. RECONSTRUCTION IN 350 PATIENTS WITH SLIDING HERNIAS**

| Types of Methods | No. of Patients |
|---|---|
| Halsted | 201 |
| Bassini | 129 |
| McVay | 16 |
| Ferguson | 4 |

were used in only four operations, but their use has been steadily increasing.

### Operative Procedures

For every patient in this study, the inguinal approach was selected as the repair technique. The currently favored procedure was described earlier in this chapter.

In operations performed between 1940 and 1952, the practice of incising the peritoneum on either side of the sliding component was used infrequently. I have used this method more recently and have been satisfied with its effectiveness. Table 18–5 lists the method of reconstruction.

Currently, the practice of transplanting the cord, as advocated by Halsted, is being used infrequently. A sliding hernia must be repaired before the surgeon reaches the external oblique fascia.

The Bassini reconstruction is completely adequate in repairing the average indirect sliding inguinal hernia. It is currently the most popular method of repair of sliding inguinal hernias. I am interested in the strength of the floor of Hesselbach's triangle after repair, since many of the patients I am called upon to treat are industrial workers and must perform heavy work.

The Ferguson operation was performed in only four infants. Closure of the internal oblique over the cord has little, if anything, to do with a successful outcome. Fundamentally, high ligation of the sac is the most important detail in this operative procedure.

The McVay repair was used in large hernias and in direct, femoral, and recurrent inguinal hernias.

In summary, the operative approach to sliding hernias includes recognition of the pathologic condition, excision of the cre-

master muscle, and high ligation of the peritoneal sac after freeing the sac from the cord. To accomplish high ligation, it is necessary to replace the viscus in the peritoneal cavity. This is done by incising the peritoneum medially and laterally to the viscus. Closure of the peritoneum is accomplished with a pursestring suture of heavy silk. In infants, sliding hernias are cured at this point. It is always important to replace the viscus deep to the transversalis fascia so that it may be closed accurately over the particular sliding component. Reconstruction of a snug internal ring is absolutely necessary. Repair beyond this point should be individualized to correct any additional problem at hand.

### Complications

A most serious complication is wound infection. It occurred in 10 of 350 patients for an incidence of 3.5 percent of wound infections. Several of the serious infections occurred during the early years of the study when less exacting aseptic precautions were in vogue.

Seromas are collections of serum; they result in an obvious swelling, which gives the patient cause for concern. In four patients, aspiration of seromas was necessary.

Hematomas were encountered in seven patients. With a hematoma, large collections of blood must be evacuated. The skin is again carefully prepared as for an operative procedure. The area is draped with sterile towels. Using gloves and aseptic technique, the wound margins are gently separated. If liquid blood is present, it is easily removed. Blood clots must be evacuated if healing is to be prompt. The wound edges are loosely approximated with sterile adhesive strips, and a pressure dressing is applied. All such wounds are cultured, of course.

Scrotal swelling occurred in nine patients. In large scrotal hernias, some accumulation of fluid in the scrotal sac is not surprising. In such instances, a hydrocele support is usually all that is necessary. Venous obstruction, caused by the dissection necessary to free large hernial sacs, may result in edema of the testicle. In such instances, the testicle is large, firm but not severely painful. Eventually, the testicle will return to its normal size. If the arterial supply is severely compromised, the testicle becomes painful and swollen, and the patient experiences a febrile course. The testicle then slowly decreases in size over a period of several months. This is likely to happen if a given patient has a poor collateral circulation to the testicle. Two of our patients developed testicular atrophy. The testes became small, resembling an almond in shape and size. The remaining seven patients with scrotal swelling did not develop atrophy.

Seven patients complained of postoperative incisional pain. Careful re-examination and reassurance will satisfy most such patients. A few may require analgesics, hot tub baths, and suspensories. Rarely, a nerve may be entrapped in a cicatrix, giving justification for the patient's complaints. In such patients, a nerve block may be of diagnostic aid. If this fails to give relief from pain, then it is likely that excision of the neuroma will also be unsuccessful. At other times, the patient will insist that heavy work causes the discomfort, even in the absence of local pathology.

Pulmonary complications included atelectasis in two patients and pneumonia in one. Early ambulation has done much to decrease the incidence of such complications. Pulmonary embolism occurred in one individual.

It is not surprising that patients with sliding hernias may have urinary tract complications. Fifty-three had significant prostatic hypertrophy initially. Eight patients developed urinary tract infections requiring antibiotic therapy. Cultures of the urine are indispensable in the proper management of such cases. Urinary retention requiring catheterization was present in five patients, while the obstruction was so severe and protracted in two that prostatic surgery was necessary before urine flow was re-established.

Thrombophlebitis was encountered in three patients. In two, the thrombosis developed in the veins of the legs, requiring heparin therapy. For an acute thrombophlebitis of the arm, warm compresses and elevation were recommended.

Headaches causing significant disability in two patients after spinal anesthesia required hydration, bed rest, and analgesics.

Other complications included sensitivity to adhesive tape and to the antiseptic used in skin preparation. Iodine was the irritant in two patients. At present, paper adhesive tape is available; it causes little or no skin irritation. If the skin reaction is severe, antihistaminics may be necessary; otherwise, a local application of 0.25 percent hydrocortisone cream will give much relief.

### Significant Operative Complications

In one elderly patient, severe and continuous hemorrhage from an aberrant obturator artery injured during repair required transfusions and reoperation. This patient had a large sliding hernia with a weakness in the floor of Hesselbach's triangle. He is one of the patients who developed a recurrent hernia in the abdominal component of the incision made at reoperation.

Three patients with sliding hernias had inadvertent colotomies. In two of these patients, prompt recognition and early repair of the opening without spillage of feces resulted in an uneventful recovery. These hernias were repaired with catgut and wire and the wounds well drained; antibiotics also were given.

The third patient had a large hernia, and the surgeon performed a Mikulicz exteriorization of the injured bowel through a McBurney incision. The operative wound was closed with catgut and wire and again drained. Recovery was uneventful after the procedure, but the colostomy later required closure.

There is always some danger of an operative complication in dealing with complex and recurrent sliding hernias. Prompt recognition of the problem should direct the surgeon to take corrective steps. If an inadvertent cystotomy is made, the bladder should be closed and catheter drainage and antibiotic therapy instituted. If a colotomy is accidentally performed, it may be closed if the colon is clear of fecal material. Adequate drainage and antibiotics are recommended. I advise the use of monofilament wire and catgut for closure in the complicated situations just discussed. If the colon is devitalized, a colostomy may be necessary.

## Recurrences

In 350 sliding hernias, there were seven recurrences. Four of the seven recurred as indirect inguinal hernias and two as direct hernias. The remaining one recurred as a ventral hernia; this was observed in a patient having a secondary abdominal incision for control of operative hemorrhage. All seven recurrences were noted within four years following surgical repair; six recurred within two years. Of the total 350 patients, 148 were followed up for five years or longer. A recurrence rate of 2 percent for this series is acceptable but could be improved.

## *Deaths*

All 350 patients, regardless of condition, were operated upon without a death.

However, many of these patients were elderly and have since died of various diseases. Two died of colonic carcinomas, while bronchogenic carcinoma, brain tumor, bladder carcinoma, and carcinoma of the esophagus accounted for other deaths. In one patient the source of the neoplasm was undetermined. Seven other patients died of advanced cardiovascular disease. Four individuals perished of myocardial infarctions.

Eight additional patients have confirmed carcinomas but were still alive at the time of publication of this study.

## REFERENCES

Allen, R. P., and Condon, V. R.: Transitory extraperitoneal hernia. Radiology 77:979, 1961.

Banks, W. M.: Some statistics of the operation for the radical cure of hernia. Br. Med. J. 2:1259–1262, 1887.

Bevan, A. D.: Sliding hernias of the ascending colon and caecum. The descending colon and sigmoid and of the bladder. Ann. Surg. 92:754–760, 1930.

Burton, C. C., and Blotner, C.: Sliding and other large bowel herniae: Development, classification and operative management. Ann. Surg. 116:384, 1942.

Brown, K.: Sliding or paraperitoneal hernia of the pelvic colon. Surg. Gynecol. Obstet. 76:91, 1943.

Carnett, J. B.: Inguinal hernia of the caecum. Ann. Surg. 49:491, 1909.

Criley, C. H.: Parasaccular or sliding hernia. Surg. Gynecol. Obstet. 31:611, 1920.

DeBoer, A.: Inguinal hernia in infants and children. Arch. Surg. 75:920, 1957.

Eccles, W. M.: *Hernia: Its Etiology, Symptoms and Treatment* (2nd ed.). London, William Wood & Co., 1902.

Erdmann, J. F.: Accidents in hernia operations. Ann. Surg. 49:208, 1909.

Gans, S. L.: Sliding inguinal hernia in female infants. Arch. Surg. 79:109, 1959.

Goldstein, I. R., and Potts, W. J.: Inguinal hernia in female infants and children. Ann. Surg. 148:819, 1958.

Graham, R. R.: The operative repair of sliding hernia of the sigmoid. Ann. Surg. 104(4):784, 1935.

Hotchkiss, L. W.: Large sliding hernias of the sigmoid. Ann. Surg. 50:470, 1909.

Kirchner, W. C. G.: The treatment of sliding hernia. Trans. Am. Assoc. Obstet. Gynecol. 64:758, 1911.

Koontz, A. R.: The operation for difficult sliding hernia of the large bowel. Am. Surg. 18(1):78, 1952.

La Roque, G. P.: Intra-abdominal method of removing inguinal and femoral hernia. Arch. Surg. 24:189, 1932.

Mackid, L. S.: Inguinal hernia: With special reference to sliding hernia and a new treatment. Can. Med. Assoc. J. 34:269, 1936.

Maingot, R.: Operations for sliding herniae and for large incisional herniae. Br. J. Clin. Pract. 15(12):993–996, 1033, 1961.

Moretz, W. H. *In* Nyhus, L. M., and Harkins, H. N.: *Hernia.* Philadelphia, J. B. Lippincott Co., 1964, pp. 128–145.

Morris, H.: Two cases of inguinal hernia presenting unusual characters. Lancet 2:979, 1895.

Moschcowitz, A. V.: The rational treatment of sliding hernia. Ann. Surg. 81:330, 1925.

Ponka, J. L.: Surgical management of large bilateral indirect sliding inguinal hernias. Am. J. Surg. 112:52, 1966.

Roberto, A. E.: Unusual inguinal hernia in infancy. N.Y. J. Med. 53:3044, 1953.

Ryan, M. A.: An analysis of 313 consecutive cases of indirect sliding inguinal hernias. Surg. Gynecol. Obstet. 102:45, 1956.

Sensenig, D. V., and Nichols, J. B.: Sliding hernias. Arch. Surg. 71:756, 1955.

Shaw, A., and Santulli, T. V.: Management of sliding hernias of the urinary bladder in infants. Surg. Gynecol. Obstet. 124:1314, 1967.

Snyder, W. H., and Greaney, E. M., Jr.: Inguinal hernia. *In* Benson, C. D., et al.: *Pediatric Surgery* (Vol. I). Chicago, Ill., Year Book Medical Pubs., Inc., 1962, pp. 2, 572–587.

Treves, F.: Hernia of the Caecum. Br. Med. J. 1:382, 1887.

Walton, A. J.: Extrasaccular hernia. Ann. Surg. 57:86, 1913.

Watson, L. F.: *Hernia* (2nd ed.). St. Louis, C. V. Mosby Co., 1938, pp. 514–531.

Wiley, J., and Armando Chavez, H.: Uterine adnexa in inguinal hernia in infant females: Report of a case involving uterus, both uterine tubes and ovaries. West. J. Surg. Obstet. Gynecol. 65(Sept–Oct.):283–285, 1957.

Williams, C.: Repair of sliding inguinal hernia through the abdominal (LaRoque) approach. Ann. Surg. 126(4):612, 1947.

Zimmerman, L., and Laufman, H.: Sliding hernia. Surg. Gynecol. Obstet. 75:76, 1942.

## Supplemental Readings

Barrow, D. W.: Bilateral sliding hernia. Am. J. Surg. 87:932, 1954.

David, V. C.: Sliding hernias of the caecum and appendix in children. Ann. Surg. 77:438, 1923.

Hoguet, J. P.: Direct inguinal hernia. Ann. Surg. 72:671, 1920.

Koop, C. E.: Inguinal herniorrhaphy in infants and children. Surg. Clin. North Am. 37:1675, 1957.

Lamson, O. F.: Sliding hernia. Northw. Med., 39:175, 1940.

La Roque, G. P.: The permanent cure of inguinal and femoral hernia. Surg. Gynecol. Obstet. 29:507, 1909.

La Roque, G. P.: An improved method of removing hernia from within. Ann. Surg. 79:375, 1924.

Stoesser, P. N., and Piedad, O. H.: Simplified method for repair of sliding inguinal hernia. Am. J. Surg. 118:472, 1969.

Watson, L. F.: Sliding hernia. Inter. Clin. 4(Dec.): 155, 1925.

# 19

# Recurrent Inguinofemoral Hernia

The type of recurrent groin hernia that I have chosen to call the recurrent inguinofemoral hernia is not common and is difficult to describe or define simply; nevertheless, it should be identifiable to the surgeon. This particular type of hernia occupies the lower abdomen and upper thigh and is usually on one side of the body. It occurs as a result of previous operative treatment in the area leading to heavy scar formation, to loss of some part of the internal oblique and transversus abdominis muscles and the transversalis fascia, and to destruction of the inguinal ligament.

As a rule, recurrent inguinofemoral hernias are poorly managed. This type of defect must be considered as something more than an ordinary recurrent femoral, inguinal, or ventral hernia if it is to be repaired successfully (Fig. 19–1); therefore, I feel that a better description of the hernia and some recommendations as to its repair are in order.

## DESCRIPTION

Inguinofemoral recurrent hernias have a number of common features, which may be summarized as follows:

1. This type of hernia is recurrent — one that has been repaired several times previously and often at a number of different institutions.

2. It is usually quite large and

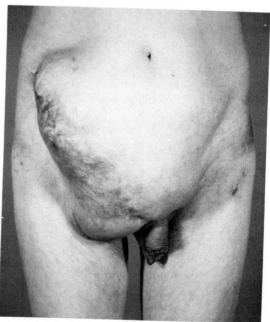

**Figure 19–1.** The large defect shown here is the result of three previous operations for inguinal hernia. The testicle has been removed. The protrusion is huge and occupies the lower abdomen and upper thigh. The inguinal ligament had been destroyed. Surgical repair was performed by reconstruction with a synthetic mesh; this held until the patient died of heart disease, three years later.

occupies the lower abdomen and thigh.

3. The inguinal ligament has been more or less completely destroyed by either inadvertent surgical procedure or deliberate therapeutic effort.

4. The testicle located on the same side of the body as the hernia has often been removed. The indication for the orchidectomy might have been tumor or, more often, atrophy secondary to trauma of repeated surgical procedures. The testicle might also have been removed to facilitate repair. In some cases, the testicle is present but atrophic.

5. A variety of underlying etiologic factors contribute to the formation of such hernias. Hernia repairs, excision of vulvar tumors or malignant testicular tumors with groin dissections, excision of sarcomas, or vascular operations in the inguinofemoral area may result in large hernias in the lower abdomen and upper thigh.

6. The recurrent inguinofemoral hernia is large and reducible and is not commonly associated with either intestinal obstruction or strangulation.

7. The patient is sometimes discouraged by the physician and is told that nothing can be done and that he must learn to live with his disability.

## HISTORICAL BACKGROUND

Recognition for being the first to recognize the general type of hernia under consideration here is rightfully given to Georg Lotheissen. It is fortunate for surgeons that Lotheissen described his initial procedure for the repair of a specific type of recurrent inguinofemoral hernia with great clarity, as the method has been successfully employed by a number of surgeons since his time.

Lotheissen was an assistant to Professor von Hacker in Innsbruck, Austria, when he published his paper, "On the Radical Operation for Femoral Hernias," in May, 1897. At this time, he planned to perform a Bassini repair of an inguinal hernia in a 45-year-old woman; the hernia had recurred after two previous attempts at repair. Because of its fundamental importance to surgeons today, the operative procedure that he used will be described, following his own account.

The skin incision was made directly above Poupart's ligament; the fascia of the external oblique muscle was split 1 or 2 mm above this ligament. According to Lotheissen, the hernial sac could be managed from above Poupart's ligament, as in an inguinal hernia, or from below it. If the procedure was carried out from below the inguinal ligament, then the sac was freed, ligated, and the stump pushed upward until the ligament of Cooper became visible.

Lotheissen recognized that placement of the sutures through Cooper's ligament was technically the most difficult part of the procedure and advised that, in order to secure better exposure, the femoral vein should be identified and retracted laterally with a vein retractor. He then placed four or five sutures of strong silk through the muscular layers (referring here, no doubt, to the "conjoined tendon," or the transversus abdominis arch). All sutures were placed, then tied, beginning with the medial suture — since the tension would be the least — and continuing in order to the most lateral suture.

Mahorner and Goss have confirmed the observation that Lotheissen, in 1898, was the first to recognize that Poupart's ligament could be destroyed by repeated failures at surgical repair of inguinal hernias. No doubt, Lotheissen also was the first surgeon to deal successfully with a recurrent hernia following destruction of the inguinal ligament and unsuccessful earlier repair. In this instance, there was no suitable structure to serve as an anchoring point to which the abdominal wall could be attached. He improvised an operation, not previously described, for a recurrent hernia in which the inguinal ligament had been damaged. Lotheissen acknowledged that Professor Narath of Utrecht, Holland, had obtained very good results using a similar method. Along with his description of the history-making operation, Lotheissen reported that he had performed the operation in 12 cases.

Chronologically, the next outstanding contribution was made by McVay and Anson (1942). They called attention to the anatomic arrangements in the area, demonstrating that the inguinal ligament was not a suitable anchoring structure in the repair of large direct and indirect inguinal hernias since it was not the site of normal insertion for the abdominal wall strata. They emphasized the fact that the superior pubic ligament was the normal place of insertion for the inguinal strata and, furthermore, was strong and readily available. Thus, McVay and Anson contributed an anatomic basis for an operative technique devised by Lotheissen. In addition, McVay made the valuable contribution of popularizing the repair known as the Lotheissen-McVay repair.

A more recent contribution was made in 1962 by Mahorner and Goss who described in some detail their patients with recurrent inguinofemoral hernias. One patient, aged 64, had bilateral recurrent hernias after three attempts at repair. The left recurrent hernia was large, and the hand could be slipped over the pubic ramus. The second patient was 56 years old and worked as a keeper of whooping cranes in the Audubon Park Zoo in New Orleans. He had had two attempts at bilateral repair and later had third and fourth repairs on the left side. In the process, he lost both testicles. The similarities between these cases and those which I have encountered are striking.

Both hernias were repaired with dermal grafts. Mahorner and Goss attached the graft to transversalis fascia, the iliopsoas fascia, and the lateral remnants of Poupart's ligament. Both repairs were considered successful. While I agree with the principles of repair, I consider the use of dermal grafts obsolete in hernia repair.

In the remainder of the chapter, the focus of the discussion will be on the clinical and surgical aspects of recurrent inguinofemoral hernias, as demonstrated by 12 patients operated upon at the Henry Ford Hospital, along with a description of recommended repair techniques. Case histories of four individuals with this type of hernia are also provided.

## CLINICAL FEATURES OF RECURRENT INGUINOFEMORAL HERNIA

Certain aspects of large recurrent inguinal, femoral, and lower abdominal hernias are of interest. The sex incidence among the 12 patients being considered in this chapter is that usually seen in hernia cases. Of the total operated upon, 10 were men and only two were women.

The age incidence reveals that this type of hernia occurred most often in adult males. The ages of the 12 patients ranged from 42 years to 80 years; six of them were in the sixth decade of life.

The initial diagnoses leading to the first operation were as follows: inguinal hernia in eight patients, femoral hernia in two patients, carcinoma of the vulva in one patient, and malignant testicular tumor in the remaining patient.

## Initial Operative Procedures

The initial operative procedure most commonly performed was repair of an inguinal or femoral hernia. No single operative procedure appeared to be dominant. Some of the repairs had originally been performed at other hospitals, and the precise method of reconstruction could not be determined. I could not implicate any single operative technique of repair as contributing to the eventual formation of a recurrent inguinofemoral hernia. Destructive operative procedures, on the other hand, appeared to be definite factors in the formation of such hernias. One patient had had a radical vulvectomy and lymphadenectomy for squamous cell carcinoma at another hospital (Fig. 19–2). Another patient had had an orchidectomy for a malignant testicular tumor performed elsewhere, and recurrence of the malignancy required local re-excision and radical lymphadenectomy. He then developed a huge inguinofemoral hernia.

## Subsequent Operative Procedures

It is impossible to describe in detail the various operative procedures employed in repairing the recurrent hernias in the 12 patients. Two of the patients had had two previous repairs, six had had three previous repairs, and three had had four repairs. The remaining patient still had a recurrence after seven repairs! (Unfortunately, some of the previous repairs in this individual had been performed at the Henry Ford Hospital.)

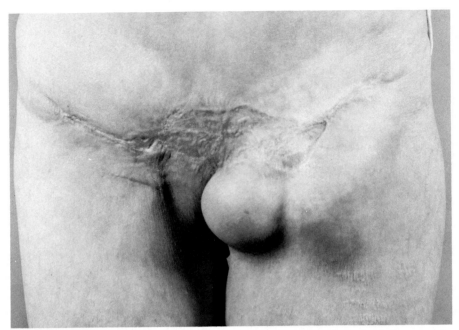

**Figure 19–2.**   Another example of a recurrent inguinofemoral hernia in which the defect occupies the lower abdomen and upper thigh. The patient had undergone a vulvectomy and lymphadenectomy 15 months earlier.

As a result of the necessary manipulation and difficult dissection that is the inevitable result of often-repeated operative procedures, seven of the nine males had lost testicles on the side in which the hernia occurred. In one patient, an orchidectomy had been deliberately performed for a malignancy.

I am of the opinion that these cases are most instructive, for they emphasize that hernia repair, in some patients, may be a formidable undertaking. The surgeon should be able to select an appropriate technique for the individual patient. The late Dr. Henry N. Harkins, one of my teachers whom I remember with fondness and gratitude, explained the situation in one of these patients. As a senior staff surgeon of Henry Ford Hospital, he described his findings and procedure in an operative note dated February, 1941, as follows:

In fact, the whole direct region had prolapsed forward and downward so it was impossible to tell whether this recurrence was a new femoral or whether it was a new direct recurrence. We could find no trace of Poupart's ligament whatsoever. Of all the cases that I have seen, this is certainly an argument for the McVay procedure.

This patient's repair remained secure throughout a follow-up period of 17 years.

In four patients, the Lotheissen-McVay procedure proved effective in curing their complicated hernias. However, in the remaining eight patients, a synthetic mesh was required to replace the destroyed portion of the abdominal wall. Follow-up observations continue, covering periods of time from one to 17 years. There have been two known recurrences.

## GENERAL PRINCIPLES OF REPAIR

Repairing the recurrent inguinofemoral hernia requires improvisation. I can think of three possible methods of repair. In one method, the smaller hernias that protrude through the abdomen and into the upper thigh may be repaired satisfactorily by the Lotheissen-McVay technique. This procedure is described in Chapter 15, on the femoral hernia. A properly made relaxing incision is an important adjunct. In some cases, the second method—the preperitoneal approach—may be applicable, but only if the abdominal wall is in reasonably good condition. The third method, which I have used with success in the treatment of the largest and often-recurring inguinofemoral hernia, calls for the use of a synthetic mesh. Fascia probably could be used as well. I will confine my remarks to the huge recurrent inguinofemoral hernia in which the loss of tissue is so great and scarring so heavy as to preclude the Lotheissen-McVay repair or the preperitoneal approach.

### Recommended Technique for Repair of Large Recurrent Inguinofemoral Hernias

Particular care must be given to preparation of the skin of the lower abdomen and groin, since at times maceration and ulceration are present. Bed rest, compresses, exposure to a drying light, and antibiotics may be used in individual cases. Bathing with pHisoHex on several occasions during the preoperative period is insisted upon. Prior to operation, the skin is prepared with 70 per cent alcohol and one other germicide.

The skin incision is made so as to excise the heavy excess skin and cicatrix. This is always an individual matter, and a decision as to the specific type of incision must be made at the time of the operative procedure. Scalpel dissection is mandatory, since tissue planes have largely been obliterated, and heavy scarring is usually present. Careful hemostasis is essential. All vessels must be secured with fine suture material. I prefer number 4–0 silk, but fine catgut is acceptable.

Exploration is completed before any further decisions can be made. The inguinal ligament is typically absent. The hernial sac extends over Cooper's ligament into the upper thigh (Fig. 19–3). Medially, the rectus abdominis and rectus sheath are usually intact. Above, the laminae of the abdominal wall are strong, but the distance between these layers and Cooper's ligament is often too great to permit their coadaptation. There is no semblance of the normal transversus abdominis arch or the conjoined tendon.

The periotoneal sac is freed from all surrounding structures and closed with interrupted figure-of-eight chromic catgut.

At this point, the important anatomic structures must be visualized. Medially and inferiorly, Cooper's ligament and the pectineus muscle must be clearly identified. The dissection is carried to the femoral vein. A good length of the external iliac artery and vein may be easily seen. The dissection is carried out laterally, where the relatively thin fascia may be seen overlying the iliacus muscle. The lateral margin or fragment of the inguinal ligament may or may not be seen, depending upon the extent of its destruction. The region of the anterior superior iliac spine is easily identified. Throughout the dissection, the use of touch is not to be forgotten. The dissection is completed so that an effective anchoring surface is provided above and toward the midline.

The peritoneum and transversalis fascia are first closed with number 3–0 chromic catgut. Anteriorly and medially, the mesh must be attached beneath the rectus, the rectus abdominis muscle, and the anterior sheath, because these structures provide an excellent barrier and effective anchoring structure. Superiorly, some portions of the transversus abdominis and internal oblique muscles contribute strength and serve as anchoring structures. Inferiorly, the mesh is easily anchored to Cooper's ligament and to the fibrous periosteum over the symphysis pubis. The structures are strong, usually available, and serve as formidable anchoring structures. As the attachment proceeds laterally, the transversalis fascia must be used. The placement of the sutures must be accurate. The femoral nerve and the lateral femoral cutaneous nerve must not be injured. Since the transversalis fascia is rather attenuated here, wide but superficial placement of sutures in the transversalis fascia and fascia overlying the iliopsoas muscle is essential.

Either chromic catgut or synthetic sutures, number 2–0 or number 3–0 in size, are acceptable. Laterally, the mesh is attached to the anterior superior iliac spine. It can be seen that the mesh is attached firmly under slight tension from the anterior superior iliac spine to Cooper's ligament and to the pubic tubercle medially (Fig. 19–4).

The prosthesis that is implanted extends below from the anterior superior iliac spine to the pubic tubercle inferiorly. It is anchored to Cooper's ligament as well. Medially, it nearly reaches the midline

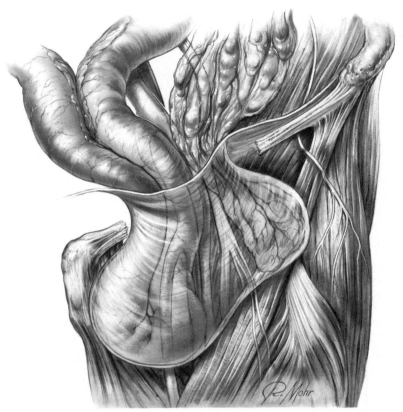

**Figure 19–3.**    This illustration shows the relationship of the hernia to the upper thigh. The femoral vessels, the femoral nerve, and the lateral femoral cutaneous nerve are structures to be identified and preserved.

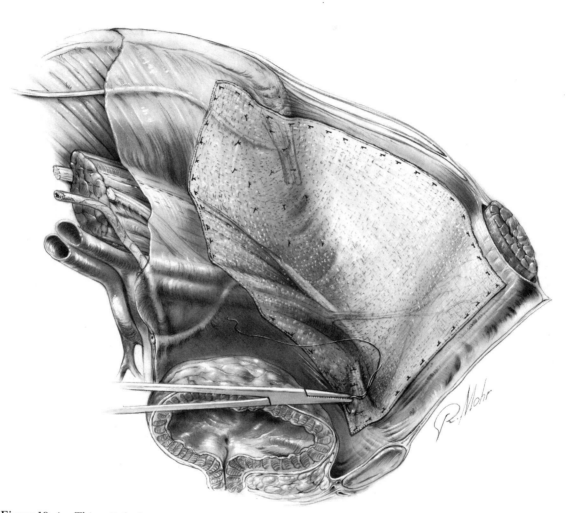

**Figure 19–4.** This artist's drawing shows the extent of the defect and its repair with mesh. Attachment is made below to the anterior superior iliac spine, the pubic tubercle, and Cooper's ligament. Laterally, numerous interrupted sutures are carefully placed into the iliopectineal fascia. Superiorly, the mesh is sutured to available musculoaponeurotic structures. Medially, the rectus abdominis fascia provides a strong anchoring structure. The mesh is placed in a retroperitoneal position whenever possible.

and is attached beneath the rectus muscle. Above, or superiorly, it lies on the peritoneum and is sutured to the remains of the transversus abdominis and internal oblique muscular layers. Laterally, it lies on the peritoneum and is sutured to available musculoaponeurotic structures of the transversus abdominis and internal oblique muscles.

## CASE HISTORIES OF RECURRENT INGUINOFEMORAL HERNIA

The clinical course of the patient with recurrent inguinofemoral hernia is so complicated that the use of typical individual case reports may prove instructive.

### Case History 1

The patient, a male 74 years of age, had previously undergone surgery elsewhere for repair of right and left inguinal hernias. The left inguinal hernia had been repaired 20 years after a surgical repair of the right groin hernia. When first seen at the Henry Ford Hospital, the patient had a left recurrent indirect, direct, and femoral hernia. He was found to have generalized arteriosclerosis, benign prostatic hypertrophy, emphysema, and diverticulosis.

The combined type of groin hernia was repaired by the Bassini-Halsted technique. No master stitch was used, and no relaxing incision was made in the anterior sheath of the rectus abdominis muscle. The patient developed a wound hematoma postoperatively, which required drainage.

The hernia reappeared within three years as a direct and femoral recurrence. The protrusion near the pubic spine was of moderate size. A definite femoral hernia was present as well. The scarring in the area was extensive. The testicle was atrophic. Orchidectomy was performed and the Lotheissen-McVay principle was utilized in the repair. The patient again developed a wound hematoma, which required drainage, and also developed a moderately severe anginal attack, which responded to therapy.

He developed a third recurrence of the left groin hernia at the age of 84, requiring a fourth repair. Now the problem was acute, with incarceration being present.

At this time, I was consulted, and implantation of polypropylene mesh (Marlex) was advised. It was attached inferiorly to the anterior superior spine, to the pubic tubercle, and to Cooper's ligament. Superiorly, it was implanted beneath the transversus abdominis and the internal oblique muscles. Medially, it was placed beneath the rectus abdominis muscle. The external oblique aponeurosis was sutured over the mesh. Atelectasis and ileus required treatment in the postoperative period. This repair remained strong until the patient died, three years later, of advanced cardiovascular disease secondary to arteriosclerosis.

### Case History 2

This patient was referred for repair of a recurrent inguinofemoral hernia after her surgeon had been forced to repair an incarcerated right femoral hernia. His referring letter described the operative situation and genesis of the hernia as follows:

A great deal of difficulty was encountered in trying to reduce the incarcerated bowel. It was necessary to transect the inguinal ligament in order to free the darkened and edematous bowel. The question arose as to whether resection should be done, but with the application of warm packs the pink color returned, and it was determined that the viable bowel could be safely returned to the peritoneal cavity. A repair was then accomplished but in view of the fact that the inguinal ligament was transected there was some difficulty in reapproximating it and getting an adequate repair.

The surgeon was called upon to repair a right recurrent femoral hernia in the same individual within two years. When the hernia again recurred, I had the opportunity of seeing the patient.

In this healthy woman, 42 years of age, repair was not technically complicated. A Lotheissen-McVay repair was performed with success and was still intact at a follow-up examination nine years later. It was this type of hernia that Lotheissen first described in his method of repair in 1897.

Coincidentally, his patient also had undergone hernia repairs on two previous occasions.

## Repair with Synthetic Mesh: Case History 3

This patient was a 62-year-old female who had undergone radical vulvectomy and inguinal node dissection for squamous cell carcinoma. In less than one year, she had had two attempts at repair of a large hernia occupying the left lower abdomen and upper thigh (see Fig. 19–2). The repair will be described in some detail.

The skin of the abdomen and the upper left thigh were thoroughly prepared with hexachlorophene, ether, and alcohol. The incision was made, approximately 5 cm above the inguinal ligament, from a point above the anterior superior iliac spine to the midline. Skin towels were clipped in position in order to protect the wound against contamination. Bleeding points were ligated with fine silk. The incision was developed through the external oblique muscle and fascia and the anterior sheath of the rectus. The remaining portions of the internal oblique and transversus abdominis muscles were divided. The anterior sheath of the rectus muscles was divided. This permitted division of the posterior rectus sheath after retracting the rectus muscle medially.

The peritoneal cavity was entered and the abdomen explored. The viscera were normal, and the rest of the exploration was aimed at discovering residual or metastatic malignancy. None was found.

The peritoneal sac was dissected free. It extended over Cooper's ligament into the medial aspect of the left thigh. There was no identifiable inguinal ligament; it had been sacrificed at the time of the previous vulvectomy and radical groin dissection. The dissection of the sac in some areas was at the level of the dermis. In other areas, the sac was overlain by subcutaneous fat in the upper thigh (see Fig. 19–3).

Laterally, the large sac found its way under the deep fascia of the thigh and under the iliacus and psoas muscles and their fascial layers. The peritoneal sac extended into the thigh for a distance of 6 cm medially and 8 to 10 cm laterally. Small intestine was adherent to the sac in one area, but separation was easily accomplished.

After complete separation of the sac, a part of the iliacus muscle could be seen laterally, and the psoas and pectineus muscles could be seen medially. Cooper's ligament was easily identified, as were the femoral vein, femoral artery, and femoral nerve from the medial to the lateral positions (Fig. 19–4). The lateral femoral cutaneous nerve and the deep circumflex iliac artery were easily identified and preserved.

Repair commenced by closure of the peritoneal sac. This was accomplished with interrupted sutures of number 2–0 chromic catgut. It was essential to provide support for the lower left abdomen so that the intestinal contents could be prevented from descending into the thigh. Marlex mesh in a sheet measuring approximately $15 \times 12$ cm was sutured in position. It was anchored medially to the pubic tubercle and Cooper's ligament (see Fig. 19–4). Care was taken to anchor the mesh, with number 2–0 chromic catgut, very near to the femoral vein to avoid a femoral recurrent hernia. Posteriorly, the mesh was sutured to the fascia overlying the iliacus and psoas muscles. Laterally, the mesh was attached to the anterior superior iliac spine. The large sheet of mesh was sutured above to the posterior rectus sheath and the transversus and internal oblique muscles. The mesh was fixed in position exterior to the peritoneum. Laterally, it was possible to attach the synthetic mesh to the remaining transversus abdominis and internal oblique muscles. The fascia of the external oblique was closed over the mesh, as was the anterior sheath of the rectus. The skin was closed with fine silk sutures.

A small rubber drain was delivered through the most dependent portion of the dissection in the thigh. A spica type of pressure dressing was then applied. The patient tolerated the procedure well. Her postoperative course was remarkably benign, and her wound healed satisfactorily (Fig. 19–5, A and B). She has been followed for three years without recurrence of her hernia or tumor. She did

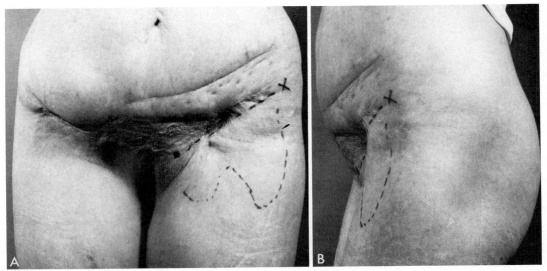

**Figure 19–5.** *A,* This postoperative view shows the anterior of the lower abdomen and upper thigh of the patient shown preoperatively in Figure 19–2. *B,* Lateral view of the postoperative result obtained in the same patient.

complain of pain in the operative site, but this was controlled with nonnarcotic analgesics.

### Case History 4

An obese male, 52 years of age, was referred with a huge inguinofemoral hernia occupying the right lower abdomen and upper thigh. He had had an orchidectomy for a malignant testicular tumor six years earlier. This was followed by a recurrence of the tumor, requiring re-excision. He subsequently had radiotherapy to the right lower abdomen. Eventually, a large hernia developed, and the loss of tissue forced the surgeons to employ a pedicle graft in order to cover the area.

With recurrence of the hernia, the patient was referred for repair. It was necessary to prepare the skin overlying the hernia that had ulcerated; this was done through the use of tub baths, pHisoHex, and exposure to the drying effects of a bedside light.

The operative procedure consisted of excision of a portion of the redundant skin and placement of the Marlex mesh. Dissection of the bladder was difficult, and the bladder was inadvertently entered during the operative procedure. The defect was carefully closed, and an indwelling cath-

eter was placed in the bladder postoperatively. The mesh was sutured below to the pubic tubercle, to Cooper's ligament, and to the anterior superior iliac spine. Because of poor vascularity in the area, a pedicle was fashioned from the omentum and delivered through a transverse opening in the abdominal wall, lateral to the umbilicus. The mesh was sutured beneath the rectus muscle medially, and under the transversus abdominis and internal oblique muscles laterally and superiorly. The omental pedicle was sutured in place over the mesh. The skin was then closed with number 4–0 nylon sutures. Suction drainage was employed to continually aspirate the area of operation.

The postoperative course was complicated by a vesicocutaneous fistula, which required operative repair. Healing was slow but quite satisfactory. The repair of this huge hernia was secure one year after repair, although a small ulcerated area remained.

### RESULTS

The 12 hernia cases that I have described in this chapter were difficult to repair. Two patients have died, one of arteriosclerotic heart disease and one of carcinoma. There had been no recurrence of the hernia in either individual. Two more patients were followed for one year without recurrence. Other patients were followed for periods of five, five, six, seven, nine, and 17 years without reappearance of herniation. Unfortunately, in the remaining two patients, the repairs did not remain secure, but the subsequent protrusions were much smaller in size when compared to the original hernias.

## SUMMARY

The type of hernia occurring in the inguinoabdominal area and resulting from numerous previous operative repairs or excisional therapy in the groin is designated a recurrent inguinofemoral hernia. This hernia was first recognized by Lotheissen, and an appropriate method of repair was devised. McVay placed the principles of repair on a sound anatomic basis. The Lotheissen-McVay technique of repair, properly performed, offers excellent prospects of cure. Once excessive destruction of tissue has occurred, placement of a synthetic mesh is unavoidable if repair is to be secure. The recurrent inguinofemoral hernia should be recognized for what it is. Too often it is simply designated as a "recurrent hernia," whereas, in truth, it has both an inguinal and a femoral component. Only those methods of repair dealing with both defects should be utilized.

## REFERENCES

Lotheissen, G.: Zur Radikaloperation der Schenkelhernien. Centralbl. Chir. 25:548, 1898.

McVay, C. B., and Anson, B. J.: Fundamental error in current methods of inguinal herniorrhaphy. Surg. Gynecol. Obstet. 74:746, 1942.

Mahorner, H., and Goss, C. M.: Herniation following destruction of Poupart's and Cooper's ligaments: A method of repair. Ann. Surg. 155:741, 1962.

# 20

# Wound Disruption

One might question the purpose of including a chapter on wound disruption in a book on hernia. It is useful, however, to consider the disrupted abdominal wound as a most dramatic type of "hernia," since in many ways the genesis of wound disruption is similar to that of postoperative herniation. Hence, a better understanding of both these conditions can be achieved through an appreciation of the mechanisms involved in the failure of postoperative wounds to heal normally. Of course, in the patient with complete wound disruption, there is no sac; and, therefore, this entity is not ordinarily considered in works on hernia. On the other hand, innumerable abdominal wounds undergo partial disruption, with skin and subcutaneous tissues remaining intact, and eventually become recognized and accepted as ventral or postoperative hernias. Approximately one-third to one-half of all patients with wound disruptions ultimately develop incisional hernias; the so-called sacs in such hernias often are omentum that has modified its appearance. Incisional hernias are largely iatrogenic in nature; not infrequently, they require repeated operative procedures before being successfully repaired.

In the vast majority of cases, there are many factors contributing to disruption of the postoperative incision. In the exceptional case, a single cause for disruption may exist, but more often the causes are numerous, complex, and interrelated. Thus, an attempt should be made to organize the numerous factors into a comprehensible and useful form that approaches the problem with a "wide-angle lens." For example, carcinoma may lead to malnutrition, hypoproteinemia, and anemia. Nutrition may also be impaired when intestinal, pancreatic, or biliary tract fistulae develop. Infection from any source interferes with wound healing locally, but it may also cause ileus and distention.

## DEFINITION AND DESCRIPTION

A number of terms have been applied to the disconcerting phenomenon of postoperative wound disruption. Among those most commonly used are wound disruption, wound dehiscence, wound separation, and evisceration. In the British literature, one encounters the distressingly clear term of "burst abdomen" for the same event. The term "wound evisceration" is not entirely accurate, since it connotes some degree of disembowelment — certainly prolapse of abdominal viscera through the wound is not always present. I prefer the designation *wound disruption*, since it implies discontinuity of the wound owing to some force.

In *wound disruption*, there is a failure of the postoperative wound to remain anatomically approximated for a sufficient amount of time to permit effective healing; and, because of unusual demands upon such a wound, discontinuity results following increased intra-abdominal and intrathoracic pressure. This disruption may be *partial*, and include only skin and subcutaneous tissues or only the deeper fascial layers. On the other hand, the disruption may be *complete*, and involve all layers. In some instances, intestines protrude through the gaping wound; for these cases, the terms "intestinal prolapse" and "disembowelment" are applicable. Thus, postoperative wound separation may be superficial only in extent, and in such instances the deeper portions of the wound may heal soundly. If the deeper layers (including the peritoneum and transversalis fascia) become separated, then a hernia will follow. The result may not become evident until late in the recovery period; in obese patients, for example, small disruptions may be overlooked for many months. Although wound disruption, wound dehiscence, wound separation, and evisceration are used interchangeably by most surgeons, I am of the opinion that a more accurate definition of terms would be desirable. It is becoming increasingly clear that disruptions occurring within the first four days are largely the result of faulty wound closure techniques. Thus, early disruptions are actually gross failures of the suture technique or the suture material. Disruptions that occur later — i.e., after 10 to 12 days — often appear in the presence of infection, with dissolution of suture material and tissue destruction as the contributing factors.

## INCIDENCE OF WOUND DISRUPTION

The precise incidence of wound disruption or wound dehiscence is difficult to determine accurately. At the Henry Ford Hospital, I have found a number of records in which the description of the immediate postoperative clinical course strongly suggested that the wound had separated beneath the skin; however, since complete disruption had not occurred, these cases were never indexed as "wound disruption." In a few instances, taping of the abdomen was performed on the in-patient floor, and again there was no record of the event in the medical records department. Thus, I suspect that the actual incidence of wound disruption is greater than that indicated by most publications.

Some authors point out that, even with advancement in the knowledge of wound healing and antibiotic therapy, the incidence of wound disruption has not decreased and might even have increased. It should be pointed out that in the past three decades, the magnitude of operative procedures has increased. Older patients with degenerative diseases are being operated on, and the incidence of gunshot and stab wounds has given the surgeon more extensively infected wounds to contend with. Some of the available statistics relative to the incidence of wound disruption are summarized in Table 20–1.

The incidence of disruption was extremely high in patients with carcinoma, as reported by Mendoza and his colleagues (1966). They found 21 wound disruptions in 291 patients for an incidence of 7.0 percent. Campbell and Swenson (1972) found the incidence of disruption in infants and children to be significant. In 2,692 operations there were 26 dehiscences in pediatric patients for an incidence of 0.97 percent. In the brief survey shown in Table 2–1, the reported incidence of wound

### Table 20–1.  INCIDENCE OF WOUND DISRUPTION

| Authors (Selected at Random) | Year | Laparotomy Incisions | Dehiscence Reported | Percent | Percent Mortality |
|---|---|---|---|---|---|
| FALLIS | 1937 | 7,903 | 50 | 0.64 | 34.0 |
| NORRIS | 1939 | 2,316 | 13 | 0.56 | — |
| GLENN AND MOORE | 1941 | 6,417 | 43 | 0.66 | — |
| DEL JUNCO AND LANGE | 1956 | 11,334 | 40 | 0.35 | — |
| MANN ET AL. | 1962 | 3,988 | 109 | 2.73 | 23.0 |
| HAMPTON | 1963 | 30,610 | 120 | 0.39 | 23.0 |
| GUINEY ET AL. | 1964 | 37,888 | 235 | 0.61 | 15.0 |
| FISH | 1964 | 7,235 | 64 | 0.90 | 19.0 |
| MENDOZA ET AL. | 1966 | 291 | 21 | 7.00 | — |
| LEHMAN | 1968 | 2,081 | 53 | 2.50 | 17.7 |
| HIGGINS ET AL. | 1969 | 2,377 | 51 | 2.20 | — |
| CAMPBELL AND SWENSON | 1972 | 2,692 | 26 | 0.97 | — |
| KEILL ET AL. | 1973 | 4,242 | 47 | 1.11 | 29.8 |

disruption was found to vary from 0.39 percent to 7.0 percent. Many authors place the incidence at approximately one percent. It is important to remember that in selected patients with advanced malignancies, the incidence is much higher.

## CLINICAL CONDITIONS SEEN IN PATIENTS WITH POSTOPERATIVE WOUND DISRUPTIONS

There are a number of diseases and clinical conditions often seen in patients who eventually suffer from wound disruption. These conditions are operative, in varying degrees, in individual patients — making it difficult to assess precisely what part they play in dehiscence. In most cases a number of factors contribute to the complications. As a result, there is some controversy as to the exact significance of certain diseases and clinical states in the genesis of wound dehiscence. These conditions, which are listed for quick reference in Table 20–2, will be discussed only briefly.

### Age Incidence

Without exception, investigators agree that wound dehiscence occurs far more frequently in elderly patients than in other age groups. Wolff (1950) divided his patients into two groups consisting of those above or below 45 years of age. In the group under 45 years of age, there were 14 disruptions in 1,115 operative procedures for an incidence of 1.3 percent. In patients

**Table 20–2. CLINICAL CONDITIONS OFTEN SEEN IN PATIENTS WITH WOUND DISRUPTIONS**

| | |
|---|---|
| 1. Age | 7. Gastrointestinal tract |
| 2. Sex |    diseases |
| 3. Malnutrition |   A. peptic ulcer |
| 4. Infection |   B. inflammatory |
|   A. wound |      disease |
|   B. intra-abdominal |   C. carcinoma |
| 5. Respiratory tract |   D. biliary tract disease |
|   Infection | 8. Obesity |
| 6. Malignancies | 9. Laennec's cirrhosis |
|   A. colon | 10. Diabetes Mellitus |
|   B. stomach | 11. Cardiac Diseases |
|   C. pancreas | 12. Hypothyroidism |
|   D. pelvic organs | |

above 45 years of age there were 31 wound dehiscences among 585 operations for an incidence of 5.4 percent. Thus, older patients were found to suffer wound disruptions four times more often than younger patients. Reitamo and Möller (1972) found that most dehiscences occurred in the fifth, sixth, and seventh decades of life. Glenn and Moore (1941) found that the majority of disruptions occurred in the fifth and sixth decades. Hartzell and Winfield (1939) reported a similar age incidence. Nevertheless, wound dehiscences do occur in infants and children. Campbell and Swenson (1972) studied the problem in 2,692 patients and found the incidence of disruption to be 0.97 percent.

It can be concluded that any patient, under the appropriate conditions, might suffer from disruption of an operative wound, but the event is far more likely to occur in the older or aged patient. Advanced disease, malignancies, malnutrition, and pulmonary disease may coexist in the geriatric patient whose wound-healing potential is impaired because of aging.

### Sex Incidence

Many studies consistently report that wound dehiscences occur most frequently in males. Wolff has correctly pointed out that the total number of operations performed in males and females is not available ordinarily; hence, the validity of the reported higher incidence in males is questionable. Nevertheless, from a practical point of view, the surgeon should be aware of the danger of wound disruption following operative procedures in men. The incidence will vary somewhat, depending upon the type of patient being operated upon. For example, Veterans' Administration hospitals can certainly be expected to report a higher incidence of disruption in men than in women or children.

Fallis (1937) reported that 55 percent of 49 wound disruptions occurred in males. Alexander and Prudden (1966), in studying 200 wound disruptions, found that 112, or 56 percent, occurred in men. Guiney, Morris, and Donaldson (1966) reported 76 percent of their cases of wound dehiscences occurred in men. Keill, Nichols, and De Weese (1973) analyzed 47 patients with "burst abdomens" and found that 33, or 70.2 percent, were seen in males. Hampton (1963) studied the problem in somewhat more detail; in 30,610 operations, he found 120 "burst abdomens." There were 13,650 operations with 82 disruptions in men for an operative incidence of 0.60 percent and 16,900 operative procedures with 38 disruptions in women for an incidence of 0.19 percent. Culp (1934), Glenn and Moore (1941), Meleny and Howes (1934), and Hartzell and Winfield (1939) all reported a preponderance of wound disruptions in men. Reitamo and Möller found the male/female ratio to be 2.8:1.

It becomes very clear that the danger of disruption of laparotomy wounds is significantly and consistently greater in males than in females. It has been suggested that the greater muscular strength of males is a factor, since the disrupting force due to coughing or straining is enormous. This knowledge indicates that heavier suture material and retention sutures are needed for closing incisions in muscular male patients.

serving as an Army Medical Officer in Manila, Philippine Islands, during World War II, I saw returning prisoners of war who were so gaunt and thin that they had the appearance of a skeleton, yet their operative wounds healed. This does not mean that serious and prolonged starvation has no adverse effect on the healing of wounds and on patient recovery. There are specific deficiencies that occur in some patients with malnutrition, including anemia, hypoproteinemia, and vitamin depletion (Fig. 20–1). These deficiencies are so important that they will be considered individually in this chapter.

According to del Junco and Lange (1956), constitutional disease would have little effect on wound healing, provided that malnutrition, dehydration, anemia, hypoproteinemia, or vitamin deficiencies were not present. Supporting this view in another study, Joergenson and Smith (1950) found a catabolic state in 48.3 percent of 97 patients with wound disruption. Moore (1959) noted that wounds will heal to completeness, even in the presence of preoperative starvation.

## Malnutrition

The term "malnutrition" is so all-inclusive as to be unsatisfactory. We have all seen patients who are practically cachectic recover from operative procedures. While

## Infection

The informed surgeon should be aware of the destructive effects of bacteria on the operative wound as identified by Altemeier (1966) and by Meleny and Howes (1934).

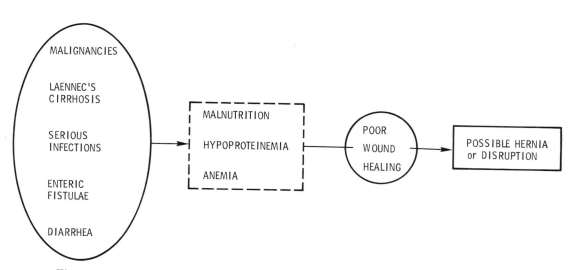

**Figure 20–1.** Several disease states interfere with nutrition and affect the healing wound.

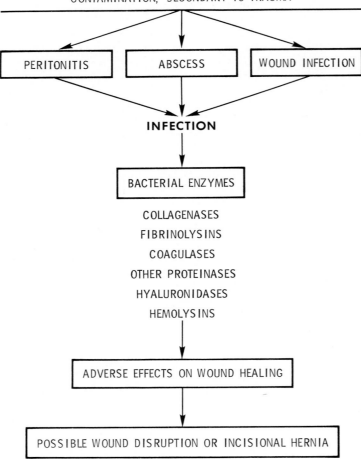

Figure 20-2. Infection seriously interferes with the healing wound through a number of destructive enzymatic actions.

In the context of this discussion, I cannot describe these effects in detail, but a few must be recalled (Fig. 20–2).

Bacteria produce a variety of enzymes that are deleterious to the healing process. Necrotizing enzymes cause death of tissues; collagenases may decrease the production of or actually destroy collagen. Fibrinolysins or streptokinases interfere with a fundamental process in wound healing through the destruction of fibrin. To aid in dissemination of the organisms, bacteria produce hyaluronidases. While these processes are in force, other enzymes, such as coagulases, cause thrombosis of blood vessels in the infected wound, further interfering with repair. In addition, bacteria produce hemolysins, which cause hemolysis of red blood cells, and other enzymes that interfere with the ability of hemoglobin to deliver oxygen.

In general, there are two distinct avenues by which bacteria establish themselves in the surgical patient. One group of organisms reaches the operative wound as a result of contamination of the site with skin flora. Staphylococci may enter the wound from the patient's skin in the operative area or from the surgeon's skin through a perforation in the glove. The other group of organisms are of enteric origin. The organisms cultured from these wounds include *Streptococcus fecalis, Escherichia coli, Klebsiella, Pseudomonas* and *Proteus* species. These organisms may appear in the wound from gross contamination that occurs during intestinal surgery, following perforated viscera, or following gunshot wounds or traumatic rupture of hollow viscera.

The exact incidence of wound infection is difficult to determine because of the great variation in reported statistics. Keill and colleagues (1973) reported infection to be present in 34, or 72.3 percent of 47 patients with wound disruption. Fallis (1937) found the incidence of infection to be 20 percent, while Reitamo and Möller (1972) reported an incidence of 37 percent. Del Junco and Lange (1956) found that 14.7 percent of their patients with disruption had infections, and Tweedie and Long (1954) reported the incidence to be 13 percent. Guiney and coworkers (1966) reported a low incidence of 11 infections in 87 wound disruptions. Marsh, Coxe, Ross, and Stevens (1954) reported that dehiscence occurred in 9.3 percent of contaminated vertical incisions, but 5 percent of clean vertical incisions also disrupted.

There is little doubt that the contaminated or grossly infected wound heals more precariously than the clean one. In any patient with gross contamination, such as occurs in a perforated viscus or a gunshot wound with visceral injury, particular care must be taken in wound closure. Nonabsorbable and retention sutures are indi-

cated. Delayed closure of the skin and subcutaneous tissues is good practice in selected cases.

**Respiratory Tract Disease**

The adverse effects of coughing on the healing wound are well appreciated by many investigators. A number of conditions may result in wound disruption brought on by great increases in intra-abdominal pressure (Fig. 20–3). Lam (1939) studied the problem, as did Kewenter and Koch (1969). The two colleagues investigated the effects of coughing by placing a balloon in the peritoneal cavity during an operative procedure. Highest pressures were recorded during bronchial toilette prior to extubation after general anesthesia. Increased intra-abdominal pressures were recorded during coughing and straining.

Light and Routledge (1965) studied the intra-abdominal pressure in 50 male surgical patients. The method was an ingenious one in which a balloon was attached to a rectal tube inserted at least 15 centimeters into the rectum. The balloon was inflated, and various maneuvers were carried out in order to increase the intra-abdominal pressure. The two researchers found that the Valsalva maneuver and coughing consistently produced the highest pressures.

Drye (1948) placed a rubber condom that

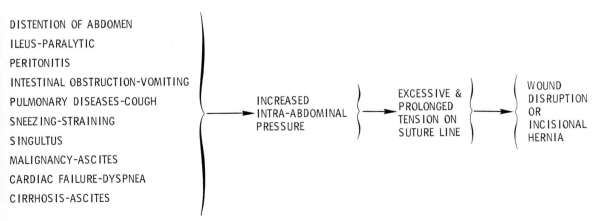

**Figure 20–3.** Exciting causes of wound disruption are numerous; they result in an increased intra-abdominal pressure, which places an additional distracting force upon the closed incision.

was connected to a manometer via a urethral catheter into the peritoneal cavity at abdominal laparotomy. During vomiting and coughing, the pressure reached from 80 to 150 centimeters of water. Getting out of bed resulted in a recorded pressure of 29 centimeters and walking produced a pressure of 18 centimeters of water.

Lord, Pfeffer, and Golomb (1969) pointed out that at the time of recovery and during the ensuing struggle, great stress was placed upon an abdominal incision. They suggested that the most important disruptive forces are coughing, sneezing, and vomiting. Paralytic ileus with distention also added to the stress placed upon the wound closure. Tweedie and Long noted coughing, distention, and vomiting to be the causes of increased intra-abdominal pressure in approximately 75 percent of their cases of disruption.

Patients with acute or chronic lung disease, such as pneumonia, atelectasis, emphysema, bronchitis, and asthma, are commonly found in statistical studies dealing with wound disruption. The adverse effect of a severe chronic cough on the healing wound is recognized by students of the subject. Sedgwick and Sullivan (1957) found that the pre-evisceration symptom of coughing occurred in 73 out of a total 170 patients. They found atelectasis in 24, bronchitis in 12, pneumonia in 5, and emphysema in 4 patients. Joergenson and Smith found respiratory disease to be present in 12.3 percent of their patients with wound evisceration. Alexander and Prudden found pulmonary complications in 24 percent of their patients prior to disruption. Guiney and colleagues found the incidence of tracheopulmonary disease to be 13 percent in patients who suffered from wound dehiscence, while in a control group of patients, the incidence was only 2 percent.

Pulmonary dysfunction or infection is a relatively common finding in patients who are about to disrupt abdominal incisions. The exact incidence is difficult to determine, but reports in the literature range from 12 to 75 percent. Careful investigations should be carried out to determine the presence of pulmonary disease prior to performance of major operative procedures, and treatment should be instituted before carrying out elective surgical operations.

## Malignancy

It is extremely difficult to indict malignancy per se as a cause of wound disruption. Nevertheless, carcinoma is a common pathologic state found in patients with wound disruptions. Patients with advanced malignancies may be suffering from hypoproteinemia, anemia, dehydration, and weight loss due to inadequate food intake.

Sedgwick and Sullivan found that of 217 patients with wound dehiscence, 93 had malignant diseases. Glenn and Moore (1941) noted that wound disruption occurred almost three times more often in patients with malignancies. Marsh and his colleagues (1954) were convinced that nutritional deficiencies incident to carcinoma were important predisposing factors to wound dehiscence. In a study by del Junco and Lange (1956), malignancy was present in 32.5 percent of 40 patients who suffered from postoperative wound dehiscence. Additional reported figures concerning the incidence of malignancy in patients with wound disruption are as follows: Hartzell and Winfield (1939), 22 percent; Wolff (1950), 38 percent; Mann and colleagues (1962), 20 percent; Reitamo and Möller (1972), 39 percent; Tweedie and Long (1954), 21 percent; and Joergenson and Smith (1950), 27.8 percent.

Malignancy of some type is found in 20 to 40 percent of patients who eventually develop the "burst abdomen." A combination of factors have a bearing on this complication. Generally, patients with malignancies are likely to be elderly. They may be malnourished and anemic. Furthermore, if the tumor is large, extensive and prolonged operations may be necessary. These patients also are likely to have pulmonary disease.

Strong nonabsorbable sutures and nonabsorbable retention sutures are both recommended to reduce the incidence of disruption in patients with malignant disease.

## Gastrointestinal Tract Disease and Wound Disruption

Diseases of the gastrointestinal tract lead to operative procedures that too often lead to wound disruption. Surgical operations of the stomach, colon, and biliary tract, performed for a variety of reasons, may be followed by dehiscence.

Mann and coworkers found that more than 50 percent of 109 patients with disruption had operations performed upon the upper gastrointestinal tract (e.g., stomach, duodenum, and biliary tract). Del Junco and Lange found that 45 percent of disruptions in their study occurred in patients operated upon for gastroduodenal pathology and biliary tract disease. In Fallis' series, 35 percent had biliary tract or gastric surgical procedures, while Reitamo and Möller found that 77 percent of their patients with disruptions had undergone surgical operations of the gastrointestinal tract.

There are a number of reasons why patients who undergo operations for gastrointestinal tract disorders might suffer from wound disruption. Nutrition may be impaired in prolonged illnesses. Infection is not a rare event following operations upon the stomach, colon, or biliary tract. If peritonitis develops, ileus causes an increase in intra-abdominal pressure. Pulmonary complications further increase the possibility of disruption.

Care in closure of vertical upper abdominal operations is essential if the danger of dehiscence is to be minimized. Use of nonabsorbable retention sutures and mass closure techniques with wire or synthetic nonabsorbable sutures are measures that will reduce this serious complication.

## Obesity

Whether obesity of itself affects wound healing adversely can be debated. Surgeons are conscious of the frequency of incisional hernias and wound complications in obese individuals. However, there is no proof that obesity per se interferes with the biologic process of healing. Reitamo and Möller found obesity to be present in 14 percent of their patients with disruption. Del Junco and Lange found that 30 percent of their patients with dehiscence were overweight.

There is no doubt that it is technically more difficult to approximate wound edges in a patient with a heavy pendulous abdomen. It actually requires considerable physical strength to draw together the wound edges in a patient whose vertical incision gapes under the distracting force of a heavy panniculus. The thick layer of adipose tissue makes closure of the dead space somewhat more difficult in the obese patient than in the thin patient. Serum and blood may accumulate in the depths of the wound, thus providing optimal conditions for bacterial growth.

In obese patients, particular care must be given to the technique of wound closure. I strongly recommend the use of both nonabsorbable and retention sutures.

## Cirrhosis

Laennec's cirrhosis affects the recovery potential of a patient in several ways. If bleeding is severe, such as from esophageal varices, anemia may be present. If the liver is severely damaged, hypoproteinemia will result. In any series of wound disruptions studied, the relative number of patients with cirrhosis of the liver appears deceptively small, since the overall incidence of Laennec's cirrhosis is not great. Fallis found that 6 percent of the patients he studied had hepatic cirrhosis. Nevertheless, postoperative wounds of cirrhotics are known to heal poorly, since anemia and hypoproteinemia are so often present. Abdominal distention and ascites may create additional problems. Transverse incisions should be used whenever possible. Great care in wound closure, with use of both nonabsorbable sutures and retention sutures, is essential. Caution should be taken against premature removal of sutures.

## Diabetes Mellitus

The surgeon about to operate on a patient with diabetes should be aware of several associated problems. First, the patient is likely to be obese, and this makes the wound closure technically more difficult. Second, diabetics develop wound infection easily, particularly when the diabetes is difficult to control. Third, infection is more difficult to treat in the diabetic, once established. Reitamo and Möller found the incidence of diabetes mellitus to be 10 percent among the patients they studied.

### Hypothyroidism

There is no valid reason today for the existence of a hypothyroid state in a patient, since treatment is easily available and curative. Nevertheless, occasionally a patient with severe hypothyroidism is seen, and an operative procedure may be indicated. Such patients should be treated with thyroid extract until a normal metabolic state is achieved, if possible. The patient's postoperative recovery will be more successful once the metabolism level has reached normal.

### Cardiac Disease

The presence of cardiac disease creates several problems for the surgeon. In all elective operative cases, heart disease is treated to a point of maximal improvement before surgical treatment is initiated.

Patients with heart disease may have edema, ascites, and respiratory difficulty, with resultant increased intra-abdominal pressure. Poor oxygenation of the tissue at the site of the incision is the result of inadequate circulation (Fig. 20–4). The matter of circulation to the operative site and the adequacy of oxygenation to the

healing wound are currently subjects of great interest to research workers as well as clinical surgeons.

## WOUND HEALING AND WOUND DISRUPTION

The surgeon cannot possibly treat hernias and wound disruptions without an appreciation of not only how but also when operative incisions heal. Hence, I will briefly review the most important and recent ideas on the subject and provide a bibliography for further reading.

The surgeon must take advantage of the propensity of each patient to heal wounds and incisions. He must acknowledge that he has a great capability to interfere with the healing process but little or no ability to accelerate it. Therefore, it behooves the surgeon to provide the optimal circumstances for healing of the operative wound. In some patients, such as those undergoing deep x-ray therapy, healing is definitely impaired as a result of radiation changes in the tissues.

We must consider two facets of the phenomenon of wound healing: the biologic events of healing and the effect of those events on the tensile strength of the incised

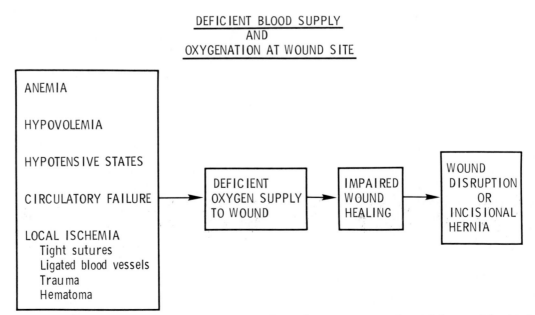

**Figure 20–4.**   The interrelationship of anemia, hypovolemia, hypotension, circulatory failure, and local ischemia is complicated, but a deficient delivery of oxygen at the site of the wound interferes with healing.

### Table 20–3. PHASES OF WOUND HEALING

PHASE I   SUBSTRATE

Duration: first to fourth day

Also referred to as *lag, exudative,* or *inflammatory phase.*

PHASE II   FIBROBLASTIC

Duration: fifth to twentieth day

Also referred to as *proliferative, connective tissue,* or *incremental phase.*

PHASE III   STAGE OF DIFFERENTIATION

Duration: twenty-first day up to years

Also referred to as *remodeling, resorptive,* or *plateau phase.*

For practical purposes, the phenomenon of wound healing has been divided into three recognizable phases (Table 20–3); however, the process itself is a continuous one, with one phase proceeding into the next until healing has been achieved. Studies and observations on wound healing carried out by Howes and Harvey (1929), Howes and colleagues (1929), Localio and colleagues (1948), Sandblom (1944), Douglas (1972), Dunphy (1960), and Peacock (1962). Two excellent works have been recently published on the subject of wound healing; Peacock and Van Winkle (1970) have written on the surgery and biology of wound repair, and Dunphy and Van Winkle (1969) have considered repair and regeneration in some detail. Both texts are highly recommended.

and sutured wound. In regard to healing of abdominal wounds, we are essentially considering the healing of fascial and aponeurotic layers—structures that heal effectively but slowly.

### Substrate Phase

During the first four days, the abdominal wound has practically no holding strength. The wound simply falls apart if the sutures are removed (Fig. 20–5). Nevertheless,

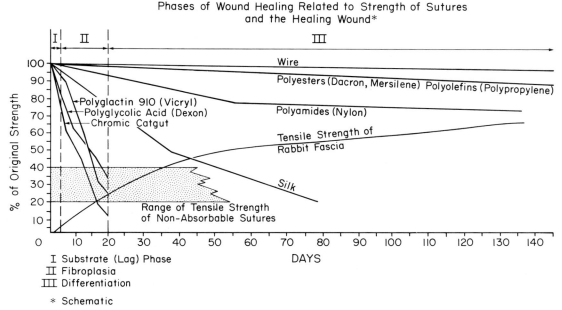

**Figure 20–5.** This complicated schematic illustration is designed to correlate the phases of wound healing with the durability of sutures. Certain sutures—catgut, polyglactin (Vicryl), and polyglycolic acid (Dexon) are absorbed fairly rapidly. They are not to be depended upon where enduring strength is needed. Wire remains strong unless, after a time, it undergoes fragmentation. Silk buried in the wound undergoes gradual loss of strength over a period of weeks. Polyamide sutures (nylon) are intermediate between silk and sutures of polyesters and polyolefins in durability. (Modified after Dunphy, Postlethwait, VanWinkle and Salthouse and Herrmann: "Practical applications of experimental studies in the care of the primarily closed wound. p 276, fig. 3).

during this lag, or inflammatory, period, many changes have occurred in preparation for fibroplasia. Vasoconstriction is followed by vasodilatation, and exudation of plasma protein occurs. Hemostasis takes place with the initial participation of the surgeon, but blood vessels are capable of retraction. The usual mechanisms of blood clotting are operative. Platelet aggregation occurs, fibrinogen is converted to fibrin, and clotting results. In addition, leukocytes enter the area and, through phagocytosis and enzymatic action, remove debris, bacteria, and devitalized tissue. Gross, rough technique, such as using large crushing clamps, encompassing large masses of tissue in hemostats, and ligating with heavy suture material, prolong the substrate phase.

### Fibroblastic Phase

This period lasts from approximately the fifth to the twentieth day. Douglas (1972) called this period the *incremental phase*, while Dunphy (1960) referred to it as the *proliferative phase*. During this period fibroblasts proliferate and are responsible for the increasing strength of the sutured wound. Surgeons must appreciate that during this period the gain in strength of the closed incision is approximately 25 to 30 percent of the original tensile strength of the intact tissues. Douglas (1975) found that 100 days after the wounding occurred, the incision had reached only 30 percent of the strength of normal tissues. Even after one year, the wound had not attained the strength of normal fascia. This point should be emphasized; greater care must be taken in the choice of suture material for those patients in whom wound healing might be expected to proceed slowly. Not many years ago it was taught that wounds heal in three to four weeks. Yet Lichtenstein and his fellow workers (1976) found that after two months of healing the wound regained 70 percent of intact tissue strength. In abdominal incisions, where the closed incision is subjected to pressure, to distention, or to the explosive forces of coughing or vomiting, strong nonabsorbable sutures are needed, since fibroplasia alone cannot provide full holding-strength during the early stages of healing. Abdominal incisions require more than six weeks for

substantial healing. In the meantime, nonabsorbable sutures must provide the needed strength.

### Stage of Differentiation

This stage is also known as the *remodeling phase* and commences after the third week of wounding. During this period, there is reorganization and maturation of the cicatrix. Even after 100 days of healing, the wound has not regained its original tensile strength. It must be repeated that aponeurotic and fascial wounds heal more slowly than is generally recognized. At least three to five months are required to achieve substantial resistance against spreading of the cicatrix. These facts lead us to the use of nonabsorbable sutures, since catgut loses most of its strength in three to four weeks. Even if the period were extended to six weeks, the duration of effective strength would still be too short. Hence, the need for nonabsorbable suture material in closure of abdominal wounds becomes increasingly clear. Furthermore, obese patients and those patients with pulmonary diseases continue to apply great stress to the operative incision. In these situations, nonabsorbable sutures, which possess enduring strength, are essential.

## NUTRITIONAL AND CHEMICAL FACTORS IN WOUND HEALING

There are certain nutritional and chemical factors that have a bearing on wound healing. Their levels in various patients can be influenced by a number of diseases. In some patients, certain therapeutic agents, such as steroids and antimetabolites, may adversely affect wound healing. Specific factors bearing on wound healing include hypoproteinemia, anemia, ascorbic acid deficiency, available oxygen supply, steroid therapy, and antimetabolites. Although important, the clinical role of these factors in wound dehiscence has been overemphasized, in some instances. I will point out the background for some of the opinions held in the past.

Although many individual clinical conditions can be listed as contributing to wound disruption, the number of fundamental metabolic processes that are affected by these diseases is quite small. For instance, carcinoma may cause anemia, hypoproteinemia, and depletion of vitamin C reserves. Ulcerative colitis, severe infections, and intestinal fistulae may cause similar deficiencies. It is important to consider in some detail the effects of anemia, hypoproteinemia, and ascorbic acid deficiency on wound healing, as well as those of massive steroid therapy and chemotherapy.

## Hypoproteinemia

In the experimental laboratory, definite impairment of wound healing under severe depletion of blood protein has been demonstrated by a number of investigators. Clinically, we have observed that even the wounds of poorly nourished patients will heal. Fibroplasia proceeds slowly, likewise the gain in tensile strength of the wound.

Thompson, Ravdin, and Frank (1938) employed an unusual method to induce hypoproteinemia in dogs. Using plasmapheresis, they were able to reduce serum proteins to low levels — a condition that can hardly be duplicated in man. Patients with large intestinal fistulae or with extensive burns might be considered in somewhat comparable circumstances. Thompson and colleagues found that in hypoproteinemic dogs, abdominal wounds healed much more slowly when closed with both silk and catgut. Disruption occurred more often in wounds sutured with catgut.

Abbott and Mellors (1943) have pointed out that determination of blood protein levels does not necessarily reflect the state of nutrition of the patient, since it cannot reflect the severity of depletion of the total body reservoir of protein. Progressive weight loss is a good clinical indication that protein stores are being depleted.

Localio and colleagues (1948) found that wound healing approaches normal in protein-depleted animals, provided that the amino acid, methionine, is supplied. Moore (1959) has pointed out that wounds will heal in the face of preoperative starvation. They will heal completely when there is negative nitrogen balance. In protein starvation, wounds will heal, although slowly. These observations contradict the theory that wound dehiscence is specifically due to hypoproteinemia. The experimental models used in laboratory testing on the effect of hypoproteinemia on wound healing have been severe and cannot be readily duplicated in clinical practice.

## Anemia

I suspect that the role of anemia in wound disruption has not been fully appreciated in the past. Anemia may be systemic as a result of blood loss or local, owing to strangulation of tissue and severance of blood vessels. It generally refers to a lack or deficient amount of blood in the circulatory system. Yet circulation may be impaired because of poor cardiac function, even though there is no blood loss. In addition, poor wound closure, in which large amounts of tissue are strangulated, further impairs circulation to the incisional site, so that again, the delivery of blood and oxygen locally is inadequate.

Bains, Crawford, and Ketcham (1966) produced chronic anemia in rats and studied its effect on the tensile strength in these animals. They found that the average wound tensile strength was lower in anemic animals than in an iron-supplemented group.

Heughan (1975) studied the effect of anemia on experimental wounds in rabbits. He concluded that mild or moderate normovolemic anemia in otherwise healthy animals did not interfere with the delivery of oxygen to the wound and was of no consequence to wound healing.

In trying to assess the effect of anemia on healing wounds in patients, certain problems arise. There is a lack of agreement as to which hemoglobin values should justify the diagnosis of anemia. Reitamo and Möller found hemoglobin of less than 11 grams per 100 milliliters to be twice as common in patients with wound dehiscence. Guiney and colleagues considered that a hemoglobin value of less than 12 grams per 100 milliliters was an indication of anemia. Using this rather high value, they found that 50 percent of their patients who suffered wound disruptions were anemic. Only 20 percent of a comparable group with normal healing had similar values. Other observers (including Marsh et al., 1954; Mann et al., 1962; and Alexander and Prudden, 1966) were of the opinion that in the absence of other deficiencies anemia did not interfere significantly with wound healing.

Basic studies on the healing of wounds indicate that deficiencies in circulation and in oxygen supply definitely interfere with wound healing. In hypovolemia, blood oxygen partial pressure at the wound site falls to low levels. It has been shown that in induced normovolemic anemia, wound healing is relatively normal; however, hypovolemia has an adverse effect on the healing process. It appears that adequate flow of blood is of greater importance than anemia or reduced oxygen-carrying capacity. Unfortunately, in the clinical situation patients may present with anemia, hypovolemia, and circulatory impairment simultaneously. Treatment of anemia, replacement of body fluids, and maintenance of circulation at optimal levels are objectives to be attained preoperatively and pursued postoperatively.

## Ascorbic Acid Deficiency

It has been well established that a deficiency of vitamin C will interfere with wound healing. The exudative phase is prolonged, and an excess of serum glycoproteins persists in the wound. There is severe inhibition of collagen synthesis, and large numbers of fibroblasts are present in the wound. Wound contraction will occur. The ground substance is abnormal, and there is a failure of normal fiber formation. There is no doubt that severe depletion of ascorbic acid seriously interferes with the healing process, particularly in experimental models. It is important to review the experimental background that supports these observations. The information obtained must be cautiously interpreted, since certain laboratory animals are able to synthesize ascorbic acid.

An extremely important study was carried out by Lund. He showed that immediately following operation, plasma vitamin C level quickly drops to zero without signs of scurvy. Lund and Crandon (1941) then studied the problem of vitamin C deficiency in man. A vitamin C-free diet produced scurvy in a man at the end of five months. Ascorbic acid levels in the blood plasma fell to zero in 42 days. The amazing observation was that wounds healed well when individuals were on a scorbutigenic

diet for three to six months. They concluded that vitamin C deficiency may be a factor in the failure of some wounds to heal in man.

Lund discussed a paper by Hartzell and Winfield (1939), and pointed out that although vitamin C deficiency is capable of producing absolute failure of healing, it is uncommon in clinical cases. He referred to the work of A. O. Whipple and his associates (1940), who were able to reduce the incidence of disruptions by 80 percent through improvement of their surgical technique.

Based on the study I carried out on our cases of wound disruption, I believe that wound disruption as a result of ascorbic acid deficiency is a rare event in surgical practice today.

## Oxygen

Hunt and Zederfeldt — in their contribution to the book, *Repair and Regeneration*, by Dunphy and Van Winkle (1969) — considered the role of oxygen in wound healing. They stressed the fact that the oxygen tension is extremely low at the advancing edge of granulation tissue during the first 10 days of healing. They were of the opinion that oxygen is necessary for energy production and protein synthesis. They calculated that at least 1000 molecules of oxygen are needed to form a collagen molecule from amino acids. It has been observed that fibroblasts replicate optimally at oxygen tensions between 15 to 30 mm Hg. Collagen synthesis proceeds favorably as oxygen tension rises and diminishes as it falls.

The role of oxygen in the healing wound is currently of interest to surgeons and other people interested in wound healing. However, the problem becomes somewhat complicated. In anemia, oxygen delivery to the tissues is compromised. When the blood volume is diminished, circulation is interfered with, and blood $pO_2$ decreases at the site of the incision. While wounds in normovolemic animals heal normally, wounds in hypovolemic animals show impaired healing. Inadequate blood flow at the site may be more deleterious to the healing wound than either anemia or reduced oxygen-carrying capacity. The surgeon may find anemia, hypovolemia, and circulatory impairment to be present simultaneously. Treatment of anemia, replacement of body fluids, and maintenance of circulation at optimal levels are essential.

## ACTH and Steroid Therapy

Peacock and Van Winkle (1970) have noted that although large doses of steroids were ordinarily necessary to interfere significantly in healing, low doses have this capacity in conditions of starvation or protein depletion. Indeed, this observation often has a practical application.

Cole, Grove, and Montgomery (1953) and Creditor and his coworkers (1950) found that ACTH and cortisone exerted an inhibitory effect on proliferation of fibroblasts. Capillaries develop poorly, and formation of granulation tissue is impaired. It has been observed that steroids given several days following the operative procedure have little effect on the healing wound.

Cortisone interferes with wound healing by decreasing the inflammatory response; hence, it reduces protocollagen and proline hydroxylase, with a reduction of collagen synthesis. Hunt and coworkers have shown that vitamin A reduces some of the effects of cortisone in the healing of an open wound.

In the practice of clinical surgery, patients on massive doses of steroids, such as individuals with ulcerative colitis or lupus erythematosus, often show impaired wound healing. Particular care must be taken in the choice of incision and technique of closure in these patients. In addition, sutures must not be removed prematurely.

## Antimetabolites

Cytotoxic drugs present definite problems to surgeons, since they interfere with cell proliferation and, therefore, with wound healing. This statement is difficult to support experimentally, but the practicing surgeon is aware that wound healing is anything but normal in many of the patients receiving these drugs. Peacock and Van Winkle (1970) pointed out that rats on mechlorethamine hydrochloride (nitrogen mustard) therapy suffer from malnutrition and show a decrease in tensile strength of experimental wounds. Cyclophosphamide also has deleterious effects on the healing wound.

Mass closure techniques or the use of retention sutures are indicated in patients who must be treated with chemotherapeutic agents. Retention sutures should be removed after two to three weeks or whenever danger of disruption has passed.

The healing of a wound is a complicated process and involves many substances and mechanisms. Protein and ascorbic acid must be provided if healing is to proceed normally; oxygen is also necessary if normal fibroplasia is to occur. In addition, carbohydrates and adequate doses of insulin must be present. Since the B vitamins are involved in carbohydrate metabolism, these, too, are important. Cortisone interferes with wound contraction, but this action may be reversed by the administration of vitamin A.

## SUTURE MATERIALS AND SUTURE TECHNIQUE

Much research has been done concerning sutures, and we are provided with excellent suture material; however, the matter of suture material and suture technique is not frequently subject to careful scrutiny by surgeons. Much of what the surgeon has learned about suture material had been acquired during residency training. Choice of suture material too often depends upon habit rather than on sound scientific basis. Since wound disruptions and incisional hernias can be prevented or greatly decreased by the proper selection of suture material and proper suture technique, I believe a discussion of the matter is relevant. A number of deficiencies in choice of sutures and suture technique can contribute to wound disruption (Fig. 20–6). Surgeons create wounds daily and are responsible for the ultimate result following closure; therefore, it is appropriate that surgeons familiarize themselves with currently available suture materials. In this section we will consider sutures as they are applied to closure of abdominal incisions. A wide variety of excellent sutures is available, and a simple and useful classification is presented in Table 20–4. This

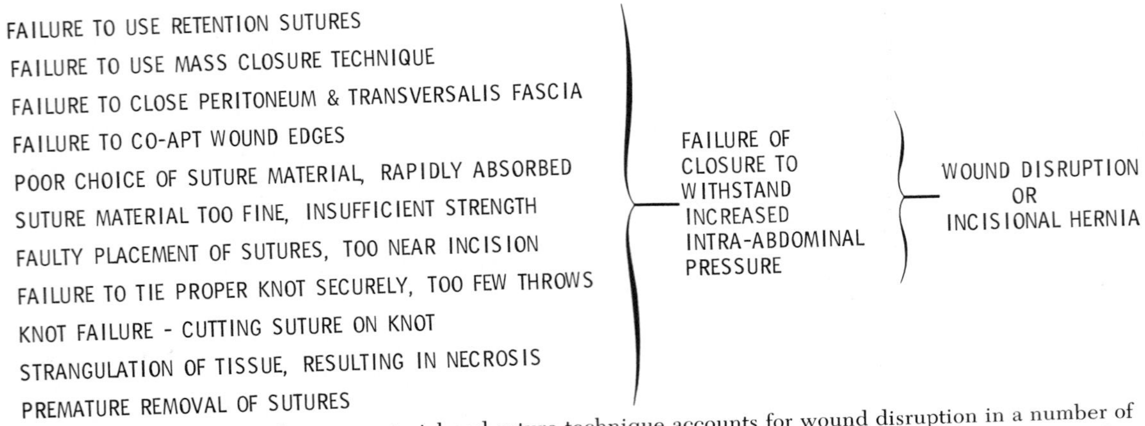

FAILURE TO USE RETENTION SUTURES
FAILURE TO USE MASS CLOSURE TECHNIQUE
FAILURE TO CLOSE PERITONEUM & TRANSVERSALIS FASCIA
FAILURE TO CO-APT WOUND EDGES
POOR CHOICE OF SUTURE MATERIAL, RAPIDLY ABSORBED
SUTURE MATERIAL TOO FINE, INSUFFICIENT STRENGTH
FAULTY PLACEMENT OF SUTURES, TOO NEAR INCISION
FAILURE TO TIE PROPER KNOT SECURELY, TOO FEW THROWS
KNOT FAILURE - CUTTING SUTURE ON KNOT
STRANGULATION OF TISSUE, RESULTING IN NECROSIS
PREMATURE REMOVAL OF SUTURES

} FAILURE OF CLOSURE TO WITHSTAND INCREASED INTRA-ABDOMINAL PRESSURE } WOUND DISRUPTION OR INCISIONAL HERNIA

Figure 20–6. Failure of suture material and suture technique accounts for wound disruption in a number of patients; this applies especially to those patients in whom disruption occurs within the first four postoperative days.

classification has practical merit but also some limitations. For example, silk had long been considered "nonabsorbable," but we now know that in time it disappears completely from the wound. Phagocytosis plays a part in this phenomenon. Catgut is the established absorbable suture material, but polyglycolic acid sutures (Dexon) and polyglactin sutures (Vicryl) are being used with increasing frequency in special situations.

Even though a number of excellent sutures are available, the search for the perfect suture material continues. The ideal suture material would have great and enduring strength in small diameter. Enduring strength of the suture material is a quality that has not, in my opinion, received enough attention in the past. An acceptable suture for abdominal wound closure must retain its strength over many months. It would be easy to manage; after a knot is tied, it would remain secure. Ease of handling and threading are important features to the nurse as well as the impatient surgeon. A desirable suture material would cause little or no tissue reaction and would be nonallergenic. Organisms would not find the interstices a haven in an otherwise hostile environment. The perfect suture material should be inexpensive and easily produced. It should be easily sterilized without loss of strength.

The criteria that are described here for an ideal suture material are not complete, but most of the desirable qualities have been noted. It is important to remember that I am directing attention to the qualities needed in a suture that is expected to maintain the abdominal wall in approximation following laparotomy. Of great importance is the need for apposition of the fascial and aponeurotic layers. It is necessary to ap-

### Table 20–4. A CLASSIFICATION OF SUTURE MATERIALS

*Nonabsorbable*
A. *Natural*
   1. Cotton
   2. Silk
B. *Synthetic*
   1. Polyamide
     a. Nylon
     b. Nylon-braided (Nurolon) (Surgilon)
   2. Polyester
     a. Multifilament (Dacron) (Mersilene)
     b. Teflon-coated (Etheflex) (Deknatel)
                 (Tevdek)
                 (Polydek)
     c. Silicone-treated (Tycron)
   3. Polyolefins
     a. Polypropylene (Prolene)
     b. Polyethylene
   4. Metallic
     a. Steel
        1. Monofilament
        2. Braided
     b. Tantalum

*Absorbable*
A. *Natural*
   1. Catgut
     a. Plain
     b. Chromicized
     c. Iodized
   2. Reconstructed collagen
B. *Synthetic*
   1. Polyglycolic acid (Dexon)
   2. Polyglactin (Vicryl)

Table 20–5.  QUALITIES OF VARIOUS SUTURE MATERIALS*

| | Ease of Handling | Knot Security | Absorb-ability | Inflam-matory Response | Refuge for Organisms | Strength Immediate | Strength Long-Term |
|---|---|---|---|---|---|---|---|
| SILK | 5 | 3 | 1–2 | 3–4 | 5 | 2–3 | 1–2 |
| COTTON | 3 | 3–4 | 0–1 | 3 | 3 | 2 | 2–3 |
| POLYAMIDE (Nylon) | 2 | 1–2 | 0 | 1 | 1–2 | 3 | 3 |
| POLYESTER (Dacron) | 2–3 | 2–3 | 0 | 2 | 1–2 | 4 | 4 |
| POLYPROPYLENE (Prolene) | 2–3 | 2–3 | 0 | 2 | 1–2 | 3 | 2–3 |
| STEEL WIRE | 1 | 5 | 0 | 1 | 1 | 5 | 5 |
| CATGUT, PLAIN | 2 | 1–2 | 5 | 5 | 0 | 1–2 | 0 |
| CATGUT, CHROMIC | 2 | 2 | 5 | 4 | 0 | 2 | 0 |
| POLYGLYCOLIC ACID (Dexon) | 3 | 3 | 5 | 1–2 | 0 | 3–4 | 0 |
| POLYGLACTIN (Vicryl) | 3 | 3 | 5 | 1–2 | 0 | 3 | 0 |

*0 to 1 = Complete absence or minimal evidence of quality. 5 = greatest evidence of quality.

proximate these layers accurately with sutures of enduring strength.

In Table 20–5, I have attempted to summarize the various attributes of different suture materials on a quantitative basis and to demonstrate the relative advantages that some suture materials possess over others. It is impossible to provide a completely accurate summary in chart form. It is well known that coating synthetic sutures with Teflon or silicone modifies their characteristics. Braiding also alters the qualities of suture materials. The comments that follow have been taken from the surgical literature on the subject of sutures. Although individual experiments may be criticized for various reasons, much of the information is sound and can be applied to clinical situations.

### Ease of Handling

Silk has long been recognized as a suture material that is easily managed whereas other single stranded, nonabsorbable sutures are somewhat stiff to touch, and knots are likely to slip under pressure. Wire in single strands is somewhat difficult to manipulate. It is obvious that surgeons become adept at handling various suture materials and, hence, ease of handling becomes a matter of experience. Many surgeons are educated in the use of silk and come to appreciate its ease of management. On the other hand, the surgeon experienced in the use of wire has found little difficulty in its use. Silk as well as

cotton enjoyed great and deserved popularity in the past, but its pre-eminent position in the world of sutures is slowly being challenged. Synthetic nonabsorbable sutures are gaining in popularity in modern surgical practice. The well-motivated surgeon can learn to use any suture material adeptly if he so desires.

### Knot Slippage

Although surgeons tie an enormous number of knots, it is interesting to observe that there are comparatively few publications on the subject. It may be that tying a knot is considered a simple technical maneuver that is unworthy of more than a fleeting thought and a minimal effort. Yet I agree with Taylor, who pointed out in 1938 that often the least reliable part of any suture is the knot.

Knot slippage is partly a function of the suture material and partly of the technique of forming the knot. Nylon and Dacron require special effort if knots are to remain intact. Wire is relatively difficult to manage; however, once properly tied, it provides the greatest strength and security of all currently available suture materials. Silk is well recognized for ease of tying, but the knot must be carefully tied with four throws as a square knot.

Taylor found the triple throw knot to be the safest when all throws are tied square. He found that chromic catgut produced a more secure knot than did plain catgut and only with the triple throw knot did it approach 100 percent dependability. He pointed out that wet catgut is more slippery than dry, and when wet with saline or serum, there is an increase in elasticity and swelling occurs. This may result in a loosening of the knot or in knot failure. Knots of silk sutures are more secure than those of catgut.

Taylor noted that when it is difficult to pull the surgeon's knot down tightly, it may be less dependable than the triple throw knot. He cautioned against cutting the suture ends too short and advised that a length of 5 millimeters be left beyond the knot if catgut sutures are used and of 3 millimeters if silk is employed. I strongly endorse the application of these details. The house officer must be aware of the importance of this technique.

The studies of Herrmann (1973) have been well planned and carefully performed, and his results are consistent with clinical experience. He found that metallic sutures provided the greatest knot security. Impregnation of Polyamide (Nylon) or Polyester (Dacron) sutures with wax, Teflon, or silicone impaired knot security significantly. Herrmann confirmed many of the same observations reported by Taylor. They both found that knots of catgut showed loss of strength when exposed to body fluids.

More recently, Thacker and colleagues (1975) carefully studied the mechanical performance of sutures. They noted that the degree of force required to produce knot breakage varied with the following: (1) the size of the loop, (2) the type of suture, and (3) the diameter of the suture. It is also known that tissues have the ability to cause a rapid decline in the knot-breaking strength of synthetic absorbable sutures and catgut. The loss of strength of polyglycolic acid sutures is exceedingly rapid. Postlethwait (1970) found that approximately 80 percent of the tensile strength of these sutures was lost in two weeks.

As noted by Thacker and colleagues, knot integrity is known to depend upon diameter of the suture, type of knot, length of the cut end (or "ears") of the suture, and presence of moisture. They studied knot integrity of silk and Teflon-coated sutures of Dacron (Tevdek). In tying silk, the granny knot was the least dependable. Four throws were necessary to reach knot-

break-holding strength; whereas, with surgeon's knots or square knots, three throws were necessary to achieve comparable knot security. Thacker and his coworkers pointed out that the length of the ears of the knot have a bearing on knot security. Obviously, if the amount of slippage at the knot exceeds the length of the cut ends (or ears), the knot will become untied. They prefer the cut ears to measure 3 millimeters in length. In obese patients and in those patients with pulmonary diseases, I increase this slightly.

Thacker and coworkers found that all three-throw knots of silk that were tied loosely required cut-ear lengths of more than 3 millimeters before the knots reached knot break. On the basis of their studies, they recommended four-throw square knots if number 4–0 waxed braided silk is being used. Each throw is tightly tied. When number 4–0 Teflon-coated synthetic sutures (Tevdek) are being used, Thacker and colleagues recommended a five-throw knot. Each throw must be securely placed against the preceding throw. Knots of five tightly placed throws are dependable, whether granny, square, or surgeon's knots are being employed. Magilligan and DeWeese (1974), in studying knot security, used a variety of synthetic nonabsorbable sutures. They found that four throws, all square, gave the most secure knot. Comparable security of the knot can be achieved with five throws—two slip and three square.

### Refuge for Organisms

Surgeons have learned that when infection is a potential problem, certain suture materials are less desirable than others. Silk sutures, especially those of large diameter, provide a haven for organisms. The extrusion or "spitting of silk" sutures is annoying to the patient as well as the surgeon. Organisms "hide in the braids" and are protected from body defenses and antibiotics. Since silk is made up of a number of braided strands and provides a refuge for organisms, it is not the suture material of choice in potentially infected wounds.

Monofilament wire sutures are popular in contaminated cases, but organisms may still find shelter in the knot. The need for both numerous throws in tying the knot and lengthy ears increases the amount of foreign materials in the wound.

Catgut sutures and synthetic absorbable sutures, such as polyglycolic acid or polyglactin sutures, are eventually absorbed. The absorption rate of catgut and polyglycolic acid sutures may be rapid, so that they may fail to hold the wound in approximation long enough to permit healing when infection is present. In patients with infection, sutures of enduring strength are essential. At the present time, monofilament wire and synthetic nonabsorbable sutures are acceptable for use in potentially infected wounds.

### Strength

The immediate strength of suture material varies with its nature and diameter. Besides the quality of immediate strength, another desirable attribute is the quality I call "enduring strength"; this subject will be considered later on in this section. Standards for suture materials are described in the *United States Pharmacopoeia*. Wire possesses the greatest strength and causes the least tissue reaction; however, it may fragment and migrate. It is well tolerated in most contaminated wounds. Wire is difficult to manage, however, unless the surgeon employs it regularly and be-

comes adept in its use. Another objection to wire is that it occasionally causes local pain. Also, wire quickly destroys the sharp edge of a scalpel, e.g., when it is necessary to enter the abdomen through an incision previously closed with it.

Herrmann (1971 and 1973) studied the tensile strength of suture materials extensively (Fig. 20–7). He found that metallic sutures were the strongest, synthetic polyester and polyolefin sutures the next strongest, and silk, cotton, and catgut the weakest.

In selecting suture material for abdominal wound closure, the surgeon must consider the greatest stress that might be placed on the incision. Furthermore, the entire thickness of the abdominal wall, rather than an individual layer, must be maintained in apposition until adequate healing takes place. Hence, sutures that are rapidly absorbed, such as catgut, polyglycolic acid (Dexon), or polyglactin (Vicryl), even though of adequate strength, are not suitable for closure of abdominal wounds when prolonged strength is required.

### Tissue Reaction

All implanted suture materials are foreign to the body; therefore, its defense mechanisms respond to the challenge. The degree and duration of the response varies

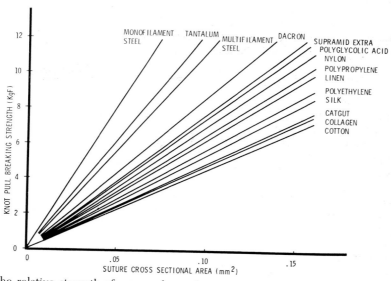

**Figure 20–7.** The relative strength of commonly used suture materials as determined by Herrmann. From Herrmann, J. B.: Tensile strength and knot security of surgical suture materials. Am. Surg. 37:215, 1971. (Reproduced with permission of the author and the publishers of The American Surgeon.)

with the type of suture material, and this has been studied in considerable detail.

Postlethwait, Willigan, and Ulin (1975) studied the response of the human body to various suture materials. They found that fibrous tissue formed about wire sutures and monocytes lined the connective tissue capsule. They also found that silk and cotton caused the appearance of a connective tissue capsule, with histiocytes interposed between the silk and the fibrous tissue capsule. Giant cells and lymphocytes were present in variable numbers. In some areas, capillaries were present. It is important to note that silk is eventually absorbed and disappears from the wound. The cellular response is responsible for removal of the silk.

Polyester sutures (Dacron), uncoated or coated with Teflon, were also studied by Postlethwait and colleagues. The uncoated suture material caused a similar but less intense tissue reaction than was seen with silk. Teflon coating shed off the suture material and provoked a greater tissue response.

Herrmann, Kelley, and Higgins (1970) studied polyglycolic acid (Dexon) sutures through implant studies in animals and surgical patients. They found that tissue reaction to the polyglycolic suture was minimal, in comparison to the active inflammatory response caused by catgut. Phagocytosis is active when catgut is cleared from wounds, while enzymatic action is sufficient to achieve dissolution of polyglycolic acid sutures. Catgut creates a much greater cellular response than that of the synthetic absorbable sutures, which are hydrolyzed.

## Absorbability

Absorbability is a quality that may be desirable in a suture or may seriously limit its usefulness. For example, intestinal suture absorbability is beneficial in mucosal approximation. When closing abdominal aponeurotic layers, the quality of enduring strength is highly desirable. The feature of absorbability should receive careful attention from the surgeon about to select sutures for abdominal wound closure.

Of all the sutures, only stainless steel wire and a few synthetic sutures remain unabsorbed in wounds. Silk, which is ordinarily considered to be nonabsorbable, loses approximately one-half of its strength in one year and has no strength after two years, according to Postlethwait and colleagues. In time, it is completely absorbed. They also found that cotton lost one-half of its strength in six months, retaining about 40 percent at the end of two years.

Catgut has been a popular absorbable suture material for many decades. In many situations its absorbability is a desirable quality. Catgut, even when chromicized, loses its strength rapidly over a period of four weeks. The deterioration is even more rapid when infection is present. It should not be depended upon where long-term strength is needed, as in patients with pulmonary diseases or in obese individuals. Nor should catgut be depended upon when the danger of infection is great, such as in cases of peritonitis or gross contamination.

Polyglycolic acid sutures undergo dissolution rapidly. Postlethwait (1970) found that these sutures lose 33 percent of their tensile strength in 1 week and 80 percent in 2 weeks. Thus, care must be taken when choosing this material for abdominal wound closure.

## Enduring Strength

In selecting a suture, it is becoming clear to surgeons that the long-term effectiveness of the material is important. Wounds of the abdomen simply do not heal completely in three to four weeks, contrary to earlier beliefs. By that time, the wound has regained only 30 to 40 percent of the strength of the intact abdominal wall. The margins of the incised musculoaponeurotic structures should be approximated by individually selected sutures. For instance, sutures with great and enduring strength should be used in obese patients. It must be recalled that healing continues during the remodeling phase of wound healing and for several months thereafter.

Enduring strength in a suture material is a quality that is increasingly being recognized as important by those individuals engaged in research on suture materials. Clinical surgeons, of course, should select suture materials according to both the immediate and long-term needs of the individual patient. In patients whose wound healing is likely to proceed slowly, such as the aged or those patients in steroid therapy or on antimetabolites, the use of a suture material that retains its strength over many months is essential. In this section, we are specifically interested in sutures as they hold aponeurotic or fascial structures in apposition.

Wire has great strength that is maintained over long periods of time, but even this material undergoes fragmentation and migration in time. Nevertheless, wire is a useful material in situations where prolonged strength is needed and when there is a possibility of infection. Polyester sutures, such as Dacron, Mersilene, and Tycron, cause comparatively little reaction in tissues and retain their strength for well over one year. However, coated synthetic sutures do cause more reaction than the smooth individual strands. Postlethwait (1970) found that after 18 months, Dacron caused little reaction other than fibrosis. Coated Tevdek sutures shed fragments of Teflon. Nylon sutures were identifiable easily after two years.

In a discussion of the paper by Postlethwait, Dr. Joseph M. Miller of Fort Howard, Virginia, reported an extensive experience with polypropylene (Prolene) sutures. He found that polypropylene was well tolerated and remained intact for periods of 180 days in experimental animals. The enduring strength of polypropylene and its nonreactivity makes it a desirable suture material.

Sutures of polyamide material, such as nylon, cause little tissue reaction and are well retained in tissues for periods of over two years, during which there is little or no loss of strength.

On the basis of clinical and experimental studies, it can be concluded that the synthetic nonabsorbable sutures are second only to wire in immediate suture strength. Furthermore, they retain their strength for longer periods of time than do silk and cotton.

Silk and cotton have been popular suture materials, but both are currently under increasing scrutiny. Surgeons appreciate its ease of handling, but silk lacks the quality of enduring strength. When strength of suture must be maintained over several months or even years, silk cannot be depended upon. It has been found unacceptable in vascular surgery for this reason. In fact, silk may be absorbed as early as six months. We have operated upon patients who had undergone hernia repairs with silk one or two years previously without being able to find a trace of silk suture material. Postlethwait found that silk lost approximately 50 percent of its strength in 1 year. Cotton lost 50 percent of its strength after 6 months, but still retained 30 to 40 percent of its strength at the end of 2 years. Silk continues to enjoy popularity among many surgeons because of its ease of handling and has adequate strength for most abdominal operations.

Catgut has been a popular suture material for several decades. Its absorbability has been a desirable quality as, for instance, in intestinal surgery. Catgut, even when chromicized, loses its strength rapidly over a period of four weeks. The deterioration is even more rapid when infection is present. Since it is becoming increasingly clear that wounds do not heal to completion for many months, a more permanent suture is needed to hold tissues in apposition during the prolonged remodeling phase of wound healing.

Where long-term strength is needed in wound closure, the abdominal surgeon may choose stainless steel wire, polyamide (Nylon), Polyester (Dacron), (Mersilene), (Ethiflex), (Tycron), polypropylene (Prolene), silk, or cotton. Currently introduced absorbable sutures, such as polyglycolic acid (Dexon) or polyglactin (Vicryl), do not retain sufficient strength for long periods of time and, hence, are not recommended for use in closure of aponeurotic and fascial layers of the abdomen. In closing vertical abdominal incisions, a suture that retains its strength for several months is highly desirable, especially in patients whose wounds are likely to heal slowly while exposed to unusual stress.

## FUNDAMENTAL PRINCIPLES OF OPERATIVE TECHNIQUE

Important basic principles in the performance and care of operative incisions have been enumerated and described by Halsted, Reid, Whipple, and Dunphy. It is amazing that the critically important subjects of abdominal incisions, wound closure, and wound care have been treated lightly in some textbooks and almost neglected in others. Even today, dangerous practices, such as delivery of a drain through a midline incision, are endorsed by some authors. Although principles of wound care should be learned in the operating room, I have found that constant and enthusiastic repetition is needed if important details are to be learned, appreciated, and implemented. The availability of antibiotics has not reduced the need for asepsis and precise operative technique in abdominal operative procedures.

## Asepsis

The surgeon should be aware that organisms find their way into the operative wound via two important pathways; i.e., from the skin or the viscera.

The patient's skin, poorly prepared, may be the source of staphylococci, which might be introduced into the wound by a surgeon who places his hand first on the skin and then into the wound. The organisms can originate from the surgeon's hand and enter the operative field by way of a punctured glove. Careless technique or accidental mishap sometimes results in a defective glove. I have seen a surgeon palpate for the location of a deeply imbedded needle, which, in this instance, had been placed in Cooper's ligament, with a gloved finger! A hazardous practice like that should not be tolerated, since it easily leads to wound infection. Needles should always be placed under direct vision and controlled with instruments, not searched for with gloved fingers!

Asepsis implies the exclusion of disease-producing bacteria from the operative field. It is impossible to "sterilize" the viable skin; hence, the objective is to reduce the number of organisms to a point where the body defenses can cope with the few microbes that remain. Besides careful preparation of the skin, everyone in the operating room must adhere rigidly to principles of asepsis. Hands and instruments that touch the skin should be kept out of the operative wound as completely as practicality will permit. The wound site should be protected from skin contaminants through the use of towels or drapes.

Skin preparation, performed with thoroughness, is not a minor part of an operation. The presence of excoriation,

folliculitis, dermatitis, or furunculosis necessitates delaying elective operative procedures until a cure or an optimal improvement has been achieved.

The patient about to have an abdominal operation is advised to take a leisurely tub bath, preferably with a surgical soap, the evening of operation. Physical cleanliness must be achieved by whatever means necessary. All traces of adhesive tape or other adhesive agents used in the application of appliances must be removed before antiseptics are applied. In elective cases, the umbilicus often harbors a variety of gross debris, which must be physically removed before skin preparation is applied. This is followed on the next morning with a wet shave. The area is again washed with a surgical soap. If a soap is to be used in skin preparation, the temporal factor is important, and the abdomen must be washed for a period of ten minutes.

In skin preparations, I prefer the routine application of a tincture of iodine solution and its subsequent removal with 70 percent alcohol. Thorough application of the iodine solution followed with removal will require some time, and this time factor is important. If the surgeon prefers a surgical soap, thorough surgical scrubbing for a minimum of ten minutes is recommended. After preparation of the operative field, double thicknesses of sterile drapes must be placed about the immediate area to be operated upon. The basic principles described above will reduce wound infections due to skin contaminants to a minimum.

There are situations in which organisms have been liberally and unavoidably implanted in the peritoneal cavity and subcutaneous tissues. Blunt abdominal trauma and penetrating wounds due to bullets or knives cause visceral perforation. Even worse are shotgun injuries inflicted at short range. Antibiotics should be given as early as possible following the trauma. Other conditions in which infection can be expected include operative procedures for drainage of abdominal, pelvic, subphrenic, or perirenal abscess. Adequate drainage and appropriate antibiotic therapy are essential if recovery is to be expected.

Wound infection too often occurs in a dirty, contaminated, or infected operative wound as no surprise to the surgeon, such as, for instance, when an acutely inflamed appendix has ruptured or a duodenal ulcer or sigmoid diverticulum perforates resulting in peritonitis. Organisms can commonly be identified, in these situations, by culture. Whenever any part of the gastrointestinal, genitourinary, or reproductive tract is operated upon, organisms can find their way into subcutaneous tissues. This is particularly true if spillage of urine, bile, and intestinal or colonic contents is permitted or if it occurs after trauma. It is essential to control the luminal contents by application of clamps or rubber bands about the viscera. The wound can be further protected by utilization of a waterproof drape. When gross contamination occurs, the contents must be carefully controlled and aspirated. The wound must be locally irrigated and closed with nonabsorbable sutures. The skin and subcutaneous tissues should be loosely approximated and drained; later, the wound may be safely closed.

## Sharp Dissection

Sharp dissection means that most of the dissection is performed cleanly with the curved portion of the belly of the scalpel. Tearing or ripping of tissues with the scalpel handle or hemostat should not be tolerated. Scissors should not be used to incise the skin or any other structures accessible to the scalpel. Precise knowledge of anatomy, gained through the process of cadaver dissection, allows the surgeon to use the belly of the scalpel blade in a safe, decisive, and gentle fashion. Master surgeons (such as Halsted, Reid, Zollinger, and Dunphy) all stress the need for clean, precise, and sharp dissection with scalpel.

## Gentleness

Avoidance of unnecessary trauma or injury is implied in the word gentleness. Using care in retraction, protecting the wound against the drying effects of room air, and gentle sponging with moist sponges are important details. If retaining retractors are used, they should be released and reapplied from time to time. Hemostats with fine points are just as effective as those with large crushing surfaces in the control

of bleeding vessels. After ligatures are placed about the fine-pointed hemostat, much less tissue is devitalized. Only fine suture material, such as number 4-0 silk, should be used as ligatures. Use of large crushing clamps, such as Kocher clamps, should not be tolerated when other, less injurious instruments, which are just as useful, are available. Large clamps crush the vitality out of the tissues. Sharp, precise dissection performed with the scalpel is, in effect, the surgical art.

## Removal of Devitalized Tissues

During dissection, if any obviously devitalized muscle, fascia, or fat is seen, it should be removed or excised. During extensive dissection of the layers of the abdominal wall, the margins may become devitalized. Tissue of questionable viability should be excised. Similarly, large masses of tissue located beyond a ligature should be excised. Left behind, this tissue must undergo liquefaction necrosis and thus may serve as a nutrient for bacteria. careful débridement of shotgun wounds or crushing injuries is obviously extremely important.

Heavy scar tissue does not add to the strength of the wound upon closure. It may be excised to advantage in many cases.

## Hemostasis

Postoperative bleeding and hematomas are avoided by painstaking attention to detail. Every blood vessel, either bleeding or "oozing," should be clamped precisely with a fine-pointed hemostat and ligated with fine suture material. I want to emphasize that the surgeon must seek out and clamp each blood vessel, not a large mass of adipose tissue in the vicinity of the blood vessel. Poor hemostasis leads to hematoma formation, and extravasated blood that is left behind in the operative wound is, in effect, a dead tissue. Surgeons are taught early that devitalized or necrotic tissues should not be permitted to remain in operative or traumatic wounds; yet they often make an exception to this principle when dealing with hematomas. Hematomas are too often antecedent to wound disruption or postoperative ventral herniation by causing pressure to form upon the suture line and by providing an excellent culture medium for bacterial growth. Hemorrhage in an operative wound provides nutrition for any bacteria that, in turn, may gain access to the wound. Pressure develops in the wound, further decreasing circulation and oxygenation to the area. As a consequence, healing is interfered with and wound disruption may occur. Healing of a wound containing a hematoma is, at best, a slow process. Prevention of hemorrhage and hematoma formation by painstaking hemostasis contributes to prompt and effective wound healing. The word "ooze" should not be used to excuse poor hemostasis technique.

### Avoidance of Dead Space

First of all, creation of dead space should be avoided by eliminating unnecessary dissection. Large fascial flaps or skin flaps should not be fashioned unless they contribute directly to the effectiveness of the operative procedure. If a one-layer closure achieves satisfactory closure of a ventral hernial defect, no further and unnecessary dissection should be performed.

Second, the problem of dead space can be minimized by reapproximating subcutaneous tissues with careful placement of absorbable sutures in the subcutaneous fat. Another method, which I have utilized in obese patients, is placement of vertical mattress sutures at a distance of 2 to 3 centimeters from the wound edges.

Third, negative suction applied to a catheter placed in the wound depths is a valuable adjunct (Fig. 21–10, p. 388). A Steadman pump or one of the other devices currently available provides the negative pressure. This technique has worked better for me than have pressure dressings. Withdrawal of blood and serum from wide areas of dissection, as occurs in repair of ventral hernias, resulted in improved wound healing in my experience.

### Secondary Closure

Complete approximation of the skin and subcutaneous tissue may not be advisable in infected wounds or in wounds that have been grossly contaminated, as in those following a shotgun blast. It is necessary to close the fascial layers, but the skin and subcutaneous space may be left unapproximated or loosely closed to effect drainage. The surgeon, on subsequent inspection, can make the decision to close the wound secondarily. This approach is not used as often as it should be.

In summary, the surgeon who carries out the principles of careful asepsis, gentleness, and thorough hemostasis and who uses precise surgical technique will enjoy the best results for his operative endeavors. Use of fine suture material, sharp dissection, débridement, and avoidance of dead space in the operative area are important details. Secondary closure is a useful technique when dealing with grossly contaminated or infected wounds.

## ABDOMINAL INCISIONS

Surgeons have now been making abdominal incisions with great frequency for nine decades. After countless opportunities to observe the healing of such wounds, one would think there would evolve universal agreement on the choice of an appropriate abdominal incision for each type of abdominal operation. Unfortunately, there is no general agreement on how the surgeon can best perform laparotomy. The justification for this statement can be found in the number of ill-conceived incisions seen in practice. There are, nevertheless, a number of valid and useful observations recorded in the literature. These should aid the surgeon in his choice of abdominal incision for each patient.

The transverse incision is less disruptive of the nerve and blood supply to the musculature than are the pararectus, paramedian, or long subcostal incisions. Since the line of force exerted by the transversus abdominis, internal, and external oblique muscles is in a lateral direction, the tendency is for the wound edges to approximate each other when a transverse incision has been made.

The use of the transverse incision is highly recommended whenever the intended procedure can be expeditiously performed through its use.

Many surgeons have been able to confirm that transverse incisions are inclined to heal without disruption.

Merscheimer and Winfield (1955) pointed out that even when disruption occurs in transverse incisions, the occurrence of actual evisceration is lower. They noted the low incidence of disruption following McBurney's, Pfannenstiel's, and Kocher's incisions. Campbell and Swenson (1972) studied the problem of disruption in infants and children and found the incidence of disruption to be 3.37 percent in vertical midline incisions and only 0.2 percent in transverse incisions. Tweedie and Long (1954) found that not a single disruption was seen following McBurney's incisions and only 4 disruptions among 113 occurred in transverse or paracostal incisions. Keill, Nichols, and De Weese (1973), Fish (1964), and Lehman, Cross, and Parkington (1968) also stressed the fact that transverse incisions tend to heal with little or no tendency to disruption.

The vertical incision has certain disadvantages by nature of its anatomic location. A substantial lateral distracting force is exerted upon it as a result of contraction of the transversus abdominis, internal oblique, and external oblique muscles. If the incision is made in error at the site of entry of the nerves and blood vessels, there is serious impairment to sound healing. If a vertical incision must be used, the vertical midline incision results in minimal destruction of the blood supply and innervation to the abdominal wall. Several surgeons have shown that disruptions occur with the greatest frequency in vertical upper abdominal incisions. Hartzell and Winfield (1939), Tweedie and Long (1954), Sedgwick and Sullivan (1957), Lehman and colleagues (1968), and Joergenson and Smith (1950) were among those who found that vertical incisions have an increased vulnerability to disruption. I have been able to confirm these observations.

In spite of its limitations, the vertical incision is extremely useful in certain situations when wide exposure is needed, extending from the xiphoid process to the symphysis pubis, as is seen in gunshot wounds, in abdominal trauma, or in resection of an abdominal aortic aneurysm. No other incision will permit the needed exposure. When rapid entry into the peritoneal cavity is required, as in hemorrhage following trauma, the midline incision is desirable, since it can be performed quickly. Furthermore, it may be enlarged easily in either direction. Midline incisions provide ease of entry to and excellent exposure of pelvic viscera. If an umbilical hernia is present, it also may be repaired.

In order to offset the disadvantages of the vertical incision — namely, evisceration and herniation — greater care in closure becomes necessary. Use of nonabsorbable sutures of sufficient strength as well as retention sutures will reduce the incidence of disruption to an acceptable level.

The practice of making new and separate incisions with repeated entry into the abdomen often seriously weakens the abdominal wall. This subject is discussed in more detail in Chapter 21. Whenever repeated incisions are necessary to gain access to the peritoneal cavity, if at all possible, the previous incision site should be utilized so that minimal injury of the abdominal wall occurs. When choosing the abdominal incision, the needs of the individual patient must be considered. Good exposure is a necessity if an effective and safe procedure is to be performed. For instance, a longer incision is necessary in an obese patient. In a thin patient with a narrow costal margin, the vertical incision between the xiphoid process and the umbilicus may be just as desirable as the subcostal incision for cholecystectomies, gastroduodenal surgical procedures, and operations upon the pancreas. Transverse incisions are to be preferred when they serve the objective of exposure. Vertical midline incisions are indispensable in certain patients; however, the surgeon must compensate for their use by means of nonabsorbable sutures, retention sutures, and greater care in closure.

In my experience, I have found that whenever drains are used, they should be delivered through small, separate stab wounds. Drains delivered through the full thickness of the abdominal incision will often result in a weakness at the point of exit. It is unfortunate that in certain modern textbooks, one may find support for drainage of the peritoneal cavity through a midline incision! As a principle, intestinal stomas should also be delivered through the abdominal wall at a site different from the incision. Even if disruption of the wound does not occur, drains delivered through abdominal incisions leave an area of weakness that may later become the site of an incisional hernia. The surgeon should carefully consider which incision will best serve his purpose without sacrificing the future welfare of his patient. Suture material and method of closure should be selected on an individual basis. Certainly, primary consideration must be given to the amount of exposure obtained with an incision, but the effect of that incision on the integrity of the abdominal wall must not be overlooked. Preferred incisions are shown in Figure 20–8.

Among the incisions that I recommend are:

1. **TRANSVERSE INCISION** (Fig. 20–8,*C*): The great advantage in using this incision is that it heals well with little tendency to disruption. Injury to nerves and blood vessels is minimal. The disadvantage is that it takes longer to open the abdomen and to close the incision. Exposure may be limited, since it can be easily extended in a lateral direction only.

2. **SUBCOSTAL INCISION** (Fig. 20–8,*A*): It has many of the features of the transverse incision when used in patients with wide costal angles. It affords excellent exposure to the right or left upper quadrants, including the biliary tract, liver, and spleen. Drains should be delivered through a small separate stab wound rather than through these incisions. The incision requires more time in its performance than do other incisions, for instance, a midline incision.

3. **VERTICAL MIDLINE INCISION** (Fig. 20–8,*B*): This is a useful incision since it can be made quickly as well as extended in either direction to provide excellent exposure. It provides adequate exposure of the viscera in the epigastric area when made above the umbilicus and excellent exposure of the pelvic viscera when made below the umbilicus. Minimal injury to nerves and blood vessels occurs with its use. The incision is easily closed, but it must be closed with retention sutures or mass closure techniques, since disruption occurs most frequently in this incision.

4. **RECTUS INCISION** (Fig. 20–8,*D*): This is a vertical incision over the midrectus sheath. The rectus muscle is retracted laterally; then, the posterior rectus sheath is incised vertically. Theoretically, this incision should provide greater strength following closure. This incision requires more time for performance and closure. It does not offer any great advantage over the vertical midline incision. I am currently using the rectus incision infrequently.

## PREFERRED INCISIONS

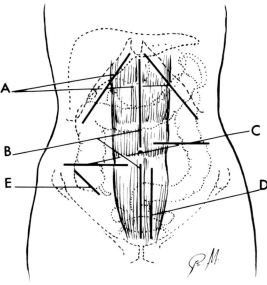

**Figure 20–8.** Transverse incisions are preferred when they serve the purpose of exposure. Vertical incisions are less disruptive but more difficult to maintain in apposition.

*A.* The subcostal incision on the right gives access to the gallbladder, duodenum, head of the pancreas, and the stomach. On the left side the spleen, pancreas, splenic flexures of the colon, and the kidney may be exposed.

*B.* The midline supraumbilical incision gives quick access to the organs in the epigastric area and the aorta as well. The midline incision below the umbilicus gives excellent exposure to the pelvic organs and rectosigmoid. A long midline incision from the xiphoid process to the symphysis pubis gives excellent and rapid exposure of abdominal vicera, which may be injured in gunshot wounds, penetrating wounds, and severe trauma.

*C.* The transverse incision is useful in operations on the colon. It is particularly desirable for right colectomy.

*D.* The paramedian incision is made through the anterior sheath of the rectus. The rectus muscle is retracted laterally, sparing nerves and blood vessels. Then entry is gained to the peritoneal cavity through an incision in the midportion of the posterior rectus sheath.

*E.* The McBurney or muscle-splitting incision is preferred for appendectomy.

5. MCBURNEY'S INCISION (Fig. 20-8,E):
The McBurney muscle-splitting incision is an ideal incision for areas to appendiceal lesions. The disruption to the abdominal wall is minimal, since the muscles and aponeurotic layers are being spread apart rather than divided. Access to the appendix is adequate. If greater exposure is needed, the incision may be enlarged medially.

SITE OF PREVIOUSLY MADE INCISION. If care is taken in performing the incision, the site of a previous incision provides an excellent reentry route to the abdomen, with minimal injury to the nerve and blood supply. If the incision is lengthened slightly at either end, the danger of encountering adherent bowel is minimal. This approach results in minimal disruption to the integrity of the abdominal wall.

*The most destructive incisions are:*

1. PARARECTUS INCISION: This incision, made just lateral to the rectus abdominis muscle, destroys the intercostal nerves and blood vessels as they course medially. It has no advantage over the midline or the rectus incision. (See Fig. 21-4, p. 376.)

2. EXCESSIVELY LONG SUBCOSTAL INCISIONS: If this incision is unduly long, it will sacrifice three or more intercostal nerve trunks and vascular pedicles, with resultant weakness in the abdominal wall (Fig. 21-4, F).

3. LONG OBLIQUE INCISIONS: These incisions are destructive to nerve and blood supply.

4. MULTIPLE INCISIONS: When a paramedian incision is followed by a midline incision, an area of weakness may develop between them. Another example, which I have seen, is a right paramedian incision followed by a left paramedian incision. A number of hernias have developed at the angle formed by a vertical midline incision followed by a subcostal incision (Fig. 21-4).

Great care should be taken in the performance of the abdominal incision. Vertical midline incisions, which are prone to disruption and herniation, require proper closure with suture materials of enduring strength.

# CLOSURE OF ABDOMINAL WOUNDS

It is, of course, impossible to improve upon the integrity of the normal abdominal wall with suture techniques. An ideal closure would restore all layers to precisely the same anatomic relationships and strength as existed in the intact abdominal wall prior to the incision. The surgeon should recall that after 20 days the laparotomy incision regains approximately 20 to 30 percent of its original strength and that even after 100 days the original strength has not been attained; hence, the need for careful selection of suture material is clear. The cicatrix should be kept to a minimum by careful surgical technique since it is a poor substitute for the original tissue.

Although many surgeons exercise great care in wound closure, this is not always evident from operative notes. A description such as "the wound was closed in layers with fine sutures" could be elaborated upon to good advantage. Another expression used in recording is "wound closure was routine." In my opinion, there is nothing routine about wound closure. Martyak and Curtis (1976) advocate the use of systems analysis and flow-charting techniques for procedure on laparotomy incisions and closure. Thus, a complete view of objectives and alternatives would be available for the surgeon's scrutiny. Every operative wound closure should be given the same individual attention that is applied to the definitive procedure. For instance, obese or muscular patients and patients with cardiopulmonary disease will require heavier suture material, such as number 2 chromic catgut or 28 gauge stainless steel wire. When contamination is a consideration, wire or synthetic nonabsorbable monofilament sutures are advisable. In clean wounds, either synthetic nonabsorbable or silk sutures may be used. Retention sutures of number 2 nylon are invaluable in selected subcostal incisions and in all long vertical midline incisions. Generally, nonabsorbable braided sutures should not be used to suture potentially infected wounds. Fine sutures, such as number 4-0 chromic catgut or silk, do not possess sufficient strength to hold the wound in approximation, especially in obese patients or in those with ileus and bronchitis.

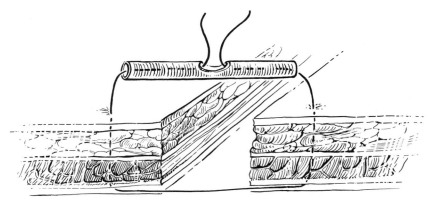

**Figure 20-9.** The retention suture of number two nylon is placed through the full thickness of the abdominal wall but just anterior to the peritoneum. It is tied over a piece of tubing, which prevents or minimizes the cutting effect of the suture. It is the simplest of "mass-closure" sutures.

As a principle in the closure of transverse abdominal wounds, I favor closure of layers individually. Closure of the peritoneum and transversalis fascia is essential, since all eviscerations and herniations must egress through them. Before closing the aponeurosis in a vertical incision, retention sutures of number two nylon are placed at intervals of approximately 3 centimeters (Fig. 20-9). These sutures are particularly helpful in obese patients and in those patients with liver, cardiac, or pulmonary diseases. They are well indicated in patients with inflammatory bowel diseases or with malignancies and should always be used when healing is likely to be less than optimal. In vertical incisions, both above and below the umbilicus, retention sutures are placed at a distance of 2 to 3 centimeters from the wound edge, depending upon the thickness of the panniculus. They are passed through the full thickness of the abdominal wall and guided to the wound margin between the peritoneum and aponeurosis. Thus, the retention suture is essentially extraperitoneal in location. With the technique just described, adhesions are less likely to develop, and entrapment of bowel in the suture is avoided.

A number of surgeons have found the Smead-Jones suture technique highly effective for situations in which two layers of the abdominal wall are identified (Fig. 20-10). Jones, Newell, and Brubaker (1941) attribute this suture to Dr. Louis Smead of Toledo, Ohio, who devised it while serving as a resident under Dr. John Finny, Sr., of Baltimore. The method calls for placing the suture a good distance away from the wound margin, then approximating the edge of the aponeurosis. It has been called the "far and near" suture technique.

In closure of midline incisions below the umbilicus, retention sutures of number 2 nylon are placed as indicated in Figure 20-9. If the peritoneal layer is closed separately below the umbilicus, a continuous suture (such as number 0-chromic . . .) or a synthetic absorbable suture may be used. In approximating the anterior sheath of the rectus abdominis below the umbilicus,

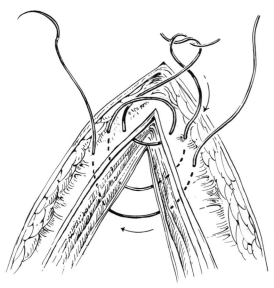

**Figure 20-10.** The Smead-Jones suture is another technique for achieving "mass-closure" of tissue.

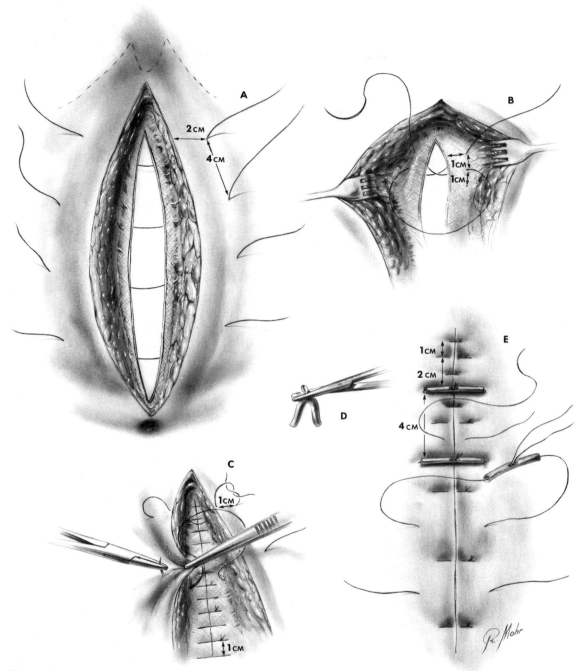

**Figure 20–11.** Details of effective wound closure are shown.
A. Retention sutures are placed at intervals of 4 centimeters, 2 centimeters from the wound edge.
B. Wound closure is achieved by placing sutures 1 centimeter apart and 1 centimeter from the wound edge. Wire or nonabsorbable sutures are recommended.
C. Nonabsorbable sutures are placed to approximate the full thickness of the wound and to eliminate dead space.
D. A small portion of the circumference of the catheter segment is excised at its midportion to permit passage of heavy, nonabsorbable sutures prior to tying.
E. Appearance of wound after complete closure.

nonabsorbable sutures are strongly recommended. Wire, Dacron, or silk may be chosen and placed as interrupted sutures. In approximating the tissues in the midline, the transaponeurotic sutures are placed at intervals 1 centimeter apart and 6 to 10 millimeters from the wound margin (Fig. 20–11). Every suture placed through aponeurotic tissue is carefully secured with a minimum of four throws. When using nonabsorbable synthetic sutures, I place five throws to each knot and make a surgeon's knot of the first two throws. Excessive pressure during ligature should be avoided, since strangulation of tissue may result. Tightly tied sutures act as a tourniquet and may result in ischemia and gangrene at the site. A great deal of instruction and discipline is demanded before the house officer becomes adept at approximation of tissue without strangulation occurring.

After the knot is tied, care must be taken in cutting the suture. Intense abdominal pressure develops during recovery from anesthesia, and knot slippage may occur, especially with synthetic nonabsorbable sutures. Hence, it is important to leave a small portion of suture beyond the knot when strength is a consideration. As mentioned previously, these projections of the suture at the knot are known as suture "ears." I prefer to leave a segment of 3 to 5 millimeters beyond the knot at each individual suture. Silk sutures may be cut safely at 3 millimeters from the knot; however, with catgut or the synthetic nonabsorbable sutures placed in aponeurotic structures, a segment with a length of 4 or 5 millimeters is safer. Supervision is essential if the neophyte surgeon is to respect these principles.

Subcutaneous tissues may be approximated with number 3–0 plain catgut or a synthetic absorbable suture.

In certain wounds, like those resulting from dissection of large ventral hernias, I insert plastic catheters into the depths of the wound and apply negative suction by means of a Steadman pump or one of the commercially available devices (Fig. 21–10, p. 388).

Skin closure is accomplished with number 3–0 and number 4–0 nylon. Contaminated wounds are not closed tightly, and small rubber drains are placed at intervals of 5 centimeters to facilitate drainage.

In some contaminated wounds, it is wise to loosely close the wound and place soft rubber drains in the subcutaneous space, extending down to the aponeurotic layer. If infection does not occur, these drains can be removed in three to four days.

## CLINICAL STUDY

In the hope that more could be learned concerning the nature of wound disruption and, possibly, the genesis of incisional hernias, I reviewed the available clinical records of 266 patients who had suffered wound disruptions at the Henry Ford Hospital from 1948 through 1972. In many instances, the records of older or deceased patients had been transferred to microfilm tapes. It was not possible to locate the record of every patient who might have suffered from this complication, since it might not have been indexed for retrieval. Some patients, who had their disrupted wounds taped or strapped received treatment on the in-patient floor, with the progress note recording the event and treatment. While studying incisional hernias, I found several of these records. Nevertheless, worthwhile practical information was recovered from available records.

### Sex

In this study, 171 males and 95 females suffered from wound dehiscence. The male-to-female ratio was 1.8:1. This incidence is consistent with other reports in the literature.

### Age Incidence

Wound disruption was found to occur twice as often in patients over 50 years of age than in younger individuals (Fig. 20–12). Wound dehiscence is comparatively rare in infants and children but does occur in unusual cases. In one infant, dehiscence occurred following an operative procedure for Hirschsprung's disease, 23 days after delivery. Two other children suffered the complication following operations for megacolon. One child, eight years old, suffered from a disruption following an

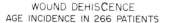

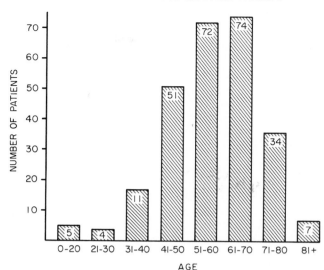

**Figure 20–12.** The age incidence of 266 patients with disruption shows that adult and elderly patients are more often afflicted.

appendectomy through a right rectus incision. Only 10 percent of the wound dehiscences occurred in patients under 40 years of age.

In this study, most wound disruptions occurred by far in the fifth, sixth, seventh, and eighth decades. This is not surprising, since many of these patients suffer from prolonged illnesses, debilitating diseases, or neoplasms. Many have pulmonary disorders such as bronchitis or emphysema and cardiac disease is quite common in aging patients.

## Clinical Picture

The clinical picture associated with wound dehiscence is extremely variable. The reason for this is obvious, since patients with a great variety of serious illnesses had initially required the surgical treatment. The effects of the presenting diseases take their toll of the patient's reserves. Weight loss, anemia, and malnutrition may be evident. Obesity is, however, not rare in patients who disrupt operative incisions. Among the primary diseases, we found carcinoma of various organs, such as uterus, cervix, colon, stomach, and pancreas. Peptic ulcer disease, especially with complications of bleeding

and obstruction, is also rather commonly found in patients who have disrupted postoperative incisions. Inflammatory diseases of the bowel, such as diverticulitis, ulcerative colitis, and regional enteritis were other diseases seen in this group of patients.

The state of the patient immediately proceeding actual disruption varied enormously. In some instances, the patients were gravely ill with severe peritonitis, ileus, and pulmonary complications. In other cases, the patient appeared to be progressing so well that the sutures were removed; however, a sudden increase in intra-abdominal pressure, such as a cough, resulted in wound disruption, even evisceration.

## Signs and Symptoms

The signs and symptoms of wound disruption are numerous and depend upon the preoperative condition of the patient, the operative procedure, and the postoperative complications. It is impossible to formulate a list of all possible signs and symptoms found in these patients, but the important ones are summarized in Table 20–6. Since a given patient will often have more than one

Table 20–6. SYMPTOMS AND SIGNS OF WOUND DISRUPTION (266 PATIENTS)

| Description | No. of Patients |
|---|---|
| Serosanguineous discharge | 140 |
| Cough | 122 |
| Nausea, vomiting, distention | 76 |
| Infection | 91 |
| Ileus | 114 |
| Straining | 13 |
| Seen at dressing change | 28 |
| Seen following suture removal | 17 |
| Hematomas | 13 |
| Fistulae | 9 |
| Hiccups | 12 |

sign or symptom, the total number exceeds by far the number of patients.

The list in Table 20–6 does not exhaust all of the signs and symptoms, but most of the important manifestations are mentioned.

Three extremely significant groups of symptoms are evident. First, infection of the wound or of the peritoneal cavity, or of both, appears as a significant factor in eventual wound disruption. The incidence of wound infection has been reported to vary from 11 to 31 percent in patients with wound disruption. These patients often have ileus and distention as well. Second, distention has an adverse effect upon the recently closed incision and has been observed in from 14 to 57 percent of wound eviscerations studied by various authors. Third, severe and recurrent coughing is seen consistently in patients whose abdomens are about to burst. The underlying diseases are numerous and include bronchitis, bronchopneumonia, atelectasis, asthma, and emphysema.

Although the appearance of a profuse serosanguineous drainage is strong evidence that the wound is not healing well, it occurs in connection with a variety of conditions. The unexpected appearance of unduly large amounts of serosanguineous fluid in a patient apparently making a satisfactory postoperative recovery should alert the surgeon to the possibility of wound disruption. Over one-half of the patients in this study presented the surgeon with a serosanguineous discharge from their operative wounds. The appearance of an abnormal amount of pinkish or sanguineous liquid from the postoperative

wound is an ominous sign. At times, the discharge may be quite bloody; at other times, it may be serous and even resemble blood-tinged urine. The appearance of such a discharge may precede wound infection. It implies that the wound was perhaps closed under excessive tension, resulting in strangulation of tissue. Wounds that occur with either postoperative bleeding or hematomas must always be regarded seriously, for healing is likely to be less than perfect. A significant number of patients with discharge of bloody fluid from the wound no doubt had less than perfect hemostasis.

## Temperature and Pulse

The disruption of the wound, per se, had far less effect on the patient's temperature and pulse than did the underlying disease. For instance, patients with severe sepsis characteristically had rapid pulse rates and febrile courses. This group was gravely ill. Other patients appeared to be doing quite well but disrupted their wounds following premature suture removal. In this group, there was no significant temperature or pulse elevation. Temperature and pulse variations in patients with dehiscence were consistent with the severity of the initial disease and the nature of associated postoperative complications.

## Date of Dehiscence

Some conclusions insofar as the date of dehiscence is concerned are warranted in my opinion. If wound disruption occurs prior to the fourth postoperative day, it is strong evidence that closure has been faulty. Either the sutures were of insufficient strength to hold the wound together or they were carelessly placed or there was knot slippage. Of course, there is a remote possibility that the suture material was faulty and fractured as a result of stress. Even though the thought is discouraging, wounds that disrupt before the fourth day must be considered technical failures in wound closure. It is interesting that 238, or nearly 90 percent, of 266 wound disruptions occurred between the fourth and fifteenth days. Wound infection becomes an increasingly important factor in wound

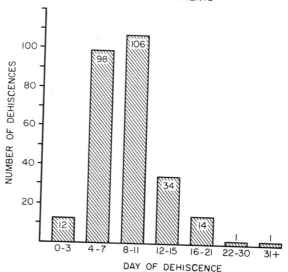

POST-OPERATIVE DAY OF WOUND DEHISCENCE
IN 266 PATIENTS

**Figure 20–13.** Dehiscences rarely occur prior to the fourth postoperative day. Most wound disruptions occur between the fourth and eleventh postoperative day.

disruption after the eighth day. It is noteworthy that wound disruption is rarely seen after the third postoperative week. It is interesting that other workers — including Fallis (1937), Mann and colleagues (1962), Reitamo and Möller (1972), and Eisenstat and Hoerr (1972) — have found the date of disruption to be quite similar to that depicted in Figure 20–13.

### Wound Infection

It is unfortunate that bacteriologic studies of the wounds following disruption were not done uniformly. In cases of disruption that occurred early in the study, cultures had been infrequently obtained. In my opinion, these wounds should be promptly and, if necessary, repeatedly cultured to identify the bacterial flora. Ninety-one of the wounds appeared to be clinically infected. Staphylococci were responsible for a number of infections. Enteric organisms were obtained upon culture of a number of wounds, following operations upon the gastrointestinal tract and complicated biliary tract procedures. Wound infection following trauma and gunshot wounds to the abdomen yielded similar organisms. *Escherichia coli, Pseudomonas, Proteus, Bacterioides,* and anaerobic streptococci were cultured from such wounds. Wound infection is more commonly a factor in wound disruption than is generally recognized. Cultures are often taken at night with cotton swabs, which dry out. This results in at least a few false negative reports.

### Organ Systems Operated on Followed by Wound Dehiscence

A consideration of the organ systems operated on prior to dehiscence in 266 patients is of practical value (Table 20–7). The female genitourinary tract was most frequently the site of operative procedures. Seventy-six females required a variety of pelvic operations for carcinoma of the uterus and cervix and for fibroids, ovarian lesions, and urinary tract disorders. There

**Table 20–7. ORGANS OPERATED UPON FOLLOWED BY DISRUPTION**

| | |
|---|---:|
| Female pelvic organs | 76 |
| Colon surgery | 49 |
| Gastroduodenal surgery | 45 |
| Biliary tract surgery | 37 |
| Genitourinary tract | 19 |
| Appendix | 12 |
| Small bowel | 5 |
| Pancreatic surgery | 4 |
| Splenectomy | 3 |
| Miscellaneous and multiple organ systems | 16 |
| Total | 266 |

were 45 dehiscences following gastroduodenal surgical procedures, commonly performed for bleeding or gastric outlet obstruction. A few gastric neoplasms were also included. Wound dehiscence followed extensive colon operations, such as total colectomy, abdominal perineal resections, and pull-through procedures. Carcinoma, ulcerative colitis, and congenital megacolon were the common diseases requiring these operations.

Miscellaneous operations that were eventually followed by wound disruptions include such procedures as resections of aortic abdominal aneurysms, explorations for gunshot wounds or for abdominal trauma with multiple organ injuries, and repairs of ventral incisional hernias and for clipping of the inferior vena cava.

It is clear that most reported series find the incidence of wound disruption to be greatest following gynecologic operative procedures, gastroduodenal surgery, biliary tract surgery, and surgery of the colon. The exact incidence of the various operative procedures will vary from one institution to another, depending upon the available specialists and the patient population.

## Site of Disruption

The location and specific type of wounds that are prone to disruption can be learned from a review, as included in this chapter. The incidence of the various incisions with postoperative disruption is shown in Table 20–8.

It can be seen that insofar as the threat of wound dehiscence is concerned, vertical incisions are the most dangerous. I was surprised that the left rectus incision was not as effective in prevention of dehiscence

**Table 20–8.  INCISIONS COMPLICATED BY POSTOPERATIVE DISRUPTION IN 266 PATIENTS**

| | |
|---|---|
| Lower abdominal midline | 88 |
| Upper abdominal midline | 57 |
| Left rectus incision | 52 |
| Right rectus incision | 20 |
| Right subcostal | 21 |
| Left subcostal | 2 |
| Xiphoid to symphysis (midline) | 14 |
| Miscellaneous | 12 |

**Table 20–9.  FINDINGS AT TIME OF DISRUPTION IN 266 PATIENTS**

| | | |
|---|---|---|
| Disruption (Without prolapse) | | 154 |
| Disruption (With prolapse) | | 112 |
| Small bowel | 56 | |
| Small bowel and omentum | 32 | |
| Omentum | 24 | |

as I had previously thought. In this procedure, the skin incision is made over the rectus abdominis muscle, then, the rectus muscle is retracted laterally to preserve the nerve and blood supply of the muscle. Disruptions that occurred following appendectomy presented through right paramedian or right rectus incisions. Acute infection and even peritonitis were encountered uniformly in these patients.

In most cases of disruption of operative incisions in this study, prolapse did not occur (Table 20–9). Small intestine was the single viscus most commonly recognized and reported as being extruded through the disrupted wound. Omentum was reported as being present in 37 disruptions; however, I suspect that omentum was present in more instances than the operative notes indicate because of the greater concern for the prolapsed intestine. Colon was uncommonly present in the disrupted wound.

## Management of Patients with Wound Disruption

Prevention of disruption of abdominal incisions is far more rewarding than treatment of the catastrophe. Once evisceration has been recognized, prompt action at several levels is necessary.

It is essential to cover the prolapsed or exposed viscera with a sterile dressing. A small sterile towel, moistened with normal saline solution, is effective and of a sufficient size. The tape and binder should be applied in a manner that will prevent further prolapse of viscera and will hinder greater distraction of the wound edges. If the patient experiences severe pain, a narcotic analgesic is administered. Nasogastric intubation is essential to relieve any further distention. Intravenous fluids are given, and if there is evidence of anemia or hypovolemia, blood transfusions are indicated. The critically ill patient may be moved to the operating room in his bed, without the trauma of transfer to a stretcher. Broad-spectrum antibiotics should be administered.

I favor early repair of the disrupted wound, as soon as the patient's general condition had been treated to a point of optimal improvement. Walton (1948), del Junco and Lange (1956), and Mersheimer and Winfield (1955) also favor immediate resuture of the wound.

## Anesthesia

The surgeon has a number of options in dealing with the disruption. He can choose to avoid an operative procedure on critically ill patients, especially if prolapse has not occurred. He can elect to apply broad strips of adhesive tape and a scultetus binder over an appropriate dressing in selected patients, without anesthesia. If the patient is adequately sedated and cooperative, local anesthesia may be adequate. In gravely ill patients, this may be the anesthesia of choice, though patience on the part of the surgeon is necessary if this method is to be used. If the patient is in reasonably good condition, spinal anesthesia is ideal, since relaxation of the abdominal wall is highly desirable. Finally, general endotracheal anesthesia, expertly administered, offers advantages when operating upon apprehensive patients. The type of anesthesia selected for 266 patients is summarized in Table 20–10.

## Correction of Dehiscence

Once the patient has been prepared and anesthesia established, dressing and adhesive tape are removed. The skin is gently washed for at least ten minutes with a surgical soap to the margin of the incision, the wound itself and prolapsed viscera being protected. After the area has been cleansed, the prolapsed omentum and in-

**Table 20–10. ANESTHESIA FOR 266 PATIENTS WITH WOUND DISRUPTION**

| | |
|---|---|
| General | 88 |
| Local | 71 |
| Spinal | 52 |
| None – taping only | 55 |
| | 266 |

testine are generously lavaged with lukewarm normal saline. Any suture material is, of course, removed. Fibrin and obviously devitalized tissue is removed. I do not favor dissection of the layers of the abdominal wall at this point, since infection so often is present or poses a serious threat. Furthermore, surgeons have learned that sutures must be placed through the thickness of the abdominal wall at a distance from the wound edge.

It has been consistently observed in this study that when a surgeon is called upon to repair a wound dehiscence, he invariably resorts to heavier suture material and retention sutures. The reason for reluctance on the part of the surgeon to initially place retention sutures in appropriate cases escapes me. After I commenced this study, I began using retention sutures in all vertical incisions and in selected cases where subcostal or transverse incisions were used.

In the repair of dehiscence, I currently advocate use of nylon retention sutures placed at intervals of approximately 2 to 3 and 3 to 4 centimeters from the wound edge. These sutures are placed through the entire thickness of the abdominal wall and tied over measured segments of a rubber catheter to minimize the cutting or constricting effect of the suture.

After retention sutures are placed, interrupted sutures of wire or synthetic nonabsorbable may be placed in the fascia between the retention sutures. Many surgeons favor closure with thru-and-thru mass sutures, using the Smead-Jones technique.

In closure of the skin and subcutaneous tissue of wounds that had disrupted, the surgeon must avoid the urge to achieve a tight closure. Since infection is common, it is prudent to place some type of drain at intervals through the subcutaneous fat to the fascia. I use small sections of a soft rubber drain placed at intervals of 5 to 8 centimeters.

Many investigators favor placement of heavy suture material, such as stainless steel or nonabsorbable sutures, placed through the entire thickness of the abdominal wall at some distance from the incision. Wolff (1950), Walton (1948), McCallum and Link (1964), Pratt (1973), and Lehman and colleagues (1968) pointed out the advantages of this technique.

Why is it that a technique, useful in the treatment of wound disruption, is not applied initially in its prevention? The question deserves careful thought, and the answer becomes obvious.

## Mortality

Although the complication of wound dehiscence is frightening to the patient and annoying to the surgeon, it is not the direct cause of death in the great majority of cases. Wound disruptions usually occur in patients who have serious underlying diseases, which result in death of the patient. Often the patient is aged and has diseases involving more than one system.

Perforations of the gastrointestinal tract (e.g., perforated peptic ulcers and perforations of the colon or small bowel, secondary to inflammatory bowel disease) were responsible for most cases of peritonitis and sepsis. Complications of biliary tract lithiasis resulted in pancreatitis, which necessitated operations upon the biliary tract.

It is evident from Table 20–11 that deaths following wound disruption are essentially due to complications arising from treatment of the underlying disease. The mortality rate of approximately 10 percent in this series is lower than that reported by other researchers. Fallis reported a mortality rate of 34 percent in 1937, while Guiney and colleagues reported a mortality rate of 15 percent. One possible explanation is that since sepsis is a major factor in causing fatalities, the availability of antibiotics has resulted in steadily improving survival statistics. More effective treatment of the underlying disease and control of infection will further reduce mortality rates in this group of patients.

Table 20–11. CAUSES OF DEATH IN 266 PATIENTS WITH WOUND DISRUPTION

| | |
|---|---:|
| Sepsis | 10 |
| (Peritonitis, intra-abdominal abscess, subdiaphragmatic abscess, enteric fistulae) | |
| Cardiac failure and pneumonitis | 4 |
| Pancreatitis | 3 |
| Malignancy | 3 |
| Pulmonary embolus | 2 |
| Cerebrovascular accidents | 2 |
| Liver failure; Laennec's cirrhosis | 1 |
| Total | 25 |

## Taping and Closure for Wound Disruption

Taping has been advocated as a method of management of the wound in the desperately ill, postoperative patient. This study supports the suspicion that the method is unsatisfactory, since the incidence of incisional hernia was a staggering 66 percent. Of 35 patients whose wounds were taped, 23 had subsequently developed hernias. Taping should be used only temporarily, until the patient's general condition can be improved on by supportive measures. Repair may be done under local anesthesia.

On the other hand, closure was accomplished in 206 surviving patients and 49 developed incisional hernias. The incidence of incisional hernia following closure of disrupted wounds was 24 percent. The over-all incidence of postoperative hernias was 30 percent in this study. The great importance of wound closure and management for every patient undergoing laparotomy is clear to those who deal with the problem of hernias.

## Prevention of Wound Disruption

The prevention of wound disruption is a highly desirable but complex goal. It demands knowledge of anatomy, physiology, nutrition, and bacteriology, and of the effect of various local and systemic conditions on the healing wound. Furthermore, the surgeon must be informed about sutures and suture techniques. He must recognize and treat postoperative complications, such as cough and ileus, promptly and vigorously. Table 20–12 is an abbreviated list of steps to be implemented in the prevention of wound disruptions.

The propensity of every wound, even in gravely ill patients, is to heal. If the suture is strong enough and suture technique sufficiently effective, disruption will be rare. Use of mass closure, retention sutures, or Smead-Jones closure will all but eliminate the complications of wound disruption and evisceration. Mass closure techniques, properly performed, will radically reduce the incidence of "burst abdomens," even in seriously ill patients. The surgeon who performs the operative incision has a great deal to do with its ultimate fate. Through

## Table 20–12. PREVENTION OF WOUND DISRUPTION

I. *Improve Nutrition*
  A. Intravenous feeding
  B. Tube feeding
  C. Reduce obese patients—Obesity is a hazard for mechanical and technical reasons.
II. *Correct Disease States*
  A. Cardiac
  B. Pulmonary
  C. Metabolic
    1. Diabetes
    2. Hypothyroid
III. *Control Infection*
  A. Implement sound principles of control
  B. Prompt use of antibiotics
IV. *Use of Sound Surgical Principles*
V. *Choice of Incision*
  A. Use transverse incisions
  B. Avoid vertical incisions
  C. Spare nerves
  D. Preserve blood supply
  E. Use previous incision
VI. *Choice of Suture in Closure*
  A. Use mass closure techniques, retention sutures of number 2 nylon or Smead-Jones technique of closure with wire or synthetic nonabsorbable sutures.
  B. Use sutures of sufficient strength, number 2–0 nonabsorbable or 28 gauge wire.
  C. Use nonabsorbable sutures in infections, such as wire or monofilament synthetic sutures.
VII. *Treat*
  A. Postoperative ileus
  B. Postoperative pulmonary complications
  C. Operative and postoperative blood loss

use of proper materials and technique, he can minimize his complications almost to the point of elimination.

## SUMMARY

Wound disruption is a serious complication of abdominal surgical operations because of a significant mortality rate, variously reported to be 15 to 35 percent and an incidence of 30 to 50 percent of incisional hernias following recovery. The burst abdomen often results in prolonged morbidity, and patients often spend three to five weeks in the hospital.

The surgeon should appreciate that a number of clinical conditions have a direct bearing on the patient's ability to heal an operative incision.

A sound knowledge of wound healing is essential if proper wound care is to be exercised. The metabolic needs of a heal-

ing wound must be recognized, and where deficiencies exist they must be corrected.

Wound surgical principles must be painstakingly carried out, using expert operative technique.

In making an abdominal incision, the surgeon should follow sound anatomic principles. The transverse incision—in the event an incisional hernia does occur—heals with a smaller defect. Furthermore, this type of defect is technically more easily repaired. In my experience, the transverse incision results in fewer incisional hernias. Nevertheless, even with the risk of incisional hernia, the vertical incision can be made rapidly and provides necessary exposure—and, hence, is indispensable.

In the final analysis, the key to prevention of wound disruption lies in the closure. Of course, the surgeon must consider all the numerous, complex, and interrelated factors involved in wound healing and wound care. Mass closure techniques, such as using retention sutures of number 2 nylon (or a similar material) or employing the Smead-Jones suture technique with 28 to 32 gauge wire (or synthetic nonabsorbable sutures), will largely prevent disruption. Even should disruption occur, evisceration is largely prevented by mass closure techniques.

The surgeon should always critically reassess his wound care, choice of incision, choice of suture material, technique of closure, and method of management of every wound dehiscence. Provided with such information, the surgeon will inevitably improve his technique and, thus, his results.

## REFERENCES

Abbott, W. E., and Mellors, R. C.: Total circulatory plasma protein in surgical dehydration and malnutrition: Indications for intravenous alimentation of amino acids. Arch. Surg., 46:277, 1943.
Alexander, H. C., and Prudden, J. F.: The causes of abdominal wound disruption. Surg. Gynecol. Obstet., 122:1223, 1966.
Altemeier, W. A.: Control of wound infection. J. Royal Coll. Surg. Edinb., 11:271, 1966.
Bains, J. W., Crawford, D. T., and Ketcham, A. S.: An effect of chronic anemias on wound tensile strength: Correlation with blood volume, total red cell blood volume and proteins. Ann. Surg., 164:243, 1966.
The burst abdomen. (Editorial) J.A.M.A., 195(7):170, 1966.
Campbell, D. P., and Swenson, O.: Wound dehis-

cence in infants and children. J. Ped. Surg., 7:123, 1972.

Closure of wounds. Br. Med. J., 1:129, 1970.

Cole, W. H., Grove, W. J., and Montgomery, M. M.: The use of ACTH and cortisone in surgery. Ann. Surg., 137:718, 1953.

Creditor, M. C., Bevans, M., Mundy, W. L., and Ragan, I. C.: Effect of ACTH on wound healing in humans. Proc. Soc. Exper. Biol. Med., 74:245, 1950.

Culp, R.: Disruption of abdominal wounds. Ann. Surg., 99:14, 1934.

Del Junco, T., and Lange, H. J.: Abdominal wound disruption with eventration. Am. J. Surg., 92:271, 1956.

Douglas, D.: Bursting of wounds after abdominal operations (Letter to Editor). Lancet 2:437, 1972.

Douglas, Sir Donald: Wounds and their problems. Roy. J. Surg. Edinb., 20:77, 1975.

Drye, J. C.: Intraperitoneal pressure in the human. Surg. Gynecol. Obstet., 87:473, 1948.

Dunphy, J. E., and Van Winkle, W.: Repair and Regeneration: The Scientific Basis For Surgical Practice. New York, Blakiston Division of McGraw-Hill Book Co., 1969.

Dunphy, J. E.: On the nature and care of wounds. Ann. R. Coll. Surg., 26:69, 1960.

Eisenstat, M. S., and Hoerr, S. O.: Causes and management of surgical wound dehiscence. Clev. Clin., 39:33, 1972.

Fallis, L. S.: Postoperative wound separation: Review of cases. Surgery 1(4):523, 1937.

Fish, J. C.: The prevention of wound disruption and evisceration. Am. Surg., 30:458, 1964.

Glenn, F., and Moore, S. W.: Disruption of abdominal wounds. Surg. Gynecol. Obstet., 72:1041, 1941.

Guiney, E. J., Morris, P. J., and Donaldson, G. A.: Wound dehiscence. Arch. Surg., 92:47, 1966.

Halsted, W. S.: Ligature and suture materials. J.A.M.A., 60:1119, 1913.

Halsted, W. S.: The treatment of wounds. Johns Hopkins Hosp. Rep., 2:255, 1891.

Hampton, J. R.: The burst abdomen. Br. Med. J., 5364:1032, 1963.

Hartzell, J. B., and Winfield, J. M.: Disruption of abdominal wounds. Intern. Abstr. Surg., 68:585, 1939.

Herrmann, J. B.: Tensile strength and knot security of surgical suture materials. Am. Surg., 37:209, 1971.

Herrmann, J. B.: Changes in tensile strength and knot security of surgical sutures in vivo. Arch. Surg., 106:707, 1973.

Herrmann, J. B., Kelley, R. J., and Higgins, G. A.: Polyglycolic acid sutures. Arch. Surg., 100:486, 1970.

Heughan, C.: Some aspects of wound healing research: A review. Can. J. Surg., 18(2):118, 1975.

Higgins, G. A., Jr., Antkowiak, J. G., and Esterkyn, S. H.: A clinical and laboratory study of abdominal wound closure and dehiscence. Arch. Surg., 98:421, 1969.

Howes, E. L., and Harvey, S. C.: Strength of healing wound in relation to holding strength of catgut suture. N. Engl. J. Med., 200:1285, 1929.

Howes, E. L., Sooy, J. W., and Harvey, S. C.: Healing of wounds as determined by their tensile strength. J.A.M.A., 92:42, 1929.

Hunt, T. K., Ehrlich, H. P., Garcia, J. A., and Dunphy, J. E.: Effect of vitamin A on reversing the inhibitory effect of cortisone on healing of open wounds in animals and man. Ann. Surg., 170:633, 1970.

Joergenson, E. J., and Smith, E. T.: Postoperative abdominal wound separation and evisceration. Am. J. Surg., 79:282, 1950.

Jones, T. E., Newell, E. T., and Brubaker, R. E.: The use of alloy steel in closure of abdominal wounds. Surg. Gynecol. Obstet., 72:1056, 1941.

Keill, R. H., Nichols, W. K., and De Weese, M. S.: Abdominal wound dehiscence. Arch. Surg., 106:573, 1973.

Kewenter, J., and Koch, N. G.: Wound separation and intra-abdominal pressure. Acta Anaesth. Scand., 13:97, 1969.

Lam, C. R.: Intra-abdominal pressure. Arch. Surg., 39:1006, 1939.

Lehman, J. A., Jr., Cross, F. S., and Parkington, P. F.: Prevention of abdominal wound disruption. Surg. Gynecol. Obstet., 126:1235, 1968.

Lichtenstein, I. L., Irving, L., Herzkoff, S., and Shore, M.: The dynamics of wound healing. Surg. Gynecol. Obstet., 130:658, 1970.

Light, H. G., and Routledge, J. A.: Intra-abdominal pressure: Factor in hernia disease. Arch. Surg., 90:115, 1965.

Localio, S. A., Morgan, M. E., and Hinton, J. W.: Biological chemistry of wound healing: Effect of dl-methionine on the healing of wounds in protein depleted animals. Surg. Gynecol. Obstet., 86:582, 1948.

Localio, S. A., Casale, W., and Hinton, J. W.: Wound healing—Experimental and statistical study. Surg. Gynecol. Obstet., 77:369, 459, 1943.

Lord, J. W., Pfeffer, R., and Golomb, F. M.: Elimination of disruption of abdominal incisions. Surg. Gynecol. Obstet., 129:758, 1969.

Lund, C. C., and Crandon, J.: Human experimental scurvy and the relation of vitamin C deficiency to postoperative pneumonia and to wound healing. J.A.M.A., 116:663, 1941.

Magilligan, D. J., and DeWeese, J. A.: Knot security and synthetic suture materials. Am. J. Surg., 127:355, 1974.

Mann, L. S., Spinazolla, A. J., Lindesmith, G. G., LeVine, M. J., and Kuczerepa, W.: Disruption of Abdominal Wounds. J.A.M.A., 180:1021, 1962.

Marsh, R. L., Coxe, J., W., III, Ross, W. L., and Stevens, G. A.: Factors involving wound dehiscence. J.A.M.A., 155(14):1197, 1954.

Martyak, S., and Curtis, L. E.: Abdominal incision and closure. A systems approach. Am. J. Surg., 131:476, 1976.

Meleny, F. L.: Infection in clean operative wounds: A nine year study. Surg. Gynecol. Obstet., 60:264, 1935.

Meleney, F. L., and Howes, E. L.: The disruption of abdominal wounds with protrusion of viscera. Ann. Surg., 99:5, 1934.

Mendoza, C. B., Jr., Watne, A. L., Grace, J. E., and Moore, G. E.: Wire versus silk: Choice of surgical wound closure in patients with cancer. Am. J. Surg., 112:839, 1966.

Mersheimer, W. L., and Winfield, J. M.: Abdominal wound disruption: A review of the etiology, recognition and management. Surg. Clin. North Am., 37:471, 1955.

McCallum, G. T., and Link, R. F.: The effect of closure technique on abdominal disruption. Surg. Gynecol. Obstet., 119:75, 1964.

Moore, F. D.: Metabolic care of the surgical patient. Philadelphia, W. B. Saunders Co., 1959, pp. 130–133.

Norris, J. D.: Review of wound healing and mechanics of dehiscence. Surgery, 5:775, 1939.

Peacock, E. E.: Some aspects of fibrinogenesis during the healing of primary and secondary wounds. Surg. Gynecol. Obstet., 115:408, 1962.

Peacock, E. E., and Van Winkle, W.: *Surgery and biology of wound repair.* Philadelphia, W. B. Saunders Co., 1970.

Mack Publishing Co., *Pharmacopaeia of the United States, Vol. 17.* Easton, Penna., 1965, p. 921.

Postlethwait, R. W.: Further study of polyglycolic acid sutures. Am. J. Surg., 127:617, 1974.

Postlethwait, R. W.: Polyglycolic acid sutures. Arch. Surg., 101:489, 1970.

Postlethwait, R. W.: Long-term comparative study of nonabsorbable sutures. (Paper presented at the Southern Surgical Association Meeting, Dec. 8–10, 1969.) Ann. Surg., 171:892, 1970.

Postlethwait, R. W., Willigan, D. A., and Ulin, A. W.: Human tissue reaction to sutures. Ann. Surg., 181:144, 1975.

Pratt, J. H.: Wound healing—Evisceration. Clin. Obstet. Gynecol., 16:126, 1973.

Reid, M. R.: Some considerations of the problems of wound healing. N. Engl. J. Med., 215(17):753, 1936.

Reitamo, J., and Möller, C.: Abdominal wound dehiscence. Acta Chir. Scand., 138:170, 1972.

Sandblom, P.: Tensile strength of healing wounds. Acta Chir. Scand., 90:1, 1944.

Sandblom, P.: Effect of injury on wound healing. Ann. Surg., 129:305, 1949.

Sedgwick, C. E., and Sullivan, J. T.: Abdominal wound disruption: Analysis of 217 cases. Surg. Clin. North Am., 37:731, 1957.

Taylor, F. W.: Surgical knots. Ann. Surg., 107:458, 1938.

Thacker, J. G., Rodeheaver, G., Moore, J. W., Hauzlarich, J. J., Kurtz, L., Edgerton, M. T., and Edlich, R. F.: Mechanical performance of surgical sutures. Am. J. Surg., 130:374, 1975.

Thompson, W. D., Ravdin, I. S., and Frank, I. L.: Effect of hypoproteinemia on wound disruption. Arch. Surg., 36:500, 1938.

Tweedie, F. J., and Long, R. C.: Abdominal wound disruption. Surg. Gynecol. Obstet., 99:41, 1954.

Walton, F. E.: Prevention and treatment of wound dehiscence. Arch. Surg., 57:217, 1948.

Whipple, A. O.: The essential principles of clean wound healing. Surg. Gynecol. Obstet., 70:257, 1940.

Wolff, W. I.: Disruption of abdominal wounds. Ann. Surg., 131:534, 1950.

## Supplemental Readings

Altemeier, W. A.: Postoperative infections. Surg. Clin. North Am., 25:1, 1945.

Altemeier, W. A., and Furste, W. L.: Studies in virulence of clostridium welchii. Surgery 25:12, 1949.

Babock, W. W.: Metallic sutures and ligatures (Symposium on Modern Trends in Surgery). Surg. Clin. North Am., 27:1435, 1947.

Backer-Gröndahl, N.: The influence of "early rising" on the postoperative complications. Acta Chir. Scand., 91:193, 1944.

Blomstedt, B., and Welin-Berger, T.: Incisional hernias. Acta Chir. Scand., 138:275–8, 1972.

Bruin, T. R.: Prevention of abdominal disruption and postoperative hernia. Inter. Surg., 58:408, 1973.

Carrel, A.: Process of wound healing. Proc. Inst. Med. (Chicago) 8:62, 1930.

Caulfield, P. A., and Madigan, H. S.: Fundamentals of healing. Am. J. Surg., 86:249, 1953.

Conolly, W. B., Hunt, T. K., Zederfeldt, B., Cafferata, H. T., and Dunphy, J. D.: Clinical comparison of surgical wounds closed by suture and adhesive tapes. Am. J. Surg., 117:318, 1969.

De Bruin, T. R.: Prevention of abdominal disruption and postoperative hernia. Inter. Surg., 58(60):408, 1973.

Douglas, D. M.: Acceleration of wound healing produced by preliminary wounding. Br. J. Surg., 46:401, 1959.

Dunphy, J. E., and Jackson, D. S.: Practical application of experimental studies in the care of the primarily closed wound. Am. J. Surg., 104:273–282, 1962.

Efron, G.: Abdominal wound disruption. Lancet 1:1287, 1965.

Echeverria, E., and Jimenez, J.: Evaluation of an absorbable synthetic material. Surg. Gynecol. Obstet., 131:1, 1970.

Edlich, R. F., and Kuphal, J. E.: Bioengineering analysis of sutureless wound closure. Inter. Surg., 58:246, 1973.

Ehrlich, H. P., and Hunt, T. K.: Effects of cortisone and vitamin A on wound healing. Ann. Surg., 167:324, 1968.

Elman, R.: Protein metabolism and the practice of medicine. Med. Clin. North Am., 27:303, 1943.

Ferrer, R. O.: Wound disruption after abdominal laparotomies. Maryland Med. J., 18:57, 1969.

Fisher, W. J., and Tolins, S.: Spontaneous evisceration through a suture sinus. Am. J. Surg., 119:749, 1970.

Fox, M., and Young, W.: Experimental evaluation of a new synthetic polymer suture material, supramid extra. Surgery 52:913, 1962.

Freeman, L.: The cause of postoperative rupture of abdominal incisions. Arch. Surg., 14:600, 1927.

Gallitano, A. L., and Kondi, E. S.: The superiority of polyglycolic acid sutures for closure of abdominal incisions. Surg. Gynecol. Obstet., 73:794, 1973.

Goldenberg, I. S.: Catgut, silk and silver—The story of surgical sutures. Surgery 46:908, 1959.

Grace, R. H., and Cox, S. J.: Incidence of incisional hernia following dehiscence of the abdominal wound (Editorial). Proc. R. Soc. Med., 66:1091.

Hartzell, J. B., Winfield, J. M., and Irvin, J. L.: Plasma vitamin C and serum protein levels in wound disruption. J.A.M.A., 116:669, 1941.

Harvey, S. C.: The velocity of the growth of fibroblasts in the healing wound. Arch. Surg., 18:1227, 1929.

Henzel, J. H., and Stephenson, H. E., Jr.: Postoperative rectus hematoma. Am. J. Surg., 116:882, 1968.

Herrmann, J., and Woodward, S. C.: An experimental study of wound healing accelerators. Am. Surg., 38:26, 1972.

Hoerr, S. O., Allen, R., and Allen, K.: The closure of abdominal incisions: A comparison of mass closure with wire and layer closure with silk. Surgery 30:166, 1951.

Howes, E. L.: Strength studies of polyglycolic acid versus catgut sutures of same size. Surg. Gynecol. Obstet., 137:15, 1973.

Howes, E. L., and Harvey, S. C.: The age factor in the velocity of the growth of fibroblasts in the healing wound. Jr. Exp. Med., 55:577, 1932.

Howes, E. L., Mazens, M. F., and Ellison, L. H.: Healing strength of rectus and midline wounds of the abdominal wall corrected for square area. Surg. Gynecol. Obstet., *134*:387, 1972.

Jennings, W. E.: Disruption of abdominal wounds in a 100 bed community hospital. J. Ark. Med. Soc., 69:187, 1972.

Johnson, R.: Hemorrhage from the inferior epigastric artery. Ill. Med. J., 83:187, 1943.

Jurkiewicz, M. J., and Garrett, L. P.: Studies on the influence of anemia on wound healing. Am. Surg., 30:23, 1964.

Kirk, R. M.: The incidence of burst abdomen: Comparison of layered opening and closing with straight through one layered closure. (Abstract) Proc. Roy. Soc. Med., 66:1092, 1973.

Kirk, R. M.: Effect of method of opening and closing the abdomen on incidence of wound bursting. Lancet 2:352, 1972.

Kraybill, W. G.: Total disruption of surgical wounds of the abdominal wall with reference to plasma proteinemia and plasma ascorbic acid. Am. J. Surg., 66:220, 1944.

Kronenthal, R. L.: *Wound Healing and Absorbable Sutures.* Ethicon, Inc.

Lanman, T. H., and Ingalls, T. H.: Vitamin C. Deficiency and wound healing. Ann. Surg., *165*:616, 1937.

Liu, M., and Hennessy, E.: Clinical study of a new absorbable suture material — Polygolic acid. Med. J. Austr., 2:873, 1970.

Localio, S. A., Chassin, J. L., and Hinton, J. W.: Tissue protein depletion: Factor in wound disruption. Surg. Gynecol. Obstet., 86:107, 1948.

Lord, J. W., Freidman, I. H., and Pfeffer, R. B. A.: A new stay suture technic. Surg. Gynecol. Obstet., *114*:249, 1962.

Lund, C. C., and Crandon, J.: Ascorbic acid and wound healing. Ann. Surg., 114:776, 1941.

Madden, J. W., and Smith, H. C.: The rate of collagen synthesis and deposition in dehisced and resutured wounds. Surg. Gynecol. Obstet., *130*:487, 1970.

Markgraf, W. H.: Abdominal wound dehiscence. Arch. Surg., *105*:728, 1972.

Matsumoto, T., Soloway, H. B., Cutright, D. E., and Hamit, H. F.: Tissue adhesive and wound healing. Arch. Surg., 98:266, 1969.

McMinn, R. M. H.: The cellular anatomy of experimental wound healing. Ann. Roy. Coll. Surg., 26:245, 1960.

Moore, S. W., Conn, J., and Guida, P. M.: Recurrent abdominal incisional hernias. Surg. Gynecol. Obstet., *126*:1015, 1968.

Pareira, M., and Serkes, K. D.: Prediction of wound disruption by the use of healing ridge. Surg. Gynecol. Obstet., *115*:72, 1962.

Patterson, W. B.: *Wound Healing and Tissue Repair.* Chicago, Ill., University of Chicago Press, 1958.

Postlethwait, R. W., et al.: Wound Healing. Surg. Gynecol. Obstet., *108*:555, 1959.

Postlethwait, R. W.: Tissue reaction of surgical sutures. *In*: Dunphy, J. E., and Van Winkle, W., Jr.: *Repair and Regeneration.* New York, McGraw-Hill Book Co., 1968.

Price. P. B.: Stress, strain and sutures. Ann. Surg., *128*:408, 1948.

Ramsdell, E. G.: The prevention of wound disruption. South. Surg., 9(7):495, 1940.

Rhoads, J. E., Fiegelman, M. J., and Panzer, L. M.: Mechanism of delayed wound healing in the presence of hypoproteinemia. J.A.M.A., *118*:21, 1942.

Savlov, F. D., and Dunphy, J. E.: The healing of the disrupted and resutured wound. Surgery 36:362, 1954.

Sisson, R., et al.: Comparison of wound healing in various nutritional deficiency states. Surgery 44: 613, 1958.

Sloan, G. A.: A new upper abdominal incision. Surg. Gynecol. Obstet., 45:678, 1927.

Slome, D.: *Wound Healing: Proceedings of a Symposium.* New York, Pergamon Press, 1961.

Slome, D.: The tensile strength of healing wounds in aponeurosis. *In* Douglas, D. M.: *Wound Healing.* New York, Pergamon Press, 1961, p. 62.

Spencer, F. C., Sharp, E. H., and Jude, J. R.: Experiences with wire closure of abdominal incisions in 293 selected patients. Surg. Gynecol. Obstet., *117*:235, 1963.

Taylor, F. W., and Jontz, J. G.: Fixed figure-of-eight type of retention suture. Surg. Gynecol. Obstet., *109*:387, 1959.

Thorngate, S.: Effect of tension on healing of aponeurotic wounds. Surgery 44:619, 1958.

Udupa, K. N., and Chansouria, J. P. N.: Studies on wound healing. Part II — Role of suture materials in healing of skin wounds. Ind. J. Med. Res., 57:442–448, 1969.

Van Winkle, W., Jr., and Hastings, J. C.: Considerations in the choice of suture material for various tissues. Surg. Gynecol. Obstet., *135*:113, 1972.

Van Winkle, W., and Salthouse, T. N.: Biological response to sutures and principles of suture selection. San Francisco, Scientific exhibit — ACS Clinical Congress, 1975.

Williams, M. B. (ed.): *The Healing of Wounds.* New York, McGraw-Hill Book Co., 1957.

Worsfield, D. C.: Knots for nylon twices and nets. Nylon Outlook, *11*:24, 1961.

Young, D.: Repair of burst abdominal incisions. Br. J. Surg., *61*:456, 1974.

# 21

# Incisional Hernias

## INTRODUCTION

Unexpected complications detrimental to a patient's welfare sometimes accompany advances in scientific knowledge. Incisional hernias fall into this undesirable sequelae to surgery, since they must be considered as largely iatrogenic problems. As a result of the increase in the variety and number of abdominal incisions dictated by surgical progress, the incidence of postoperative incisional herniations increased rapidly. The development of a knowledge of bacteriology and anesthesia enabled surgeons to enter the peritoneal cavity with increasing safety and, in turn, led to increased numbers of operative procedures. Advancements in preoperative and postoperative care made extensive operative procedures common events. Fluid replacement and blood transfusions further enhanced the possibility of even more extensive and complicated intra-abdominal operations. These accomplishments increased the number of possible operative procedures, thus contributing to the number of incisional hernias. This, in turn, stimulated the surgeon's interest in the mechanics of incisional hernia formation.

In the early years of this "March of Progress," emphasis was placed more on mortality than on morbidity. Incisions were at first designed simply to gain entry into the abdominal cavity. Then surgeons became aware that certain incisions were followed by disruptions and incisional hernias; and it was soon recognized that vertical midline incisions were the most common site of postoperative incisional herniation. Because of this awareness, more consideration was given to choice of incisions, suture selection, wound closure, and wound healing.

## HISTORICAL SUMMARY

The rapid increase in the number and types of intra-abdominal operations performed in the last 100 years can be appreciated from this brief historical summary taken largely from the books by Garrison (1929) and Talbott (1970). The report by Rees and Coller (1943) also provided interesting facts on the origin of the transverse incision.

1809  Ephraim McDowell excised a large ovarian cyst.
1847  Baudelocque performed cesarean sections using transverse incisions.
1873  Tait performed his first hysterectomy for myoma.
1876  Porro introduced cesarean section.
1881  Partial gastrectomy performed by Billroth.
1883  Billroth and Senn anastomosed ileum and colon.
1882  Langenbuch performed a cholecystectomy.
1883  Tait operated for extrauterine pregnancy.
1884  Billroth excised a portion of the pancreas; (however, the patient died).
1884  Mikulicz operated for perforated typhoidal ulcer.
1887  By the year 1887 John Homans of

Boston was able to report on 384 laparotomies for a variety of diseases. He noted with surprise that in over 300 patients, nearly 10 percent had ventral hernias.

1900   Wertheim introduced the radical operation for uterine malignancy.

1906   Miles developed a combined, one-stage, abdominal-perineal resection of the rectum for carcinoma.

When the need for entry into the abdomen had been established, surgeons gave more thought as to how this goal could best be achieved.

1894   McBurney described the gridiron incision for appendectomy after Fitz had described the pathology of appendicitis in 1886.

1900   Pfannenstiel described his incision, which combined features of both transverse and vertical incisions. The skin incision was made transversely, approximately 5 centimeters above the symphysis. The aponeurosis of the external oblique and the rectus sheath was also incised transversely, but the transversalis fascia and peritoneum were opened vertically. The incision was recommended for gynecologic operative procedures.

Czerny made an abdominal incision similar to that described by Pfannenstiel; however, Czerny detached the tendinous attachments of the rectus abdominis muscles at their pubic attachment and then made the incision in the transversalis fascia and peritoneum transversely.

1895   Kocher described his subcostal incision for use in biliary tract operations.

1899   Mayland used a transverse incision to enter the upper abdomen.

As a result of the enormous increase in the variety of abdominal incisions, the incidence of postoperative incisional herniations increased rapidly. It was recognized that vertical midline incisions were the most common site of postoperative incisional hernias.

From this increased incidence of incisional hernias came a variety of techniques for their repair. Iason (1941) states that even as early as 1836, Gerdy successfully repaired an incisional hernia. He also gave credit to Maydl for closure of an incisional hernia in layers in 1886. The musculoaponeurotic layers were identified and closed separately, even at that comparatively early date.

In 1899 Mayo described the transverse overlapping technique for repair of umbilical hernias; this method was soon successfully adapted to repair of incisional hernias.

Judd in 1912 described a method in which flaps consisting of peritoneum, muscle, fascia, and scar tissue were overlapped over a similar flap on the opposite side.

Gibson in 1920 described a useful method for repair of midline incisional hernias that he had first used six years earlier, with success. After the sac was dissected and excised, the peritoneal layer was closed. Then, remains of the rectus abdominis muscle was approximated. Generous "relieving incisions" were then made vertically in the midportion anterior sheath of the rectus abdominis, permitting closure of the aponeurosis in the midline (Fig. 21–1). The relaxing incision was made long enough to avoid undue tension at the suture line. Variations of the Gibson technique that were designed to avoid excessive tension at the site of repair continue to be used today, for the method is sound in principle; however, the need for approximation of the rectus muscle in the midline can be questioned.

Maguire and Young (1976) also used lateral relieving incisions in the anterior of the rectus to decrease tension at the suture line following repair of epigastric incisional hernias. Their recurrence rate following repair was 16 percent.

Between 1913 and 1932, incisional hernias were seen in increasing numbers. Branch (1934) noted that during this period, 3142 patients were admitted to Peter Bent Brigham Hospital in Boston for treatment of a variety of hernias. Three hundred, or nearly 10 percent, were incisional hernias.

Freeman in 1927 offered a hypothesis that postoperative rupture of wounds often follows inadequate closure of the peritoneum. Omentum, or bowel, is able to force itself between sutures—especially when exudation and suppuration are present. Rupture may be completed by the patient's vomiting or through distension from many causes. Cave in 1933 and Allen and Wallace in 1942 advocated that abdominal drains be delivered through stab wounds in the flank.

Singleton and Blocker observed that drainage of the peritoneal cavity through an abdominal incision predisposes to disruption and hernia. In 1939, they stressed the need for placement of abdominal incisions properly. They advocated use of a subcostal incision for cholecystectomy in which the rectus muscle was retracted medially.

In 1943 Rees and Coller strongly advo-

cated the use of transverse incisions. They based their recommendations on anatomic and physiologic observations.

Prosthetic materials have played an important role in the surgeon's attempts to replace portions of the abdominal wall, which have been weakened by infection or previously repeated surgical procedures. The historical aspects of the use of prosthetic materials in surgery of the abdominal wall are dealt with in some detail in Chapter 26.

## INCIDENCE OF INCISIONAL HERNIAS

In 1887 Homans stated that 10 percent of all abdominal operations were followed by incisional hernias. Watson, in a review of the subject (1948) found that incisional hernias occurred in 2 to 5 percent of uninfected abdominal operations; however, when infection supervened, the rate of incisional hernias jumped to between 15 and 30 percent. Watson cited the statistics of Warren, who reported the incidence of incisional hernias to be only 2 percent following appendectomy in which the McBurney incision was used.

It is generally recognized that the incidence of incisional hernias will be greater when vertical incisions are employed, especially if infection occurs as a complication.

When considered from another viewpoint, it is found that incisional hernias constitute a rather small percentage of all hernias facing surgeons.

Zimmerman and Anson (1967) compiled statistics on 100,114 hernias. They found that incisional hernias numbered 1,724, or 1.7 percent of the total. Inguinal hernias accounted for 81.4 percent of the total number of hernias. They also noted that incisional hernias constituted anywhere from 1.3 to 10.8 percent of the various types of hernias studied by a number of authors. Cave (1933) found the incidence of incisional hernias to be 6 percent among 928 patients studied.

The incidence of incisional hernias is steadily decreasing in the practice of modern surgery. Proper care in selection of suture materials and, incisions; use of excellent surgical techniques, including mass closure techniques; drainage of subcutaneous spaces, in selected cases; elimi-

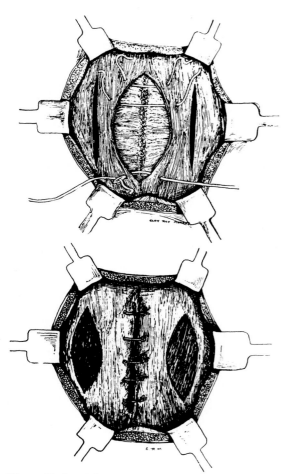

**Figure 21-1.** Gibson's original illustration showing the relaxing incision made vertically in the anterior sheath of the rectus. (Reproduced by permission of J. B. Lippincott Company. From Gibson, C. L.: Operation for cure of large ventral hernias. Ann. Surg. 72:214B, 1920.)

nation of the practice of placing drains
through the full thickness of abdominal
wounds; and proper use of antibiotics have
all been contributing factors.

## DEFINITION

It should be a simple matter to identify an
incisional hernia correctly; and, ordinarily,
both the surgeons and medical records
department do manage to label the postoperative hernia properly. In a number of
cases, however, the accuracy of the diagnosis remains in doubt and thus a clear
definition of a hernia that develops at the
site of an operative incision is essential.

One area of concern involved the question of whether a hernia that is found at the
umbilicus following an earlier infraumbilical hernia should be considered an umbilical hernia or a postoperative incisional
hernia. When earlier physical examinations included descriptions of a previous
umbilical hernia, this was no problem.
Another source of confusion was the indexing of other hernias (such as epigastric
or lumbar) as being included under the
category of "ventral hernias," without
qualification. Specifically, a ventral postoperative incisional hernia is one that
develops at the site of a previously made
incision through the thickness of the abdominal wall. Many factors — such as faulty
closure, infection, unusual stress on the
sutured wound, or impaired healing — cause imperfect healing of the incisional site; and, therefore, protrusion
occurs at the site. The defect can be huge
giving the appearance of a well-advanced
pregnancy; or, in the rare patient, a very
small defect at the suture line may result in
a Richter's hernia. The two terms, ventral
incisional hernia and postoperative hernia,
are used interchangeably.

"Ventral hernia" should be employed as
a collective term for all protrusions through
the anterolateral abdominal wall, excluding groin hernias. It is essential to identify
all hernias of the abdominal wall specifically as to their location and nature. For
instance, those hernias at the umbilicus
should be designated as *umbilical hernias;*
midline protrusions are designated as *epigastric hernias.* In certain instances, protrusion of the abdominal wall carries an

**Table 21–1. A CLASSIFICATION OF
VENTRAL HERNIAS**

1. Postoperative incisional hernias
2. Umbilical hernia (Chapter 22)
3. Epigastric hernias (Chapter 23)
4. Omphalocele (Chapter 22) and Hernia
   into the umbilical cord (Chapter 22)
5. Lumbar hernia (Chapter 14)
   a. Superior lumbar triangle and
   b. Inferior lumbar triangle
6. Spigelian hernia (Chapter 24)
7. Hypogastric hernia (Chapter 23)
8. Gastroschisis (Chapter 24)
9. Diastasis recti (Chapter 23)
10. Interparietal hernia (Chapter 24)

eponym — the Spigelian hernia is a good
example.

If "ventral hernia" is considered to
include all protrusions through the anterolateral abdominal wall (exclusive of groin
hernias), this large category of protrusions
should then be subdivided into a more
specific classification. A classification that
has practical merit is offered in Table 21–1.
The terms "incisional" or "postoperative
hernia" should be reserved solely for those
protrusions of the anterior abdominal wall
occurring at the site of earlier operative
procedures.

The only common denominator shared
by the hernias listed in Table 21–1 is their
gross anatomic locations. They vary significantly in pathogenesis, pathology, and
method of management. As a result, each
type of ventral hernia listed in Table 21–1
will be dealt with individually in those
chapters listed. Because of their unusual
nature of rarity, interstitial hernias will be
treated in the chapter on unusual hernias
(Chapter 24).

## CLINICAL STUDY

In order to better understand the nature
of incisional hernias, I personally reviewed
the records of 794 patients who underwent
repair of incisional hernias during the
period of time between 1948 and 1973
(inclusive) at Henry Ford Hospital. The
hernias occurred following an initial
operation that had been performed at
various institutions, including our own. It
was often difficult to determine the exact
postoperative course in some patients.
Surprisingly, many patients could describe

postoperative wound disruptions, and wound infections were generally recognized and described by patients as well. Unfortunately, follow-up observations on many patients were limited.

## Age and Sex Incidence

There was no significant difference in the incidence of incisional hernias in males versus that in females in this study. Postoperative hernias were seen in 383 males and 411 females. However, it should be noted that 184 hernias in this study occurred in females undergoing a variety of pelvic operative procedures. If one considers only those operations performed on both sexes, then incisional hernias occurred more frequently in males than in females by a ratio of approximately 3:2.

It is interesting that Obney (1957) found the incidence of incisional hernias to be 53.6 percent in males and 46.6 percent in females, while Fischer and Turner (1974) found an incidence of 57 percent in males and 43 percent in females. Seidel and

colleagues (1972) found the incidence to be equal among males and females.

The great preponderance of incisional hernias in older patients, as shown in Figure 21–2, is easily explained, since aged patients are subject to a great variety of diseases requiring operative procedures. Furthermore, they are afflicted with other metabolic and degenerative diseases. Inflammatory diseases, such as inflammatory bowel disease and complicated biliary tract disease, are also common problems among patients who develop incisional hernias. The same individual may have cardiac, renal, pulmonary, or metabolic diseases as well. In addition, arteriosclerosis and arteriosclerotic heart disease are often present.

It can be seen that 728 of 794 incisional hernias (92 percent) occurred after the age of 40 years. Viljanto and Vänttinen (1968) noted that incisional hernias are rare in persons under 40 years of age. Obney found that the peak incidence of incisional hernias occurred in patients 40 to 70 years of age. Seventy-two percent, or 568, incisional hernias occurred in patients older than 50 years of age. The need for greater

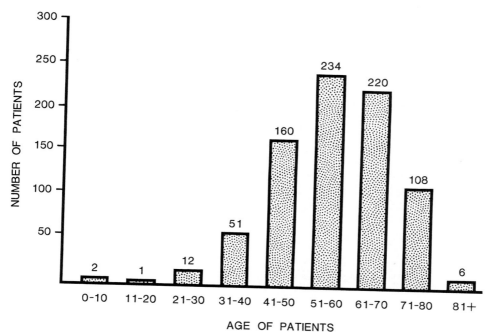

AGE INCIDENCE OF INCISIONAL HERNIA IN 794 PATIENTS

Figure 21–2. Age incidence of 794 patients with incisional hernias.

care when operating on older individuals is clear.

## Clinical History

Obviously, most patients with incisional hernias will present with a protrusion of the abdominal wall, with or without pain. In a few obese patients, the protrusion may be hidden from sight by a heavy panniculus. Many of the largest incisional hernias cause no pain at all while others merely cause discomfort. Incarceration leads to some pain, but intestinal obstruction leads to nausea, vomiting, and further distension. Intestinal obstruction following initial surgery developed in 75 (9 percent) of 794 patients whose records were reviewed.

The surgeon should always elicit details of the history. Patients with incisional hernias are often able to describe the events preceding the development of their protrusions with acceptable accuracy. They recall indications for the original operative procedure and can often describe the postoperative course in some detail. For instance, patients who suffered wound disruptions are able to recognize and describe the event. Wound disruption had occurred in 90, or 11 percent, of 794 patients studied. Grace and Cox (1976) were able to study 70 patients with postoperative wound disruption. Of their patients, 49 or 47.6 percent developed hernias and 20.4 percent healed satisfactorily. Those who developed pain and prolonged drainage from the wound recognized that infection was present following the initial operative procedure. Patients may also be aware of postoperative bleeding and incisional hematomas.

It is worthwhile to develop the clinical history in every patient with incisional hernia. The surgeon can learn the circumstances leading to the development of hernia in each case and, hence, may be able to minimize any occurrence in the future.

## Physical Examination

*Fat people are the bane of the surgeon's existence.*

*Koontz, 1963*

Koontz stated that obesity as an important factor cannot be overemphasized. He noted that obese individuals find it difficult to lose weight and many of them do not recognize the relationship between food intake and their obesity. Trace and colleagues (1950) found that 95.5 percent of such patients carried excessive amounts of adipose tissue. Obney (1957) found that of the patients he studied with incisional hernias, 96.3 percent of them were overweight. Branch (1934) noted that 48 percent of his patients with incisional hernias were obese. Thus, the prevalence of obesity among patients with incisional hernias is clearly established. Furthermore, the recurrence rate following repair of incisional hernias is much higher for obese individuals (Fig. 21–3).

The size of the hernia varied greatly—as described in general terms such as large, medium, or small—in the 794 patients studied. The largest hernias were seen in the epigastrium and lower abdomen, particularly when long midline or paramedian incisions were used. Small hernias were seen at drain site incisions in the right lower quadrant, following appendectomy and peristomal protrusions. Signs of obstruction were present in 9 percent of the patients studied. These patients had nausea, vomiting, and abdominal distention. Hyperactive bowel sounds were present in patients who had not yet developed peritonitis. The presence of a tender, distended abdomen with absent bowel sounds indicated the presence of peritonitis.

The physical examination of the hernia, unfortunately, was often performed in a perfunctory manner. The observer too often noted the presence of a hernia with little description of details. For a more accurate report, the length and width of the defect should be noted. The presence of a widened cicatrix with loss of substance of the abdominal wall should also be noted. Multiple incisions and their locations should be recorded on a "map" of the abdomen. Such observations will result in a better appreciation of the pathogenesis of certain incisional hernias.

## Initial Operative Procedures

Any abdominal incision can be followed by subsequent herniation—given a number of unfortunate circumstances and misdirected surgical efforts. Poor place-

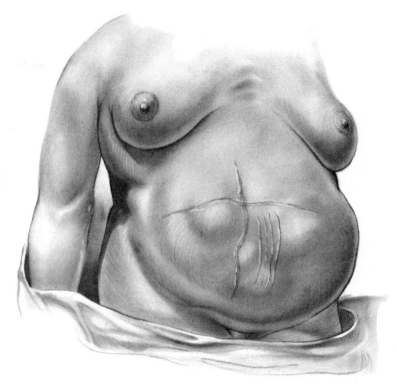

Figure 21–3. Obesity and numerous operative procedures weaken the abdominal wall.

ment of incisions, postoperative infection, and improper closure are examples of conditions predisposing to incisional hernias. Some operative procedures are more likely than other ones to be complicated by the appearance of hernias. It can be seen in Table 21–2 that operations on female pelvic organs are the most frequent antecedant procedures. In my opinion, this

incidence is due, in part, to the fact that operations on the female generative tract are so common. (Cholecystectomies and biliary tract operations are also popular.) Two circumstances predispose to the development of incisional hernias in patients requiring biliary tract operations: infection is occasionally a factor; but, more commonly, the placement of a drain through the incision is a direct factor in eventual hernia formation (see Fig. 21–4, E; p. 376). When absorbable sutures are loosely placed at the drain site, the result may be herniation.

Appendectomies were followed by the development of smaller hernias in a surprisingly large number of patients. In these cases, infection was a common contributing factor, the delivery of the drains (often more than one) through the McBurney or transverse incision was again an important factor.

Gastric operations were carried out mostly for patients with complications of duodenal ulcer through an epigastric midline incision. Multiple factors (such as infection, wound disruption and poor technique of closure) entered into the genesis of postoperative hernias in this group. Furthermore, the patients were often el-

## Table 21–2. INITIAL OPERATIVE PROCEDURES AND ORGANS OPERATED UPON

| | |
|---|---|
| Hysterectomy and female pelvic organs | 170 |
| Cholecystectomy and other biliary tract operations | 166 |
| Appendectomy | 126 |
| Gastric operations | 90 |
| Colectomy, abdominoperineal resections and colostomies | 72 |
| Laparotomy for abdominal trauma | 29 |
| Resection—small bowel | 18 |
| Bladder | 17 |
| Cesarean section | 14 |
| Vascular operations | 12 |
| Prostatic resections | 7 |
| Others | 73 |
| Total | 794 |

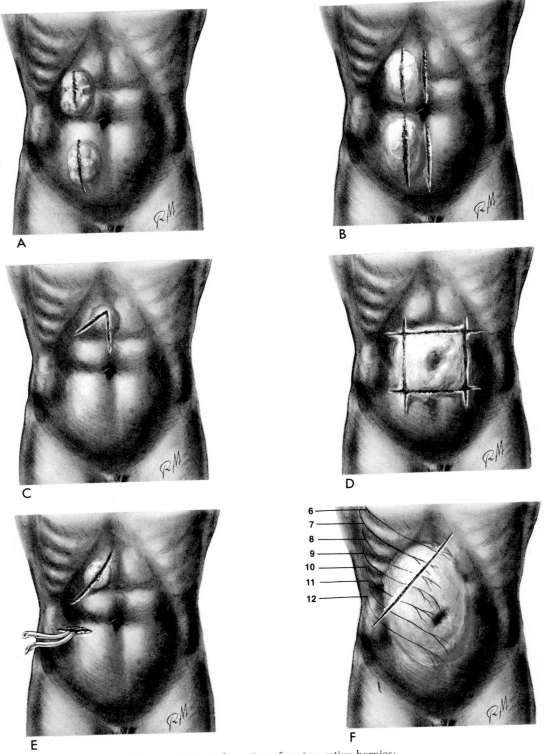

**Figure 21–4.** Incisions that contribute to formation of postoperative hernias:

A.  Vertical incisions at lateral margin of rectus abdominis muscle that destroy nerve and blood supply to the abdominal wall.

B.  Midline and pararectus incisions have a devastating effect on the abdominal wall.

C.  Subcostal and vertical midline incisions weaken the abdomen at the apex.

D.  Two transverse and two vertical incisions produce the "tic-tac-toe" abdomen with a central hernia.

E.  Delivering a drain through the subcostal incision weakens the abdomen at the site. A hernia may appear years later. A large stab site for egress of the drain may eventually result in a hernia.

F.  Section of three or more intercostal nerves will too often result in an extensive diffuse protrusion.

derly and had cardiac or pulmonary diseases, or both. Bleeding from a duodenal ulcer and obstruction were among the common indications for operative treatment of patients studied. I was surprised that operations on the colon and rectum were not more frequently followed by herniation. We do not place drains through midline incisions, nor do we place such drains when a rectus incision is made with lateral retraction of the rectus abdominis muscle. I also expected to find more hernias in those patients operated on following trauma—for example, involving gunshot wounds, penetrating abdominal wounds, and blunt abdominal trauma. For this group of patients, a vertical midline incision was preferred. Such incisions are regularly closed with wire plus the additional insertion of retention sutures. Thus, the principle of mass closure technique is consistently employed. Drains are frequently inserted into selected areas (such as the subhepatic space, subphrenic space, or right lower quadrant) but invariably are delivered through separate stab wounds. Finally, patients with suspected visceral injuries are promptly placed on broad-spectrum antibiotics, which are continued into the postoperative period.

Urinary bladder and prostate infections often appeared as contributing causes to the development of incisional hernias following operations on the small bowel.

Vascular operations are often performed on patients who are extremely ill, either chronically or acutely. The elderly patient with arteriosclerotic heart disease or chronic pulmonary disease may require resection of a ruptured aortic aneurysm. The vertical midline incision from the xiphoid to the symphysis is preferred. This incision is regularly closed with either synthetic nonabsorable or wire sutures, together with retention sutures. I believe that the technique of closure is directly responsible for the good results obtained in these chronically ill patients who have additional, acute problems.

It was surprising that 14 incisional hernias developed following Cesarean section. In these patients, the abdomen is obviously most relaxed after delivery with little tendency to separation of wound edges. Nephrectomy, splenectomy, and repair of umbilical hernias were followed

by incisional hernias in a smaller number of patients.

## Known Complications Following Initial Operation

There was great difficulty in accurately establishing the occurrence rate of complications following the initial operative procedure. Even such dramatic events as postoperative wound disruptions were occasionally lost in the obscure recesses of the medical record—or through the failure of the Medical Records Department to achieve accurate indexing. This responsibility must fall to the operating surgeon if more accurate records are to be achieved. Nevertheless, it was possible to obtain some information regarding the events that preceded the development of incisional hernias in a number of patients. If we are to decrease the incidence of incisional hernias, we must become aware of every factor that could be important in their production.

The complications following the initial procedure in 794 patients are summarized in Table 21–3. Many of these individuals had operative procedures performed elsewhere, hence, valuable information was not available. Certain information obtained from this study merits serious reflection.

The precise incidence of wound infection as an important factor in the genesis of incisional hernias has not been determined. In this study, it was present in 190, or one-fourth, of the patients who eventually developed incisional hernias. Peritonitis was initially present as well in 67, or 8 percent, of patients studied. Irvin and colleagues (1977) also found that infection was a prominent contributing factor to wound dehiscence and hernia.

Table 21–3. COMPLICATIONS FOLLOWING INITIAL OPERATION IN 794 PATIENTS WITH INCISIONAL HERNIAS

| Type | Number | Percent |
|------|--------|---------|
| Wound infection | 190 | 24 |
| Wound disruption | 90 | 11 |
| Peritonitis | 67 | 8 |
| Hematoma | 23 | 3 |

In 90 (or 11 percent) of the patients, wound disruption could be established as a complication following the original operation.

Hemostasis is obviously an important technical goal for every surgeon. Furthermore, it was obvious to me that surgeons are, in fact, accomplishing this objective with reasonable fidelity. Hematomas or bleeding occurred in only 3 percent of the 794 patients studied. The explanation for occurrence of incisional hernias must be sought elsewhere, even though hematomas are contributing factors to herniation in an occasional patient.

As indicated in Table 21–3, wound infections, wound disruptions, and hematomas were present in 303, or 38 percent, of 794 patients with incisional hernias.

## Onset of Incisional Hernias

The duration of time elapsing from the time of the operative procedure is both interesting and informative (Table 21–4).

Of 475 patients in whom incisional hernias developed early in the postoperative period, reasonable explanations were evident in 303 patients (Table 21–4). By far, the greatest percentage of incisional hernias occur within the first year following the operative procedure. In 615 patients, or 77 percent, the hernia was discovered within the postoperative year. This observation suggests to me that the technic of wound closure has much to do with appearance of incisional hernias and use of non-absorbable sutures is important in the prevention of incisional hernias.

### Table 21–4. INCISIONAL HERNIAS

| Time of Onset Following Operative Procedure | Number of Hernias |
|---|---|
| First month | 124 |
| 2 to 6 months | 351 |
| 7 to 12 months | 140 |
| 2 to 3 years | 83 |
| 4 to 5 years | 46 |
| Longer | 50 |

Others have observed the early development of incisional hernias following surgical procedures. King in 1935 observed that 40 percent of incisional hernias developed and were diagnosed in the first four weeks of the postoperative period. He noted that 75 percent of these hernias were present in the first postoperative year. Cave (1933) noted that 60 percent of postoperative ventral hernias developed in a period of two months following the initial operative procedure. Akman (1962) found that 50 percent of the hernias he studied developed during the first six months and, furthermore, 66 percent were identified during the first year. Seidel and colleagues (1972) found that more than 50 percent of incisional hernias developed within 6 months postoperatively.

It is clear that the surgeon—through choice of incision and suture material, careful surgical technique, adequate control of infection, and sound preoperative preparation of the patient—has the necessary knowledge and information to minimize the incidence of incisional hernias. Use of gastrointestinal intubation and vigorous treatment of ileus should not be overlooked.

## Site of Incisional Hernias

It is reasonable to expect that incisional hernias will be found in those portions of the abdominal wall most often subjected to surgical incisions. The midline incision below the umbilicus is often used as an operative technique; thus, it is the site of more incisional hernias. Also, it is a well-known fact that vertical incisions are followed by a greater incidence of postoperative hernias than are transverse incisions. My study of 794 incisional hernias confirmed the observations of others—i.e., that more incisional hernias are seen after subumbilical midline incisions than after other types incisions (Table 21–5).

Obney (1957) found that 84.4 percent of the cases that he studied had incisional hernias of the lower abdomen. Fischer and Turner (1974) found that a vertical incision had been used in 65 percent of 169 postoperative hernia cases that had undergone initial hernia repairs.

It is impossible to obtain accurate statis-

Table 21–5.  SITE OF INCISIONAL
HERNIAS—794 PATIENTS

| | |
|---|---:|
| Midline—Lower abdominal | 206 |
| Midline—Upper abdominal | 126 |
| Subcostal—Right and left | 126 |
| Rectus—Right and left | 86 |
| Transverse and muscle splitting— Right lower quadrant | 67 |
| Peristomal incisional | 31 |
| Vertical—Right upper quadrant (Type of incision uncertain) | 30 |
| Vertical—Right lower quadrant (Type of incision uncertain) | 23 |
| Vertical, midline—xiphoid to umbilicus | 12 |
| Miscellaneous and poorly described | 87 |

tics on the exact frequency of incisional hernias following various procedures. Precise records as to the number of various procedures followed by incisional hernias are not available. Yet some generalizations are possible. The observation can be made that incisional hernias are more often seen in the midline below the umbilicus. In this study, 206 of the incisional hernias, or 26 percent, occurred in the midabdomen below the umbilicus. Hysterectomies and various pelvic operations were performed on 170 of these patients.

Upper abdominal midline incisional hernias occurred in 126, or 16 percent, of the patients whose records were reviewed. Such hernias also occurred in 90 individuals who had had gastric operations (usually for complications of duodenal ulcer). A variety of other operations were also performed through the midline epigastric incision. Cholecystectomy, hiatal hernia repair, pancreatic surgery, and exploration for trauma were other operations performed through this incision.

The subcostal incision was utilized for operations upon the gallbladder, bile ducts, stomach, pancreas, spleen, and kidneys. Biliary tract procedures were most often performed through the subcostal incision. Incisional hernias occurred at the site of subcostal incisions in 126, or 16 percent, of 794 patients with postoperative hernias. In this group of patients, I am convinced that the practice of delivering drains through the incision contributed directly to the appearance of the incisional hernia. Infection of some degree occurred in the majority of patients. I have discontinued this practice for the past 10 years. Drains, if needed, should be delivered

through a small stab wound remote from the incision in the lateral abdominal wall.

The right rectus incision was used for a variety of procedures. Appendectomies and operations on the female pelvic organs were among the most common of these. The left rectus incision was typically employed in operations on the sigmoid colon and rectosigmoid. Rectus incisions were complicated by incisional hernias in 86, or 11 percent, of 794 incisional hernias studied.

It was noteworthy that incisional postoperative hernias were seen in 67 patients with right lower quadrant muscle-splitting or transverse incisions. These patients were operated on for either acute suppurative appendicitis or gangrenous appendicitis with peritonitis, both of which required the use of drains. The drains were invariably delivered through the abdominal incision, with resultant weakness at that site. Such drains should be delivered farther laterally in the flank through a separate stab wound. The musculoaponeurotic structures should be closed with wire or monofilament synthetic nonabsorbable sutures. The subcutaneous portion of the wound should be loosely closed, and small drains placed superficially in the subcutaneous space for drainage. It is unusual that 67 hernias, or 8 percent, of the incisional hernias occurred after transverse or muscle-splitting incisions in the right lower quadrant. Postoperative infection and delivery of drains through the incision explain this unusually high incidence of incisional hernias. These hernias were usually of small size and comparatively easily repaired.

A wide variety of "peri-stomal" hernias was encountered. The pericolostomy hernia was most common, but a few such hernias were seen about ileostomy incisions. Improper placement of the stoma site and poorly placed abdominal incisions were two common factors in the genesis of the peri-stomal hernias seen in 31, or 4 percent, of the 794 patients with incisional hernias.

There were a number of incisions made vertically in the region just lateral to the midline. The exact location of these incisions was difficult to determine. They usually resulted in hernias that presented as large bulges in the right upper and right lower quadrants, and it was difficult to determine which incision was later followed by hernation. Infection was not a prominent complication in these cases. It appeared that faulty closure was a common factor in causation of the hernia in these patients.

It was surprising that the long, vertical midline incision was not followed by incisional hernia more frequently. These incisions were utilized often for vascular operations or abdominal trauma. The incision was usually closed with heavy retention sutures and nonabsorbable sutures (such as wire or synthetic nonabsorbable sutures.

Miscellaneous incisions included laparotomy incisions, which were made after one or more previous entries had been attempted into the peritoneal cavity. One extraordinary patient had a total of 10 cesarean sections. Several patients had eight abdominal entries that ultimately resulted in the appearance of large incisional hernias.

Transverse incisions at areas other than the right lower quadrant infrequently resulted in hernias. Drains were not placed in such wounds but, instead, were delivered through a separate wound in the flank.

## Number of Previous Laparotomies

One annoying aspect of incisional hernias is their tendency to recur. Of 794 patients, 578 of them, or 73 percent, developed incisional hernias following a single laparotomy. One hundred twenty-seven patients had undergone abdominal section on two previous occasions for an incidence of 16 percent. Forty-eight patients required 3 abdominal operative procedures; 21 patients required 4 operations, while 20 patients required more than 4 laparotomies — in other words, 216 patients required a total of 606 incisional hernia repairs or laparotomies. The importance of the problem of incisional hernias cannot be overemphasized. Seidel and colleagues (1972) found the incidence of recurrent incisional hernias to be 20 percent, and the chance of a third relapse was 40 percent. The morbidity is unduly prolonged, and financial losses from repeated hospitalizations are enormous.

## Size of the Incisional Hernia

The exact size of the protrusion was recorded in approximately three-fourths of the cases reviewed. Hernias were considered large when the defect measured more than 10 centimeters at its greatest diameter. Medium hernias measured between 6 and 10 centimeters in diameter, while those under 6 centimeters were considered to be small. Using the above criteria, 198 incisional hernias were large; 234 were medium, and 149 were considered to be small hernias.

The largest incisional hernias were seen at or near the midline, both above or below the umbilicus. A few large hernias were encountered following long midline incisions from the xiphoid to the symphysis pubis. Large hernias were also common in those patients having multiple operations and in those who developed wound infection as a postoperative complication.

Generally, smaller hernias were located at drain sites, at the site of transverse or McBurney incisions, and around intestinal stomas.

## Etiologic Factors in Incisional Hernias

In reviewing the medical records of 794 patients, I concluded that better results could be achieved through a more critical attitude toward the choice of incision, method of closure, choice of suture material, suture technique, and control of infection. In many cases, it was impossible to ascribe the appearance of an incisional hernia to a single cause, since so often more than one factor was operative.

The summary of etiologic factors listed in Table 21–6 is unorthodox perhaps, but it does contain a number of truths. The reduplication of etiologic factors in postoperative hernias becomes evident, and this, I believe to be a valid observation. For example, an individual patient may be obese, may have had multiple operations, may develop a wound infection, and subsequently may suffer a wound disruption. The ultimate appearance of an incisional hernia in such a patient is to be expected unless every contributing factor has been recognized and taken into account during the operative procedure.

Table 21-6.   ETIOLOGIC FACTORS IN
794 INCISIONAL HERNIAS*

| Type | Number | Percent |
|---|---|---|
| Faulty closure | 338 | 43 |
| Drain in incision | 189 | 24 |
| Infection | 190 | 24 |
| Wound disruption | 90 | 11 |
| Ileus | 60 | 8 |
| Pulmonary disease | 48 | 6 |
| Hematoma and bleeding | 26 | 3 |
| Multiple operations | 196 | 25 |
| Obesity | 319 | 40 |
| Undetermined | 157 | 20 |

*Multiple factors were often found to be operative
in the same patient.

One might ask, "Where are the factors of
anemia and malnutrition in relation to the
genesis of incisional hernias?" The answer
is relatively simple and clear. Since it is a
policy at our institution to avoid elective
surgery for patients with a hemoglobin of
less than 10 grams/%, measures are taken to
correct any anemia prior to surgery. A few
patients with acute blood loss may be
operated on in the anemic state when the
loss of blood is more rapid than that
replaced. Traumatic vascular injury and
bleeding from viscera are examples of such
cases. Here, the cause of blood loss is
remedied, and the blood volume appropriately restored. Similarly, malnutrition is
corrected with tube feedings or intravenous hyperalimentation prior to elective
surgical intervention. In my experience,
anemia and malnutrition are only minor
factors in the etiology of incisional hernias
(although this was not the case as recently
as 50 years ago).

Faulty closure was easily the most common deficiency detected that resulted in
eventual herniation. The particular deficiency or deficiencies in closure that ultimately result in incisional hernia are
sometimes difficult to identify. Faulty closure includes such deficiencies as the use
of suture material that is too delicate. The
technique of closure itself might be ill
conceived. I have found a number of
hernias occurring after wound closure in an
obese patient—with continuous number
3-0 and number 4-0 chromic catgut used
for closure of the aponeurotic layers! The
use of catgut sutures without heavy retention sutures in patients with infected or

potentially infected wounds is another example.

The technique of drain placement
through the full thickness of any abdominal
wall incision is to be condemned. If a
postoperative wound is held open by a
drain or drains while suppuration continues, hernia is an almost inevitable result.
I would suggest that Chapter 20 on wound
disruption be reviewed at this point and
that Figures 20-1 through 20-8 be re-
considered. Some fault could be found
with wound closures in 338, or 43 percent,
of the cases studied. I must add that most
of the deficiencies in technique have been
corrected and that the incidence of wound
disruption and postoperative herniation is
declining in our practice.

Drains were placed in the incisions of
189, or 24 percent, of the cases reviewed.
This practice is considered faulty closure.
In the cases I reviewed, the subcostal
incision and the right lower quadrant
transverse (or McBurney), incisions were
the two areas where drains were too often
placed through the full thickness of the
abdominal wall. Incisional hernias at these
sites were uncomfortably common, considering that such incisions should heal
soundly.

It must be admitted that infection at the
site of the drain was an important added
factor contributing to poor healing and
eventual herniation.

I believe that the incidence of postappendectomy incisional hernias could be
reduced by delivering the drains through a
separate stab wound, lateral to the appendectomy incision. Closure of the abdominal wall in infected cases should be performed with nonabsorbable sutures. Wire
or monofilament synthetic sutures are recommended. The subcutaneous tissues
should be drained and loosely approximated.

Three definite reasons for herniations
following appendectomy are evident: (1)
Infection, usually severe, was present.
Acute suppurative appendicitis, perforated
appendicitis, and appendiceal abscess
were the common causes for appendectomies in these cases; (2) Drains were
regularly delivered through the incisions;
(3) The incisions were uniformly closed
with catgut.

Wound infection, was considered to be

an important factor that interfered with wound healing (see Chapter 20; Fig. 20–2, p. 334). In 190, or 24 percent, suppuration was seen at the incision site. Acute appendicitis, biliary tract disease, perforated ulcer, duodenal fistulae, enteric fistulae, anastomotic leaks, diverticulitis, ulcerative colitis, and traumatic visceral injuries were the most common sources of mixed bacterial flora. The skin of either the patient or the operating room staff was considered to be the source of staphylococcal infection.

Wound disruption was a direct contributing factor in the development of incisional hernias in 90 patients, or somewhat more than 11 percent of the total. The problem of wound dehiscence is far more serious than most surgeons appreciate (see Chapter 20).

Ileus was not considered to be a sole factor in the etiology of incisional hernia. It occurred most often after extensive bowel surgery and following an exploratory procedure to locate visceral perforation in cases of peritonitis. Ileus contributes to poor healing through increased intra-abdominal pressure, with resultant impairment of circulation to the incision site. Increased stress upon a poorly healing wound results in incisional hernias. Ileus was an annoying problem in 60, or 8 percent, of the patients studied. Underlying peritonitis was common among these patients.

Severe pulmonary disease – including emphysema, bronchitis, and asthma – was observed in a number of patients who developed incisional hernias. Forty-eight individuals, or six percent, were found to have well-advanced pulmonary pathology. Diseases of the respiratory tract place increased stress on the suture line by increasing intra-abdominal pressure. Proper suture techniques will diminish the incidence of incisional hernias in such individuals.

Hematoma and postoperative bleeding were less of a contributing factor than I had anticipated. Slightly more than three percent of 794 patients with incisional hernias could be considered to have had less than perfect hemostasis. Thus, our surgical staff generally practiced effective hemostasis. It is to be recalled that bleeding is more likely to occur in patients with blood dyscrasias, liver disease, and advanced malignancy with hepatic metastases.

Multiple operations and poorly con-

ceived incisions contributed substantially to the incidence of incisional hernias. Almost 25 percent of the patients had undergone more than one operative procedure. Furthermore, the incisions in many were poorly planned, if any planning at all preceded the abdominal incisions. The proper selection of incisions is largely a matter of experience, but it is based on a sound knowledge of anatomy. Some examples are illustrated in Figure 21–5.

The Pfannenstiel incision is desirable for pelvic operations. I discovered two patients who had two transverse and two vertical abdominal incisions. This entity has been appropriately designated as the "tic-tac-toe" abdomen (Fig. 21–4, D, p. 376). I have seen a vertical midline inci-

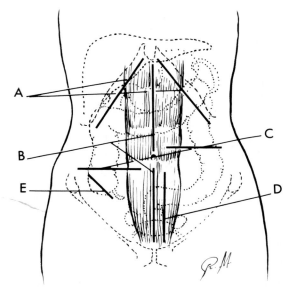

**Figure 21–5.** Preferred incisions for entry into the peritoneal cavity.
A. Subcostal incisions permit access to organs in the upper abdomen – including stomach, liver, gallbladder, spleen, pancreas, kidney, and transverse colon.
B. The midline incision permits operative procedures upon most of the organs noted in A. If made below the umbilicus, pelvic organs are accessible to a midline incision. The entire peritoneal cavity is best reached through a midline incision from the xiphoid process to the symphysis pubis.
C. The transverse incision may be used to gain access to the right colon and the appendix; and, on the left side, the descending colon may be reached through a transverse incision.
D. Paramedian incisions, above or below the umbilicus, give much the same access to the peritoneal cavity as do midline incisions.
E. The McBurney incision is preferred for appendectomy.

sion, above or below the umbilicus, which was later followed by a parmedian or rectus incision (Fig. 21–4, *B;* p. 376). Occasionally, an unusually long subcostal incision is followed by a vertical midline incision, resulting in an area of weakness at the apex of the triangle created by the incision (Fig. 21–4, *C;* p. 376). I have also seen a remarkable patient with five separate vertical infraumbilical incisions: one midline, two paramedian, and two incisions laterally over the rectus muscles.

A critical analysis of each patient's problem will result in more appropriate selection of incisions when repeated entry into the abdomen is necessary.

Obesity is a common problem in those individuals who develop incisional hernias. The problem, in my opinion, is largely mechanical. When vertical incisions are necessary in obese patients, the lateral distracting force is great. As has been noted, it requires a measure of physical strength to approximate the wound, and extra strength on the part of the suture material to maintain that approximation. Retention sutures are indispensable in wound closure in obese patients. When weight reduction is possible in elective surgical procedures, it should be insisted on by the surgeon. In obese patients with visceral perforation, the subcutaneous tissues superficial to the musculoaponeurotic layers should be drained.

## Method of Repair

In this study of 794 incisional hernia cases, there was a great variation in the technique selected for repair, however, some consistencies in treatment method can be seen (Table 21–7).

**Table 21–7. INCISIONAL HERNIAS – TECHNIQUE OF REPAIR IN 794 PATIENTS***

| | |
|---|---|
| Repair with prosthetics | 267 |
| Two-layered closure | 199 |
| Mayo principle | 107 |
| One-layered closure | 104 |
| Three-layered closure | 81 |
| Side-to-side overlap | 36 |

*In 31 patients combinations of above techniques and transplantation of enteric stomas were performed.

The surgeons of Henry Ford Hospital prefer to repair incisional hernias without implantation of a prosthetic material. Such adjuncts have been found useful in the repair of large hernias with loss of abdominal wall tissue. In 267 patients, or 34 percent, a prosthetic was considered desirable—especially in those patients with huge hernias and multiple recurrences, Tantalum mesh, Marlex mesh, and fascia lata were used with some frequency. Cutis grafts were used in very few repairs. At the present time, Marlex mesh appears to be superior to other materials used as implants. The use of prosthetics in hernia repair is further discussed in Chapter 26.

The two-layer technique of closure was utilized more frequently than any other single technique. The method was used in 199 patients, or approximately 25 percent of the total. Midline incisional hernias in which the anterior and posterior rectus sheath could be identified were repaired by this technique. This principle was also applied to other areas where both a peritoneal–transversalis fascia layer and a second aponeurotic layer could be identified. The technique has been popular with surgeons for over five decades (Fig. 21–6).

An important adjunct to a two-layer repair of incisional hernias is the judicious use of relaxing incisions, placed laterally and vertically in the anterior sheath of the rectus abdominis, as recommended by Gibson in 1920. (See Fig. 21–1, p. 371.)

The Mayo principle in repair of incisional hernias refers to the technique of transverse closure, in which the upper layer is imbricated over the lower in a "vest-over-pants" manner; this method is suitable if the defect is not too large in a vertical direction. One hundred seven incisional hernias were repaired in this manner (Fig. 21–7).

The one-layer closure technique was utilized in 104 individuals. This method was used most frequently in midline incisional hernias. It is a desirable method when the margins of the defect can be approximated without undue tension. It has the advantage of simplicity, plus it avoids opening up tissue spaces. Koontz (1953) used this method and illustrated an effective mass-closure technique in his book on hernia (Fig. 21–8).

The three-layer closure was used in the

*Text continued on page 387*

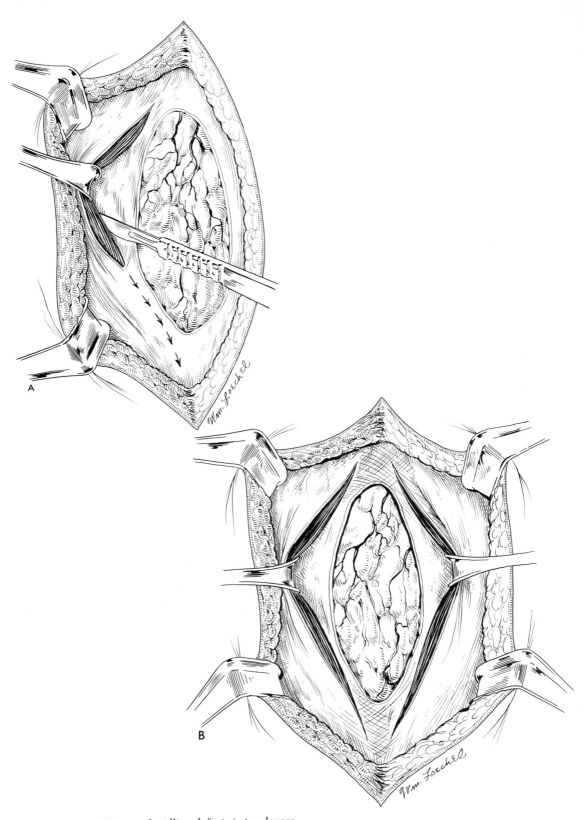

**Figure 21–6.** Closure of midline defects in two layers.

A. The hernial sac has been excised. The posterior rectus sheath is being identified. Only enough dissection is carried out to clearly identify normal structures.

B. The posterior rectus sheath has been identified.

*Legend continued on the opposite page*

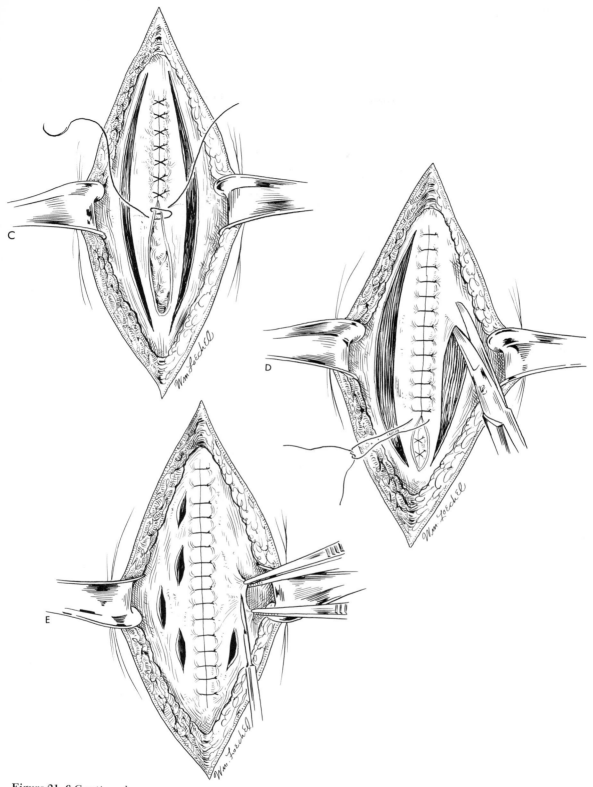

**Figure 21–6** *Continued*

C.  The posterior rectus sheath is closed with interrupted figure-of-eight sutures. Absorbable sutures may be used for this layer.

D.  A vertical relaxing incision is made in the anterior sheath of the rectus.

E.  Numerous small incisions in the anterior rectus sheath may be utilized as an alternate means of avoiding tension. Nonabsorbable synthetic sutures or monofilament wire is preferred for closure of this layer.

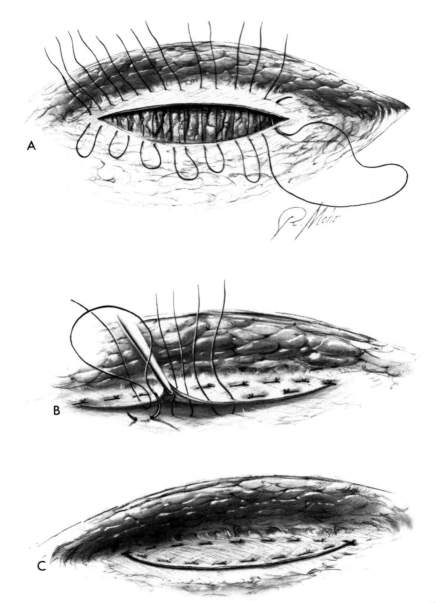

**Figure 21-7.** *A.* The margins of the defect have been identified. Imbrication with sutures of number 2–0 nonabsorbable material are placed.
*B.* The sutures are being tied, showing minimal overlapping.
*C.* Closure of the incisional hernial defect is completed.

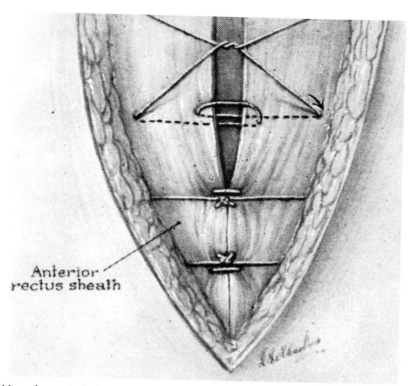

Anterior
rectus sheath

**Figure 21–8.** Mass closure technique in a single layer as described by Koontz. (See also Smead-Jones suture – Fig. 20–10, p. 356.) Reproduced with permission from Koontz, A. R.: Failures with Tantalum gauze in ventral hernia repairs. Arch. Surg. 70:125, 1955. Copyright 1955, American Medical Association.

repair of incisional hernias in the lower abdominal quadrants. In such cases, hernias developed most frequently following appendectomy. Repair of a postappendectomy incisional hernia through a muscle-splitting incision is a comparatively simple matter. The abdomen is carefully prepared and draped as usual, and the previous cicatrix is excised. The incision is developed about the defect at the level of the external oblique. Hemostasis is achieved with number 4–0 suture material. We often use silk, but catgut or synthetic sutures may be used just as well.

The external oblique is opened, in the direction of its fibers, well beyond the hernia both medially and laterally. Both the upper and lower leaflets of the external oblique are clearly identified. The dissection is carried out at the level of the hernial sac; this may be done with the sac opened and with the index finger inserted into the peritoneal sac. Dissection can then be easily carried out over the finger. Upon dissection of the sac, the internal oblique and transversus abdominis layers are more or less recognizable. Thus, three layers for closure are identified – the peritoneum and transversalis fascia, the transversus abdominis and internal oblique, and the aponeurosis of the external oblique.

The peritoneum and transversalis fascia are first closed, using interrupted sutures of number 2–0 or number 3–0 suture material. Chromic catgut is sufficiently strong for this closure. The internal oblique and transversus abdominis layers are approximated gently with number 2–0 chromic catgut. Care must be taken not to crush the muscle in a strangulating ligature. The external oblique aponeurosis is the third and final layer of closure, and for this procedure number 2–0 nonabsorbable suture material is used. This layer may be overlapped for a distance of approximately one centimeter, is used. Subcutaneous tissues are closed with number 3–0 plain catgut or absorbable synthetic sutures, and skin may be approximated with a monofilament nonabsorbable suture. Eighty-one, or ap-

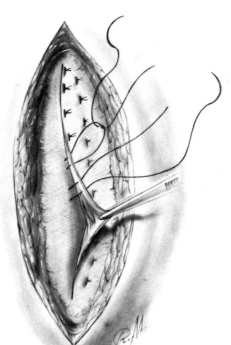

**Figure 21–9.** Side-to-side overlapping technique is occasionally useful. Nonabsorbable sutures must be used, and minimal overlapping is recommended.

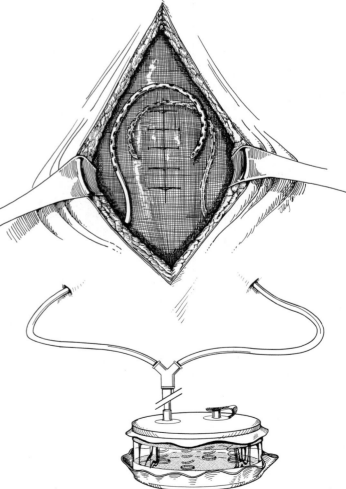

**Figure 21–10.** One of the significant technical contributions toward better management of operative wounds is the use of synthetic suction catheters to which negative suction is continuously applied. Blood and serum may be aspirated thereby decreasing the incidence of seromas and hematomas.

proximately 10 percent, of the postoperative hernias were repaired in this manner.

The side-to-side overlapping method of closure was used in only 36 patients. This closure is used in highly selected cases (Fig. 21–9).

One useful adjunct in management of postoperative wounds is the application of continuous suction through plastic tubes inserted into the depths of the wound (Fig. 21–10). I place one small tube deep to the muscular layer and a second tube over the aponeurosis. Negative suction applied to wounds, which have been implanted with mesh, is especially desirable. Negative suction also cancels the need for tightly applied pressure dressings, thereby facilitating respiration and lessening the probability of atelectasis as a complication.

### "Peri-stomal" Hernias

The problem of the peri-ileostomy or peri-colostomy herniation is far too common. There are two common causes for such herniations: first, the size of the initial opening in the abdominal wall is too large; and second, the opening in the abdominal wall is not placed in the optimal location. Peri-stomal hernias have been described by Ray and colleagues (1960) as inherent complications of delivering the intestine through the abdominal wall. Delivery of the bowel through the primary abdominal incision predisposes to such hernias. The presence of obesity or increased intra-abdominal pressure further increases the possibility of peri-stomal herniation. Such hernias may become quite large, and their bulk alone justifies repair. At other times, smaller hernias may become incarcerated. Burns (1970) found 16 paracolic hernias among 307 colostomy patients, for an incidence of 5 percent; however, obstruction was present in only one patient. Saha and coworkers (1973) found 2 peristomal hernias in 21 patients. Obstruction was present in one individual.

Prian and colleagues (1975) described peri-stomal hernias in 9 patients who underwent surgical repairs. Three of the nine developed recurrences in from six to eight months after repair. Six patients underwent surgery for relocation of the stoma, with success in follow-up examinations extending from four months to six years. Prian and his coworkers advocate transposition of the stoma in recurrent peri-stomal herniation. This is generally sound advice.

For the repair of peri-stomal hernias, the patient must be prepared much the same as for other intestinal operations. The stoma is closed with a purse-string suture of number 2–0 silk, and the abdomen is carefully prepared with pHisoHex. After appropriate drapes are applied, an incision is made in the skin about the stoma. The skin incision is extended either transversely or vertically, depending on the previous incisions; and the plan for the neo-stoma in the current situation depends on the condition of the abdominal wall. Transplantation of the stoma is preferred if the defect about the bowel is large and the strength of the abdominal wall is compromised. The new location may be near the site of the original stoma if the abdominal wall is of good strength. In general, delivery of the bowel through the rectus abdominis muscle and its sheath is preferred since the strength of the abdominal wall will be least compromised by this method. Generally, midline locations for intestinal stomas are to be avoided, since complications following such placement are too common. However, some surgeons have been enthusiastic about results obtained following placement of the stoma at the umbilicus.

Occasionally, the strength of the wall has been seriously compromised by a number of previous abdominal operations. In such cases, the length of the available bowel may not permit shifting of the stoma to a new site. It then becomes necessary not only to mobilize the stoma as described but also to enter the abdomen through a separate incision. The intestine can be mobilized by dividing and ligating appropriate vessels near their origins. For example, the inferior mesenteric artery may be ligated and divided near its origin, permitting mobilization of the left colon up to and somewhat beyond the splenic flexure. Thus, the added mobility of the remaining colon will permit shifting of the stoma to a desirable location.

Whenever the stoma of an ileostomy or colostomy is moved to a new locaton, the same attention must be given to those details already described. The size of the stoma must be precisely measured: if it is two centimeters or less in diameter, it is too tight and dysfunction will result; if it is larger than four or five centimeters, it is too large and herniation will most likely develop. The proper size of a desirable stoma is approximately 3.5 centimeters in diameter. Transfer of the stoma to a new location is usually successful, provided care is taken in fashioning the new stoma.

## Performance of Ileostomy and Colostomy

Abdominal surgeons often encounter hernias about ileostomies and colostomies that cause malfunction of the stomas and perhaps, obstruction. The presence of large protrusions makes it difficult to fit an appliance. Repair of peri-ileostomy and peri-colostomy hernias then becomes necessary.

The *Atlas* written on the subject of intestinal stomas by Turnbull and Weakley (1967) is highly recommended. The volume is brief but informative and is well illustrated.

The appearance of peri-stomal hernias is largely due to the technique of performance of the stomas. As is so often true in medicine, prevention is better than cure; and this applies to peri-stomal hernias. The abdominal incision should be carefully selected according to each patient. If it is planned to place the stoma on the right, then a left rectus incision is acceptable. Planning of the location of the stoma should be deliberate and precise. The face plate of the pouch should be used as a guide in locating the position for the stoma. The upper margin of the face plate is placed just below the umbilicus and the medial margin at the linea alba; this ensures that the ileum or colon must exit through the anterior sheath, the rectus abdominis muscle, and the posterior sheath. The stoma lies approximately one-third of the distance between the umbilicus and the anterior superior iliac spine. This will serve as a most favorable location for fitting the ileostomy appliance, from the functional aspect. Naturally, the location of the stoma will vary with the patient's physique, and weight.

After the location of the stoma has been selected, size is the next important detail for the surgeon to determine. The size of the intestine to be delivered through the opening is an important factor to be considered. In general, the opening is larger than the size of one finger, but slightly smaller than two digits. If the surgeon has large fingers, then the size should be such that it will not quite accommodate two fingers. The aperture in the abdominal wall should measure approximately 3.5 centimeters. I would like to repeat that the anterior rectus sheath is incised vertically after a button of skin has been excised and subcutaneous fat has been incised. The rectus muscle fibers are spread apart with a hemostat, then, the posterior sheath is also incised vertically.

The mesentery of the intestine is carefully sutured to the abdominal wall to prevent withdrawal of the bowel into the free peritoneal cavity and to prevent internal herniation.

Experience has taught us the advantages of everting the mucosa over the protruding stoma at the time of performance of the ileostomy. By everting the mucosa, the period for maturation of the stoma is largely eliminated and stomal function is excellent. Furthermore, suture of the mucosa to the epidermis has resulted in excellent healing.

In the performance of abdominoperineal resection, I favor the midline incision. The location of the colonic stoma is carefully planned and the technique is executed similarly to that used for performance of an ileostomy; however, instead of excising the skin (as for a ileostomy), I divide it transversely at the colostomy site. The end of the colon must be delivered through the abdominal wall at the site of the rectus abdominis muscle in order to minimize the danger of herniation. The mesentery of the colon must be attached to the abdominal wall to prevent internal herniation, obstruction, or intestinal volvulus. At present, the end of the colon is sutured to the epidermis with number 4–0 chromic catgut, thus approximating skin to colonic mucosa.

## Anesthesia

A variety of methods were used to achieve anesthesia in patients undergoing incisional hernia repair. Spinal anesthesia was generally preferred, being used in 452,

**391**

or nearly 57 percent, of 794 repairs. General anesthesia was selected for 234, or nearly 30 percent; and local anesthesia was administered to 104, or 13 percent, of the cases.

Spinal anesthesia provides excellent relaxation and, hence, is appropriate for repair of incisional hernias. Local anesthesia was used in aged patients with severe cardiovascular, pulmonary, and metabolic disorders. These patients often had a number of infirmities occurring simultaneously.

## Suture Material Selected for Repair of Incisional Hernias

Silk has traditionally been the suture material of choice for clean operative procedures at the Henry Ford Hospital since its founding. Silk was the suture material of choice in 249, or 31 percent, of the patients. Nonabsorbable sutures (including silk, wire, and synthetic nonabsorbable sutures) were used in the repair of postoperative hernias in 557, or 70 percent, of 794 repairs.

Catgut was used in 237 patients, or 30 percent, of the total; however, this suture material is currently being displaced by synthetic nonabsorbable sutures, such as coated Dacron (Tevdek) and by wire. It is expected that catgut will continue to decline in popularity as a suture material for hernia repair, and results can be anticipated to improve as better synthetic nonabsorbable sutures become available.

## Location of Implanted Material

As a general principle, I prefer to implant the prosthetic material deeply within the abdominal wall but superficial to the peritoneum. When Tantalum mesh was used in the late 1950s and early 1960s for implantation in the peritoneal cavity, dense adhesions between the metallic mesh and the intestine often made dissection hazardous, if not impossible. Inadvertent enterotomies were common at reoperation.

In 13 patients, the mesh was placed in the subcutaneous space; that is, external to the musculoaponeurotic layers. I am not convinced of the value of this method of repair, especially if the peritoneal transversalis

fascial layer has not been properly identified and closed.

One method which I believe to be desirable is placement of the mesh in an intraperitoneal position, overlying the omentum when it is present. This method is useful when generous portions of the abdominal wall have been destroyed by numerous previous operations or by severe infection. In these situations, it is unwise to attempt to bring the edges of the defect together because of the resultant excessive tension. A large portion of mesh is sutured about the defect in a manner so as to place slight tension upon the implanted material.

The aponeurotic layer and available cicatrix is closed over the implanted material. Obviously, this method is selected for difficult cases in which there is destruction of substantial portions of the abdominal wall. Intraperitoneal placement of the mesh was considered desirable in 52, or 7 percent, of the incisional hernias repaired.

Placement of a synthetic mesh superficial or just external to the peritoneal layer was the preferred method in repair of 202, or 25 percent, of 794 hernias repaired. However, of those hernias repaired with a prosthesis the material was placed in the extraperitoneal location in 202 (76 percent) of 267 repairs.

It is not necessary to cover the mesh entirely with aponeurosis or cicatrical tissue. In 168 patients, the mesh was completely covered by connective tissue; but in 99 patients, the coverage was not complete. Prosthetic materials (such as Marlex) are well tolerated by subcutaneous tissue. It is preferred that the material not be covered with aponeurosis if the result is excessive tension on the suture line.

## Complications

As might be expected, wound complications outnumber other problems associated with incisional hernias by a wide margin (Table 21–8). Fortunately, most of the complications are of a minor nature, and many of them are comparatively simple to manage.

**SEROMA:** Collection of abnormal amounts of serous fluid occurred in 54, or

**Table 21–8.   INCISIONAL HERNIA COMPLICATIONS IN 794 PATIENTS**

| Type | Number | Percent |
|---|---|---|
| Wound complication | | |
| Seroma | 54 | 7.0 |
| Wound infection | | |
| Major | 22 | 3.0 |
| Minor | 18 | 2.0 |
| Wound induration | 16 | 2.0 |
| Abdominal wall sinuses | | |
| Suture | 5 | 0.6 |
| Mesh | 15 | 2.0 |
| Pulmonary | | |
| Atelectasis, Pneumonitis | 48 | 6.0 |
| Phlebothrombosis | 18 | 2.0 |
| Pulmonary embolism | 3 | 0.4 |
| Genitourinary (Retention, infection) | 16 | 2.0 |
| Miscellaneous | 23 | 3.0 |

nearly 7 percent, of the patients who underwent surgery.

Accumulation of fluid in the area of repair varied in amount and duration from patient to patient. The degree of dissection appeared to be a factor as did the implantation of mesh. The problem seemed to be greater when Tantalum and fascia lata were used together in the same individual. The use of two prosthetic materials was discontinued after a comparatively short period of time. The high complication rate was unacceptable.

Treatment of seromas consists of aspiration under aseptic conditions when the collection is large and troublesome. Smaller collections are not withdrawn, for in a few weeks they disappear.

Sharp dissection, avoidance of excessive dissection, and use of suction catheters postoperatively are preventive measures. I have not found pressure dressings really helpful, since they often result in painful excoriation of the skin following tight application of adhesive tape.

**HEMATOMAS:** Excessive collection of blood in the operative areas was seen in 21, or nearly 3 percent, of patients whose incisional hernias were repaired. Hematomas obviously result from imperfect he-mostasis. Dissection is sometimes extensive. When retention sutures are placed more or less blindly, injury to blood vessels can occur. At other times, bleeding may occur in an area previously considered to be dry. Small hematomas need not be disturbed, but it should be recalled that blood outside the vascular system is a type of necrotic or dead tissue. Any large hematomas should be "debrided" or evacuated, as is any other devitalized tissue.

Evacuation of hematomas must always be performed with strict adherence to aseptic principles. The larger hematomas and postoperative bleeding require treatment in the operating room. The incision should be opened; all blood and clots evacuated; and hemostasis re-established. Small subcutaneous drains are desirable. Broad-spectrum antibiotics are administered.

One of the significant advances in modern surgery is the availability of plastic drainage tubes and portable appliances, which provide constant negative suction at the operative site. These mechanical devices provide enough negative pressure in the wound area to aspirate much of the blood and plasma, which might otherwise accumulate in the wound. Proper placement of the tubes is essential (Fig. 21–10). If a prosthesis is used, one suction tube should be placed deep to the mesh and the other tube may be placed in the subcutaneous tissue anterior to the aponeurosis.

**WOUND INFECTION:** Wound infection is a substantial threat to the successful repair of incisional hernias. Obese patients, wide areas of dissection, and the presence of cicatrix are conditions favoring the development of infection. Some degree of infection was observed in 5 percent of 794 patients, but the infections were considered major in somewhat over two percent. What are minor infections? These are superficial infections associated with minor skin loss at the margins of the wounds; for example, an obese patient with a huge hernia often has atrophic skin over the herniated mass, with little subcutaneous tissue over the hernia. After dissection and closure, necrosis of the skin and a minor infection are occasionally seen. Other minor infections are those occasionally associated with retention sutures. Treatment consists of debridement of the necrotic skin, application of warm, sterile compresses, and removal of those sutures which are troublesome.

Major infections are those in which suppuration occurs in the depth of the wound. These patients are often ill with pain and swelling in the operative area. Chills, fever, and leukocytosis accompany the onset of infection. Drainage of the wound is essential, and antibiotic irrigations may be used as well. Cultures, both aerobic and anaerobic, should always be obtained. Warm sterile compresses are helpful. Systemic antibiotics are essential. Infection in the postoperative wound is a real threat when strangulating obstruction of the bowel is present along with the hernia. Antibiotics should be administered promptly and continued in the postoperative period.

WOUND INDURATION: When mesh is used in incisional hernia repair, a small number of patients will complain of postoperative pain. In this group of 794 patients, 2 percent had an unusual amount of pain and induration in the operated area. Infection was not a factor in these cases. Reassurance, use of warm applications, tub baths, and analgesics were helpful. The pain gradually diminishes in nearly every patient.

ABDOMINAL WALL SINUSES: Two mechanisms account for abdominal wall sinuses following incisional hernia repair. Minor problems arise when a suture (such as silk, wire, or synthetic) is present along with a low-grade superficial infection. In such cases an area of redness, swelling, and eventual drainage develops about the suture, which continues to serve as a nucleus of infection until it is extruded or removed surgically; this describes the first mechanism.

The second mechanism involves sheets of implanted material that subsequently become infected. In most cases the problem of infection manifests itself early in the postoperative period. A number of patients will continue to be plagued with recurrent episodes of infection. Ultimately, removal of the mesh becomes necessary. In a few patients, infection and abdominal wall sinuses develop in the recovery or late postoperative period without early evidence of infection. In any case, the infected area must be adequately drained. Nonabsorbable, braided suture material must be removed. Many early infections will re-

spond to drainage, irrigations, compresses, and antibiotic therapy, but in a few cases, the infection will not be cured until the mesh is removed. Infection occurred in nearly 2 percent of 794 patients who had incisional henias repaired, 250 of whom had mesh implantations. Removal of synthetic mesh was necessary in only 1 percent of 794 patients. We had more difficulty with tantalum mesh than with Marlex mesh, although the former was used far less frequently.

Other complications and their incidence are listed in Table 21–8. The management of these complications is detailed in Chapter 27 on postoperative management.

## Recurrences

The recurrence rate was found to be approximately 9 percent in 794 repairs. The follow-up studies were limited; 53 percent of the patients were followed for up to five years. Many patients, having moved to other cities and states, were lost to follow-up studies. During the period of the study being discussed here, the recurrence rate was higher than I thought it would be; with the passage of time, other recurrences would have undoubtedly developed.

Others have observed the high incidence of recurrences following repair of incisional hernias. The recurrence rate of 9 percent, which I have identified in cases at Henry Ford Hospital, is probably being improved at the present time. Branch in 1934 found the rate of recurrence to be 19.6 percent. As recently as 1940, Shelly found that hernias reappeared in 17.8 percent of 207 cases. Five years later, Singleton and Stehower found the recurrence rate to be 18.2 percent. In 1962 Akman reported a surprisingly favorable recurrence rate of 1.2 percent among 500 repairs. With the current knowledge available to surgeons, it is reasonable to expect a decreasing rate of relapses following incisional hernia repair.

As I have observed, most of the recurrent incisional hernias were recognized within the first year of the repair, and many of these occurred within six months.

The numerous factors that lead to incisional hernias have been considered, and often in the same patient a number of etiologic factors are responsible. An obese patient may be suffering from severe pulmonary disease when faced with a troublesome incisional hernia.

The technique of repair is obviously of the greatest importance. Most failures can be attributed to an ineffective technical performance, which encompasses a great variety of possibilities. For example, in one patient with a recurrence, number 3–0 chromic catgut and number 4–0 silk were used in the repair. At other times, retention sutures were not utilized when they might have been helpful. In a few recurrences, the protrusion occurred above or below the inserted prosthetic material, indicating that the implanted material should have been of a more generous size.

Further scrutiny of the use of chromic catgut in the repair of incisional hernias is in order. Healing proceeds more slowly in heavily scarred tissue, with its impaired blood supply and loss of elastic fibers; and catgut sutures may fail to maintain approximation long enough. Nonabsorbable sutures and mass closure techniques are advised.

Infection seriously interferes with wound healing; and, when it occurs following incisional hernia repair, recurrences are common. Every measure should be taken to avoid contamination with organisms from the skin or the gastrointestinal tract. Asepsis is no less important today than it was before the era of antibiotics.

Hematomas are detrimental to optimal wound healing, since they interfere with circulation to the operative area and predispose to infection. Even when healing occurs, the process proceeds at a greatly retarded rate. Since at times wide dissection is necessary, the effort for a perfect hemostasis must be redoubled. Even the smallest vessels must be clamped and tied with fine suture material; for, by their numbers alone, they can cause considerable extravasation of blood.

The need for precise surgical technique with sharp scalpel dissection cannot be overemphasized. It takes a certain amount of courage to excise generous amounts of a cicatrix that cannot replace normal tissue. Excessive disruption of tissue planes should be avoided when such exercises serve no useful purpose. This is especially true for a number of midline hernias, which may be closed in a single layer.

In my experience, seromas have not been as detrimental to wound healing as have hematomas. Nevertheless, use of suction catheters placed in the depths of the wound have proved useful in minimizing the subcutaneous collection of serum. Pressure dressings used in past years have not proven as effective in controlling seroma formation. Furthermore, large, tightly applied, bulky dressings often limited respiration leading to atelectasis and pneumonitis.

Pulmonary complications and ileus also have an adverse effect on the healing wound by increasing intra-abdominal pressure. Severe coughing and emphysema both put additional stress on the closed incision. Illeus increases intra-abdominal pressure through distention, which, in turn, interferes with circulation at the incision and compromises healing.

## Mortality

Incisional hernias can be repaired with remarkable safety. In 794 patients, there were 5 deaths — a mortality rate of 0.63 percent.

Two of the five patients who died had neglected strangulated obstructions with resultant gangrene of the bowel, peritonitis, and sepsis. In one of these individuals, the hernia had been present for 32 years.

Two patients died of cardiac failure; one of these patients was 89 years of age.

The fifth patient died on the fifth postoperative day of pulmonary embolism.

## FACTORS IN PREVENTING RECURRENCE OF INCISIONAL HERNIAS

If the surgeon is to decrease the recurrence rate following incisional hernia repair, he must:

1. Accomplish repair through use of sound surgical principles — this includes gentleness in handling of tissues, sharp dissection and careful hemostasis.
2. Employ sound technical maneuvers — e.g., use of nonabsorbable suture materials and proper technique. Excessive tension must be avoided.

3. Avoid infection—but when it occurs, treat it properly and vigorously. Therapy must be instituted preoperatively when infection is evident or anticipated.

4. Use plastic tubes and suction apparatus to aspirate blood and serum.

5. Avoid ileus through the use of gastrointestinal intubation and suction.

6. Treat pulmonary complications before and after repair.

7. Combat ileus (once it develops) through early use of appropriate decompressive measures.

8. Achieve weight reduction in the obese patient. Obesity is an added hazard to the patient with incisional hernias; however, weight reduction—as a desirable goal in the patient with incisional hernia—is more easily identified than implemented.

9. Use mass closure techniques and retention sutures in appropriate cases (such as those involving obesity, pulmonary disease, or peritonitis).

10. Learn to use a synthetic mesh judiciously when there is destruction of a portion of the abdominal wall.

It is recommended that Figures 20–1 through 20–4, pages 333 to 335, and page 338, be reviewed again.

## REFERENCES

Akman, P. C.: A study of five hundred incisional hernias. J. Int. Coll. Surg. 37:125, 1962.

Allen, A. W., and Wallace, R. H.: Drainage of the common hepatic duct with special reference to bile peritonitis, wound infection and other complications. Surg. Gynecol. Obstet. 75:273, 1942.

Bartlett, W.: A clinical and experimental study of postoperative ventral hernia. Trans S. Surg. Assn. 38:453, 1915.

Bevan, A. D.: Postoperative ventral hernia. Surg. Clin. Chicago 4:775, 1920.

Blomstedt, B., and Welin-Berger, T.: Incisional hernias: A comparison between midline, oblique and transrectal incisions. Acta Chir. Scand. 72:275, 1972.

Boerema, I.: Case and repair of large incisional hernias. Surgery 69(1):111, 1971.

Branch, C. D.: Incisional hernia. New Engl. J. Med. 211:449, 1934.

Burns, F. J.: Complications of colostomy. Dis. Col. Rect, 13(6):448, 1970.

Carlucci, G. A.: Incisional hernias following gallbladder operation. Am. J. Surg. 58:97, 1942.

Cave, H. W.: Incidence and prevention of incisional hernias. J.A.M.A. 101:2038, 1933.

Chiene, G.: Notes on an operation for large midline ventral hernias. Edinb. Med. J. 24:402, 1920.

Coley, W. B.: Postoperative ventral hernia. Prog. Med. 11:36–46, 1921.

Fischer, J. D.,Turner, F. W.: Abdominal incisional hernias: A ten year review. Can. J. Surg. 17:202, 1974.

Freeman, L.: The cause of postoperative rupture of abdominal incisions. Arch. Surg. 14:600, 1927.

Garrison, F. H.: History of Medicine (4th ed.). Philadelphia, W. B. Saunders Co., 1929.

Gibson, C. L.: Operation for cure of large ventral hernia. Ann. Surg. 72:214–217 (August), 1920.

Glenn, F., and Moore, S. W.: The disruption of abdominal wounds. Surg. Gynecol. Obstet. 72:1041, 1941.

Grace, R. H., and Cox, S.: Incidence of incisional hernia after dehiscence of the abdominal wound. Am. J. Surg. 131:210, 1976.

Homans, J.: Three Hundred and Eighty-Four Laparotomies for Various Diseases. Boston, Nathan Sawyer & Son, printers, 1887.

Iason, A. H.: Hernia. Philadelphia, The Blakiston Co., 1941, p. 895.

Irvin, T. T., Stoddard, C. J., Greaney, M. G., and Duthie, H. L.: Abdominal wound healing: A prospective clinical study. Br. Med. J. 2:351, 1977.

Jenkins, H. P.: Clinical study of catgut in relation to abdominal wound disruption. Surg. Gynecol. Obstet. 64:648, 1937.

Judd, E. S.: The prevention and treatment of ventral hernia. Surg. Gynecol. Obstet. 14:175, 1912.

Karipineni, R. C., Wilk, P. J., and Danese, C. A.: The role of the peritoneum in the healing of abdominal incisions. Surg. Gynecol. Obstet. 142(5):729, 1976.

King, E. S. G.: Incisional hernia. Br. J. Surg. 23:35, 1935.

Kocher, T.: Textbook of Surgery (translated by H. J. Stile from 2nd rev. ed.). London, A & C Black, 1895, p. 140.

Koontz, A. R.: Failures with Tantalum gauze in ventral hernia repairs. Arch. Surg. 70:123, 1955.

Kozoll, D. D.: In Nyhus, L. M., and Harkins, H. N.: Hernia. Philadelphia, J. B. Lippincott Co., 1964, pp. 330–390.

Lucas-Championnière, J.: La hernia ombilicale. J. Med. Chir. 60:609, 1895.

Magee, B. A., Rodeheaver, G. T., Golden, G. T., Fox, J., Edgerton, M. T., and Edlich, R. F.: Potentiation of wound infection by surgical drains. Am. J. Surg. 131:547, 1976.

Maguire, J., and Young, D.: Repair of epigastric incisional hernia. Br. J. Surg. 63:125, 1976.

Marburg, W. B.: Postoperative hernia. Am. J. Surg. 59:60, 1943.

Masson, J. C.: Postoperative ventral hernia. Surg. Gynecol. Obstet. 37:14, 1923.

Mayo, W. J.: Radical cure of umbilical hernia. Ann. Surg. 34:276, 1899.

Obney, N.: An analysis of 192 consecutive incisional hernias. Can. Med. Assoc. J. 77:463, 1957.

Pfannenstiel, J.: Ueber die vortheile des suprasymphysärer fascienquerschnitt für die gynäkologischen köliotomien zugleich ein beitrag zu indikationsstellung der operationswege. Samml. Klin. Vortr. Leipz. 1900 N268 (Gynäk No. 97) 1:1735–1756, 1900.

Prian, G. W., Sawyer, R. B., and Sawyer, K. C.: Repair of peristomal colostomy hernias. Am. J. Surg. 130:664, 1975.

Ray, J. E., Hines, M. O., and Hanley, P. H.:

Postoperative problems of ileostomy and colostomy. J.A.M.A. *175*(17):48, 1960.

Rees, V. L., and Coller, F. A.: Anatomic and clinical study of the transverse abdominal incision. Arch. Surg. *47*:136, 1943.

Saha, S. P., Narasihma, R., and Stephenson, S. E., Jr.: Complications of colostomy. Dis. Col. Rect. *16*(6): 515, 1973.

Seidel, von W., Spelskerg, F., and Sauer, K.: Genese und rezidivneigung von narbenhernien. Munch. Med. Wochenschr. *114*:1533, 1972.

Shelley, H. J.: Ventral hernia. South. Surg. *9*:617, 656, 1940.

Singleton, A. O., and Blocker, T. G., Jr.: The problem of disruption of abdominal wounds and postoperative hernia. J.A.M.A. *122*, 1939.

Singleton, A. O., and Stehower, O. D.: The fascia patch transplant in the repair of hernia. Surg. Gynecol. Obstet. *80*:243, 1945.

Sloan, H. P.: Physiologic abdominal incisions. Am. J. Surg. *45*:515, 1939.

Smith, C. H., and Masson, J. C.: Results of the repair of ventral hernias with sutures of fascia lata: Review of eighty-five hernias. Surgery *7*:204, 1940.

Talbott, J. H.: *A Biographical History of Medicine.* New York, Grune & Stratton, Inc., 1970.

Trace, H. D., Kozoll, D. D., and Meyer, K. A.: Factors in the etiology and management of postoperative ventral hernias. Am. J. Surg. *80*:531, 1950.

Turnbull, R. B., and Weakley, F. L.: *Atlas of Intestinal Stomas.* St. Louis, C. V. Mosby Co., 1967.

VanWinkle, W., and Salthouse, T. N.: Biological response to sutures and principles of suture selection: Scientific exhibit. Clinical Congress of American College of Surgeons, San Francisco, 1975.

Viljanto, J., and Vänttinen, E.: Incisional hernias as a function of age. Ann. Chir. Gynaecol. *37*:246, 1968.

Watson, L. F.: *Hernia.* (3rd ed.). St. Louis, C. V. Mosby Co., 1948, pp. 366–386.

Zimmerman, L., and Anson, B. J.: *Anatomy and Surgery of Hernia.* Baltimore, Williams & Wilkins Co., 1967, pp. 20, 272–294.

## Supplemental Readings

Aren, A. J., and Madden, J. W.: Effects of stress on healing wounds: I. Intermittent noncyclical tension. J. Surg. Res. *102*:93–102, 1976.

Faxen, A., Meurling, S., and Borkowski, A.: A new kind of "deep retention suture." Acta Chir. Scand. *142*:13, 1976.

Lichtenstein, I. L., and Shore, J. M.: Repair of recurrent ventral hernias by an internal "binder." Am. J. Surg. *132*:(1):121, 1976.

Martyak, S. N., and Curtis, L. E.: Abdominal incision and closure: A systems approach. Am. J. Surg. *131*:476, 1976.

Priebe, C. J., Jr., and Wichern, W. A., Jr.: Ventral hernia with a skin covered silastic sheet for newborn infants with a diaphragmatic hernia. Surgery *82*(5):569, 1977.

Tera, H., and Aberg, C.: The strength of tissue against individual sutures in structures involved in the repair of inguinal hernia. Acta Chir. Scand. *142*:309, 1976.

Thorlakson, R. H.: Technique of repair of herniations associated with colonic stomas. Surg. Gynecol. Obstet. *121*:347, 1965.

Van Winkle, W., and Hastings, C.: Considerations in the choice of suture material for various tissues. Surg. Gynecol. Obstet. *135*:113, 1972.

# 22

# Umbilical Hernia in Infants and Adults and Omphaloceles

## INTRODUCTION

It is useful to consider the subject of umbilical hernia as it relates to infants, children, and adults, since there are important prognostic differences in these groups. The generalization can be made that infant umbilical defects, if not too large, tend to close spontaneously; however, I have never seen this happen in adults. Umbilical hernias are rarely the site of strangulation obstruction in infants and children; in adults, it is not unusual to see painful incarceration of bowel or omentum. Strangulation obstruction of intestine is not rare in older patients; not infrequently, these patients are obese, hypertensive, and diabetic as well. Therefore, the urgency for repair of umbilical hernias is much greater for adults than it is for infants.

Umbilical hernias in adults generally are acquired lesions. It is conceivable that in many individuals, a relative weakness occurs at the umbilical ring; when intra-abdominal pressure rises (as in extreme obesity or numerous pregnancies), a protrusion appears at the thin and poorly supported umbilical ring. I have found that 6.5 percent of adults had their umbilical hernias from infancy; this figure is significant as an indication that not all umbilical hernias will undergo spontaneous closure.

Omphalocele will also be considered in this chapter, since the protrusion occurs at the site of the umbilicus. Although physicians and medical records personnel at times use the term "omphalocele" interchangeably with umbilical hernia, this is an error. An omphalocele is an abnormality that carries a much more serious prognosis. In the material that follows, other differences between umbilical hernia and omphalocele will be pointed out.

In reviewing large numbers of records of patients with umbilical hernias, I became convinced that a thorough understanding of umbilical protrusions is less than universal. In the Medical Records Department, umbilical hernia has been too frequently indexed as "omphalocele." The pathologic anatomy of umbilical hernia is unlike that of omphalocele. Furthermore, some differentiation of omphaloceles based on size is useful. The problem presented to the surgeon and the prognosis to the infant vary with the specific abnormality. Omphalocele is a serious developmental abnormality in a newborn infant.

An umbilical hernia is a protrusion through a defective umbilical ring occurring in infants, children, or adults. The abdominal wall is otherwise well developed, and the protruding mass is covered with relatively normal skin. The difference in external covering between an omphalocele and an ordinary umbilical hernia is of prognostic and therapeutic significance. Umbilical hernias may occur at birth—through an opening that has failed to obliterate normally—or they may appear later in life. Although the intestine may prolapse into the umbilicus in children, it is readily reducible in the great majority of cases.

An omphalocele, amniocele, or exomphalos is a type of developmental anomaly characterized by a variable-sized defect of the umbilical ring and adjacent abdominal wall. By definition, intestine is present in the protruding mass. The protrusion at the umbilical area, which is covered by a thin transparent avascular membrane, is continuous with the umbilical cord of which it is a part. The largest protrusions with associated anomalies present numerous difficult technical problems, and the prognosis for these is guarded. Smaller omphaloceles have been designated as hernias into the umbilical cord.

A hernia into the umbilical cord is one in which the protrusion of viscera, usually small intestine, occurs through a defect at the umbilical ring and into the umbilical cord. The covering of the herniation is the same as in omphalocele; however, herniation into the umbilical cord differs from an omphalocele in that the development of the abdominal wall itself is essentially normal in other respects.

The greater the deviation from normal development, the larger and more complicated will be the omphalocele and associated anomalies; this obvious generalization is a practical one for the clinician who is called upon to treat newborn infants with omphalocele. The largest omphaloceles have been found to contain the liver, gastrointestinal tract from the duodenum to the lower descending colon, and even the spleen. The smallest abnormalities of this type may simply consist of a single loop of small intestine that has herniated into the umbilical cord. It is necessary to appreciate that in the largest omphaloceles, the surgeon will encounter maldevelopment of the abdominal wall, malrotation of the midgut, and a number of other possible developmental anomalies.

## HISTORY

Although umbilical hernias have been recognized for well over 19 centuries, effective surgical treatment is a comparatively recent achievement. According to Watson (1943), Celsus in the first century A.D. recommended that "a bandage must be made trial of before the knife" in the management of umbilical hernias in children. This was sage advice, indeed; because of a lack of knowledge concerning bacteriology, the danger of infection was enormous. Without analgesics, operative pain would have been unbearable.

Celsus has been given credit by Watson for use of the elastic ligature in the treatment of umbilical hernia. Watson also stated that the method was practiced by Paulus Aegineta in Alexandria in the seventh century; Avicenna, in the eleventh century; Guy de Chauliac in the fourteenth century; and Paré, in the sixteenth century. Others whom Watson credited with the use of the elastic ligature included de Garengeot, Saviard, and Petit. In the early literature few cases were reported, but in 1803 Hey reported on three patients with umbilical hernia. It is obvious that for 18 centuries, little progress was made in the treatment. One type of treatment consisted of draining inflammatory umbilical lesions; as might be expected, this usually resulted in peritonitis and, at times, fecal fistulas. Death from peritonitis was always a threat. Two famous anatomists who recognized umbilical hernias were Cooper in 1807 and Scarpa in 1809. Scarpa also realized that a lobe of the liver could find its way into a hernia at the umbilicus.

Operative treatment for umbilical hernia, according to Watson, evolved slowly; significant progress had to await the development of anesthesia and the science of bacteriology. Berard operated for a congenital type of umbilical hernia in 1841. Watson noted that even as recently as 1890, McDonald was able to collect only 19 operated cases from the literature. Two of the patients died. Storer, in 1864, is credited with performing the first successful repair of an umbilical hernia in the United States.

Elisabeth Altpeter reviewed the problem of hernia into the umbilical cord in a doctoral thesis in 1930. She noted the impact of Lister's antiseptic principles on this anomaly. Prior to this era, all infants with omphaloceles died. According to Altpeter, Lindfors was able to identify 30 cases of omphalocele treated successfully prior to 1882, only two of which were operated on. It is obvious that prior to the era of asepsis and antisepsis, only the conservative approach offered some hope for survival. Altpeter states that Lindfors in 1882 performed the first laparotomy for this anomaly. He opened the sac, freed the intestine from the area, reduced the contents into the abdomen, and closed the abdominal wall in two layers. Altpeter pointed out that failure to perform a laparotomy might result in overlooking co-existent pathology.

Modern surgical treatment of umbilical hernias really began in 1895, when Lucas Championnière attempted to strengthen umbilical hernia repairs by overlapping the linea alba from side to side. Other surgeons during that period also utilized the same method.

W. J. Mayo made his significant contributions in four separate publications. He read a paper entitled, "Remarks On the Radical Cure of Hernia," before the American Academy of Railway Surgeons in October, 1898. He presented the need for adherence to basic principles in hernia repair — asepsis, care in tying sutures, and avoidance of tension. Discussing umbilical hernias, he stated that "this form of hernia has been the hardest to cure. Usually found in corpulent people with small muscular development, the conditions are naturally unfavorable." While operating upon two difficult umbilical hernias, Mayo was unable to effect a vertical closure and, consequently, was compelled to close the wound transversely. He was pleasantly surprised at the good result. Because of the fundamental importance of the principle of transverse closure and the introduction of the transverse overlapping technique, I will quote Mayo directly:

Mattress sutures of silver wire are introduced an inch and a half from the margin of the aponeurosis on one side, and one-fourth of an inch from the margin on the opposite side; when these are tightened it draws one side beneath the other, the overlapping edge being sutured to the surface of the opposite aponeurosis.

In 1903 Mayo reported further experience with the transverse overlapping operation for repair of umbilical hernia. He had performed the first of the overlapping operations in 1895. But by 1903, he had accumulated 25 such operations without mortality and with only one relapse. The discussion of the paper presented by Mayo at the 54th Annual Session of the American Medical Association was most informative. A. J. Ochsner of Chicago, in discussing Mayo's paper, noted that in umbilical hernias there is a "dragging of the abdominal wall transversely, causing the opening to assume an elliptical form." J. B. Murphy of Chicago, in discussing this same paper, pointed out the danger of impaired cardiopulmonary function following repair of large umbilical hernias. He referred to the operation for umbilical hernia described by Mayo as being a "very simple, complete and perfect operation." In discussing Mayo's paper, Ferguson of Chicago, a renowned herniologist, first called the procedure the "Mayo Operation."

By 1907 Mayo reported his additional experiences with attempts at radical cure of umbilical hernia. Since his initially performed operation, in 13 years he had performed 126 umbilical herniorrhaphies. He was able to trace 75 patients and found only one relapse. The operation as described by Mayo thus set a new standard for surgeons who were to repair umbilical hernias. The fundamental contributions of Mayo resulted in great improvement in results obtained with surgical treatment of umbilical hernia. More recently, the contributions of Farris and colleagues (1959) should result in still further improvement. Farris noted that in the transverse closure, sutures were placed at right angles to the direction of the aponeurotic fibers; whereas, in vertical closure the sutures would be of necessity placed parallel to the direction of the fibers. Obviously, sutures placed at right angles to the connective tissue fibers are more effective in maintaining approximation than are sutures placed parallel to the fibers.

Farris also compared the effectiveness of overlapping or imbrication of aponeurotic abdominal layers in rabbits with simple approximation. He found in his experiments that the bursting strength was not improved by imbrication. In fact, he observed that the bursting strength could actually be impaired to a degree almost proportional to the amount of overlapping. Excessive overlapping is not recommended, since increased tensions at the suture line impairs blood supply and, consequently, healing.

## NATURAL HISTORY

It is remarkable how much umbilical hernias in neonates, infants and children differ from umbilical hernias in adults even though they are located at the same anatomical site. The tendency for spontaneous closure of umbilical defects in infants is generally better recognized by pediatricians and pediatric surgeons than it is by other physicians. Only surgical repair can eliminate the umbilical hernia in adults.

Grace E. Woods published a signficant report, *Some Observations on Umbilical Hernia in Infants*, in 1953. She carried on her studies at the University of Bristol, basing her data on 283 infants. She found the incidence of umbilical hernia to be 1 in 5.4 infants. She commented on treatment of umbilical hernia with adhesive taping and application of trusses. She referred to an observation made by Richet in 1856, stating that forcible apposition of the rectus muscles will not alter the size of the umbilical orifice and can hardly accelerate the natural healing process. According to Woods, taping tends to cause loss of tone of the abdominal wall, and trusses may enlarge the umbilical orifice. As a result, she abandoned treatment by these modalities in 122 infants. All but three resulted in spontaneous cures with the passage of time. She also observed a number of other infants with umbilical hernia and found that spontaneous disappearance occurred in 93 percent of the children. She pointed out that symptoms directly attributable to umbilical hernia are rare and, more significantly, that no case of strangulation has been recorded. The rarity of strangulation as a complication of umbilical hernia in infants is striking. Benson, as recently as 1962, reported that he had never seen an instance of strangulation due to umbilical hernia. Gibson and Gaspar in 1962 studied 198 patients with congenital umbilical hernias. There was obstruction in one case—but not a single instance of strangulation. Halpern had no record of strangulation occurring in 147 premature infants, whom he had observed over a ten-year period.

In 1961 Karlström of Sweden asked the question: "Should infantile umbilical hernias be treated with navel emplastra?" Among 124 infants with small- and medium-sized hernias, healing occurred in 95 percent within one year. He divided his patients into two groups: in one group, the individuals were taped; in the other group,

they were left untreated. He could find no differences in healing in the treated or untreated infants and concluded that taping was unnecessary in the management of small and moderately large umbilical hernias in infants.

Halpern in 1962 studied the problem of umbilical hernias over a ten-year period in 118 of 147 outpatient infants. He found that spontaneous healing was the rule, although in some cases it required two to five years. Surprisingly, the size of the defect or magnitude of protuberance did not influence the result. He concluded that taping of umbilical hernias had no advantage. Others have noted that taping causes skin irritation and superficial infection about the umbilicus.

Heifetz and colleagues (1963) made observations on the disappearance of umbilical hernias in infants and children. Of 78 infants with fascial rings over 0.5 centimeter in diameter, the deficit disappeared completely in 72 of them—in 31, during the first year postpartum. The healing was one of gradual contraction of the fascial ring. Heifetz and his coworkers noted that larger defects took longer to close. They felt that, given sufficient time, practically all umbilical hernias disappear spontaneously. This observation coincides with the fact that as infants grow into childhood and become young adults, umbilical hernias are seen in decreasing numbers.

Walker in 1967 studied the natural history of umbilical hernia in 314 Negro children. The incidence of umbilical hernias in one family is striking (Fig. 22–1). In a study of infants under three months of age, Walker could offer an absolute prognosis based on repeated measurements of the umbilical hernias. His study was conducted on a continual basis for six years. He observed that the larger the size of the defect, the less likely spontaneous closure will occur. The hernial defects that are likely to close spontaneously will do so by the time the child reaches six years of age; a few will close later. Walker noted that defects less than 1 centimeter in diameter almost always healed spontaneously but defects greater than 1.5 centimeters rarely healed before the age of six years. He recommended repair in these patients so as to avoid embarrassment once they enter school. He

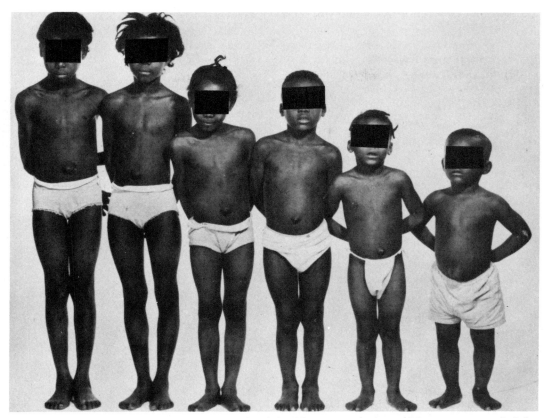

**Figure 22–1.** A remarkable familial incidence of umbilical hernia in which six siblings present with defects. (Reproduced with permission of authors and the *South African Medical Journal*. From Neves-e-Castro, M., and Saavedra, A. B.: A pregnant uterus protruding through an umbilical hernia sac. S. Afr. Med. J. *49*:1774, 1975.)

also recommended repair of occasional smaller hernias of 1.0 and 1.5 centimeters in diameter that persist after a period of observation. He did not encounter a single instance of incarceration in 314 patients observed. Thus, the danger of incarceration or strangulation cannot be advanced as a strong reason for repair of umbilical hernia in infants.

Morgan and coworkers (1970) advocated prophylactic umbilical hernia repair in childhood to prevent adult incarceration. They found 108 cases of incarcerated umbilical hernias; 101, or 94 percent, occurred in adults while 7 or 6 percent, occurred in children. The mortality was 7 percent, mostly involving patients over the age of 60 years who did not undergo surgery. Morgan and colleagues advocated repair of all umbilical hernias in girls under the age of two years and in all children over four years of age. The object of this plan was to prevent incarceration of umbilical hernias in adults.

Need (1972) reported two instances in which children with umbilical hernias developed obstruction. In one child, the mass became reduced with anesthesia; the bowel was viable at operation. In the second patient, the physician was able to reduce the incarceration prior to surgical repair.

Lassaletta and colleagues (1975), in considering the management of umbilical hernias in infancy and childhood, reviewed the records of 590 children under the age of 12 years. Their observations were unusual in that they found a 5.1 percent incidence of incarceration, strangulation, or evisceration. This is a much higher incidence than other researchers have found. Lassaletta and coworkers recommended that in fascial defects greater than 1.5 centimeters incarceration would be an indication for operative repair under the age of four years.

In spite of the great propensity for most umbilical hernias to heal spontaneously, a small number continue into adulthood. The healing that occurs spontaneously is adequate for most children who do not participate in strenuous activity; however, some of these individuals may indulge in active sports or perform heavy labor, and the defect reappears. Others may become obese or pregnant, or both; and, again, umbilical hernias might appear. I have found that in 6.5 percent of 520 adults with umbilical hernias, the defects were present since infancy. Other researchers have noted that umbilical hernias persist into adulthood. Castro and Saavedra (1975) saw a spectacular patient with a pregnant uterus in an umbilical hernial sac (Fig. 22–2).

Once an adult develops an umbilical hernia, it remains unless repaired. Obesity and pregnancy are two prominent factors that contribute to the development of umbilical hernias in adults. Furthermore, I suspect that even those umbilical hernias which cause little difficulty for many years can reappear later under the stressful activities of adulthood, obesity, and pregnancy.

### CLINICAL STUDY OF UMBILICAL HERNIA IN INFANTS AND CHILDREN

In order to better understand the hernia problem as it affects infants and children, I reviewed the available records of those patients who had umbilical hernias repaired at Henry Ford Hospital between 1950 and 1972, inclusive. During this period 318 operations were performed—an average of approximately 14 repairs per year. Of course, a great many more infants and children were seen with umbilical hernias during this time, both as inpatients and outpatients; however, operative treatment was recommended for certain selected cases. Small asymptomatic hernias were observed and, consistently, presented no problems.

### Age Incidence

Selection of patients for operative correction of umbilical hernias was based on a number of considerations: age of the patient, size of the hernia, presence of symptoms, presence of other diseases or anomalies, and progress of the hernia with the passage of time. The age incidence of those patients who underwent surgery is shown in Figure 22–3. One hundred eighty-six of 318 umbilical hernias, or 58 percent of the total, were repaired within the first two years of life. The decrease in the number operated on drops precipitously during the first five years of life.

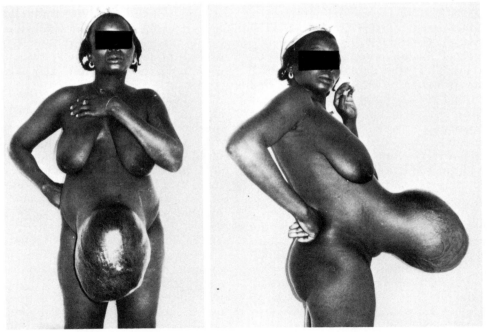

**Figure 22–2.**   Umbilical hernia in which the pregnant uterus is dislocated into the defect. (Reproduced with permission of the author and Appleton-Century-Crofts, Publishing Division of Prentice-Hall, Inc., Englewood Cliffs, N.J. From Swenson, O.: *Pediatric Surgery* (3rd ed.), Vol. I. New York, Appleton-Century-Crofts, 1958, p. 544.)

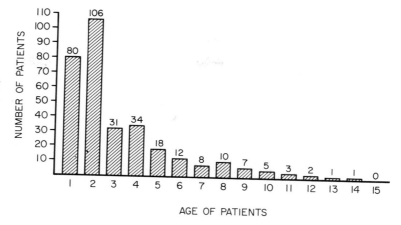

**Figure 22–3.** Age incidence of umbilical hernia in infants and children.

Operations for repair of umbilical hernia are rarely necessary during late childhood and adolescence.

## Sex

I was surprised that male infants and children were operated on somewhat more frequently than were females. Operative procedures were performed on 183 males and 135 females; thus, 58 percent of the operations were peformed on males and 42 percent, on females. These statistics are at variance with others reported in the literature.

## Race

The significantly greater incidence of umbilical hernias in blacks is confirmed in this study. Eight-five percent of the hernias repaired were present in black children. This increased incidence of umbilical hernias in black children is striking. Crump in 1932 and Jones in 1941 discussed the great preponderance of umbilical hernias in black infants at length. The ratio of umbilical hernias in blacks versus whites has been variously reported to range from 2.5:1 to 15:1. Mack, writing in the *East African Medical Journal* (1943), found the incidence to be 60 percent among black infants in the territory of Tanganyika.

At times, the incidence of umbilical hernia in a single black family is truly remarkable. In Figure 22–1 (p. 401), six siblings all required repair of their umbilical hernias. There are a number of theories, but no universally satisfactory explanation for the frequency of umbilical hernias in blacks.

## Clinical Features

The symptoms and signs resulting from umbilical hernias in neonates and children are comparatively few in number. Almost without exception, the hernia had been present and recognized at birth or shortly thereafter. In only 17 patients out of 318 was the hernia recognized later. For instance, in one boy, 14 years of age, the hernia was identified after he began playing football.

Protrusion or herniation at the umbilicus was the single major complaint in 261 patients, while pain as well as protrusion was present in 57 additional patients. The pain was seldom severe; discomfort was far more common. Mothers generally expressed great concern over the umbilical protrusion and described the circumstances under which the umbilical herniation increased in size. Certain activities—such as crying, straining or coughing—caused the protrusion to enlarge in a substantial number of patients. Children with asthma, bronchitis, or repeated upper respiratory tract infections often required repair of umbilical hernias. Whooping cough resulted in increasing discomfort at the umbilicus in five children.

I have been unable to confirm the great danger of umbilical hernias as a cause of intestinal obstruction in children. Although small intestine finds its way into umbilical hernias in young patients, it is easily reduced in nearly all of them. In this study of 318 patients, only 21 felt nauseous and 16 had vomited. Sixteen complained of cramping abdominal pain.

As is increasingly recognized, many umbilical hernias in infants and children tend to diminish in size with the passage of time. It was felt on examination prior to surgery that there was actual enlargement of the hernia in 32 percent of those patients operated on. Important signs leading to surgical repair of umbilical hernias in children included: protrusion, pain, history of intermittent incarceration, enlargement of the hernia, and failure of the defect to decrease in size.

## Physical Findings

It is remarkable that obesity was rarely present in infants and children with umbilical hernias. This is in marked contrast to the great frequency of obesity in adults who develop such hernias. On the other hand, neonates and children are often found to have inguinal hernias and congenital anomalies. Inguinal hernias were present in 40 patients, or nearly 13 percent of the children. Congenital cardiac anomalies, mental retardation, prematurity, and orthopedic abnormalities were seen in several other infants and children with umbilical hernias. Inguinal hernias were the most common additional abnormality seen in patients with umbilical herniation.

An attempt to classify umbilical hernias as small, medium, and large was not particularly rewarding. The need for individual consideration became clear insofar as surgical correction was concerned. In general, umbilical hernias measuring up to one centimeter in diameter were considered small; those between one and two centimeters in diameter were moderate-sized and those above two centimeters in diameter were considered large. One hundred sixteen, or 36 percent, were moderate-sized, and 116 more were designated as large umbilical hernias while 188 were small. Large umbilical

hernias were repaired uniformly, since there was little hope that spontaneous closure would occur. The smaller umbilical hernias were repaired because they were symptomatic or because they failed to decrease in size with the passage of time. Many of the intermediate-sized hernias gradually decreased in size and repair was deferred.

## Indication for Operative Treatment of Umbilical Hernias

The natural propensity for most congenital umbilical defects to close spontaneously—as recognized by Grace E. Woods (1953), Karlström (1961), Halpern (1962), and Heifetz and colleagues (1963)—has been reviewed. Furthermore, the technique of taping, strapping, or application of binders has proved to be practically worthless; therefore, the practice of taping has largely been abandoned.

The single important question to be answered is, "Which umbilical hernias should be repaired in infants?" Surgical repair of umbilical hernias is reserved for a selected small group of patients. These are not simple to identify. Defects over 1.5 centimeters in diameter should probably be repaired; however, even these can be observed, since umbilical hernias rarely become incarcerated. Certainly, symptomatic hernias should be repaired.

Gross in 1953 stated that umbilical defects with a diameter equal to or less than one centimeter after the first year of life should cause little concern, since spontaneous closure will occur with growth of the child. He advocated repair of those measuring from 1.5 to 4 centimeters in diameter. He called attention to the fact that there is greater urgency to repair umbilical hernias in females, since pregnancy is an aggravating factor during reproductive years.

Kieswetter (1961) advises that up to six months of age, infants with umbilical defects smaller than the tip of the index finger should be observed only. Surgical treatment is reserved for specific symptomatic patients in this group. If the child is between six and twelve months of age, and the hernia is of index-finger–tip size, observation is continued; however, symptomatic patients are operated on. Increase in size of the defect and presence of symptoms are indications for repair in infants from one to two years of age. Kieswetter feels that repair is indicated for infants with defects persisting after two years of age.

Stanley-Brown (1961) feels that if the umbilical defect is less than one centimeter in diameter, spontaneous closure is likely. Larger defects — admitting two, three, or more fingers — are much less likely to close without surgical correction.

Morgan and colleagues (1970) stated that umbilical defects greater than 1.5 centimeters rarely close spontaneously. They cite a mortality of 7 percent in elderly patients with incarceration. They advocate prophylactic repair of umbilical hernias in girls over two years of age and in all children over four years of age.

Certainly, in view of current knowledge, small umbilical hernias ranging up to one centimeter in diameter should be observed in neonates and in children under two years of age. Decrease in size of the defect can be documented as favorable progress. Nevertheless, even in this group, hernias causing symptoms should be repaired. Symptomatic umbilical hernias and persisting defects larger than 1.5 centimeters are suitable for repair. In female infants some consideration is warranted toward earlier repair, since pregnancy in adulthood is an etiologic factor in herniation. Because umbilical hernias rarely become strangulated in infants and children, a period of observation is not hazardous.

## Anesthesia

General anesthesia was almost without exception the anesthetic of choice. Spinal anesthesia was employed in three older children, and local anesthesia was selected for three others.

In recent years, ketamine chloride has been used with increasing frequency. The agent is administered intramuscularly with resultant analgesia and amnesia; this agent has been safe and effective in children, without the side effects seen in adults. Infants and children are being discharged on the day of operative repair of hernias in increasing numbers. Most of them are discharged by the third postoperative day.

## Recommended Technique of Repair of Umbilical Hernias in Infants and Children

It is well to bear in mind that infection is a constant threat and can largely be avoided by preceding the operative procedure with a thorough bath of the patient (using a surgical soap), conducted on two separate occasions prior to the operation. The umbilical depression must be thoroughly cleansed. Skin preparation is accomplished with a surgical soap or with an iodine-containing germicide.

I feel that some thought and effort should be directed at preservation of the umbilicus in infants and children. The umbilicus serves as a badge or button indicating that the bearer belongs to a particular group in society. The presence of the "belly-button" implies to the owner, as well as to his peers, that he is normal and healthy. The child's mental well being should receive consideration, and the umbilicus should not be wantonly sacrificed.

A slightly curved skin incision is ordinarily made just below the umbilicus in a transverse direction (Fig. 22–4, A). Its length depends on the size of the hernia and the thickness of the panniculus. Bleeding vessels are grasped with a fine-pointed hemostat and ligated with fine silk or catgut sutures.

The skin flap and the umbilicus are dissected upward at the level of the anterior sheath of the rectus abdominis muscle and the linea alba (Fig. 22–4, B). The sac is identified and carefully entered so as to avoid injury to any viscera or omental vessels (Fig. 22–4, C). Excess of sac is excised (Fig. 22–4, D).

The peritoneal sac is often thin and easily torn. With care, it is possible to free the peritoneal sac so that it may be ligated with a purse-string suture or interrupted sutures of medium silk or fine nonabsorbable suture (Fig. 22–4, E). If the hernial sac is large and has been subjected to trauma of repeated visceral prolapse, it may be somewhat thickened or hypertrophied. The need for separate ligation of the sac can be argued.

Clear identification of the upper and lower aponeurotic leaflets is essential. Adipose tissue must be carefully cleared from the surfaces to be approximated or overlapped. The incision is carried later-

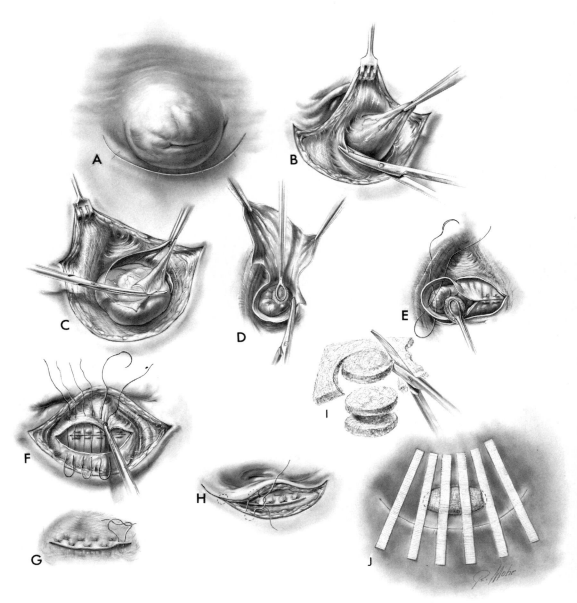

**Figure 22–4.** This illustration shows the important detail in repair of an umbilical hernia. *A*, Skin incision; *B*, dissection of peritoneal sac; *C*, opening of peritoneal sac; *D*, excision of sac; *E*, closure of peritoneum; *F*, placement of sutures through aponeurosis; *G*, tacking down free aponeurotic edge; *H*, placement of subepidermal sutures; *I*, gauze pledgets cut to fit the umbilical depression; *J*, epidermal edges held in place with strips of adhesive.

ally to each rectus abdominal muscle by incising the linea alba transversely. This more clearly identifies the upper and lower aponeurotic flaps. Accurate approximation of the superior and inferior aponeurotic margins is mandatory (Fig. 22–4, *F*). Overlapping of the aponeurotic leaflets, vest-over-pants style, has been established through use as an effective

method of repair (Fig. 22–4, *G*). It is essentially the method popularized by Mayo. In recent years, I have decreased the amount of overlapping as a result of the studies of Farris and colleagues (1959). If overlapping is omitted, precise approximation of the aponeurotic edges is essential.

In suturing the aponeurotic flaps, care must be taken to place the sutures so that the lateral margins are precisely closed and the closure is complete; otherwise, adipose tissue or omentum might insinuate itself between them and act as a wedge, leading to a recurrence of the hernia. Heavy or number 2–0 silk or another comparable nonabsorbable suture is used. In small infants and children, finer suture material is used. When closure of the aponeurotic flaps is performed in one layer, great care must be taken to achieve accurate approximation of the edges.

Subcutaneous adipose tissues are approximated with fine catgut and subcuticular number 4–0 synthetic absorbable sutures are used to approximate the epidermis (Fig. 22–4, *H*). A small rounded portion of gauze or cotton is fashioned to fit the umbilical depression (Fig. 22–4, *I*). The wound edges are held in approximation with small strips of nonallergenic adhesive tape (Fig. 22–4, *J*). If hemostasis is effective, large bulky dressings and drains are unnecessary. I do not recommend the use of drains in umbilical herniorrhaphy. The method, as essentially described here, was used in over 80 percent of repairs of umbilical hernias which I studied.

A number of techniques may be used for repair of umbilical hernias, but in this study transverse closures were performed (Table 22–1). The Mayo technique of repair was the preferred method for correction of umbilical defects in most infants and children. Transverse closure of the linea alba in a single layer is gaining in popularity as a method of repair. The vertical incision is used in situations when it is necessary to explore the peritoneal cavity or when the surgeon wishes to repair a diastasis recti.

Some comment is indicated on the need for closure of the peritoneum during umbilical herniorrhaphy. The peritoneal sac was closed separately in 61, or slightly less than 20 percent, of 318 patients operated on. Surgeons are aware that the peritoneal sac may be extremely thin and gossamer-like. Dissection can be time consuming and tedious, and the total effort may contribute little or nothing toward the final result.

Alevar and Pilling (1974) have considered the management of the peritoneal sac during umbilical herniorrhaphy in children. They found that excision of the sac prolongs the operative procedure by 10 to 15 minutes without contributing to the effectiveness of the repair. It is, however, essential to identify the aponeurotic surface clearly and to free the margin of the hernial ring of peritoneum. No serosal sac should protrude beyond the closure.

Silk has long been preferred as the suture material for repair of umbilical hernias. It was used in the repair of 250 hernias in infants and children; however, in recent years synthetic nonabsorbable sutures have gained in popularity. Although catgut was used in selected cases, it is not recommended as a suture material of choice in the repair of umbilical hernias. Wire was used only six times. This material may be palpable through the thin skin of the umbilicus, or it may cause postoperative pain and, hence, is not recommended. Nonabsorbable sutures, such as silk or Teflon-coated Dacron are preferred for repair of umbilical hernias. These materials were used in 286 or 90 percent of the repairs.

### Findings at Operation in Infants and Children

The operative findings are interesting; when the umbilical sac is entered, in most instances, it is found to be empty. Even when a protruding mass was present preoperatively, spontaneous reduction occurred commonly following induction of anesthesia with resultant relaxation of the abdominal wall.

The omentum is so thin and small in small babies that it cannot occupy a significant portion of the sac. Even in larger children the omentum is commonly poorly developed. Omentum was found in the

**Table 22–1. TECHNIQUE FOR REPAIR OF UMBILICAL HERNIA IN INFANTS AND CHILDREN**

| Technique | Number | Percent |
|---|---|---|
| Mayo repair | | |
|   Transverse overlapping | 263 | 82.7 |
| Transverse closure | | |
|   Single Layer | 34 | 10.7 |
| Vertical | | |
|   Side-to-side overlapping | 13 | 4.1 |
|   Single layer | 8 | 2.5 |
| Total | 318 | 100 |

hernial sac in only ten infants and children. Small intestine was recognized in hernial sacs of nine patients, and the transverse colon protruded through the umbilical ring in two other children. The peritoneal sac was found to contain omentum or bowel in only 19 of 318 patients. Strangulation of intestine requiring resection was not present in a single instance. It is remarkable that gangrenous intestine is rarely encountered in umbilical hernias in infants and children.

## Complications

Fortunately, the 318 operations for repair of umbilical hernias in infants and children were performed without a single death. Postoperative complications can be categorized as either major and minor. There were two major complications related to anesthesia. One child suffered from respiratory arrest following injection of ketamine hydrochloride and required resuscitation; the second child had a cardiac arrest following laryngospasm while in the recovery room. In this case, general anesthesia had been administered. Resuscitation was prompt and completely successful in both cases. These two cases emphasize the need for continuing observation of all patients undergoing operative procedures.

Postoperative wound complications included wound infections in six patients, hematomas in three patients, and seromas in five patients. One infant was seriously ill with wound infection, pylephlebitis, and gram-negative septicemia but recovered with vigorous antibiotic therapy.

Children are prone to develop upper respiratory tract or gastrointestinal infections while hospitalized. Seven patients had acute upper respiratory tract infections following surgical repair and four others had diarrhea requiring treatment.

Umbilical hernias can be repaired in infants and children, when indicated, with little danger to life. With careful operative technique, the complication rate should also be quite low.

## Recurrences

There were two recurrences following repair of 318 umbilical hernias, for a recurrence rate of 0.63 percent. One recurred within three months following a Mayo repair; this was considered to be a technical failure. A second repair utilizing the same technique in this patient was successful. A second recurrence appeared three years following transverse closure of the linea alba in one layer. If careful dissection is performed and if accurate approximation of the aponeurosis is achieved, the recurrence rate following umbilical hernia repair in infants and children should approach zero.

## UMBILICAL HERNIA IN ADULTS

Umbilical hernias in adults often cause prolonged morbidity and can lead to death in a few patients. In order to understand the problem of umbilical hernia in adults, I reviewed the records of 520 patients operated upon during the years from 1950 to 1972 at Henry Ford Hospital. Every available record in the Medical Records Department was reviewed. During this time period, many more patients were seen with umbilical hernias; however, operative repair was deferred, usually because of serious concomitant medical diseases. Elderly patients whose physical activities were limited because of advanced arteriosclerosis and severe cardiac or pulmonary disease were not operated on unless they developed potentially fatal complications (such as strangulating obstructions).

Even though I was unable to accomplish a thorough follow-up study, useful information was gained from the investigation of our case records.

## Age Incidence

In infants and children, most operations for umbilical hernia were performed during the first two years of life. The incidence continued to decline during late childhood, and the lowest incidence of umbilical hernias was found in teenagers. The incidence of umbilical hernias then increased gradually during early adulthood. In young women, umbilical hernias often develop following repeated pregnancies. A high incidence of umbilical hernias occurred in patients in the third

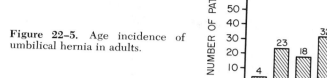

Figure 22–5. Age incidence of umbilical hernia in adults.

to the seventh decades of life (Fig. 22–5). The highest number for a single decade was 144 umbilical hernias seen in patients between the ages of 51 and 60 years. One hundred and eight umbilical hernias were seen in patients in the seventh decade of life, but the incidence dropped off rapidly thereafter.

### Duration of Hernia

The precise onset of umbilical hernias in adults is not easily determined. I was surprised to find that 34, or 6.5 percent, of the patients knew of their hernias for 30 to 50 years. Many of the umbilical hernias caused little disability, and the patient tended to ignore its presence for long periods of time. One hundred and one patients, or 19 percent, stated that their hernias had been present for "many years" but were unable to pinpoint the onset more accurately. One-hundred fifty-eight, or 30 percent, of adult patients had hernias repaired within one year of onset.

Two events appeared with striking regularity in patients with umbilical hernias—pregnancies (often repeated) and obesity.

As might be expected, the circumstances that force the patient to seek relief promptly include painful incarceration and threat of strangulation. These patients occasionally kept their umbilical hernias for many years, but acute discomfort finally drove them to seek relief.

### Number of Children

Many female patients could date the onset of their umbilical hernia to preg-

nancy. It was interesting that 178, or 62 percent, of 286 women had given birth to one or more children. Furthermore, the same patient often had several pregnancies. Fifty-two percent had given birth to two or more children, while 31 patients, or 11 percent, had given birth to five or more children.

Several of the young women with umbilical hernias had repeated pregnancies within a few years. One patient had three pregnancies by the time she reached 23 years of age. A 19-year-old girl who had borne two children also developed an umbilical hernia.

Pregnancies place additional stress on the umbilicus. Where some weakness exists initially, the distention of pregnancy can cause permanent protrusion at the umbilicus.

### Symptoms

Painful protrusion at the umbilicus causes the majority of patients to seek relief from the disability of umbilical hernia. Three hundred and two, or 58 percent, of the patients experienced both pain and protrusion prior to seeking relief. A number of descriptive terms were used by patients to describe the discomfort—including soreness, sharp pain, tenderness, and severe pain. Severe pain was present in complicated cases—as, for instance, when strangulation followed incarceration. Generally speaking, the discomfort attributable to uncomplicated umbilical hernias is not severe.

Protrusion alone was the reason for surgical repair in 197 patients, or 38 percent, of 520 adults with umbilical hernias (Fig. 22–6).

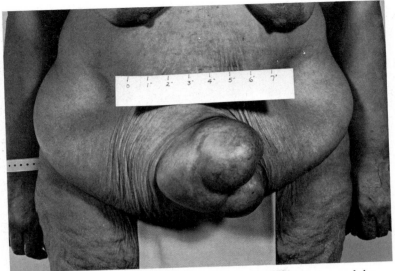

Figure 22–6.   Large umbilical hernias are often seen in obese adults.

In a few patients there was excoriation of the skin and discharge from the umbilicus.

Nausea, vomiting, and cramping abdominal pain were present in approximately 10 percent of the patients. Incarceration with intestinal obstruction accounted for these symptoms in a few patients; cholecystitis, cholelithiasis, and intestinal diseases were present in others. Patients with symptoms other than protrusion at the umbilicus (with or without discomfort) merit roentgen studies prior to repair to rule out such conditions as cholelithiasis, hiatal hernia, and gastroduodenal disorders. Gaseousness, fatty food intolerance, and bloating were other symptoms recorded, but were often due to gastrointestinal or biliary tract diseases.

Enlargement of the umbilical hernias in adults is a gradual process, with such hernias tending to enlarge slowly over a period of years. Only 57 patients, or 11 percent, were annoyed by the enlarging protrusion at the umbilicus.

### Physical Findings

Some attempt at classifying umbilical hernias as to size is useful. Umbilical defects under three centimeters in diameter were considered to be small; those measuring three to five centimeters were of moderate size, while those larger than five centimeters were considered to be large. Precise measurement was often not available, but some estimate of the size of the hernia has practical value. Three hundred twenty-one, or 62 percent, were considered to be large umbilical hernias. Nevertheless, the huge umbilical hernia is relatively uncommon in modern practice.

In records available to me, precise description of reducibility of the hernia was wanting. In 91 patients, a note was made that the hernia could be reduced, while in 93 or 18 percent incarceration had been present. Furthermore, the contents (usually omentum) had been present for many years.

Occasionally a gigantic umbilical hernia is seen that contains stomach, colon, omentum and small bowel (Fig. 22–7).

Diastasis recti was present in 36, or nearly 7 percent, of the adults with umbilical hernia. The presence of diastasis recti should be recognized and respected, and repair should not be undertaken lightly.

### Other Diseases

Certain other diseases are regularly found in patients with umbilical hernias; these should be recognized prior to repair of the hernia (Table 22–2). It must be stated that many of the patients with umbilical hernias were not exhaustively studied; hence, I am sure that in some cases

The information gathered in this study has practical value. If the patient has symptoms other than local protrusion at the umbilicus, with or without pain, other diseases should be considered before repair is advised. The patient may have hypertension, diabetes, cholecystitis, hiatus hernia, cirrhosis, or other gastrointestinal diseases. Of course, in incarceration and strangulation, obstructive symptoms will be present; and prompt repair is indicated.

### Indication for Surgical Repair of Umbilical Hernia in Adults

A few adults conceal umbilical hernias for several years—tolerating the discomfort, which is not insufferable, until incarceration or strangulation occurs. Some of these hernias reach gigantic proportions and accommodate most of the small bowel, colon, omentum, and even the stomach (see Fig. 22-7). Dr. J. P. Pratt, one of my surgical teachers, who worked with Dr. J. Bloodgood at Johns Hopkins University gave me a photograph of a patient with such a hernia (Fig. 22-8). The personal communication from Dr. Pratt is included because of its historical interest.

Umbilical hernias in adults do not heal spontaneously, and those causing symptoms should be repaired before intestinal strangulation occurs.

Gibson and Gaspar (1959) noted that 10 percent of adults with umbilical hernias will die if emergency repair becomes necessary. Eighteen percent will succumb if strangulation occurs.

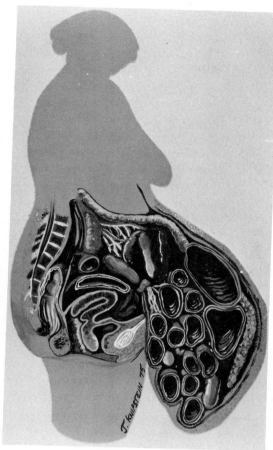

**Figure 22-7.** Lateral view of gigantic umbilical hernia containing omentum, colon, stomach, and small intestine.

one or more coexisting diseases were overlooked. Nevertheless, it is clear to me that umbilical hernia is accompanied by obesity in nearly one-half of the patients. Furthermore, other diseases commonly seen in obese patients will be found in significant numbers in patients with umbilical hernias. Cirrhosis of the liver produces ascites in some patients, with resultant increase in intra-abdominal pressure and umbilical hernia. Hiatus hernia is not rare in patients with umbilical hernia; and, in this series, such hernias were found in 2 percent of the patients. The incidence would be higher in a female population.

Other gastrointestinal diseases were present in 7 percent of 520 patients. Duodenal ulcer, gastric ulcer, diverticulitis, pancreatitis, and ulcerative colitis were seen in other patients with umbilical hernias.

**Table 22-2. OTHER DISEASES IN 520 ADULT PATIENTS WITH UMBILICAL HERNIA**

| | Number of Patients | Percent |
|---|---|---|
| Obesity | 233 | 45 |
| Hypertension | 110 | 21 |
| Arteriosclerosis | 84 | 16 |
| Arteriosclerotic heart disease | 37 | 7 |
| Diabetes mellitus | 46 | 9 |
| Cholecystitis-cholelithiasis | 37 | 7 |
| Pulmonary disease | 32 | 6 |
| Cirrhosis of liver | 17 | 3 |
| Hiatus hernia | 12 | 2 |
| Other gastrointestinal diseases | 38 | 7 |

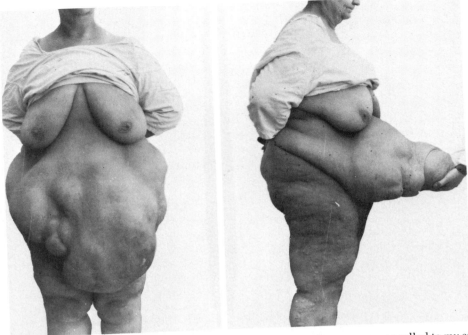

**Figure 22–8.**  A species of umbilical hernia nearly extinct. This extraordinary case was called to my attention by Dr. J. P. Pratt, who was a House Officer under Drs. W. S. Halsted and Joseph Bloodgood. The following note from Dr. Pratt is of interest:

*In appreciation of your contribution to hernias, I thought you might be interested to have these pictures of a real hernia. They were taken in 1911 during my internship at Johns Hopkins. At that time we were still seeing many neglected conditions such as hernias, ovarian tumors and so forth. I doubt that there has been a ventral hernia as large as this one. I thought you might want it for your archives. As an intern, I assisted Dr. Joseph Bloodgood and operated on this monster.*

Repair of umbilical hernias is generally advisable in adults, since they will not close spontaneously. Those hernias resulting in incarceration, ulceration, or strangulation should be repaired without delay before more serious complications ensue.

Cirrhotics, not infrequently, have umbilical hernias. The increased intra-abdominal pressure causes a gradually enlarging prominence of the navel (Fig. 22–9). This predisposition to umbilical herniation in cirrhotics was noted by Chapman and colleagues (1933). Repair is mandated from time to time due to unfavorable progress. It is always desirable to employ medical measures to control the alcoholism, to improve nutrition, and to reduce the severity of the ascites. These measures can result in a reduction in size of the hernia along with relief of symptoms.

The increased risk of umbilical herniorrhaphy in cirrhotics was also noted by Baron (1960), who recorded 5 deaths due

to bleeding esophageal varices in 16 repairs, for a mortality of 31 percent. He explained the bleeding on the basis of increased portal pressure resulting from surgical compromise of the collateral circulation about the umbilicus.

O'Hara and coworkers (1975) studied 35 patients with umbilical hernia, cirrhosis, and ascites who underwent repair; but the researchers did not find the high incidence of postoperative variceal bleeding. There were 6 deaths in the group, for a mortality of 16 percent.

Repair of umbilical hernias in patients with cirrhosis should be approached with caution.

### Operative Treatment

It is our general policy to recommend that all symptomatic umbilical hernias be repaired. Those individuals with severe pain, incarceration, or suspected strangulation should undergo surgical treatment as soon as the necessary examinations (including laboratory), have been conducted and any abnormalities in fluid and electrolyte balance have been corrected.

Nasogastric suction is employed in selected patients—as, for instance, those with vomiting or evidence of obstruction.

Anesthesia was achieved with local infiltration in 111 (21 percent), general anesthesia in 158 (30 percent), and spinal in 251 (48 percent).

The choice of suture material varied, but nonabsorbable sutures were generally preferred. Heavy or number 2–0 silk was used most often, having been employed in 305 or 59 percent of the operations. To my surprise, wire was used in 83 repairs. Postoperative discomfort might be expected, but it did not prove to be a problem. In recent years, synthetic nonabsorbable sutures, such as Teflon-coated Dacron (Tevdek), are being used with increasing frequency. These sutures should prove efficacious. Catgut was used in 75 of 520 patients, but its use is not recommended.

Umbilical hernias may be repaired successfully by a variety of techniques, and the surgeon should be aware that a number of methods in his armamentarium will provide acceptable results. The skin incision should be chosen so as to provide the desired exposure. A transverse semilunar incision below the umbilicus is preferred for most patients. It provides adequate exposure for repair of the umbilical hernia and heals as a cosmetically acceptable scar. The vertical midline incision is preferred when entry into the peritoneal cavity is desired and when repair of a coexistent diastasis recti or epigastric hernia is contemplated. The transverse skin incision was used in 414 (80 percent), while the vertical incision was used in 91 (18 percent). In some patients a vertical skin incision was used, but a Mayo repair or transverse closure in one layer was the method of repair. In general, the Mayo technique of repair was favored. The superior aponeurotic flap was imbricated, more or less depending on redundancy, over the lower flap (Fig. 22–10). In 15 patients, or approximately 3 percent, a subcostal or paramedian incision was made, and the umbilical hernia was repaired from within the peritoneal cavity.

A number of methods were used to

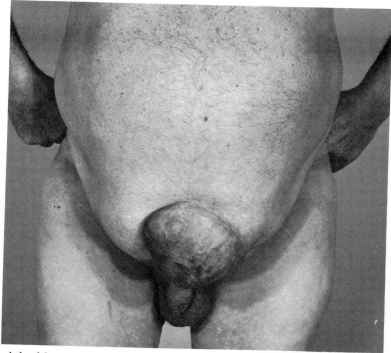

**Figure 22–9.** Umbilical hernias are potentially serious in patients with advanced cirrhosis of the liver. Prolonged drainage, wound infection, and gastrointestinal bleeding may follow repair of such hernias.

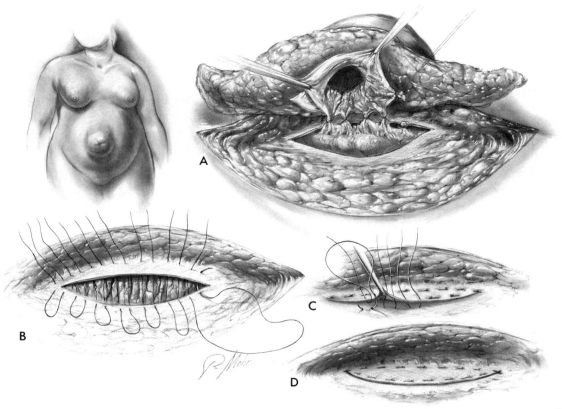

**Figure 22–10.** *A*, The large umbilical protrusion and an ellipse of adipose tissue is excised. *B*, Sutures of number 2–0 nonabsorbable material are placed to achieve a slight overlapping. *C*, The upper leaflet (vest) is being sutured over the aponeurosis below (pants). *D*, The transverse closure is completed with minimal overlapping.

repair umbilical hernias in adults at the Henry Ford Hospital from 1950 to 1972. These methods are summarized in Table 22–3.

It is seen that the transverse closure, with or without overlapping, was performed on 399, or 76 percent, of the patients; this approach to repair of umbilical hernias has been uniformly successful in our hands.

The vertical repair was selected when entry into the peritoneal cavity was desirable for other reasons such as the presence of cholecystitis. With vertical closures, retention sutures of heavy monofilament nylon were commonly used.

Vertical closure with side-to-side overlapping, as advocated by Championnière, was the method selected for 15, or 3 percent, of the patients who had diastasis recti or ventral hernias along with umbilical hernias. Although the method is useful in selected cases, it is followed by a significant number of recurrent hernias.

A simple method for closure of the defect at the umbilicus is often overlooked. During laparotomy for some other condition, it is possible to gain access to the umbilicus from within the peritoneal cavity. The peritoneum about the umbilical ring is dissected free; the sac may be removed; and the clearly identified aponeurotic edges are approximated — usually transversely, with two or three heavy or number 2–0 nonabsorbable sutures. The peritoneum may be closed over the repair if desired. This procedure is simple and has proved effective.

It is not necessary, or hardly desirable, to excise the umbilicus during repair of an umbilical hernia. The umbilicus does not really interfere with the repair, and its absence may prove upsetting to the patient—especially in young patients and those individuals whose vanity might be

**Table 22–3. METHODS OF REPAIR OF 520 UMBILICAL HERNIAS IN ADULTS**

| Technique | Number | Percent |
|---|---|---|
| Mayo repair or transverse closure | 399 | 76.0 |
| Vertical closure | 98 | 19.0 |
| Single layer | 83 | 16.0 |
| Side-to-side overlapping | 15 | 3.0 |
| Repair from within peritoneal cavity | 15 | 3.0 |
| Repair with mesh | 8 | 1.5 |
| Excision of umbilicus | 68 | 13.0 |

encroached on through needless sacrifice of this symbolic anatomic landmark. In this study, the umbilicus was excised in 68, or 13 percent, of 520 adult patients.

Some question arises as to what should be done with the peritoneal sac in an umbilical hernia. In long-standing hernias, which undergo repeated prolapse and reduction, the peritoneal sac is thickened and both dissection and closure are simple. However, in hernias of recent onset, the sac is quite thin and dissection is tedious and ineffective. Accurate identification of the aponeurosis and freeing of the peritoneum completely from the ring is essential. The peritoneum must not be permitted to protrude through the repair. The edges of the aponeurosis must be accurately approximated if a single layer of sutures is used. Clean aponeurotic surfaces must be in contact if the overlapping method is employed.

Synthetic mesh was utilized in repair of eight hernias. In those cases recurrent umbilical hernias, incisional hernias, and diastasis recti were the additional indications for use of the mesh.

Among other operations performed along with umbilical herniorrhaphy, I found cholecystectomy in 23, inguinal herniorrhaphy in 34, hysterectomy in 13, and gastrectomy in 2 patients.

## Operative Findings

Unfortunately, the findings at operation were not always well described; nevertheless, some useful observations are possible.

At times the contents of the hernial sac became reduced spontaneously with the onset of anesthesia. Most often, the umbilical hernial sac will be found to contain omentum. Its location and configuration make it possible for omentum to prolapse into the umbilical defect. Omentum was described as being present in 142, or 27 percent, of the cases.

Small intestine was present in 22 patients, or approximately 4 percent; and colon was present in 10 patients, or nearly 2 percent.

It is noteworthy that in none of the patients was the blood supply to the colon compromised. Strangulation of small intestine was present in 11 patients, or 2 percent, of 520 patients. In 8 individuals, resection of intestine was necessary.

Richter's hernias may occur at the umbilicus, since a small tight fibrous ring is present in a number of patients. In 520 patients, there were only two Richter's hernias (Fig. 22–11).

## Complications

In the repair of the largest umbilical hernias, replacement of viscera into the peritoneal cavity may interfere with venous return to the heart. Furthermore, elevation of the diaphragm may seriously interfere with ventilation and oxygenation. Hence, the blood pressure and respiratory effort must be carefully monitored in obese patients with huge umbilical hernias (see Fig. 22–7, p. 411).

Wound complications included seroma in 23 (or 4.5 percent), wound infection in 21 (or 4 percent); and hematoma in 11 (or 2 percent) of 520 operations for repair of umbilical hernias. Excessive discharge of ascitic fluid was seen in 3 patients. Wound complications occurred in a total of 58 patients, or 11 percent, of 520 patients.

Other complications occurred as follows: ileus, 9; pulmonary complications, 12; phlebothrombosis, 15; and urological complications, in 10 patients.

## Recurrences

There were 8 known recurrences in 520 patients, for a total recurrence rate of 1.54

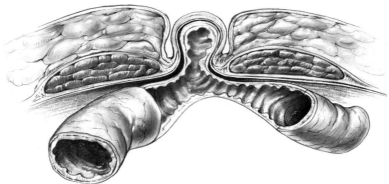

**Figure 22–11.**   Richter's type of hernia may occur at the umbilicus when a small tight fibrous ring is present.

percent. Although this rate appears to be high, it bears further examination here. Initial repairs of umbilical hernias were performed in four patients through vertical incisions. One patient had a cholecystectomy performed through a vertical midline incision with simultaneous umbilical herniorrhaphy. The second patient had an epigastric hernia repaired along with the umbilical hernia repair. The third patient was obese and had cirrhosis of the liver. His wound healed slowly, and there was postoperative draining of ascitic fluid. He developed a hematoma and a recurrence of an umbilical hernia one year later. The fourth incident of recurrence, following a vertical closure of an umbilical defect, occurred in an obese female who also had a midline incisional hernia. After repair of umbilical hernias using the vertical incision and closure, the recurrence rate was 4 patients out of a total of 106 vertical repairs—for a recurrence rate of nearly 4 percent.

On the other hand, there were four recurrences following transverse repairs, three of which were Mayo repairs with overlapping of the aponeurosis in each patient. In one patient, the recurrence appeared within one month indicating a technical failure. A second Mayo repair was successful. In one patient, recurrence was noted after transverse closure in one layer. There were 345 hernias repaired with the Mayo method. Recurrences were noted in three patients, for a rate of less than one percent. The superiority of methods utilizing transverse closure for repair of umbilical hernias is striking. The recurrence rate

of umbilical hernia repairs utilizing vertical closure was 4 percent; with transverse closures utilizing the Mayo repair or transverse closure in one layer, the recurrence rate was only one percent. Repair of epigastric hernias utilizing transverse closure also resulted in a lower incidence of recurrence. Gibson and Gaspar (1959) also obtained better results when utilizing the Mayo repair in repair of umbilical hernias. They suggested that vertical repairs of umbilical hernias be avoided because of higher recurrence rates.

Whenever the vertical incision is used, great care should be taken in the closure, and retention sutures of number one nylon or a comparable material should be used.

## Mortality

Although mortality following umbilical herniorrhaphy is low, deaths do occur. In 520 operations there were 3 deaths, for a mortality of 0.58 percent. One patient had cirrhosis of the liver and a strangulating obstruction, and it was necessary to resect necrotic small intestine. He died on the fifth postoperative day.

A second patient had undergone cholecystectomy and repair of an umbilical hernia. The patient died of aspiration pneumonitis.

The third patient was 78 years of age and died of congestive heart failure on the eighteenth postoperative day.

Repair of umbilical hernias can be performed successfully with very low morbidity and mortality. Repair should be recommended in all patients who are in reasonably good health and who have symptomatic umbilical hernias. Physicians should be aware that some patients, inappropriately, may deny symptoms even when large umbilical hernias are present.

These, too, should be repaired, since they will become troublesome as the years advance. Death most often claims those patients who have intestinal strangulation as well as severe systemic disease.

# OMPHALOCELE

*A sharp distinction exists between umbilical hernia and and exomphalos. The former is entirely skin-covered; in the latter the protruding viscera are covered by the walls of the expanded cord only—a thin translucent membrane consisting of amniotic ectoderm, with a thin layer of Wharton's jelly, and lined by the umbilical coelom. This membrane has no blood supply, and when deprived at birth of its surrounding amniotic fluid it rapidly sloughs and becomes infected. Hence the surgical treatment of exomphalos is primarily emergency work.*

*Dott, 1932*

Developmental defects of the abdominal wall at the umbilicus have not been well understood in the past. In fact, even today omphaloceles are too often indexed under umbilical hernias. It is unfortunate that the terms *omphalocele* and *umbilical hernia* are sometimes used interchangeably, since they differ so much in their pathology, treatment, and prognosis. Even the entity called hernia into the umbilical cord should be clearly differentiated from omphalocele, since the defect in the abdominal wall in the former is comparatively minor and more easily repaired.

There are other lesions occurring at the umbilicus that must be considered in the differential diagnosis; the urachus and remnants of the vitelline duct may present even though they are uncommon. Inflammatory lesions—and, less frequently, neoplasms—may be seen at the umbilicus. Gastroschisis is to be differentiated from umbilical hernia and omphalocele. No hernial sac is present in gastroschisis, and the intestine is encased in a gelatinous mass. The actual defect in the abdominal wall is situated outside the ordinary umbilical ring. Gastroschisis will be considered as an unusual hernia in Chapter 24.

In the following section we will consider omphaloceles. Other terms for this condition include: amniocele, amniotic hernia, exomphalos, and umbilical eventration. It is well recognized that infants with the largest omphaloceles frequently have anomalies of the gastrointestinal tract, heart, and thorax. Multiple and varied abnormalities tend to occur in the same individual. Hernia into the umbilical cord refers to a type of omphalocele in which the developmental defect is minimal.

## HISTORICAL BACKGROUND

The historical comments noted here are taken from the publications of Jarcho (1937), Cunningham (1956), Schuster (1967), and Wesselhoeft and colleagues (1972). The texts of Gross (1960), Swenson (1958), and the book on pediatric surgery by Benson and colleagues (1962) have been utilized. Although omphaloceles have been recognized since an early description by Paré in 1634, little had been accomplished therapeutically until 1803 when Hey performed the first primary closure of an intact omphalocele. For centuries, interest in the problem of exomphalos was negligible. This was probably due to a lack of understanding of the anomaly; also of importance was the fact that the means for surgical treatment—including asepsis and anesthesia—were yet to be developed. Aribat collected only 9 published reports of such cases prior to 1800. During the later eighteenth century, Pott and Richter described umbilical defects. Sporadic case reports appeared in the literature, but documentation was far from complete. The problem of differentiation between an omphalocele and an ordinary umbilical hernia added to the confused state of knowledge concerning omphaloceles. Nevertheless, by 1900 Jarcho estimated that less than 200 cases of congenital umbilical hernia had been reported in the world literature. Between 1900 and 1929, Altpeter had collected 109 cases.

The complicated embryogenesis of exomphalos is better understood as a result of the contributions of several investigators. The classic book by Cullen entitled *Embryology, Anatomy and Diseases of the Umbilicus*, published in 1916, adds much to our knowledge. Dott presented the embryology of intestinal rotation in 1923. Others who have made noteworthy contributions include: Pernkopf, in 1925; Sternberg, in 1930; and Margulies, in 1945. Margulies was of the opinion that a combined umbilical and supraumbilical abnormality resulted from a failure of development at approximately the third week of gestation. He believed that a simple defect at the umbilical ring alone appeared much later — in approximately the eighth to tenth week of development. Much more recently, in 1963, Duhamel presented abdominal wall defects as celosomias. He referred to the work of Geoffroy Saint-Hilaire, who in 1936 studied the morphogenetic process of closing of the body of the embryo.

Efforts at surgical correction of exomphalos came slowly. In 1803, Hey is given credit for performing the first primary closure of an omphalocele by Wesselhoeft and colleagues (1972). The same authors noted that Visick first successfully closed a ruptured omphalocele in 1873. Williams attempted the repair of omphaloceles in two patients in 1930, but neither patient survived for a significant period of time following the procedures. Modern surgical treatment of exomphalos begins with the contributions of Gross and Blodgett in 1940.

In 1967 Schuster developed a new method for staged repair of large omphaloceles. His presentation is clearly illustrated and detailed. He utilized a polyethylene film liner and Teflon mesh to cover the defect and add strength to the repair. The object of the method is to control and protect the viscera, to minimize infection, and to allow time for the developing abdominal cavity to accommodate all prolapsed viscera.

Because of several factors — improved knowledge of the anomaly and associated abnormalities, greater awareness of the peculiar physiology of neonates, application of effective fluid and electrolyte replacement, development of antibiotic therapy and of safer anesthetic agents and techniques, and utilization of effective methods of surgical management — the outlook for infants with exomphalos has improved steadily.

## EMBRYOLOGIC CONSIDERATIONS OF UMBILICAL DEFECTS

To deal exhaustively with the various anomalies and abnormalities that appear at and near the umbilicus would be outside the scope of this text; however, it is felt that an appreciation of the more common abnormalities occurring in that area is essential (Table 22–4). Details are well presented in the works of Arey (1965) and the classic book on diseases of the umbilicus by Cullen (1916). Another useful volume for surgeons is the book on congenital defects by Gray and Skandalakis (1972).

The simplified outline in Table 22–4 has practical value for the surgeon called upon to treat lesions about the umbilicus. The surgeon should be aware that a lesion at the umbilicus may involve the gastrointestinal tract. The omphalomesenteric tract may be patent with a resultant enteric fistula at the umbilicus (Fig. 22–12). A sinus, cyst, or diverticulum can be seen here in the rare

Table 22–4. **ABNORMALITIES OF THE ABDOMINAL WALL TO BE CONSIDERED IN DIFFERENTIAL DIAGNOSIS**

1. *Gastrointestinal*
   A. Patent omphalomesenteric duct
2. *Genitourinary*
   A. Patent urachus
3. *Vascular Abnormalities*
4. *Anomalies of the Abdominal Wall*
   A. Umbilical hernia
   B. Hernia into the cord
   C. Omphalocele
   D. Epigastric hernia (See Chapter 23)
      Diastasis recti (See Chapter 23)
      Gastroschisis (See Chapter 24)

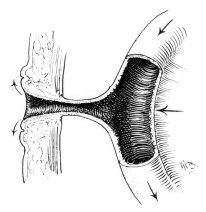

**Figure 22–12.** Patent omphalomesenteric duct with enteric fistula. (Reprinted courtesy of the W. B. Saunders Company. From Cullen, T. S.: *Embryology, Anatomy and Diseases of the Umbilicus.* Philadelphia, W. B. Saunders Co., 1916, p. 224.).

case. Similarly, a fistula at the umbilicus might communicate with the bladder (Fig. 22–13). Cysts or sinuses can appear here as well. Communications between the umbilicus and intestine or the umbilicus and bladder are rare but can exist in the exceptional newborn.

Vascular anomalies, although rare, can arise from the omphalomesenteric duct or the urachus. The umbilical vessels seldom cause serious difficulties following birth.

Abnormalities of the abdominal wall itself are among the most common at the umbilicus. The commonly found defect at this site is an umbilical hernia. An umbilical hernia results from a failure of the umbilical ring to close normally. The tendency is for the fibrous ring to close gradually; but in a small percentage of infants and children, the defect persists and may even enlarge. The protrusion at the umbilicus consists of skin, with peritoneum beneath it.

A hernia of the umbilical cord occurs when closure of the extraembryonic coelom is incomplete (Fig. 22–14). Normally during intrauterine development of the fetus, the small intestine prolapses into the umbilical cord but finds its way into the abdomen of the infant at birth. In fact, the intestine returns into the peritoneal cavity by the tenth week. Cresson and Pilling (1959) point out that technically this condition does not represent a true hernia — there is no true peritoneal sac and the ectopic viscera have never been in the peritoneal

cavity. The covering of the prolapsed bowel is made up of a thin, transparent amnion; an umbilical hernia is covered by both peritoneum and skin. Fortunately, the defect in the abdominal wall is small in instances of hernia of the umbilical cord, permitting closure in one stage. In most instances of hernia into the umbilical cord, the abdominal wall is otherwise well developed. The abnormality is usually one of a minor nature, confined to the umbilical ring; and the abdominal cavity is usually of normal size.

An omphalocele or exomphalos is an anomaly that occurs at an early stage of embryologic development. The intestines have not yet returned to the abdomen (Fig. 22–15, *A* and *B*). The gut normally remains prolapsed through the umbilical ring into the body stalk from the sixth through the ninth week of gestation, according to Patten (1968). In omphalocele, the intestines remain in this location at birth. A number of relatively recent publications have dealt with the embryology of omphalocele, and the views of Duhamel (1963) and of Izant and colleagues (1966) are of particular interest to the surgeon. Duhamel points out that exomphalos is a type of malformation resulting from a disturbance in the mech-

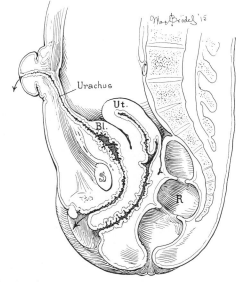

**Figure 22–13.** Patent urachus communicating with the bladder. (Reprinted courtesy of the W. B. Saunders Company. From Cullen, T. S.: *Embryology, Anatomy and Diseases of the Umbilicus.* Philadelphia, W. B. Saunders Co., 1916, p. 489.)

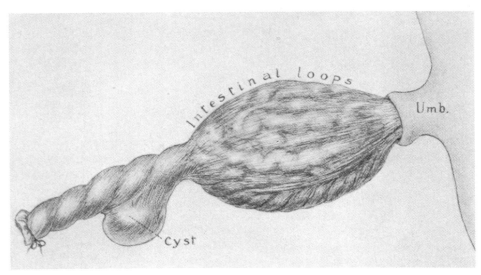

**Figure 22–14.** Hernia into the umbilical cord. (Reprinted courtesy of W. B. Saunders Company. From Cullen, T. S.: *Embryology, Anatomy and Diseases of the Umbilicus.* Philadelphia, W. B. Saunders Co., 1916, p. 460.)

anism that determines the closing of the body of the embryo. Duhamel referred to the works of Geoffroy Saint-Hilaire who in 1836 described a number of malformations called *celosomias,* which arose from failure of formation of all or some part of the embryonic folds. In order to understand the magnitude of congenital abdominal wall defects, I will refer briefly to the variety of defects that may be seen. The observations and opinions of Duhamel are helpful in explaining the abnormalities seen in certain infants. Duhamel described three categories of anomalies as follows:

1. Those arising from failure of formation of the cephalic fold.

2. Those arising from failure of formation of the caudal fold.

3. Those arising from failure of formation of the lateral folds.

Maldevelopment of the somatic layer of the cephalic fold results in complicated anomalies known as *upper celosomias.* These are characterized by the lack of the thoracic and epigastric walls. In such infants, ectopia cordis is seen along with sternal and diaphragmatic defects, and exomphalos is present as well. In 1958 Cantrell and colleagues described five cases of this type. Toyama reviewed this syndrome in 1972, adding his case to 161 cases reported in the world litera-

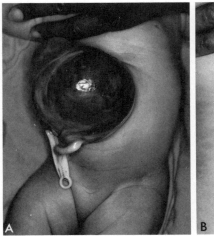
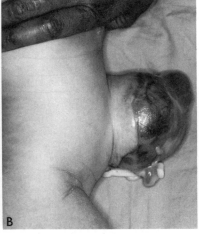

**Figure 22–15.** Large omphalocele. *A,* Anterior, and *B,* lateral view.

ture—only two survived surgical repair of omphaloceles. Spitz in 1975 added five additional cases in which thoracic, cardiac, and abdominal wall defects occurred in neonates. With a combination of conservative management and operative treatment, three of the five infants survived.

Failure of caudal fold formation can affect both the somatic and splanchnic layers, resulting in lower celosomia. According to Duhamel, when failure of the splanchnic layer formation occurs, partial agenesis of the hindgut can result in an opening into the bladder. Failure of formation of the somatic and splanchnic layers leads to a complicated anomaly consisting of exomphalos, agenesis of the hindgut, fistula between the intestine, and ectopic bladder.

Failure of formation of the lateral folds prevents the body wall from closing completely. The result is a middle celosomia, of which omphalocele is an example. This is the most common defect; Duhamel found exomphalos alone in 24 of 30 cases of congenital anomalies of the ventral abdominal wall. Hernia of the umbilical cord results from the failure in closing of extraembryonic coelom. In such cases, the small bowel is found outside the peritoneal cavity.

Thus, in those omphaloceles resulting from some degree of failure of formation of the cephalic fold, one will find a defect in the abdominal wall and nonrotation of the bowel. Actually, in such instances, the peritoneal cavity itself had never contained the intestines, which are found in the omphalocele. The normal sequence of intestinal rotation does not occur; and the portion of the intestine supplied by the superior mesenteric artery is suspended from common mesentery, making volvulus a possibility due to the mobility. The covering of an omphalocele is made up of thin, transparent, avascular amniotic membrane.

The hernia into the umbilical cord is a minimal abnormality in which the abdominal wall is well developed except for the umbilical ring. Also, the return of the intestine into a normal abdominal cavity is incomplete; however, complete intestinal rotation is possible (see Fig. 22–14, p. 420).

Gastroschisis is a rare abnormality of the ventral abdominal wall. The defect resembles an omphalocele, but no sac is found. Furthermore, the defect is not located at the umbilical ring but is most often found to the right of it. The prolapsed loops of intestine are thickened, leathery, and covered with a gelatinous substance. The term *gastroschisis* is missing from the index of Patten's *Human Embryology* (1968) and from Cullen's book on the *Umbilicus and Its Diseases* (1916); however, in recent years the defect is being recognized with increasing frequency. The defect in gastroschisis is attributed to a failure in development of the abdominal wall. The umbilicus itself is not involved in the defect. Gastroschisis will be considered in some detail in Chapter 24.

## Associated Anomalies

It has become clear that the best results in treatment management are obtained in infants with hernias into the umbilical cord or with small abdominal wall defects resulting in omphalocele. These neonates have fewer associated anomalies, making the prognosis for survival better.

The number of possible associated anomalies is truly remarkable. It is obvious that with large omphaloceles, the deviations from normal development are numerous and serious. The lack of uniform documentation of the various anomalies encountered by various contributors makes accurate estimates of the precise incidence impossible to assess. Nevertheless, useful information is available regarding the types of anomalies that the surgeon may encounter. The incidence of anomalies other than exomphalos was found to be 31 percent by Aitken (1963), over 33 percent by Firor (1975), and 42 percent by Eckstein (1963).

Soave (1963) found that associated malformations were present in 55 percent of his patients with omphalocele. Hair lip, palatoschisis, extrophy of the bladder, meningocele, inguinal hernia, and talipes were among the anomalies noted as not requiring urgent treatment. Other anomalies of utmost importance noted by Soave included atresia, duplication of the intestine, intussusception, malrotation and patent omphalomesenteric duct, and diaphragmatic hernia.

Aitken found a variety of abnormalities in the omphaloceles he studied. There were 9 amnioceles and 23 hernias into the umbilical cord. In three infants, only small bowel was present; eight Meckel's diverticula were also found. The vitellointestinal duct was patent in two instances and malrotation was present in five cases. Aitken found that 31 percent of his patients had anomalies other than exomphalos and its contents. He found malrotation to be present in 55 percent of cases with amniocele.

Hutchin and Goldenberg (1965) found the incidence of associated anomalies to be 79 percent among 16 infants with omphalocele and three with gastroschisis.

Onouchi and colleagues (1945) and Greenwood and coworkers (1974) studied the cardiovascular malformations associated with exomphalos. Tetralogy of Fallot is the most common serious cardiovascular anomaly associated with the condition.

Mahour and colleagues (1973) reviewed 27 patients with intact omphaloceles and found intra-abdominal anomalies in 10. Three, or 11 percent, had atresia of the small bowel; 7, or 25.9 percent, had malrotation with duodenal bands. He stated that such an incidence of abdominal anomalies indicates a need for surgical exploration at the time of repair.

Girvan and coworkers (1974) from the Hospital For Sick Children in Toronto found that 42 of 94 patients with omphaloceles had associated anomalies.

Thus, the incidence of associated anomalies varies with different reports; but the frequency is most impressive, ranging from 55 to 79 percent of infants with exomphalos.

Gastrointestinal anomalies associated with aberrations in rotation would show the greatest incidence in large omphaloceles; adhesive bands, stenosis, atresia, Meckel's diverticula, and tracheoesophageal fistula are also found. Cardiovascular anomalies found include: dextrocardia, patent ductus arteriosus, tetralogy of Fallot, and septal defects. Diaphragmatic abnormalities are seen in larger abdominal wall defects as well. Other important anomalies involve the genitourinary tract and the anorectum. Infants with omphaloceles require a thorough examination, since so many developmental errors exist together. Inguinal hernias and anomalies in development of the central nervous system, should be identified. A variety of abnormalities of the extremities have been reported. The exact incidence of many anomalies is difficult to ascertain, since often only the major defects receive proper documentation and attention.

## Conservative Management of Omphaloceles

There are situations in which the use of conservative measures is indicated in treatment of large omphaloceles. This technique might be utilized when a huge defect is present in a patient with multiple deformities. The patient's epithelium will grow over the defect if the thin sac can be maintained intact and free of infection. As the abdominal cavity enlarges, the contents recede into the peritoneal cavity and healing and contraction decreases the size of the defect; Grob (1963), Bozek (1953), and Cunningham (1956) were among the first to use this method, which is recognized as being helpful in certain cases.

Cunningham in 1956 reviewed various early efforts at conservative treatment, and he noted that Ahfeld in 1899 applied alcohol compresses after an attempt at reduction under light narcosis. Jarcho (1937) used a similar method. Nash in 1950 applied a dressing of penicillin and sulphonamide cream. Cunningham then described his method as it was applied to the treatment of two cases of exomphalos with large, unruptured sacs. He administered penicillin systemically and applied compresses locally. Surgical repair of the remaining umbilical defect was accomplished at six years of age in one patient. The second infant recovered, but an umbilical hernia remained.

In 1963 Drescher of Szczecin, Poland, reported his experiences in the conservative treatment of exomphalos. He advocated the use of an antiseptic solution, occasionally adding 10 percent solution of silver nitrate. Drescher reported that Bozek in 1953 treated two infants successfully using the nonoperative therapy approach. He cited these advantages of the conservative approach.

1. Avoidance of operative shock and postoperative complications.
2. Avoidance of increased intra-abdominal pressure that, in turn, exerts pressure on the diaphragm, lungs, and heart.

3. Prevention of bacterial invasion through the membrane.
4. Epithelial covering proceeds slowly but effectively.
5. Treatment is available universally in principle.

Another paper on the conservative treatment of exomphalos was published by M. Grob in 1963. In 1957 he pointed out that the method had limited application. In cases with intestinal obstruction or strangulation, surgical correction was essential. When rupture of the sac occurs, prompt surgical repair is also required. Grob used a 2 percent aqueous solution of Mercurochrome applied locally, but this is not currently recommended. Systemic antibiotics are administered during the period of local treatment. A period of six to eight weeks of treatment is required to achieve epithelial covering of the omphalocele sac. The necessity for prolonged hospitalization is a serious objection to the method.

Grob pointed out that during the period of growth the peritoneal cavity enlarges and the prolapsed organs more or less return into the peritoneal cavity. He stated that this makes it possible to cover the sac later with mobilized skin—which, according to Grob, was also recommended by Oldhausen in 1887 and more recently by Gross in 1948.

Grob treated 16 infants conservatively with three deaths among them. Two died of volvulus, and one died of pneumonia. Nine of the infants who were receiving conservative therapy developed local infection, and the sac remained intact in all patients.

Soave of Genoa, Italy, in 1963 recommended a similar method as practiced by Grob. He observed the course of the infants to be much the same as described by Grob. Soave reviewed the limitations of the staged procedure of management of larger omphaloceles as described by Williams in 1930 and Gross in 1948. The first step calls for mobilization of the skin at the subcutaneous level in order to cover the defect. The disproportion between the small size of the abdominal cavity and the large volume of viscera that must be replaced therein creates a difficult technical surgical problem. The resultant increased intra-abdominal pressure causes compression of

the inferior vena cava and the porta hepatis. Venous blood return is interfered with, and this is further aggravated by elevation of the diaphragm. Respiratory function is impaired, and cyanosis and shock may follow. It is the above sequence of events, often seen in the repair of large omphaloceles, that led to the dissatisfaction with early surgical treatment.

Seashore and colleagues (1975) have utilized biologic dressings of porcine skin and amniotic membrane.

Conservative treatment calls for protective isolation of the infant. A warm bed and some type of arrangement to protect the exomphalos from trauma is required. Local antiseptic solutions are applied to the defect. Systemic antibiotics are administered. Soave found that 8 to 12 weeks are required for healing. Utilizing the principles just described, Soave treated four infants with great omphaloceles, resulting in survival in every case. As an objection to the method, he cited the need for prolonged hospitalization.

## MANAGEMENT OF OMPHALOCELES

There is a need for individualization of treatment of omphaloceles because so much variation occurs in the magnitude of the abnormality, as well as in the number of concomitant anomalies. The defect may be limited to the umbilicus and cord where a loop of small intestine is still present in the patent umbilical cord. At the farthest end of the spectrum, the defect in the umbilical area and abdominal wall may be so large as to contain most of the small and large intestines, the spleen, and even the liver. Other anomalies, often multiple, are common in neonates with large omphaloceles. One of the more serious anomalies, atresia of the intestine, is to be recognized and corrected if the infant is to survive.

Our experience in the treatment of omphaloceles is somewhat limited, but a definite plan of management does emerge. Consideration is given to the state of the covering of the exomphalos, the size of the defect, the presence of coexisting anomalies, and the general condition of the patient.

Treatment may be operative, nonoperative, or conservative, depending upon the problem at hand. The background for nonoperative treatment has already been considered in this chapter.

At the present time, three rational methods of surgical treatment have evolved as follows:

1. Primary closure.
2. Conservative local therapy, later followed by closure.
3. Multistage operative procedures with and without prosthetic materials.

### Primary Closure

A number of omphaloceles are seen in which the abdominal wall defect is quite small, and these are recognized as hernias into the umbilical cord. The infant is usually well developed otherwise, and the abdominal cavity admits the reduced intestine without creating an excessive rise in intra-abdominal pressure. When performing primary closure, the surgeon must be reminded that forceful replacement of viscera causes elevation of the diaphragm and, thus, limits diaphragmatic excursion and pulmonary ventilation. The increased intra-abdominal pressure also interferes with return of venous blood to the heart.

Once an infant is seen with omphalocele, it is essential to protect the membrane from contamination and rupture. The patient must be carefully examined by a pediatrician or a neonatologist, who will scrutinize the infant for coexisting anomalies. Parents should be informed of the degree and type of associated anomalies.

Intravenous fluids are administered, usually via a cutdown at the ankle. Nasogastric suction is utilized to empty the stomach; this prevents gastric distention and minimizes the danger of aspiration in the postoperative period. Arrangements are made for blood transfusions. Endotracheal general anesthesia is commonly used, but small defects can be repaired under local anesthesia. Care should be taken at all times to avoid excessive loss of body heat. The skin itself is carefully prepared with an antiseptic, but the membrane is irrigated with normal saline solution. The method of repair is that advocated by Gross and Blodgett in 1940. The incision is made through the skin itself near the origin of the omphalocele sac. In the upper portion of the incision, the umbilical vein is

encountered. At this time, it is still a structure of some proportions. In the lower portion of the incision the umbilical arteries are recognized. The vein and arteries are ligated with fine non-absorbable suture material.

After the dissection has been completed about the omphalocele, the condition of the viscera is noted. Any existing abnormalities are corrected as indicated. Malrotation of the gut should be expected in larger omphaloceles.

Repair of the abdominal wall may be achieved by a two-layer closure, as advocated by Gross, approximating the peritoneum and posterior sheath together and anterior sheath of the rectus abdominis as separate layers (Fig. 22–16). The posterior layer may be closed with interrupted number 3–0 chromic catgut sutures. Silk sutures, number 3–0, and synthetic nonabsorbable sutures have been used with success to close the anterior sheath. These are placed as interrupted figure-of-eight sutures. Skin is closed with fine sutures of nylon or silk.

### Delayed Closure

This approach is applicable to small infants with the largest hernias, when the surgeon evaluates the situation at hand and finds that viscera replacement and closure would result in severe impairment of cardiopulmonary function. With the passage of time, the abdominal cavity will enlarge, and the defect in the abdominal wall will decrease in size.

Thorough preoperative evaluation by a pediatrician or neonatologist is essential. The omphalocele is carefully protected from injury with application of a sterile nonadherent dressing. Exposure to cold must be avoided and warmth provided. A number of "isolettes" are available, which constantly provide proper temperatures and humidity. Systemic antibiotics and parenteral feeding are life-saving measures in some neonates, Later, an elemental diet may be tolerated.

Local applications of various agents have been recommended. An aqueous solution of Mercurochrome was used earlier, but better agents have been discovered. Ahlfeld, in 1899, according to Cunningham, used alcohol compresses locally. His infant survived, and one year later the defect was closed. Nash in 1950 recommended that the omphalocele sac be dressed with penicillin and sulphonamide in a cream. Cunningham in 1956 reported two infants who survived after treatment of the sac with alcohol. The defect in one infant was later repaired by the Mayo technique. Firor used 0.5 percent silver nitrate in local application to the site of the defect. Other agents may be utilized, including Sulfamylon cream, Betadine dressings and various antibiotic ointments. Graivier (1974) used a triple antibiotic cream including polymyxin-B, neomycin, and bacitracin. Local applications are continued until epithelia-

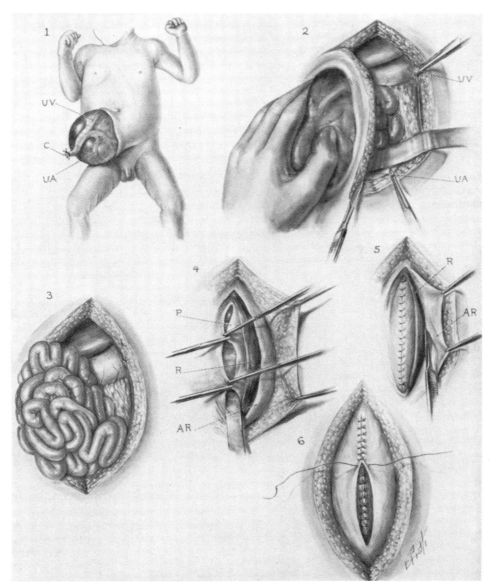

**Figure 22–16.** Gross's technique for repair of omphalocele. (1) Preoperative appearance. (2) Cutting away the sac; removing a narrow rim of the adjacent skin and abdominal wall to freshen their edges. The umbilical vein and arteries are clamped to avoid bleeding. (3) Sac removed. Umbilical vein and arteries ligated. (4) Intestines replaced in abdomen. Peritoneum freed up. (5) Peritoneum closed. Rectus muscles and anterior rectus fascia are cleared. (6) Rectus muscles are being brought together with interrupted silk sutures. *AR*, Anterior rectus fascia; *R*, rectus muscle; *C*, cord; *UA*, umbilical artery; *P*, peritoneum; *UV*, umbilical vein. (Reproduced by permission of the author and publisher. From Gross, R. E.: *Surgery of Infancy and Childhood.* Philadelphia, W. B. Saunders Co., 1960, p. 411.)

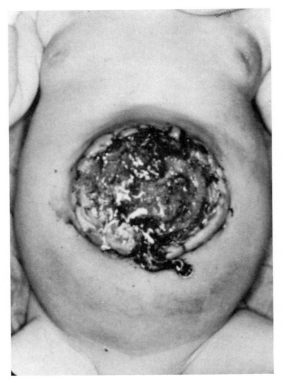

**Figure 22-17.**  This infant had a large omphalocele; two attempts at repair were unsuccessful. Local treatment with compresses resulted in gradual healing.

lization is complete. This will require approximately six to eight weeks of treatment, thus giving one basis for criticism of the method.

After a period of time (six months or longer), repair of the defective abdominal wall is carried out in layers. The contents of the sac are easily returned to the abdominal cavity without serious embarrassment of circulation and respiration.

Among our patients, we successfully treated one infant who had had two unsuccessful attempts at closure of a large defect. Infection developed at the amniocele sac, making any further efforts at repair unwarranted and extremely hazardous (Fig. 22-17). This infant had dextrocardia, malrotation of the midgut, and a hypoplastic uterus. Through systemic antibiotics and local applications of neomycin ointment, the defect slowly decreased in size (Fig. 22-18). After three months, healing was complete; and the infant was followed as an outpatient. As the child approached school

age, repair of the defect was advised (Fig. 22-19). In this patient, the defect was quite large but completely covered with epithelium. Malrotation was confirmed at the time of the operative procedure. The spleen was practically unattached to the posterior abdominal wall and floated freely on a long, mobile pedicle. We ascertained that no potentially obstructing bands were present and proceeded to repair the defect. The synthetic mesh was implanted posterior to the rectus sheath on either side (Fig. 22-20). Sutures consisting of number 2-0 silk were used to fix the mesh to the abdominal wall intraperitoneally. The abdominal wall was closed in a single layer over the implanted mesh. Healing was satisfactory, and a good postoperative result was obtained (Fig. 22-21, A and B).

## Multistaged Repairs of Omphaloceles

Currently substantial progress is being made in surgical management of the large

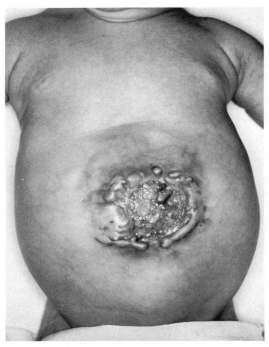

**Figure 22-18.**  The same patient shown in Figure 22-17. After six weeks of treatment, the healing, healthy wound at the umbilicus has greatly decreased in size.

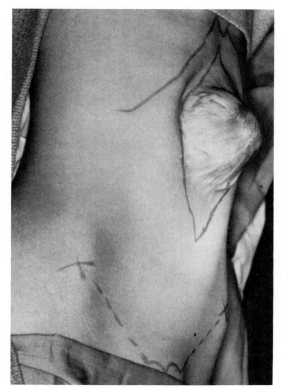

**Figure 22–19.** In the same patient shown in Figures 22–17 and 22–18, the defect at the umbilical and epigastric area is completely covered with epithelium. The child has grown normally.

complicated omphaloceles. Advances in the knowledge of pediatrics, physiology, pathology, and anesthesia have been remarkable. Antibiotic therapy and parenteral nutrition have also contributed significantly to survival of seriously ill infants.

The two-stage repair of omphaloceles was first performed by Gross in 1948. Since then, Benson, Bill, Ehrenpreis and others have utilized the method. Initial preparation essentially follows that as outlined in this section describing the single-stage repair.

During the first stage operation of a two-stage procedure, the incision is made in the skin about the omphalocele near the membrane but including a small ring of normal skin. The normal skin and its subcutaneous fat are elevated, being held with skin hooks or small retractors. Crushing clamps are not used. The dissection is carried out as widely as necessary to

achieve closure of the skin and subcutaneous tissue over the omphalocele. Dissection over the thorax itself is avoided, since blood supply to the skin flaps may be unnecessarily compromised. If the omphalocele sac is not to be excised, then the small rim of skin about the sac is excised. The mobilized skin is then closed over the omphalocele sac, which is ordinarily left intact.

New methods for multistage repair of exomphalos were presented by Schuster in 1967. The methods are clearly presented and illustrated in his publication. He utilized an impermeable polyethylene liner over which Teflon mesh was sutured to the abdominal wall. He pointed out that when skin is used for coverage, it is the skin that is distensible; hence, a large abdominal wall defect remains. When an inelastic material (such as Teflon) is used to bridge the defect, the muscular abdominal wall is forced to stretch and enlarge. When the abdominal cavity has enlarged sufficiently to accommodate the viscera

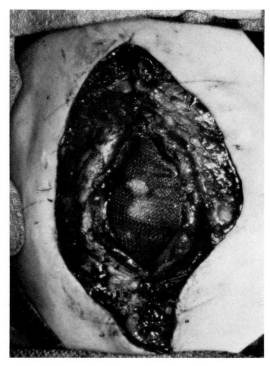

**Figure 22–20.** The hernial defect shown in Figure 22–19 is excised and repair with Marlex mesh is performed. The mesh is implanted deep to the rectus sheath on either side.

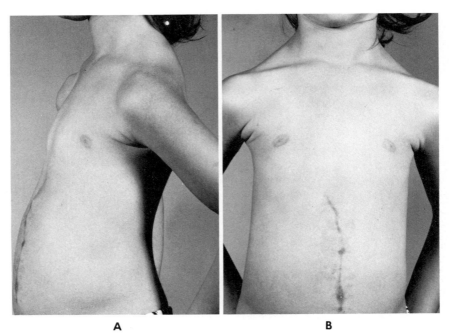

**Figure 22–21.**   Healing of the defect shown in Figures 22–18, 22–19, and 22–20 is now complete. *A*, Lateral view; *B*, anterior view.

without cardiopulmonary embarrassment, the defect is closed.

In 1969 Allen and Wrenn created a "silo" of Dacron coated with Silastic. Gradual compression of the synthetic sac resulted in return of the viscera to the abdominal cavity.

Wesselhoeft and Randolph in 1969 utilized prosthetic materials in repair of gastroschisis and ruptured omphalocele. They were impressed with the rapid enlargement of the abdominal cavity.

Gross illustrated the principles of multiple-stage closure in his atlas. He utilized sheets of siliconed Teflon over the intestine to avoid adherence to the lateral abdominal walls. His illustrations are clear, and the steps of the procedure are simple to follow (Fig. 22–22).

Not all surgeons feel it necessary to mobilize the skin. They utilize the synthetic sac as a cover until growth permits visceral replacement into the peritoneal cavity. Then, repair is achieved much as is shown in Figure 22–16.

Cross sectional views of an omphalocele repaired with silicone-Teflon sheeting is shown in sequence (Fig. 22–23; *A, B,* and *C*).

Other surgeons who have utilized syn-

thetic covering for omphaloceles include Geiger, who utilized Silastic sheeting for repair of prenatally ruptured omphaloceles. The Silastic sheeting provided a domicile for the viscera until the abdominal cavity enlarged. Seventeen days after formation of the Silastic silo the abdominal wall was successfully closed. Gilbert and colleagues utilized staged procedures in closure of both omphaloceles and gastroschisis. Firor has utilized silon sheeting for repair of both omphaloceles and gastroschisis (Fig. 24–27, p. 511).

Those surgeons who advocate the use of prosthetic materials recommend their use in infants with large defects. In such situations, forceful replacement of viscera into a peritoneal cavity would result in fatal cardiopulmonary complications.

There is a difference of opinion as to whether or not abdominal exploration is indicated in view of the significant incidence of malrotation, atresia, and stenosis. Certainly, exploration is a reasonable addition to those situations in which the omphalocele sac has ruptured. It is also a simple matter to explore those infants in whom a primary closure is to be performed.

Benson and colleagues in 1949 commented on the advisability of opening the amniotic sac at the time of the initial operative procedure. Gross advocated that the sac remain intact and inversion be carried out by closure of the skin over the protruding mass. Benson and coworkers cautioned that this method might result in overlooking associated anomalies that so often affect the midgut.

Mahour in 1974 advocated repair, excision of the sac, and thorough exploration in most cases of omphalocele. He would resort to nonoperative therapy in premature infants with multiple abnormalities who would tolerate surgical treatment poorly.

It might be worthwhile to note here that not every patient with malrotation will develop obstruction. Obstructive adhesive bands, stenosis, atresia, and meconium ileus are not present in every patient with malrotation; hence, there is a need for individualization in the management of the omphalocele sac and contents of the peritoneal cavity. When conservative treatment is used, if obstruction can be demonstrated, the need for surgical correction is clear.

Following recovery from the first stage operation, a delay of six months or more permits growth of the child and enlargement of the abdominal cavity. During the appropriate interval, it becomes possible to reduce the prolapsed contents into the peritoneal cavity. The interval of time recommended ranges from 6 to 24 months.

In the second stage of a two-stage procedure, careful preparation of the infant is repeated. A nasogastric tube is placed. The operative procedure is performed under endotracheal general anesthesia.

After abdominal preparation, the cicatrix is excised with an elliptical incision directed vertically. The dissection is carried laterally at the level of the rectus sheath, so that normal abdominal wall is identified. The sac is opened and freed laterally until peritoneum and posterior rectus sheath are identified as a first layer for repair. This layer is closed vertically with interrupted figure-of-eight sutures of number 3–0 chromic catgut. The rectus muscle itself may be gently approximated with catgut sutures. Finally, the anterior sheath of the rectus is approximated with interrupted sutures of number 2 or 3–0 silk. Fine wire or synthetic nonabsorbable sutures may be used.

The skin is closed with number 4–0 nylon sutures after redundant flaps are excised.

## Mortality

It is generally agreed that the high mortality associated with exomphalos is directly related to prematurity, number and magnitude of associated anomalies, size of the omphalocele, and presence of prenatal rupture of the sac. The rates varied among authors; but this is understandable in view of the varied patient population.

Aitken (1963) found the mortality to be 56 percent in his study. Vascular defects, intestinal obstruction, cardiac abnormalities, and gangrene of the intestine (secondary to volvulus due to malrotation) contributed to the fatalities. Respiratory embarrassment was believed to be a factor in the death of two other infants.

Schuster (1967) noted that the mortality ranged between 34 and 80 percent in different reports when large omphaloceles were encountered. He also noted that with antenatal rupture of the omphalocele sac, mortality approached 100 percent.

Wesselhoeft and colleagues (1972) found that when large, complicated omphaloceles were treated conservatively, the mortality was 20.5 percent; however, when a comparable group was treated surgically, the mortality was 62.9 percent. Finally, these authors reported a 90 percent survival rate in 20 infants with omphaloceles less than 5 centimeters in diameter and in the absence of other anomalies. They were able to achieve a survival rate of 86 percent with conservative treatment in a group of patients with defects larger than 5 centimeters.

Gross and Blodgett reported a mortality of 50 percent with primary closure in 1940; these are remarkable results considering that antibiotics were not yet available.

Benson and colleagues in 1949 noted that prematurity contributed to a fatal outcome. The mortality was 62 percent among premature infants and 33 percent among full-term infants with omphaloceles.

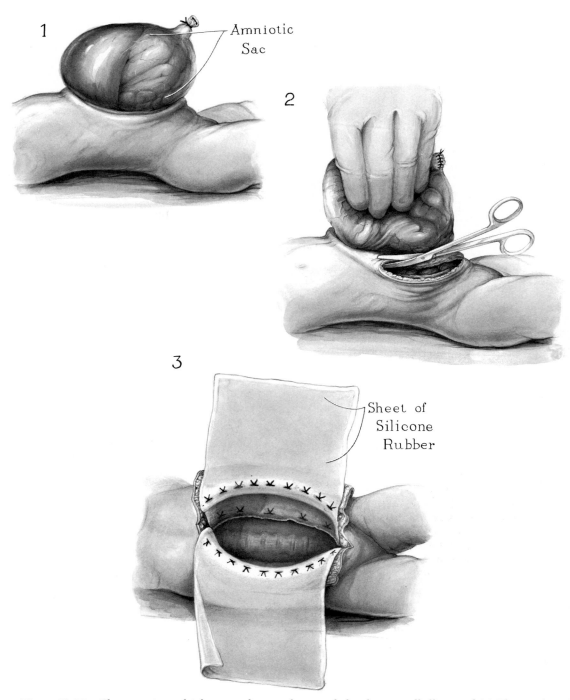

**Figure 22–22.** The steps in multiple-stage closure of an omphalocele are well illustrated (1) The ompha-locele with its contained intestine is quite large. (2) The incision is made circumferentially in the skin near the translucent amniotic sac. (3) The sheet of silicone-coated Teflon is sutured with number 2–0 silk to the margins of the rectus abdominis muscle and fascia. The margin of Teflon, which is expected to adhere to the wound margins, is free of silicone. (4) Sutures of number 2–0 silk are placed so as to provide an adequate container for the viscera. (5) The skin is now sutured over the silicone-Teflon–covered omphalocele mass. (6) Skin closure is completed with mattress sutures of number 2–0 silk. Drains are placed at the subcutaneous level. (From Gross, R. E.: *An Atlas of Children's Surgery*. Philadelphia, W. B. Saunders Co., 1970, p. 57.)

*Illustration continued on the opposite page.*

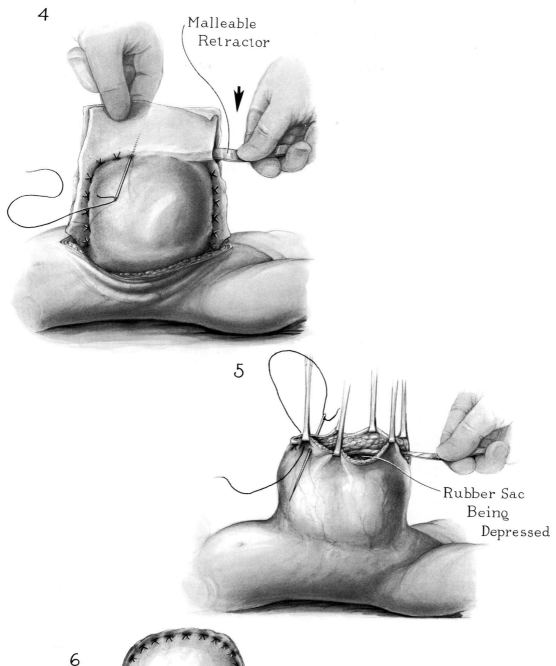

4

Malleable
Retractor

5

Rubber Sac
Being
Depressed

6

Figure 22–22.  *Continued.*

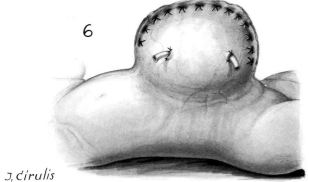

J. Cirulis

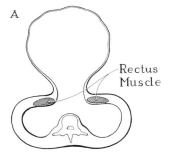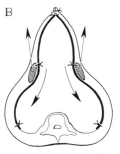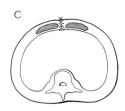

Rectus Muscle

**Figure 22–23.** These illustrations are most instructive in that they present cross-sectional views of progressive management of an omphalocele in a newborn infant. In *A*, the discrepancy between the size of the omphalocele is clearly shown. In *B*, the silicone-Teflon covering is in place and the skin covers the sheeting. Note attachment to the rectus abdominis sheath. In *C*, closure has been complete. (From Gross, R. E.: *An Atlas of Children's Surgery*. Philadelphia, W. B. Saunders Co., 1970, p. 56.)

## SUMMARY

Since 1940 great progress has been made in the understanding and treatment of omphaloceles. All writers on the subject stress the need for individualization of treatment to suit the needs of the patients at hand.

Small omphaloceles in otherwise healthy infants can be closed primarily with a success rate of over 90 percent. However, in the larger omphaloceles, a problem arises as a result of the disproportion between the volume of organs to be replaced and the capacity of the peritoneal cavity that is to receive them. Persistence at organ replacement under pressure will force the diaphragm upward and will interfere with blood flow through the vena cava. Respiratory difficulty, cyanosis, and hypotension are dangerous possibilities when excessive pressure on the viscera results from persistent efforts at immediate reduction. In such patients, the two-stage procedure may be the procedure of choice.

In certain small infants with huge defects and other serious anomalies, initial local treatment with antibacterial substances may be desirable. After growth and healing occur, the residual abdominal wall defect may be repaired.

In a few infants, the omphalocele may be treated by the method advocated by Schuster.

Rupture of the omphalocele sac and evidence of obstruction demand operative treatment. When rupture occurs, the viscera must be covered with skin or some prosthetic material.

## REFERENCES

Aitken, J.: Exomphalos: Analysis of a 10 year series of 32 cases. Arch. Dis. Child. *38*:126, 1963.

Allen, R. G., and Wrenn, E. J., Jr.: Silon as a sac in the treatment of omphalocele and gastroschisis. J. Pediatr. Surg. *4*(1):3, 1969.

Altpeter, Elizabeth: Über Nabelschnurbrüche (Inaugural-Dissertation). Druckerei der Kieler Zeitung G.m.b.H., Kiel, 1930.

Alvear, D. T., and Pilling, G. P.: Management of the sac during umbilical hernia repair in children. Am. J. Surg. *127*:518, 1974.

Arey, L. B.: *Developmental Anatomy* (7th ed.). Philadelphia, W. B. Saunders Co., 1965.

Baron, H. C.: Umbilical hernia secondary to cirrhosis of the liver—Complications of surgical correction. N. Engl. J. Med. *263*:824, 1960.

Benson, C. D., Mustard, W. T., Ravitch, M. M., Snyder, W. J., Jr., and Welch, K. H.: *Pediatric Surgery*. Chicago, Year Book Medical Pubs., Inc., 1962.

Benson, C. D., Penberthy, G. C., and Hill, E. J.: Hernia into the umbilcal cord and omphalocele (amniocele in the newborn). Arch. Surg. *58*:833, 1949.

Bill, A. H., Jr. in Benson et al.: *Pediatric Surgery*, pp. 589–598.

Bozek, J.: Observations concerning treatment of umbilical hernia. Pediat. Pol. *28*:1125, 1953.

Cantrell, J. R., Haller, J. A., and Ravitch, M. M.: A syndrome of congenital defects involving the abdominal wall, sternum, diaphragm, pericardium and heart. Surg. Gynecol. Obstet. *107*:600, 1958.

Castro e Neves, M., and Saavedra e Bruges, A.: A pregnant uterus protruding through an umbilical hernia sac. S. Afr. Med. J. *49*:1774, 1975.

Chapman, C. B., Snell, A. M., and Rauntree, L. G.: Decompensated portal cirrhosis: Report of one hundred and twelve cases. J.A.M.A. *100*:1735, 1933.

Cooper, Sir A. P.: *The Anatomy and Surgical Treatment of Crural and Umbilical Hernia*. London, Longman & Co., 1807,

Cresson, S. K., and Pilling, G. P.: Lesions about the umbilicus in infants and children. Pediatr. Clin. North Am. *6*:1085, 1959.

Crump, E. P.: Umbilical hernia. J. Pediatr. *40*:214, 1932.

Cullen, T. S.: *Embryology, Anatomy and Diseases of the Umbilicus.* Philadelphia, W. B. Saunders, 1916, pp. 459–480.

Cunningham, A. A.: Exomphalos. Arch. Dis. Child. *31*:144, 1956.

Dott, N. M.: Clinical record of a case of exomphalos: Illustrating the embryonic type and its surgical treatment. Edinb. Obstet. Soc. Trans. *39*:105, 1932.

Drescher, E.: Observations on the conservative treatment of exomphalos. Arch. Dis. Child. *38*:135, 1963.

Duhamel, B.: Embryology of exomphalos and allied malformations. Arch. Dis. Child. *38*:142, 1963.

Eckstein, H. B.: Exomphalos. A review of 100 cases. Br. J. Surg. *50*:405, 1963.

Ehrenpreis, T.: Omphalocele. *In* Nyhus, L. M., and Harkins, H. N.: *Hernia.* Philadelphia, J. B. Lippincott Co., 1964, pp. 322–333.

Farris, J. M., Smith, G. K., and Beattie, A. S.: Umbilical hernia: An inquiry into the principle of imbrication and a note on the preservation of the umbilical dimple. Am. J. Surg. *98*:236, 1959.

Firor, H. V.: Technical improvements in the management of omphalocele and gastroschisis. Surg. Clin. North Am. *55*(1):129, 1975.

Geiger, Paul E.: Prenatally ruptured omphalocele. Am. J. Surg. *116*:909, 1968.

Gibson, L. D., and Gaspar, M. R.: A review of 606 cases of umbilical hernia. Surg. Gynecol. Obstet. *109*:313, 1959.

Girvan, D. P., Webster, D. M., and Shandling, B.: The treatment of omphaloceles and gastroschisis. Surg. Gynecol. Obstet. *139*:222, 1974.

Graivier, L.: Changing concepts in treatment of ruptured omphalocele (Gastroschisis). Tex. Med. *70*:70, 1974.

Gray, W. S., and Skandalakis, J. E.: *Embryology For Surgeons.* Philadelphia, W. B. Saunders Co., 1972, pp. 409–415.

Greenwood, R. D., Rosenthal, A., and Nadas, A. S.: Cardiovascular malformations associated with omphaloceles. J. Pediatr. *8*:818, 1974.

Grob, M.: Conservative treatment of exomphalos. Arch. Dis. Child. *38*:148, 1963.

Gross, R. E.: *Surgery of Infancy and Childhood.* Philadelphia, W. B. Saunders Co., 1960, p. 423.

Gross, R. E.: A new method for surgical treatment of large omphaloceles. Surgery *24*:277, 1948.

Gross, R. E., and Blodgett, J. B.: Omphalocele (Umbilical Eventration) in the newly born. Surg. Gynecol. Obstet. *71*:520, 1940.

Halpern, L. J.: Spontaneous healing of umbilical hernias. J.A.M.A. *182*:851, 1962.

Heifetz, C. J., Bilsel, Z. T., and Gaus, W. W.: Observations on the disappearance of umbilical hernias of infancy and childhood. Surg. Gynecol. Obstet. *116*:469–473, 1963.

Hutchin, P. O., and Goldenberg, I. S.: Surgical therapy of omphalocele and gastroschisis. Arch. Surg. *90*:22, 1965.

Izant, R. J., Jr., Brown, F., and Rothmann, B. F.: Current embryology and treatment of gastroschisis and omphalocele. Arch. Surg. *93*:49, 1966.

Jarcho, J.: Congenital umbilical hernia. Surg. Gynecol. Obstet. *65*:593, 1937.

Jones, J. W.: The frequency of umbilical herniae in Negro infants. Arch. Pediat., *58*:294–300, 1941.

Karlström, G.: Should infantile umbilical hernias be treated with naval emplastras.? J. Pediatr. *59*:87, 1961.

Kieswetter, W. B.: Hernias — Inguinal and umbilical. Am. J. Surg. *101*:656, 1961.

Lassaletta, L., Fonkalsrud, E., Tovar, J. A., Dudgeon, D., and Asch, M. J.: The management of umbilical hernias in infancy and childhood. J. Pediatr. Surg. *10*:405, 1975.

Lucas-Championnière, J.: La hernie ombilicale. Thérapeutique et cure radicale. Sur. 18 Cas de hernie ombilicale et 11 cas de hernie epigastrique par 1 a cure radicale. J. Med. Chir. Prat. *66*:609, 1895.

Mack, N. K.: The incidence of umbilical hernia in Africans. E. Afr. Med. J. *22*:369, 1943.

Mahour, G. H., Weitzman, J. J., and Rosenkrantz, J. G.: Omphalocele and gastroschisis. Ann. Surg. *177*:487, 1973.

Margulies, L.: Omphalocele (Amniocele); its anatomy and etiology in relation to hernias of umbilicus and umbilical cord. Am. J. Obstet. Gynecol. *49*:695, 1945.

Mayo, W. J.: Further experience with the vertical overlapping operation for the radical cure of umbilical hernia. J.A.M.A. *41*:225, 1903.

Mayo, W. J.: Radical cure of umbilical hernia. J.A.M.A. *48*:1842, 1907.

Mayo, W. J.: Remarks on the radical cure of hernia. Ann. Surg. *34*:51, 1899.

Morgan, W. W., White, J. J., Strumbaugh, S., and Haller, J. A.: Prophylactic umbilical hernia repair in childhood to prevent adult incarceration. Surg. Clin. North Am. *50*:839, 1970.

Nash, D. F. Ellison: As cited by Cunningham, A. A.: Exomphalos. Arch. Dis. Child. *31*:144–151, 1956.

Need, A. B.: Obstructed umbilical hernia in children: Two case reports. Aust. Paed. J. *8*:152, 1972.

O'Hara, E. T., Oliai, A., Patek, A. J., Jr., and Nasbeth, D. C.: Management of umbilical hernias associated with hepatic cirrhosis and ascites. Ann. Surg. *181*:85, 1975.

Onouchi, Z., Ootsuka, T., Otabe, E., Sasagawa, H., Takada, Y., and Goto, M.: A case of the omphalocele: The discussion about these frequent combinations of the cardiac malformation and the observation at the early non-cyanotic period of Fallot's tetralogy. Jap. Heart. J. *16*:211, 1975.

Patten, B. M.: *Human Embryology* (3rd ed.). New York, McGraw-Hill Book Co., 1968, pp. 423–426.

Pratt, J. P.: Personal communication.

Russell, H. R.: The etiology and treatment of inguinal hernia in the young. Lancet *2*:1353, 1899.

Schuster, S. R.: A new method for surgical treatment of large omphaloceles. Surg. Gynecol. Obstet. *125*: 837, 1967.

Seashore, J. H., MacNaughton, R. J., and Talbert, J. L.: Treatment of gastroschisis and omphalocele with biological dressings. J. Pediatr. Surg. *10*(1):9, 1975.

Soave, F.: Conservative treatment of giant omphalocele. Arch Dis. Child. *38*:130, 1963.

Spitz, L., Bloom, K. R., Milner, S., and Levin, S. E.: Combined anterior abdominal wall sternal, diaphragmatic, pericardial and intracardiac defects: A report of five cases and their management. J. Pediatr. Surg. 10:491, 1965.

Stanley-Brown, E. G.: Hernia in infancy. G.P. 23:82, 1961.

Storer, H. B.: A new operation for umbilical hernia. M. Med. 1:73, 1866–67.

Swenson, O.: *Pediatric Surgery*. New York, Appleton-Century-Crofts, 1958.

Toyama, W. M.: Combined congenital defects of the anterior abdominal wall, sternum, diaphragm, pericardium and heart. A case report and review of the syndrome. Pediatrics 50:778, 1972.

Walker, S. H.: The natural history of umbilical hernia. Clin. Pediatr. 6:29, 1967.

Watson, L. F.: *Hernia* (3rd ed.). St. Louis, C. V. Mosby Co., 1943, pp. 334–365.

Wesselhoeft, C. W., and Randolph, J. G.: Treatment of omphalocele based on individual characteristics of the defect. Pediatrics 44(1):101, 1969.

Wesselhoeft, C. W., Porter, A., and Deluca, F. G.: The treatment of omphalocele and gastroschisis. Ann. Chir. Inf. 13(4):237 (Paris), 1972.

Williams, C.: Congenital defects of the anterior abdominal wall. Report of cases. Surg. Clin. North Am. 10:805, 1930.

Woods, Grace E.: Some observations on umbilical hernia in infants. Arch. Dis. Child. 28:450, 1953.

## Supplemental Readings

Baccari, E. M., Preiling, B., and Organ, C. H., Jr.: A study of the maturity onset of adult umbilical hernia. Am. Surg. 37:385, 1971.

Bennett-Jones, M. J.: Umbilical hernia in children with special reference to injection treatment. Br. Med. J. 1:78, 1944.

Bryant, W. M., and Griffen, W. O., Jr.: Umbilical hernia and gallbladder disease. Am. J. Surg. 117:653, 1969.

Cohen, Robert: Perforated adhesive tape for umbilical hernia. Am. J. Dis. Child. 76:44, 1948.

Deitel, M., and Friedman, I. H.: Strangulated umbilical hernia with external fecal fistula: Management by delayed definitive surgery. Arch. Surg. 95:111, 1967.

Firor, H. V.: Omphalocele—An appraisal of therapeutic approaches. Surgery 69:208, 1971.

Gilbert, M. G., et al.: Staged surgical repair of large omphaloceles and gastroschisis. J. Pediatr. Surg. 3:702, 1968.

Greenwood, R. D.: An early description of omphalocele. Maryland St. Med. J. 24(9):59, 1975.

Johnson, A. H.: Omphalocele and related defects. Am. J. Surg. 114:297, 1967.

Jones, J. W.: The frequency of umbilical herniae in negro infants. Arch. Pediatr. 58:294, 1941.

Keith, Sir Arthur: The origin and nature of hernia. Br. J. Surg. 11:455, 1924.

Kling, S.: Massive omphalocele: A method of treatment employing skin allograft. Can. J. Surg. 10:445, 1967.

Mahorner, H.: Umbilical and midline ventral hernia. Ann. Surg. 11:979, 1940.

Mahour, G. H.: Intact omphalocele: Perennial dilemma of operative or "Conservative" management. Am. J. Surg. 138(3):419, 1974.

Mayo, W. J.: An operation for the radical cure of umbilical hernia. Trans. Am. Surg. Assoc. Ann. Surg. (May, 1901).

Michelson, E., and Raffel, W.: Repair of the large umbilical hernia. Surgery 10:999, 1941.

Morton, C. B.: Symptomatic occult umbilical hernia. Ann. Surg. 169:774, 1969.

Parsons, H. H.: Infantile (Acquired) umbilical hernia in soldiers. Mil. Surg. 87:298, 1940.

Penchaszadeh, V. B.: Beckwoth-Wiedemann syndrome. (Exomphalos-Macroglossia-Gigantism: EMG syndrome.) Birth Defects 7(7):284, 1971.

Politzer, G., and Sternberg, H. As cited in Cunningham, A. A.: Exomphalos. Arch. Dis. Child. 31:144 to 151, 1956.

Prince, G. E.: The use of transparent tape in the treatment of umbilical hernia in infants. J. Pediatr. 39:481, 1951.

Reed, E. N.: Infant disemboweled at birth—appendectomy successful. Am. Med. Assoc. J. 61:199, 1913.

Rickham, P. P.: Rupture of exomphalos and gastroschisis. Arch. Dis. Child. 38:138, 1963.

Rusfeldt, O.: Umbilical hernias in children. Nordisk Med. 28:2367, 1945.

Samy, M.: Operation for radical cure of umbilical hernia. J. Egypt. Med. Assoc. 18:792, 1935.

Sharma, D. B., and Ghosh, S.: Sirenomelia with exomphalos. Ind. Pediatr. (Letter to the Editor), 12(No. 7):612, 1975.

Specht, N. W., and Shryock, E. H.: Omphalocele: Anatomical and clinical considerations. Surg. Gynecol. Obstet. 77:319, 1943.

Swenson, O.: *Pediatric Surgery*. (3rd ed.) New York, Appleton-Century-Crofts, 1969, p. 546.

Thunig, L. A.: Hernia into the umbilical cord and related anomalies. Arch. Surg. 1:1021, 1936.

Vassy, L. E., and Boles, E. T., Jr.: Iatrogenic ileal atresia secondary to clamping of an occult omphalocele. J. Pediatr. Surg. 10:797, 1975.

Watson, L. F.: *Hernia* (3rd ed.). St. Louis, C. V. Mosby Co. 1948, Chapter 21.

White, W. A., Jr.: Umbilical hernia in the bad risk patient. Surg. Gynecol. Obstet. 77:514, 1943.

# 23

# Epigastric Hernia

Epigastric hernias caused considerable difficulty for clinicians in the past. Earliest observers were slow to differentiate epigastric from umbilical hernias. A great variety of symptoms were attributed to these relatively small hernias of the linea alba; however, as their pathology became more defined, the symptoms they caused were better recognized. As a result of the contributions of many surgeons in the past, diagnostic accuracy has improved, and treatment of epigastric hernias has consequently become more effective in recent years.

## DEFINITION

An epigastric hernia is a small protrusion, usually composed of preperitoneal adipose tissue, occurring in the linea alba between the xiphoid process and the umbilicus. Unlike the groin hernia, the exceptional epigastric hernia contains a peritoneal sac. Adipose tissue protrudes through a defect in the decussating aponeurotic fibers of the linea alba with regularity. Omentum is not uncommonly found in epigastric hernias, but stomach, colon, and small intestine are rarely found in them.

The term "epigastric," when applied to supraumbilical midline hernias, is worthy of a moment's consideration. According to the earliest recorded history, it was once erroneously thought that the stomach itself was part of the herniation. Since these hernias occur in the linea alba, they are sometimes designated as "hernias of the linea alba." Midline hernias rarely occur spontaneously in the linea alba below the umbilicus; when they do, they are called "hypogastric hernias."

## HISTORICAL BACKGROUND

For a better understanding of epigastric hernias, it is useful to consider both the past and present contributions dealing with hernias in the midline of the abdomen. The early historical literature is often confusing and, at times, even inaccurate. I have consulted the publications of Watson and Iason, of Lewisohn, and of Friedenwald and Morrison for the following brief comments.

The earliest accounts of periumbilical hernias and hernias of the linea alba are confused and difficult to interpret. Arnauld de Villeneuve in 1285 apparently was the first to recognize the epigastric hernia. Guy de Chauliac in the fourteenth century observed that some hernias protrude through the umbilicus, while others follow different paths near the umbilicus. La Chausse stated in 1721 that hernias could protrude from any part of the abdominal wall, and De Garengot in 1743 recognized that they were capable of causing unusual and confusing abdominal symptoms. He thought that the stomach often herniated through the defect in the linea alba. Richter, an excellent observer, thought that the hernias actually egressed through the umbilicus in infants and to the side of the abdominal ring in adults. In 1785 he disagreed with those who held the opinion that the stomach herniated into epigastric hernias. Such famous surgeons as Cooper,

**435**

Cruveilhier, and Velpeau were of the same opinion as Richter, while De Garengot, Hoin, and Piplet were among the observers who believed that the stomach was always present in these hernias. Gunz, according to Friedenwald and Morrison, described the hernia as a gastric hernia or gastrocele in 1744. He felt that the gastric symptoms were explained by the protrusion of the stomach into the hernial sac. Pelletan in 1810 described the protrusion of preperitoneal fat with and without associated peritoneal sacs.

Maunoir in 1802 was credited with first performing a successful operation for correction of an epigastric hernia. Léviellé, ten years later, designated hernias that occurred above the umbilicus but in the midline as "epigastric."

Early contributors erroneously thought that the stomach was commonly found in midline hernias above the umbilicus; hence, the term "epigastric" was applied to them. These individuals also established the fact that operative treatment could be helpful. For many decades the subject of epigastric hernias seemed to attract little attention; this might have been owing to the infrequent occurrence of these hernias.

Even though some of the more recent contributions on epigastric hernia have been confusing, much progress has been made in the understanding and treatment of this defect. I would suggest that modern knowledge of epigastric hernias has been largely achieved in the past six decades.

Moschcowitz made a substantial attempt at explaining the pathogenesis of epigastric hernias in 1914. He described the defect in the linea alba through which some adipose tissue and a blood vessel passed. He erroneously stated that a distinct hernial sac was never present. Nevertheless, he understood the nature of the defect in the linea alba and recognized that preperitoneal fat and the falciform ligament were involved in the pathology of hernias in the linea alba. Moschcowitz refuted the idea that the stomach could enter an epigastric hernia. He felt that epigastric hernias could result in traction upon the fat and peritoneum; this rationally explained the visceral symptoms in certain patients.

In 1917 Moschcowitz presented an article before the American Surgical Association on epigastric hernia without palpable swelling. He noted that the symptoms consisted of eructations, nausea, and periodic attacks of pain localized in the epigastrium. He described the majority of epigastric hernias as being very small, rarely larger than a marble. Moschcowitz believed that the pain was a result of traction upon the falciform ligament of the liver. He stated that the principal physical sign was a sharply localized area of tenderness between the umbilicus and the xiphoid process of the sternum. In the repair of epigastric hernias, he recommended ligation of the stump with its accompanying vessel and closure of the opening in the linea alba.

In 1919 Hall reported his experiences with epigastric herniations in soldiers. He referred to the four varieties of epigastric hernia described by Keen: (1) a small mass of subperitoneal fat without any sac; (2) in addition to the subperitoneal fat, a process of parietal peritoneum attached to it without any contents; (3) a sac containing omentum; and (4) a sac containing intestine. This classification represents substantial progress in our understanding of the pathology of epigastric hernia. Hall pointed out that a lipoma in the epigastrium is more movable and less tender than a hernia. He could not confirm the observation of Bergman that the majority of these hernias contain omentum and transverse colon. Hall felt that the definite association existing between epigastric hernia and gastric ulcer was owing to reflex irritation of the stomach by the omental "drag," with resultant hyperacidity and ulceration.

In 1921 Lewisohn called attention to the need for thorough exploration of abdominal organs in operations for epigastric hernia. According to Lewisohn, Kussmaul advised Leucke in 1887 that operative repair might relieve patients with epigastric hernias of their gastric symptoms. Leucke performed two of these repairs, with favorable results. Lewisohn cited the works of Capelle in 1909, Schloffer in 1910, Ertrand in 1912 to 1913, and Leriche and Aigrot in 1914 in which these authors called attention to the coexistence of other diseases, such as carcinoma of the stomach, peptic ulcer, and even carcinoma of the colon, in patients with epigastric hernias. French surgeons were aware of the fact that patients with epigastric hernias required careful clinical evaluation of the gastric symptoms. Lewisohn correctly stated that symptoms of anorexia, sour eructations. vomiting, and abdominal pain are most frequently caused by disease of the stomach and duodenum, of the gallbladder, or of the appendix. X-ray examination of the stomach was recommended to aid in the differential diagnosis. Lewisohn also recognized the need for careful study of patients with epigastric hernia.

The suspicion that epigastric hernia with omentocele was in some way responsible for peptic ulceration led Meyer and Ivy in 1927 to take the problem to the laboratory. Their experiments failed to support this relationship; thus, they felt that any connection between gastric ulcer and epigastric hernia was coincidental. They also noted that epigastric hernia does not actually cause hyperacidity, since the results of gastric analysis are within the range of normal variation.

In 1926 Friedenwald and Morrison presented their excellent observations on 65 cases of epigastric hernia. They noted that these hernias occur more often in men who do heavy work. According to Friedenwald and Morrison, the defect is commonly acquired but occasionally appears congenitally. They recorded Terrier's classification of epigastric hernia as follows: (1) fatty hernia, with or without peritoneal diverticula; (2) fatty hernia, with sac and omentum; (3) distinctly omental hernia, without lipoma; and (4) intestino-omental hernia.

Friedenwald and Morrison added significantly to our knowledge of epigastric hernia when they noted that symptoms vary greatly among individuals. Some patients are asymptomatic, while others complain of tenderness over the hernia. The two researchers described severe symptoms, including loss of appetite, nausea, vomiting, eructations, flatulence, distention, constipation, and occasionally diarrhea, in one-half of their patients. The pain was severe in cases like these. I could not confirm their observations on the severity of symptoms, however, after studying our patients with epigastric hernias. Friedenwald and Morrison did point out that symptoms due to epigastric her-

nias could resemble peptic ulcer disease, cholelithiasis, carcinoma, and pyloric obstruction. They called attention to the need for roentgen-ray investigation and recommended surgical repair; they also reported that relapses were infrequent.

The symptomatology of epigastric hernia was investigated in 1936 by Pemberton and Curry in a review of 296 cases repaired at the Mayo Clinic from 1910 to 1933. They found that in 138 patients who underwent surgical treatment, repair of the epigastric hernia was a secondary matter.

Pemberton and Curry divided the remaining 158 patients hospitalized specifically for repair of epigastric hernias as follows:

Group I: Twenty-six patients underwent abdominal exploration at the time of hernia repair. Exploration was negative in 11 patients.

Group II: Thirty-seven patients had repairs of epigastric hernias, along with repair of other hernias.

Group III: Ninety-five patients simply had repair of epigastric hernias without exploration.

An attempt was made to evaluate the effectiveness of hernia repair in relieving visceral symptoms. They found that patients with no subjective visceral symptoms obtained good results from repair of their hernias. Patients who simply complained of pain in the abdominal wall at the hernia site prior to surgery, as a rule, obtained relief with hernia repair. In patients with numerous visceral symptoms, operative repair of the hernia was not as important a factor in relief of symptoms as was medical treatment. Proper dietary and medical management contributed more toward the relief of a variety of visceral symptoms than did operative treatment. Pemberton and Curry stated that no group of visceral symptoms was found in their study to be typical of epigastric hernia and amenable to surgical repair. However, because of the frequent coexistence of organic visceral diseases, they advised abdominal exploration at the time of hernia repair, even if preoperative diagnostic studies failed to locate abnormalities in any abdominal viscera.

As recently as 1937 Charlton of Tillamook, Oregon, raised the question of whether or not simple epigastric hernia simulated disease of the abdominal organs. He advised examination of the epigastric region and intra-abdominal organs during exploratory procedures.

In 1938 Josephus Luke reviewed the experience at the Royal Victoria Hospital of Montreal. He found that epigastric hernias occurred more frequently in men and were often associated with other types of hernias. He divided treatment into four categories. Those patients with strangulation and incarceration required prompt operation. Those patients presenting with localization of pain to a protruded hernial mass obtained good results following repair. Those in whom the protrusion occurs after heavy work or exercise but recedes at rest also obtained relief through surgical repair. Extensive investigation and abdominal exploration were not considered essential. Patients in the fourth category complained of a number of visceral symptoms. Complete diagnostic evaluation was indicated and, if negative, exploration of the abdomen was advised at the time of repair. The absence of visceral disease in these patients makes relief of symptoms a remote possibility following hernia repair.

In a more recent publication, McCaughan called attention to the fact that there may be recurrences following epigastric hernia repair. He found 6 recurrences in 64 followed cases, for a recurrence rate of 9.4 percent. Four of the six recurrences were seen in patients who had the vertical repair, with side-to-side imbrication of the linea alba. He favored the vertical incision when an umbilical hernia was also present.

## ANATOMIC CONSIDERATIONS

Although I have personally seen a great number of umbilical and epigastric hernias, I have never seen a midline hernia below the umbilicus in a patient who had not been operated upon previously. Hernias of the linea alba arising de novo

below the umbilicus must be rare indeed. Therefore, it it useful to review the anatomy directly involved with the problem of hernias occurring in the midline of the abdomen.

The linea alba extends from the ensiform cartilage to the symphysis pubis. It is much wider above the umbilicus and varies greatly from patient to patient (Fig. 23–1). In a few patients it is only a few millimeters wide, but in the majority it varies from 1 to 2 cm in width. In certain patients, it is even wider; the term "diastasis recti" is applied to this condition. The linea alba is normally wider as it approaches the umbilicus and becomes progressively narrower as the ensiform cartilage is reached.

The details of formation of the rectus sheath have been discussed in Chapter 2. We will now examine the differences in

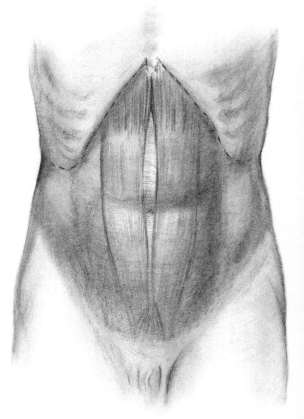

**Figure 23–1.** The linea alba is narrow below the umbilicus and becomes widest just above the umbilicus. It decreases in width as it approaches the xiphoid process.

the rectus sheath above and below the umbilicus. The aponeuroses of the external oblique, internal oblique, and transversus abdominis muscles fuse in the midline to form the linea alba. Since these structures approach the midline from different angles, there is a certain amount of decussation of fibers seen in the midline. The transversalis fascia and peritoneum are intimately attached to the rectus sheath posteriorly. There is no significant adipose tissue present, with one exception — between the leaflets of the falciform ligament and the abdominal wall, there is a variable amount of fat. In obese individuals the structure is thick and heavily infiltrated with adipose tissue. The falciform ligament is a remnant of the leaflets of the embryologic ventral mesentery of the stomach and duodenum; it is located slightly to the right of the midline and extends from the diaphragm to the umbilicus. The left umbilical vein remains recognizable in the margin of the falciform ligament and is known as the round ligament. The ligament itself extends from the liver above to the umbilicus below.

The linea alba is easily found immediately above the umbilicus, but below this structure it is so narrow that the surgeon attempting to make a midline incision invariably enters the rectus sheath.

At the medial margin of the rectus abdominis muscles and above the umbilicus, approximately five paired arterioles are seen to penetrate the fascia. These blood vessels are believed to enter into the pathogenesis of certain epigastric hernias.

Between the linea alba and the skin, there is a layer of normal adipose tissue.

## THE PATHOLOGIC ANATOMY AND THE CLINICAL PICTURE

The precise mechanism involved in the genesis of an epigastric hernia has been explained in various ways. Moschcowitz felt that the herniation occurred at the site where the blood vessels penetrate the linea alba. The fatty tissue beneath protrudes through the opening and then is further forced through the aperture by physical exertion or by any mechanism that increases intra-abdominal pressure. Other authors doubt this explanation; instead, they feel that a congenital abnormality or weakness in the linea alba leads to herniation, brought about by vigorous activities in adulthood.

The older literature on epigastric hernia abounds with inaccuracies and erroneous conclusions. In my opinion, some authors have tried to attribute every symptom in a given patient to the presence of the hernia. It is essential to recognize various types of epigastric hernias and to identify reasonable symptoms accompanying these hernias. Since most patients with epigastric hernias are adults and, in many cases, obese, they will probably have other disorders (such as peptic ulcer, hiatal hernia, biliary tract disease, and carcinoma) that are generally found in older patients. Finally, as in any patient population, there are individuals with epigastric hernias who also have functional nervous disorders. Operative repair of the hernia will not relieve the patient of his psychophysiologic malfunctions.

Although epigastric midline hernias do occur in infants and children, they are rarely seen, in the average surgeon's experience. Pentney reported 40 cases seen over a period of 6 years, but only 3 of his patients required operative treatment. He followed 33 patients for over 6 years and found that most of these small hernias disappeared in 2 to 4 years. He felt that epigastric hernias are acquired and are related to muscular effort and change in posture.

I am of the opinion that epigastric hernias are acquired and that obesity, pregnancy, and heavy work are factors in their genesis. Watson, Luke, and Pentney, and Friedenwald and Morrison, hold a similar view. The common occurrence of epigastric hernias in adults supports this concept. An epigastric hernia is, indeed, a rare event in a neonate or infant. I have never seen a preformed sac, such as the one found in an infant or neonate with indirect inguinal hernia, in a child with epigastric hernia.

In our plan of treatment of epigastric hernias, it is first essential to correlate the pathologic findings with the clinical picture. In order to understand the problem, I have divided epigastric hernias into the following categories:

1. Asymptomatic epigastric hernia, not previously recognized by the patient.
2. Painless, reducible protrusion, recognized by the patient.
3. Painful, incarcerated mass, giving rise to a sharp, burning or pulling type of epigastric pain that is well localized.
4. Protrusion appearing on physical activity or straining, giving rise to epigastric burning pain or distress with eructation, nausea, or even vomiting.
5. Protrusion with incarceration, resulting in localized pain, abdominal cramping pain, nausea, and vomiting.

This classification does much to clarify the confusion recorded in the literature regarding epigastric hernias. The symptoms elicited in a given patient will depend upon the type of hernia and its state of progression.

The first category of patients requires little elaboration. In this category, epigastric hernias are first recognized by the physician while performing a physical examination; the patients had been totally unaware of the presence of the hernia prior to the examination. In these individuals, a small amount of adipose tissue protrudes through the defect in the linea alba (Fig. 23–2,A). The small mass of the hernias makes them difficult to detect. Upon examination of a number of United States military recruits in 1919, Hall discovered this type of epigastric hernia "by the dozens." Discovery in individuals

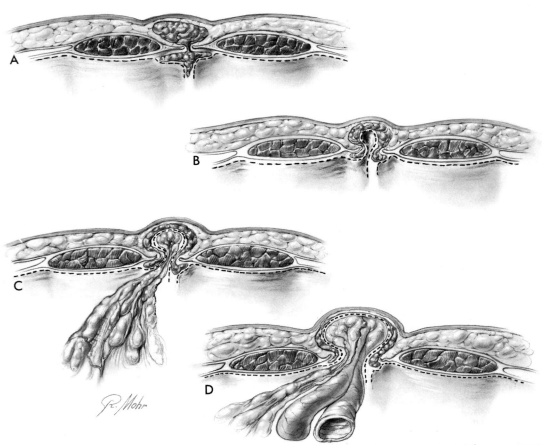

**Figure 23–2.** *A*, The small epigastric hernia consists of preperitoneal fat. *B*, A somewhat larger epigastric hernia has a peritoneal sac as well as protruding preperitoneal fat. *C*, As the hernia enlarges, the round ligament and omentum become a part of the herniated mass. *D*, In the largest epigastric hernias a sac is present and the defect occasionally permits prolapse of omentum, colon, small bowel or, rarely, the stomach.

seeking employment results in rejection of the applicant; hence, repair becomes necessary.

In the second category, the patient is aware of a painless protrusion, which is reducible, seen following activity, or which disappears when the patient lies down. In these patients, the defect in the linea alba is large enough to permit reduction of the adipose tissue (Fig. 23–2,*B*). Because the defect does not constrict the prolapsing tissue, pain is absent. A small peritoneal sac may be present in some of these patients.

In the third category of patients, we find that besides the appearance of a mass following activity, a sharp or burning type of pain is well localized to the site of the small mass. The pathology explains the symptoms; the preperitoneal fat, herniating through the small defect, is constricted during exertion at the level of the linea alba. A peritoneal sac is seen more often in this group than in the two preceding categories of patients. The fat beyond the constriction expands, giving the appearance of a small mushroom. Edema causes further swelling and discomfort. Most epigastric hernias fall into the first three categories.

The fourth category of patients gives rise to some confusion on the part of the clinician. The hernia appears following physical exertion or after coughing and sneezing. Reduction may be difficult, and some hernias remain incarcerated until an operation is performed. Symptoms include epigastric burning pain, dragging sensation, eructations with nausea, and even vomiting. The patient may feel quite ill. The anatomic defect in these cases is larger, and a peritoneal sac is present. The pathology helps to explain the visceral nature of the pain, as well as its location deep in the epigastrium and extending from the xiphoid process to the umbilicus. Traction on the falciform ligament and omentum explains the visceral type of pain (Fig. 23–2,*C*). If the prolapse of the hernia is intermittent, symptoms follow a similar pattern.

The fifth category of patients, comprising a small number in any series, includes those with larger epigastric hernias. Even these ordinarily measure only 5 to 8 cm in diameter. Incarceration of omentum, or

rarely, intestine, accounts for the nausea and vomiting. Cramping abdominal pain with vomiting suggests that intestine has prolapsed into the peritoneal sac (Fig. 23–2,*D*). The stomach is rarely found in epigastric hernias.

Thus, it is clear that the patient with an epigastric hernia may at least show the presence of a small asymptomatic epigastric mass, but in the overt case, the patient may present with protrusion, distress, epigastric pain, nausea, and vomiting. Each case must be evaluated individually and thoroughly, with an attempt at correlating the clinical history with the physical findings. Functional nervous disorders do occur in patients with epigastric hernias; however, only those symptoms produced by the hernia will be relieved following surgical repair.

It must be repeated that it is largely the adult population that develops epigastric hernias. These patients may also suffer from biliary tract, gastrointestinal, and pancreatic diseases. Hiatal hernia must not be overlooked. Fortunately, the surgeon today has a variety of diagnostic aids, such as x-rays, contrast studies, pancreatic duct cannulation, and selective arteriography, to assist in recognizing organic diseases.

## CLINICAL CHARACTERISTICS OF EPIGASTRIC HERNIAS

In order to appraise the current status of the epigastric hernia problem, I have reviewed the records of 235 patients with epigastric hernias operated upon at Henry Ford Hospital from 1950 to 1973. Every available clinical record was studied. Information gathered from these cases will provide a basis for comment and discussion. I found that the indexing of patients' records with epigastric hernias was less than ideal. For instance, several records of patients with epigastric hernias were indexed under ventral hernias, without further qualification. In other cases, the examining physician occasionally recorded the diagnostic impression of periumbilical hernia. Although an epigastric hernia is a type of ventral hernia, more precise identification is possible and highly desirable. All hernias of the anterior abdominal wall can be considered "ventral," whereas, and epigastric hernia is limited by definition to the midline between the xiphoid process and the umbilicus. Another error in indexing of records concerns incisional hernias indexed as ventral epigastric hernias. The more acceptable designation would be postoperative incisional or incisional epigastric hernias. The problems presented by postoperative midline incisional hernias are far more complicated than those caused by epigastric hernias; thus, the differential diagnosis is of fundamental importance.

## Sex and Age Distribution

Epigastric hernias occur more commonly in men than in women. The great preponderance in men reported many years ago has not been confirmed. I found that 62 of 235 epigastric hernias reviewed, or 28 percent, occurred in women. The incidence of 72 percent in men is not as high as the figures reported by others.

In this study of 235 patients seen from 1950 to 1973, epigastric hernias occurred infrequently in infants and children. Only 12 out of 235 patients were 19 years of age or younger. The youngest patient was an infant, 2 months of age, and the other young patients were 3, 3½, 6½, 7, 10, and 15 years old. There was a rapid increase in the frequency of epigastric hernias during the most vigorous years of life and a rather

precipitous drop in the advancing years, as shown in Figure 23-3. It can be seen that hernias of the linea alba are not as significant a problem in patients in the geriatric age group. An epigastric hernia proved troublesome to a 21-year-old male. Repair was successfully and safely performed under local anesthesia.

## Clinical History of Patient

The majority of patients with epigastric hernias complained of protrusion and pain, although I found protrusion to be the more common of the two. The pain was generally well localized to the epigastrium, and particularly, to the site of protrusion. In the 235 cases I studied, 141 patients experienced pain in conjunction with swelling or herniation; however, 82 of them described greater awareness of the hernia than of the pain. The pain was severe in only 19 of the 235 patients, while in the rest of the patients, it was of mild or moderate severity.

In trying to describe the pain associated with epigastric hernias, a variety of descriptive terms were used. The terms "tenderness," "soreness," "distress," and "discomfort" were most often applied to describe the subjective sensation experienced by the patients. Other terms used by patients included, "burning pain," "bloating," "gnawing," and a "pulling" or

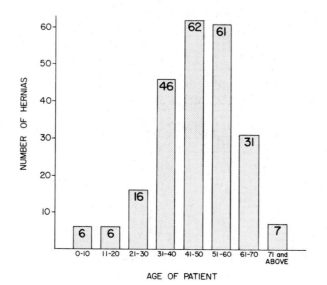

Figure 23-3. Epigastric hernias are uncommonly seen in infants and children. Such defects appear with the full vigor of life and are often precipitated by heavy physical work.

"dragging" sensation. It was not possible to correlate the size of hernia with the symptoms. At times, small epigastric hernias can cause severe and well-localized pain owing to pinching or constriction at the site of the defect in the linea alba; patients with this type of hernia seek help early. On the other hand, some of the largest epigastric hernias had been present for as long as 30 years with minimal symptoms. In fact, the only patient with both stomach and colon in his epigastric hernial sac had had the large hernia for over 30 years. These large hernias tend to be reducible for many years; when incarceration develops, help is finally sought.

The pain and protrusion were often brought on by heavy work, strenuous activity, or coughing. In two patients, the painful swelling was brought on by sneezing. Contrary to the observations of some authors, I found that the pain was often relieved upon the patient's lying down. At least 70 of the 235 patients attributed the onset or aggravation of their pain to some type of exertion.

Nausea was experienced by 20 patients, vomiting by 13, and cramping abdominal pain by 9. In this analysis, I did not include the symptoms of those patients who were clearly found to have hiatal hernia, peptic ulcer, biliary tract disease, or other organic visceral disorders. The symptoms due to these gastrointestinal diseases could hardly be attributed to uncomplicated epigastric hernias. I have observed that patients with numerous, severe visceral symptoms and negative x-ray studies seldom have significant pathology when explored through a vertical supraumbilical incision.

Patients did not seek relief promptly upon discovery of the epigastric mass. In fact, eight individuals were totally unaware of a defect; it had been discovered during a pre-employment physical examination, and repair was necessary to insure employability. Ninety-six of the 235 patients knew of the epigastric swelling for longer than a year. Twenty patients were aware of the hernia for less than one month. The fact that only 20 out of 235 patients sought medical help within one week suggests that the pain due to epigastric hernia is not severe in most patients.

The mysterious manifestations attrib-uted to epigastric herniations had originated in ancient medical history. They continued to be accepted for nearly four decades of the present century, when many of the presently available diagnostic modalities were either unavailable or infrequently used. With a careful history and physical examination and the judicious use of biliary tract and gastrointestinal contrast studies, the correct diagnostic significance of epigastric hernia can be made in nearly every patient.

## Physical Examination

Most patients with hernias of the linea alba are aware of a tender protrusion in the epigastrium. In fact, 141 of the 235 patients did have a tender epigastric mass of variable size. Epigastric hernias, completely asymptomatic, were discovered in eight patients during physical examination. A relatively asymptomatic protruding mass was present in 86 patients.

The examination for epigastric hernia must be complete. Inspection and palpation must be carried out with the patient lying down and completely relaxed. Careful examination for a visible swelling is performed with the patient's abdomen exposed to reflected light so that a small elevation might be detected. The patient is then asked to elevate his head and shoulders without the assistance of his upper extremities. The abdominal wall becomes tense, and any mass or protrusion anterior to the linea alba becomes more easily palpable. The patient's abdomen is gently palpated. The degree of tenderness is variable, but in most patients, the pain is not severe. When constriction occurs at the hernia site in the midline, extreme tenderness may occasionally be elicited upon palpation, but this is uncommon. A few epigastric hernias appeared suddenly after very heavy activity, e.g., lifting; in these patients, tenderness is precisely located at the site of herniation.

Definite identification of stomach, colon, or intestine in epigastric hernias is rare indeed on physical examination, since they are not commonly found in these hernias. The stomach was found in an epigastric hernia in only 1 of the 235 cases that I reviewed.

Table 23–1.  **LOCATION OF EPIGASTRIC
HERNIAS IN 235 PATIENTS**

| Location | No. of Patients |
|---|---|
| Upper linea alba | 32 |
| Middle linea alba | 65 |
| Lower linea alba | 137 |
| Not described | 1 |
| Total | 235 |

The examination of the abdomen should be thorough; diastasis recti, umbilical hernias, and multiple defects in the linea alba should be noted.

As can be easily seen in Table 23–1, more than half of the epigastric hernias are located in the lower linea alba near the umbilicus. They decrease in frequency as the xiphoid process is reached, but some of the largest epigastric hernias I have seen were located in the upper one-third of the linea alba. When large hernias occur near the umbilicus, they may contain colon, omentum, or small intestine and, in the exceptional patient, even stomach. In none of the patients did a midline hernia occur primarily in the midline below the umbilicus.

Diastasis recti is a common finding in patients with epigastric hernias. The degree of widening of the linea alba may be striking. In 47 of the 235 patients, the increased width and protrusion of the linea alba was noted and recorded. I suspect that diastasis recti may even be more common in patients with epigastric hernias than is indicated here.

Epigastric hernias are generally small in size, measuring less than 1 cm. In 148 of the total 235 epigastric hernias, the defect in the linea alba measured 1 cm or less in diameter, while in 50 it was estimated to be between 2 and 3 cm. It is more of a cleft or a transverse slit than a circular defect. Only 37 hernias of the linea alba were described as being large. The hernia may appear larger than the defect in the linea alba because of the "mushrooming effect" of the protruded fat. Epigastric hernias are described as larger in size by the clinician who examines the patient than they are by the surgeon who sees the actual aponeurotic defect.

Contrary to the reports in the literature, I found that multiple epigastric hernias occur infrequently. Only 17 patients had multiple midline defects, and most of these were located in the lower third of the linea alba.

Obesity was present in 48 of 235 patients. This incidence was somewhat less than I had expected.

Postoperative incisional hernias often recur, and numerous repairs in the same individual are common; however, it is unusual to find a recurrent epigastric hernia. I have found only 7 recurrent epigastric hernias out of the 235 patients. This is consistent with the observation that repair of epigastric hernias has proved highly successful in our experience and in that of many other surgeons.

## Differential Diagnosis

In spite of the fact that most patients with epigastric hernias present little difficulty in diagnosis, a small number of patients will require thorough investigation of their gastrointestinal tracts. Patients with severe epigastric pain, nausea, vomiting, and cramping abdominal pain require these studies, unless obvious incarceration is present. Those with epigastric gnawing or burning pain, bloating, and loss of appetite must also be thoroughly studied. Even if a reducible epigastric hernia is easily demonstrated in such individuals, other diseases of the gastrointestinal tract may be present as well.

**BILIARY TRACT DISEASE** may be present in the patient presenting with an epigastric hernia. Gaseousness, bloating, fatty food intolerance, and epigastric and right upper quadrant pain, radiating to the right subscapular area, all indicate a need for cholecystography.

**DUODENAL ULCERS, GASTRIC ULCERS, AND CARCINOMA OF THE STOMACH** may similarly afflict the patient with hernias of the linea alba. The symptoms resemble those of patients with midline supraumbilical hernias. Patients with ulcer disease have a rhythm and periodicity displayed in their pain patterns. The burning pain and nausea may be relieved with intake of food, milk, or antacids. Anemia and weight loss suggest the possibility of carcinoma; therefore, contrast studies of the stomach and duodenum are most important. Careful x-ray investigation will identify lesions of the stomach or duodenum. There was no increased incidence of peptic ulcer disease in our patients with epigastric hernia.

HIATAL HERNIA causes a characteristic burning pain deep in the epigastric area. The pain may also be localized to the substernal or precordial areas. At times, the pain may become more severe upon lying down. Heartburn may become a prominent complaint.

TUMORS OF THE ABDOMINAL WALL may occasionally give rise to problems in diagnosis. Lipoma may be suspected in patients having fatty tumors elsewhere (Fig. 23–4). A lipoma may be trabeculated and somewhat movable over the abdominal wall but cannot be reduced posterior to the linea alba. Unlike lipomas, many epigastric hernias are reducible. Lipomas alone do not cause the patient discomfort; however, even small epigastric hernias with a constricted defect may cause sharply localized, exquisite tenderness.

FUNCTIONAL GASTROINTESTINAL DISORDERS occur in a comparatively small percentage of patients with epigastric hernias; yet they are important and must be considered in a differential diagnosis. Unless the pathologic condition is placed in the proper perspective by considering the significance of the visceral symptoms along with the hernia, operative repair of the hernia may be considered a failure. Hence, in any patient with visceral symptoms, such as deep epigastric gnawing or burning pain, gaseousness, nausea, and vomiting, roentgen studies with contrast media are indispensable.

Eructation and aerophagia are common complaints in patients with hiatal hernia. In patients suspected of having hiatal hernia, special contrast studies are indicated. The roentgenologist should be informed that a lesion of the lower esophagus or proximal stomach is suspected. Special examinations will then reveal abnormalities that might otherwise have escaped detection. It is true, however, that such symptoms may be due to an epigastric hernia in which the falciform ligament, the omentum, the colon, or the intestine becomes incarcerated. Traction on the falciform ligament or omentum may cause such symptoms. Nevertheless, repair of the epigastric hernia should not be advised in any patient suspected of having functional complaints until the biliary tract and the gastrointestinal tract have been thoroughly investigated and found normal. Repair of an epigastric hernia will eliminate the protrusion and the associated discomfort, but any functional symptoms will remain.

MISCELLANEOUS CONDITIONS to be considered in the differential diagnosis of epigastric hernia include those disorders giving rise to deep epigastric visceral pain (e.g., pancreatitis, gastritis, colitis, appendicitis, and, in the rare patient, angina pectoris).

UMBILICAL HERNIAS are considered as separate defects from epigastric hernias. The protrusion can be seen through the umbilical ring and should present no particular diagnostic difficulty. It is noteworthy that 34 of 228 patients with epigastric hernias also had umbilical hernias. Therefore, it is important to identify any combinations of hernias, since they can be repaired simultaneously.

INGUINAL HERNIAS occur commonly in patients with epigastric hernias. Sixty-three patients presented with groin hernias during either this admission or some previous hospitalization.

DIASTASIS RECTI is, more or less, an anatomic variant that borders on a pathologic state and causes some confusion

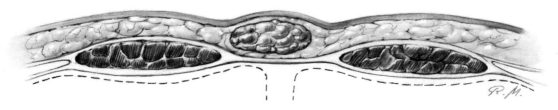

**Figure 23–4.** Lipomas occasionally can be confused with epigastric herniation. There is no defect in the aponeurosis and the mass is non-tender.

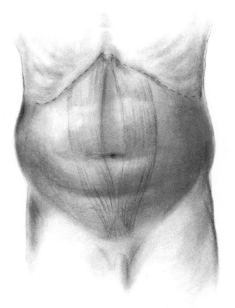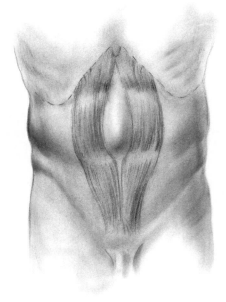

**Figure 23–5.**   Diastasis recti is a widening or attenuation of some part, or the entire, linea alba. The interval between the recti may measure from four to six centimeters. Repair should be undertaken with caution, since such divarication is not symptomatic.

among physicians as to its significance and management (Fig. 23–5). The condition has been designated by Iason as a divarication of the recti. The significant abnormality of diastasis recti is the widening of the linea alba, so that a bulge of some proportion occurs when intra-abdominal pressure rises.

The condition may be seen in children as an ovoid or elongated midepigastric swelling, which appears upon exertion. It decreases in magnitude as the child grows and as his abdominal muscles increase in size and strength.

In adults, diastasis recti may be seen in obese, hypersthenic males, in elderly men with chronic lung disease, and in women who have had repeated pregnancies. The most common type of diastasis that I have seen occurs above the umbilicus in men. In women, following repeated pregnancies, the condition is seen below the umbilicus. It may be possible to palpate the sacral promontory through the defect in some women. The separation of the rectus muscles and the widening of the linea alba may extend from the xiphoid process to the symphysis pubis, but this is rare.

I have never seen an incarceration or a strangulation as a result of diastasis recti. Repair or correction of the condition is not as simple as it might appear. Care must be taken to achieve significant weight reduction and maximum improvement in pulmonary function before attempting repair.

Forty-seven of the 235 patients with epigastric hernias had some degree of diastasis recti. This suggests that the same type of stress on the abdominal wall produces both epigastric hernias and diastasis recti in some patients.

Finally, even if diastasis recti is present as an obvious defect, other explanations should be sought in the symptomatic patient. In the following case history, diastasis recti was considered erroneously to be the cause of intestinal obstruction. The patient, aged 62, was a moderately obese female who had been ill with abdominal pain and vomiting for eight days prior to admission. The striking finding on physical examination was distention of the abdomen and extreme diastasis recti. The distended bowel loops and visible peristalsis could be seen through the attenuated linea alba between the widely separated rectus abdominis muscles. The surgeon described his findings as follows:

An incision is made which runs directly across the summit of the ventral hernia just below the umbilicus, and which extends from one anterior-superior iliac spine to the other. The subcutaneous tissues are dissected off the hernial sac for about 12 cms. both above and below. Next, the sac is opened and it is found to be filled with dilated but perfectly viable small bowel loops. It is judged that the entire jejunum and a portion of the ileum must be so involved. Now, a careful search is made to determine the cause of obstruction and it is found that the hernial sac proper has no adhesions, and that the neck of the sac is very wide, and, in fact, one can hardly speak of a neck. What one deals with here is an extremely marked diastasis recti, which, of course, consists in the extreme widening of the linea alba with a thinning and stretching of the recti muscles until the medial borders of each rectus muscle may be as much as 25 centimeters apart from the other. In such a hernia, intestinal obstruction is extremely rare if at all possible. Since this patient had no previous operation to cause adhesions intra-abdominally, it is evident at this point of the operation that the true cause of the intestinal obstruction was missed clinically. This impression is confirmed when it is found that in the right lower quadrant a loop of ileum is caught in the internal ring of the inguinal canal. The loop does not extend into the inguinal canal proper, but occupies only the upper end of this canal for a depth of about two centimeters and a width of about four centimeters.

Although the compromised portion of bowel was resected, this patient died three days after the operation. This case vividly illustrates how easily the underlying diagnosis can be missed. The patient actually had a Richter's type of indirect inguinal hernia, which caused the intestinal obstruction; the distended bowel appeared in the area of diastasis. In my judgment, the delay in treatment of this case led to the patient's death.

Diastasis recti must be an extremely rare cause of obstruction. I cannot recall seeing a single case of intestinal obstruction attributable to diastasis recti in nearly 30 years of practice. Whenever diastasis recti is present in a symptomatic patient, the surgeon must look for other explanations.

## Anesthesia

Spinal anesthesia was the method preferred for most patients with epigastric hernias. It was used in 120 patients, while general anesthesia was administered to 70 individuals. It was surprising that 45 patients had their hernias repaired under local anesthesia. These patients usually had other systemic diseases or were aged.

## AN APPROACH TO REPAIR OF EPIGASTRIC HERNIAS

Successful repair of ventral hernias of the epigastric type demands consideration of the following questions: Is the hernia simply a single, small defect through an otherwise relatively normal linea alba? If so, a simple closure, made vertically or transversely, would be effective after excision of the small protruding mass of fat. Are there multiple defects present along with diastasis recti? A vertical closure, with side-to-side overlapping of the linea alba, might be desirable. Before any attempt is made at correction of diastasis recti, weight reduction and treatment of pulmonary disease is desirable until a point of maximum improvement is reached. Is an umbilical hernia present along with the epigastric hernia? The

**Table 23–2. EPIGASTRIC HERNIA REPAIR TECHNIQUES IN 235 PATIENTS**

| Procedure | No. of Patients |
|---|---|
| TYPE OF INCISION | |
| Transverse | 117 |
| Vertical | 118 |
| | Total 235 |
| TYPE OF REPAIR | |
| Transverse closure | |
| With overlap of linea alba | 63 |
| Without overlap of linea alba | 54 |
| Vertical closure | |
| Closure of posterior and anterior sheath of rectus as separate layers | 24 |
| Vertical single layer closure of linea alba | 45 |
| Side-to-side overlap | 35 |
| With mesh | 14 |
| | Total 235 |

surgeon has a variety of techniques to utilize for this situation. It is of utmost importance to recognize any combination of defects. If the epigastric hernia is small, the defect may be closed transversely, and the umbilical hernia can be repaired by the Mayo technique.

The surgeon called upon to repair epigastric hernias should be familiar with various techniques used in the repair of midline hernias. In the treatment of 235 patients with epigastric hernias at the Henry Ford Hospital, a number of methods were used (Table 23–2). Transverse closure is favored for repair of epigastric hernias alone, but the vertical closure is used when abdominal exploration is indicated for other disease states. In general, the simple methods of repair give surprisingly good results in epigastric hernias occurring through small defects.

### Technique of Repair—Transverse Incision and Transverse Closure

In selected patients with complaints of protrusion in the epigastrium and well-localized tenderness, the simplest procedure is recommended. In these individuals, the single epigastric mass is easily demonstrable. Although other studies might be considered useful, they prove to be nonproductive of pathology. The repair may be performed under local anesthesia if so desired. A transverse but slightly curved incision is made over the mass. The incision is developed to the linea alba and to the sheath of the rectus abdominis muscle on each side. A small to moderate-sized lobulated mass of adipose tissue is easily separated from normal subcutaneous fat. The defect in the linea alba is generally quite small—usually less than 1 cm in diameter and often only a few millimeters in width. The fat then mushrooms out into a considerably larger, flattened mass of adipose tissue.

Dissection at the aponeurotic level can easily be carried down to the umbilicus and upward to the midepigastric area if multiple defects are to be detected. The herniated preperitoneal fat may be amputated; the pedicle, which regularly contains a small arteriole, should also be clamped. Care is always taken in recog-

nizing a peritoneal sac, and any contents are carefully resected. If the defect in the linea alba is small, it can be closed transversely with less than five sutures of nonabsorbable material; often, only two or three sutures are required. When larger defects are present, transverse closure with an overlapping technique is an effective method of repair. At present, I use number 2–0 silk for this purpose. Care should always be taken to approximate the edges of the aponeurosis without interposition of fat. If a thick layer of subcutaneous fat is present, sutures of absorbable material are placed to obliterate the dead space. The skin is closed with fine nonabsorbable suture material or with small strips of adhesive tape.

Larger simple epigastric hernias are similarly dissected; however, the differences are not unimportant (Fig. 23–6). If the defect is larger; more preperitoneal adipose tissue protrudes through the defect, dragging with it a portion of peritoneal lining. Omentum may find its way into the peritoneal sac. In the repair of these hernias, all vessels in the adipose tissue and in the omentum must be ligated. The omentum is then replaced within the peritoneal cavity. I enlarge the opening in the linea alba to the rectus abdominis muscle on each side, thus increasing the size of the flap available for suture. The peritoneal sac, if present, is dissected free and ligated with a number 3–0 silk suture ligature. With number 2–0 silk or synthetic nonabsorbable sutures, the upper leaflet of linea alba is sutured over the lower leaflet; this permits a slight overlapping of the two surfaces. A word of caution is necessary: excessive overlapping adds nothing to the repair and may even weaken it.

### Technique of Repair: Vertical Incision and Vertical Closure

There are a number of instances in which the vertical incision is desirable, even necessary. When the surgeon wishes to correct a diastasis recti or when multiple epigastric hernias are present, the vertical incision is preferable. Whenever the surgeon wishes to explore the abdomen in addition to repairing a hernia of the linea alba, the midline incision is convenient. I

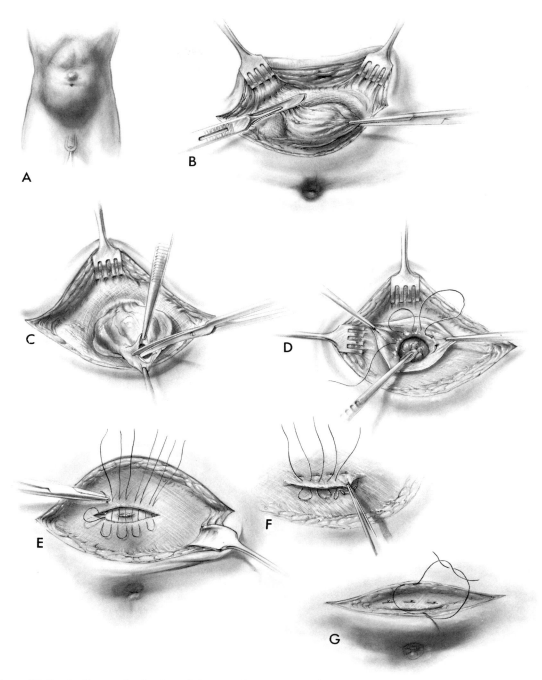

**Figure 23–6.** In the repair of epigastric hernias the transverse skin incision gives excellent cosmetic results. A, Epigastric hernial protrusion; B, dissection at aponeurotic level; C, opening of sac; D, placement of purse-string; E, placement of aponeurotic sutures; F, tacking the superior leaflet down; and G, placement of subcuticular sutures.

would add another word of caution; the vertical incision is subject to the same risk of dehiscence and herniation as it is when used for other abdominal operations.

The skin incision is made from the xiphoid process to the umbilicus (Fig. 23–7). The globular protrusion of fat is easily identified as it protrudes through the linea alba. The technique of incising the aponeurosis depends upon the findings and the proposed repair. If there is no widening of the linea alba, a midline incision is made so that a vertical single-layed closure may be achieved. If it is elected to perform a side-to-side overlapping procedure, then the incision in the linea alba is best made within one-half of a centimeter of either the right or left rectus abdominis muscle. This provides a larger flap with which to achieve the overlapping procedure. The aponeurosis is dissected clean of excess fat but not denuded of blood vessels and areolar tissue. The side-to-side overlapping technique was first recommended by Lucas-Championnière for the repair of umbilical hernias in 1895. The method is used in repair of ventral hernias and diastasis recti as

well. Synthetic nonabsorbable sutures are preferred, but number 2–0 silk sutures may be used. The free margin is always attached to the opposite rectus sheath. Although I have not used retention sutures in the past, I believe they will prove worthwhile, particularly in a vertical, single-layered closure.

Variants of the vertical closure are numerous. In some patients, the posterior rectus sheath is clearly identified and incised vertically at the margin of the rectus abdominis muscle. The posterior rectus sheath is closed as the first layer; then, the anterior sheath is approximated independently. This technique places additional tension on the suture line approximating the anterior sheath. Relaxing incisions may be made vertically in the sheath of the rectus to avoid undue tension.

The method offered by Berman is occasionally useful when a vertical midline incision is desirable. This technique may also be used for repair of incisonal hernias (Fig. 23–8).

I am of the opinion that in selected patients with large or numerous defects, with diastasis recti, and especially in those

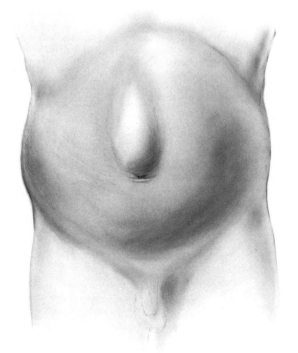 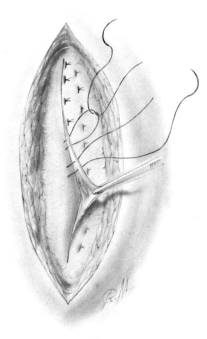

**Figure 23–7.**    An obese patient with diastasis recti is a candidate for side-to-side closure. This approach is indicated when abdominal exploration is required as well. Obese patients are expected to lose weight and those with pulmonary disease are treated first.

patients with obesity and chronic lung disease, mesh may be implanted to good advantage. Mesh can be sutured to the posterior rectus sheath after having been placed in an intraperitoneal position anterior to the omentum. I prefer placing the mesh beneath the rectus abdominis muscle after dissection and vertical closure of the posterior sheath of the rectus abdominis. The anterior sheath is then closed vertically in the midline. Relaxing incisions in the anterior sheath of the rectus may be useful in selected cases.

### Suture Material

Nonabsorbable sutures were generally preferred for repair of hernias of the linea alba. Silk was used in 156 patients, wire in

## Improved Vertical Repair Of Midline Hernias

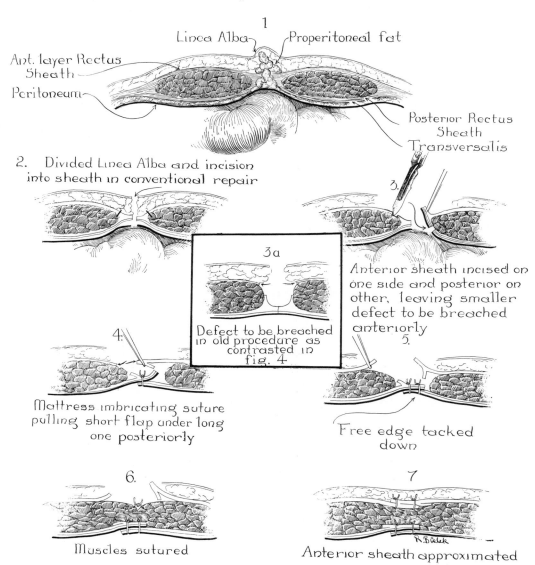

1. Linea Alba — Properitoneal fat — Ant. layer Rectus Sheath — Peritoneum — Posterior Rectus Sheath — Transversalis

2. Divided Linea Alba and incision into sheath in conventional repair

3. Anterior sheath incised on one side and posterior on other, leaving smaller defect to be breached anteriorly

3a. Defect to be breached in old procedure as contrasted in fig. 4

4. Mattress imbricating suture pulling short flap under long one posteriorly

5. Free edge tacked down

6. Muscles sutured

7. Anterior sheath approximated

**Figure 23–8.** In the occasional patient, Berman's method of closure is useful. This is true of patients with multiple defects in the linea alba. Vertical relaxing incisions in the anterior sheath of the rectus may be added. (Reproduced with permission of author and publisher. From Berman, E. F.: Epigastric hernia: An improved method of repair. Am. J. Surg. 68:84, 1945.)

46, and a variety of sutures in the remaining 33 patients. Nonabsorbable sutures are recommended for repair of epigastric hernias. Silk is extremely dependable, but synthetic nonabsorbable sutures can also be used. Wire is an excellent suture material but causes discomfort in some patients.

## Operative Findings

In this study of 235 patients with epigastric hernias, it is apparent that repair is performed to relieve the patient of discomfort and to eliminate the protrusion. In each patient, there was protrusion of preperitoneal fat. The consistent finding in these hernias is a protruded or extruded mass of preperitoneal fat, which varies greatly in size. In 143 patients, the defect was small, as was the protruding mass of adipose tissue. In these patients, the defect in the linea alba measured from a few millimeters up to 1 cm. Although preperitoneal fatty tissue was associated with all hernias of the linea alba, it was considered to be incarcerated in 94 patients. Thus, preperitoneal fat is the most common finding in these hernias.

Table 23–3 summarizes the important findings in 235 patients with epigastric hernias. There was no occurrence of incarceration followed by strangulation, while diastasis recti was a common finding among these patients. Umbilical hernias often occur with other epigastric hernias in the same patient, and their presence should always be suspected.

I was surprised to find that a peritoneal

**Table 23–3. OPERATIVE FINDINGS IN 235 PATIENTS WITH EPIGASTRIC HERNIAS**

| Findings | No. of Patients |
|---|---|
| Preperitoneal fat | 235 |
| Incarcerated preperitoneal fat | 94 |
| Demonstrable peritoneal sac | 76 |
| Incarcerated omentum | 38 |
| Incarcerated colon | 3 |
| Incarcerated small bowel | 2 |
| Incarcerated stomach | 1 |
| Diastasis recti | 47 |
| Umbilical hernia | 34 |
| Multiple epigastric hernias | 17 |

sac was identified in 76 patients; however, in most patients, this sac is small and not at all similar to that seen in inguinal hernias.

Omentum was present in 38 patients, but strangulation of incarcerated omentum was present in only 1 patient. Usually, only a small tag of omentum finds its way into the sac, which protrudes through a small defect.

The hollow viscera uncommonly find their way into an epigastric hernia. The stomach was present in a hernia in the linea alba in only one patient. This study lays to rest the erroneous idea that the stomach regularly finds its way into epigastric hernias. Furthermore, the transverse colon was found in three patients with epigastric hernias, while small intestine was found in two more patients.

In one case history of epigastric hernia containing stomach and colon, the patient was a male, 70 years of age, who had an abdominal hernia for 31 years. At times, it became uncomfortable and difficult to reduce the hernia. He wished it to be repaired because of its size and the discomfort it caused.

A vertical elliptical incision was made so as to permit excision of redundant skin. The incision was developed to the linea alba, and the large sac and defect in the linea alba were identified. The peritoneal sac contained omentum, transverse colon, and a portion of stomach. The viscera were reducible. Vertical incisions were made in each rectus sheath, permitting approximation of the posterior sheath in the midline. The anterior sheath of the rectus abdominis muscle was then sutured to the sheath on the opposite side, using number 2–0 silk sutures. Four retention sutures of heavy nylon were placed through the skin, subcutaneous fat, and anterior sheath of the rectus. These were tied over segments of rubber catheter to protect the skin.

The patient also had a small umbilical hernia, which was repaired with a vertical two-layered closure.

His postoperative course was uneventful except for a urinary tract infection, which responded to antibiotic therapy. His repair was sound in a follow-up of two years. This case is of particular interest, since it is the only one in which stomach and colon were found in a large epigastric hernia of 31 years duration. Repair was successfully accomplished in a two-layered vertical closure.

## Recurrence

A long-term follow-up examination of these patients was impossible, but all records available were personally reviewed.

Four known recurrences have been identified. Three of the four patients had vertical incisions and repairs. One patient had undergone transverse closure with overlapping of the linea alba. This individual had an epigastric and umbilical hernia. His postoperative course was complicated by a hematoma, and he eventually developed a recurrence.

One patient who had a vertical closure in a single layer developed a recurrence, while two others had side-to-side overlapping of the linea alba. One of these patients was quite obese; the other had chronic lung disease with bronchitis.

Firm conclusions cannot be reached from a small research study like this, but some observations are warranted. There was only 1 recurrence among 117 patients having transverse closure; during the same time and under similar circumstances, 3 patients with vertical closures had developed recurrent epigastric hernias. It should be pointed out that the vertical incision was made when diastasis recti was present and more extensive explorations were necessarily performed.

The overall recurrence rate following 235 repairs was 1.7 percent. Among the total number repaired, seven were recurrent epigastric hernias, indicating that other surgeons also have low recurrence rates following repair of epigastric hernias.

## Complications

There were no deaths among 235 patients operated upon for epigastric hernias.

Complications occurred more frequently when combinations of procedures were carried out and multiple hernias were present.

Postoperative seromas occurred in 11 patients, hematomas in eight, wound infection, in 2, and ileus in 3. Urinary retention occurred in seven older patients; all were repaired under spinal anesthesia. Only one patient had a post-spinal anesthesia headache. Phlebothrombosis was present in four patients and pulmonary complications were reported in eight cases. Patients who undergo repair of epigastric hernias generally recover promptly and seldom suffer from serious complications.

## SUMMARY

Epigastric hernias are not common, comprising one or two percent of hernias requiring repair. They have caused much debate and difference of opinion regarding pathology and clinical manifestations. The reasons for this earlier confusion are now understandable. The manifestations of epigastric hernia depend upon the pathology in the individual patient. Small protrusions without constriction may be asymptomatic. If there is constriction at the site of herniation, pain may be severe and well localized. Visceral symptoms are caused by traction upon and involvement of the falciform ligament and omentum in the herniation. Obstructive symptoms appear when hollow viscera become caught in the hernia. Since it is uncommon for intestine, colon, or stomach to become incarcerated in epigastric hernias, strangulation is extremely rare. It did not occur once in the 235 cases I personally studied.

The defect in the linea alba in most patients with epigastric hernia ranges in size from a few millimeters up to 1 cm. The larger epigastric hernial defects measure only 5 to 8 cm.

In patients with numerous and bizarre visceral symptoms, thorough investigation of the biliary tract and gastrointestinal tracts is essential.

The best results are obtained in patients whose epigastric hernias cause localized protrusion with pain. Patients with functional nervous disorders may obtain relief of the local discomfort, but visceral symptoms could continue.

Technique of repair should be individualized according to the particular problem at hand. Transverse closure, with or without overlapping, is fundamentally sound and gives excellent results. Vertical closure is advisable when multiple defects are present, when exploration is indicated, or when diastasis recti is to be corrected.

There were no deaths in 235 epigastric hernia repairs. Since the defect is generally small and requires minimal operative trauma, excellent survival rates can be expected.

The recurrence rate can be expected to be quite low. In this study, I found it to be less than 2 percent.

## REFERENCES

Berman, E. F.: Epigastric hernia: An improved method of repair. Am. J. Surg. 68:84, 1945.

Charlton, M. R.: Epigastric hernia causing severe symptoms. Am. J. Surg. 36:703, 1937.

Friedenwald, J., and Morrison, T. H.: Epigastric hernia: A consideration of its importance in the diagnosis of gastrointestinal disease. J.A.M.A. 87:1466, 1926.

Hall, J. N.: Epigastric hernia in the soldier. J.A.M.A. 73:171, 1919.

Iason, H. I.: *Hernia*. Philadelphia, The Blakiston Co., 1941, pp. 872–880.

Lewisohn, R.: The importance of a thorough exploration of the intra-abdominal organs in operations for epigastric hernia. Surg. Gynecol. Obstet. 32:546, 1921.

Lucas-Championnière, J.: Hernia ombilicale. Jour. Med. Chir. 66:609, 1895.

Luke, J. C.: The significance of epigastric hernia. Can. Med. Ass. J. 39:149, 1938.

McCaughan, J. J., Jr.: Epigastric hernia. Arch. Surg., 73:972, 1956.

Meyer, J., and Ivy, A. C.: Studies on gastric and duodenal ulcer: The relation of epigastric hernia to gastric ulcer—A clinical and experimental study. J. Lab. Clin. Med. 8:37, 1922.

Moschcowitz, A. V.: The pathogenesis and treatment of herniae of the linea alba. Surg. Gynecol. Obstet., 18:504, 1914.

Moschcowitz, A. V.: Epigastric herniae without palpable swelling. Ann. Surg. 66:300, 1917.

Pemberton, J. de J., and Curry, F. S.: The symptomatology of epigastric hernia. Analysis of 296 cases. Minn. Med. 19:109, 1936.

Pentney, B. H.: Small ventral hernias in children. Practitioner, 184:779, 1960.

Watson, L. F.: *Hernia* (2nd ed.). St. Louis, C. V. Mosby Co., 1938, pp. 361–369.

## Supplemental Readings

Glenn, F., and McBride, A. F.: The surgical treatment of five hundred herniae. Ann. Surg. 104:1024, 1936.

Mahorner, H.: Umbilical and midline ventral herniae. Ann. Surg. 111:979, 1940.

Pollock, L. H.: Epigastric hernia. Am. J. Surg. 34:376, 1936.

Sullivan, D. F., and Antupit, L.: Epigastric hernia in its relation to intra-abdominal disease. Ann. Surg., 86:413, 1927.

# 24

# Unusual Hernias

In this chapter, we will consider a variety of unusual hernias and defects of the ventral abdominal wall, flanks, and groin areas. Some of these derive their uniqueness through either their rare occurrence or unusual presentation; others contain visceral appendages, such as the appendix or Meckel's diverticulum. I felt that by discussing such hernias in one chapter, there would be better appreciation by the surgeon that certain hernias are unique because they are comparatively rare. Even surgeons of some experience see such hernias infrequently in a surgical lifetime. For instance, Governale and colleagues in 1941, after searching foreign and domestic literature, were able to gather only 117 instances of strangulated Richter's femoral hernias.

Most of the hernias in this chapter carry eponymic designations. I have used these terms freely for the sake of brevity and specificity, and in order to honor those persons who, in remote times and under difficult circumstances, contributed to our knowledge. To point out how cumbersome the problem of identification could become, we might cite some of the designations used to refer to the Spigelian hernia: hernia-in-the linea semicircularis; masked hernia, spontaneous lateral ventral hernia, and laparocéles spontanées. The term "Spigelian hernia," which simply refers to a particular type of hernia, has evolved through usage into a name that we all recognize.

On the other hand, identification of some hernias is best done via location, and I have designated lumbar hernias as being either *superior* or *inferior*.

Our experience at Henry Ford Hospi-

tal included a respectable number of Richter's, lumbar, and Spigelian hernias. I have personally seen only one Littre's hernia and two prevascular hernias Multilocular hernias are seen with regularity and have been reported in detail in Chapter 17.

The unusual hernias to be discussed in this chapter are listed in Table 24–1. The anatomic peculiarities of each type of hernia will be illustrated and evaluated. The pathologic implications and principles of surgical management of these unusual hernias will also be considered in appropriate detail.

Burton (1950) has identified possible hernial sites of the posterior and inferior portion of the body wall in his publication in 1951 (Fig. 24–1). The lateral vascular hernia—sometimes called inguinopelvic hernia—is extremely rare, the reason being that the musculoaponeurotic wall in this area is strong and unyielding. Prevascular hernias, arising de novo, are likewise unusual. However, I have seen two prevascular hernias that arose anterior to the femoral vessels following vascular surgical procedures. In both cases, vascular grafting

### Table 24–1. UNUSUAL HERNIAS OF THE ABDOMINAL WALL

Richter's hernia
Lumbar hernia
Spigelian hernia
Supravesical hernia
Interparietal hernia
Reduction of hernia en-masse
Littre's hernia
Gastroschisis
Herniorrhaphy and appendectomy
Hernia and colorectal carcinoma

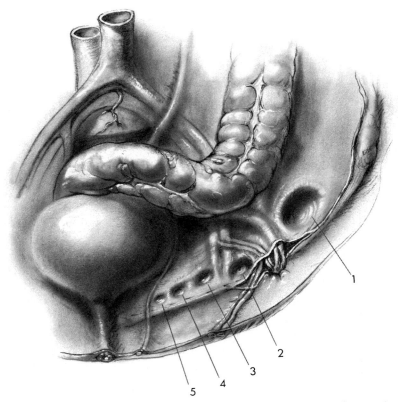

**Figure 24–1.** Illustration to show unusual hernias of the lower abdomen and pelvis as viewed from within. Some of them are rare and represent surgical curiosities: (1) lateral vascular or inguinopelvic hernia, (2) prevascular, (3) femoral, (4) pectineal, and (5) translacunar. (Modified from original by permission of J. B. Lippincott Company. From Burton, C. C.: Interligamentous inguinal hernia; classification and statistical study of 117 hernias. Ann. Surg. *134*:124, 1951.)

procedures were carried out, and the femoral sheath (transversalis fascia) was compromised The prevascular hernia, in each case, protruded between the femoral vessels and inguinal ligament. Both hernias were successfully repaired with Marlex mesh that was attached to the anterior superior iliac spine, the inguinal ligament, Cooper's ligament, and the pubic tubercle. The mesh was attached above to the aponeurosis of the internal oblique. (Femoral hernias are discussed in detail in Chapters 15 and 16.)

Other hernias identified in Figure 24–1 include the *pectineal* and the *translacunar.* Such hernias are so rare that they should be considered surgical curiosities. They are presented here for the sake of completeness; however, more important, they serve to emphasize the need for careful intraoperative digital exploration of every patient with a hernia.

## RICHTER'S HERNIA

The hernia currently recognized as Richter's hernia refers to a particular type that may occur, oddly enough, in different anatomic locations. The common denominator in Richter's hernia is the presence of a small, firm, unyielding ring, which permits incarceration and strangulation (Fig. 24–2).

Richter's hernias are deceptive because of their small size and because early in the genesis of such hernias occlusion of the lumen is partial The pathology and pathologic physiology are not universally known; hence, the treatment is less than satisfactory at times

## INCIDENCE

Richter's hernia is considered essentially an affliction of adults and older individuals, for several reasons. Infants seldom develop femoral hernias, and most Richter's hernias are located at the femoral ring. Unlike the adult situation, the infant and child have not been subjected to numerous laparotomies; hence, such hernias are rarely seen in very young patients. I have never seen Richter's hernias in an infant or child; however, they have been reported. One other reasonable explanation for the rarity of Richter's hernias in infants and children is the elasticity of their tissues, which makes entrapment of bowel unlikely.

It can be stated with confidence that Richter's hernias in infants are, indeed, rare but can occur. Rhodes (1929) reported such a case in a three-week-old infant. The observation that Richter's hernias occur most often in adults is supported by the statistics of Lyall and Loumanen (1948), who found the average age to be 61 years, and of Gillespie and colleagues, who reported the average age to be 70 years.

Richter's hernias account for a significant number of strangulated hernias. Watson (1922) found that 5 percent of strangulated hernias were of this type. Gillespie and colleagues found, in reviewing 154 incarcerated and strangulated hernias, that 13 percent were Richter's

hernias. In these cases, the bowel was viable in 8 of 20 cases; gangrene of intestine was present in 12 or 7.8 percent of 154 patients with incarcerated and strangulated hernias.

Of all femoral hernias, only a comparatively few become incarcerated and strangulated as described by Richter. Foltz (1947) found only 2 such hernias among 254 patients, for an incidence of 0.7 percent.

Richter's hernias are seen so infrequently that a precise sex incidence is not currently available. Some authors, notably Treves (1887) and Fowler (1899), found a greater incidence in females, but Gillespie and colleagues found the incidence among 20 patients to be 60 percent male, and 40 percent female.

## ANATOMIC SITES OF RICHTER'S HERNIAS

Richter's hernia, in the original concept, referred to those defects occurring at the femoral ring; however, the term is now used to refer to partial enteroceles wherever they may occur In decreasing order of frequency, I have seen Richter's hernias at the femoral ring (Fig. 15–9, p. 254), inguinal ring, umbilicus, and at incisional hernia sites In adults, I have seen two Richter's hernias at the inguinal ring (Fig.

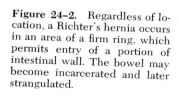
**Figure 24–2.** Regardless of location, a Richter's hernia occurs in an area of a firm ring, which permits entry of a portion of intestinal wall. The bowel may become incarcerated and later strangulated.

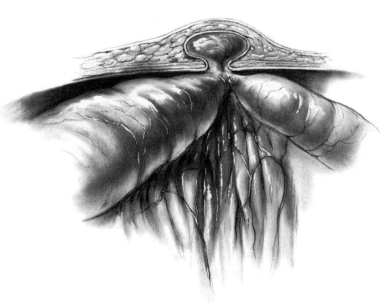

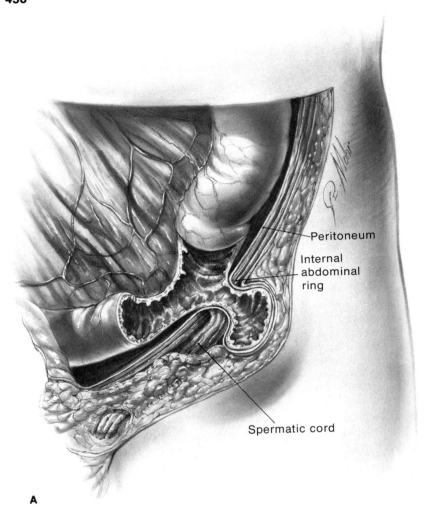

Peritoneum

Internal
abdominal
ring

Spermatic cord

**A**

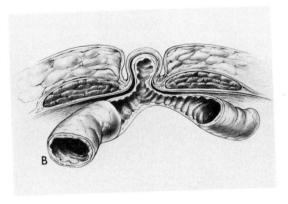

**B**

**Figure 24–3.** *A,* The internal ring may be the site of a Richter's type hernia in the presence of a small, constricted orifice at this site. *B,* The umbilicus is a possible site for a Richter's hernia because a tight firm ring permits entry of a portion of the bowel wall.

24–3, *A*) and two at the umbilicus (Fig. 24–3, *B*) but only one at an incisional hernia site. All of the others were seen at the femoral ring. These personal observations are consistent with those reported in the literature (Table 24–2).

An example of Richter's hernia reported by Bourke (1977) is of interest; the hernia occurred through a minuscule incision, which had been used to insert a laparoscope.

Naylor in 1978 encountered an extraordinary case in which a patient had a Spigelian and Richter's hernia as a single

## Table 24–2. LOCATION AND INCIDENCE OF RICHTER'S HERNIA[*]

| Site | Author | Incidence |
|---|---|---|
| Femoral | Frankau (1931) | 82% |
| | Treves (1887) | 72% |
| | Gillespie et al. (1956) | 55% |
| | Governale et al. (1941) | 90% |
| | Foltz (1947) | 90% |
| | Cattell (1933) | 90% |
| Inguinal | Frankau (1931) | 16% |
| | Treves (1887) | 25% |
| | Lyall and Loumanen (1948) | 12% |
| Umbilical | Frankau (1931) | 2% |
| Incisional Hernias | Rhodes (1929), Keynes (1956), Keeley (1937), Millard (1959), Bourke (1977), Cook and Yarington (1962) | Less than 1% (estimated) |

[*]Unusual and rare sites for Richter's hernias have been described by the following: Millard (1959), at the inferior lumbar triangle; Keynes (1956), interstitial hernia; Botsford (1977), at sacral foramen; Cook and Yarington (1962), at obturator canal; Millard (1959), in epigastrium and in a supravesical hernia; Cullen (1954), foramen of Winslow; Wilson (1934), supravesical space; Keyes (1956), supravesical space.

entity. Naylor performed a wedge cecectomy and herniorrhaphy.

From this brief survey it can be seen that Richter's hernias may occur at sites that possess certain anatomic characteristics. The defect into the abdominal wall must be quite small; furthermore, it must be surrounded by a firm or rigid ring. The size of the ring is quite small; and, significantly, the depth need not be great. Because of these features, clinical recognition of the hernia is difficult.

## DEFINITION

A Richter's hernia is one in which a portion of the antimesenteric circumference of the bowel (usually the terminal ileum) is incarcerated or strangulated—becoming caught in the unyielding structures that make up the hernial ring. The site of the constriction may be the femoral ring (Fig. 15–9, p. 254), the internal abdominal inguinal ring, or the umbilicus.

Such a small, tight ring may present in a ventral hernia and in other abdominal wall defects as well. It should be stressed that not all Richter's hernias occur in the femoral region.

### Synonyms

I agree with Treves (1887) that the particular type of hernia we are discussing is best designated by the term "Richter's hernia." Richter clearly recognized the clinical and pathologic features, and, hence, clarified much of the confusion that existed prior to his publication of 1785.

A number of synonyms are applied to this type of hernia. "Partial enterocele" is another appropriate designation for this entity. Other terms include "nipped hernia," "pinched hernia," and "masked hernia." These varied terms are helpful in understanding the nature of Richter's hernia. The French literature includes such terms as "pincement lateral," "hernie partialle," and "pincement herniaire de l'intestine." "Darmwand brüche," "lateral brüche," and "partial brüche" are the terms used in the German literature when referring to Richter's hernia. The terms in English, French, and German all convey the same ideas as to the nature of the partial enterocele.

A hernia of a Meckel's diverticulum has become known as Littre's hernia. Littre in 1700 described two instances in which Meckel's diverticula were present in hernial sacs. It is well known that the diverticulum of Meckel is a remnant of the vitelline duct, which is incompletely obliterated.

## HISTORICAL BACKGROUND

There is little to be gained from a detailed review concerning the remote past history of the partial enterocele, especially since the accuracy of some of the observations remains questionable. In the earliest descriptions, confusion as to the precise nature of a Richter's hernia was due to the fact that Meckel's diverticulum had yet to be described accurately. The similarity between a Meckel's diverticulum and the small partial enterocele on gross appearance led to erroneous conclusions as to which lesion was actually being discussed. Treves in 1887 published his report, which did much to clarify our understanding of Richter's hernia. Much of the historical data that follow is taken from his publication.

In 1598 Hildanus attended a woman with a groin hernia; the patient subsequently developed a fistula, which closed spontaneously in two months Hildanus never saw the bowel; and there was, of course, no operative procedure performed Inadequate observation and incomplete information have recorded Hildanus' name indelibly in the history of Richter's hernia. According to Treves, Littre (in 1714) described a patient with a hernia containing a portion of the wall of the colon. Strangulation was present, but the lumen of the bowel was patent. Le Dran in 1731 and George Arnaud in 1749 apparently referred to Richter's type of hernias. Louis in 1757 described a partial enterocele as well. De Haen is also given credit for recognizing such a hernia in 1761.

Morgagni discussed the problem of partial enterocele at some length in "The Seats and Causes of Disease," published in 1760 Morgagni refers particularly to Littre's work, which beautifully described the clinical and pathologic features of a partial enterocele. Littre also described two instances in which Meckel's diverticula were present in hernial sacs as well, hence adding to the confusion insofar as understanding and terminology were concerned

Richter's observations on hernia were published in 1778. Treves stated that Richter gave a "full, faithful and elaborate description of the hernia in which a part only of the circumference of the bowel is strangulated " Thus, Richter recognized a particular type of hernia before Meckel had described the congenital nature of his diverticulum

An accurate understanding and description of Meckel's diverticulum was essential if a partial enterocele was to be distinguished etiologically and pathologically from a hernia containing a Meckel's diverticulum (Littre's hernia). In 1809 Johann F. Meckel presented his explanation, stating that a certain type diverticulum located in the terminal ileum was congenital in origin.

## PATHOGENESIS

Two theories have been offered to explain the development of a partial enterocele. I have chosen to call them the "adhesive band" and the "incarceration and partial withdrawal" theories.

The Adhesive Band theory derives its name from the presence of peritoneal adhesive bands or adhesions between the hernial sac and the intestine. Under such conditions, complete reduction of the sac is impossible. Under appropriate circumstances, with an increase in either intra-abdominal pressure or intestinal luminal pressure or both, the portion of bowel over the tight hernial ring is forced into it, with incarceration and strangulation following. Gillespie and colleagues (1956) called this "White's Theory." According to Treves (1887), Riecke in 1841 and Schmidt in 1878 offered similar explanations for the onset of partial enterocele. Treves could find but few instances in which the gut was clearly attached to the sac. I have found that the intestine is comparatively easily freed from the hernial sac. White (1914) reported that he found adhesions between the gut and sac in nearly 50 percent of his Richter's hernias.

The incarceration and partial withdrawal theory was attributed to Orr by Gillespie and colleagues (1956). Orr (1950) explained that with an increase in intra-abdominal pressure, a loop of small intestine entered the hernial sac. Edema followed with resultant incarceration. Mechanical obstruction resulted in increased peristaltic activity with partial reduction of the contained intestine. The antimesenteric portion of the bowel remained caught in the tight ring, but the continuity of the intestinal lumen was restored to a greater or lesser degree. Roser in 1886 advanced a similar explanation, which was supported by Treves.

Scarpa's important observations in 1809 in regard to the flow through the intestine under various conditions were known to Treves. Scarpa performed his experiments on corpses. Occlusion of two-thirds of the lumen interfered with the passage of water, whereas occlusion of one-third usually resulted in partial obstruction. However, occasionally even this was enough to cause complete obstruction. These basic observations have application in the pathology of partial enterocele, but their accuracy should be further studied in relationship to Richter's hernia.

One additional important facet of the pathology has apparently been overlooked. How severe must the obstruction be to interfere significantly with the passage of gas? If the obstruction permits passage of gas through the constricted area, the classic radiologic features of intestinal obstruction would be absent.

Although much is known in regard to Richter's hernia, further study is required. After the pathophysiology is fully under stood, long delays in treatment will be infrequent.

More detailed reference to the works of John Baptist Morgagni is in order since few publications refer to his observations which were recorded in his work, "The Seats and Causes of Diseases," published in 1760 I have referred particularly to the translation by Alexander. Morgagni understood the problem of incarcerated and strangulated hernia very well. It might be said that he had ample opportunity to study the complications of hernia, since death from complications of hernia was common in his time. He was familiar with the works of Littre, Lavaterus, Ruysch. and Fabricius. Morgagni referred to the explanation of the pathology of such hernias as described by Littre:

. . . Symptoms of herniae of this kind proceed more slowly, are less violent than other herniae, where the whole tube of the intestine is strangulated, and they are particularly distinguished by this circumference, that a discharge of feces is never impeded.

Morgagni also stated that "the abdomen is neither tumid, nor tense, nor filled with flatus, as in common herniae." He cautioned that no maxim in medicine is so well settled but that at some time it may not mislead us.

## CLINICAL AND PATHOLOGIC CORRELATION

The pathology of Richter's hernia or partial enterocele is more complicated than it might appear. It is an oversimplification

to state that such hernias are those in which a portion of the lumen is incarcerated in a tight femoral ring. The pathology must be understood in more detail. The physical signs and roentgen findings will vary depending on how long incarceration and strangulation have been present. I will attempt first to point out where such hernias occur and then to describe the chain of events that account for the various clinical pictures that may be seen with partial enterocele.

The anatomic peculiarities involved and the pathologic events are so important that they will be presented in sequence.

1. Richter's hernias, or partial enteroceles, occur in areas where a small, tight constricting ring can be found (Fig. 24-2). The femoral ring is most commonly the site of a Richter's hernia, but it must be recognized that such small tight rings occur in other areas (Table 24-2). It is not generally appreciated that a partial enterocele may occur at the internal abdominal inguinal ring or at the umbilicus. Ventral hernias may provide such a small tight ring composed of dense connective tissue.

2. The femoral ring is surrounded by the following rigid structures: medially, the attachment of the abdominal wall to Cooper's ligament and the lacunar ligament; anteriorly, the iliopubic tract and inguinal ligament; posteriorly, Cooper's ligament and the pubis; and laterally, the distensible femoral vein and its fascial septum form its boundary. In other areas, a dense, firm cicatrix may form the unyielding ring.

3. The hernial sac is small not only in diameter but also in length of the sac, thus accounting for the ease with which it is overlooked

4. Attempts have been made to explain the pathophysiology of Richter s hernia since the time of Morgagni Scarpa, Treves and Gillespie and colleagues have also contributed to our under standing of the clinical and pathologic event. The tight femoral ring predisposes first to incarceration; then, congestion and edema follow with further compromise of blood supply and gangrene supervenes With early simple incarceration of a small portion of ileum, symptoms may be minimal and the small

femoral mass may be difficult to demonstrate. With increased congestion and edema, venous emptying is interfered with and a greater encroachment occurs on the patency of the lumen. There is pain and swelling in the groin, and obstructive symptoms develop. As long as the lumen is incompletely occluded, distention may not be marked Further interference with circulation leads to gangrene of the intestine. The patient is seriously ill, with demonstrable swelling in the groin and ileus. At this stage, vomiting is seen, and it may be feculent in nature.

5. Localized infection in the femoral region occurs after gangrene of the bowel has been permitted to occur. Pain and swelling in the groin increases and at times, leads the unsuspecting clinician to a diagnosis of lymphadenitis.

6. Although Morgagni in 1760 and Scarpa in 1809 recognized the clinical and pathologic picture of partial enterocele, there is still evidence that their contributions are not universally known. Usually the distal ileum is the portion of intestine caught in the tight femoral hernial ring or the neck of an inguinal hernial sac. The antimesenteric portion of the bowel wall is caught in the small ring. Early in the incarceration and strangulation of the intestine, only a portion of the lumen is occluded Thus, symptoms and clinical findings will depend on the duration and degree of obstruction. With partial occlusion, gas and fluid will pass along the intestinal lumen more or less efficiently. Abdominal distention will be absent or minimal, and flat films will fail to reveal air-fluid levels seen in complete obstruction. We must be reminded that some gas may pass through the lumen even with a high degree of obstruction. Thus, x-ray films of the abdomen may reveal an atypical or nonspecific gas pattern. Once inflammation and gangrene supervene, the obstruction becomes complete. Nausea, vomiting, distention, and absent bowel movements are late manifestations. The abdomen is distended; tenderness is present at the site of the hernia and may be generalized over the abdomen. Three-dimensional x-ray studies of the abdomen will now reveal air-fluid levels and distended loops of intestine.

7 In rare cases, an external fistula may develop with survival of the patient. In reviewing the literature, this was the only hope for survival before development of surgical treatment. Such an event was most likely to follow when strangulation occurred at the inguinal ring with subsequent drainage in the groin or scrotum

8. After gangrene develops peritonitis and paralytic ileus will follow. Dehydration results from the vomiting and is aggravated by the absence of oral intake. In neglected patients who have been ill for a week or more, septicemia and acidosis are common.

Thus, the clinical picture seen in Richter's hernia depends on the stage of progression of the process Early in the course of development, the surgeon may find a localized rather tender mass. The picture that is seen late in the course of incarceration, strangulation, and gangrene is very similar to that seen in intestinal obstruction due to other causes Careful exploration of the various hernial orifices is necessary if a partial enterocele is to be detected.

## CASE REPORTS

It is of practical interest to present examples of Richter's hernias occurring in areas other than the femoral ring.

### Richter's Hernia Involving the Cecal Wall: Case Report

The patient, who was a 72-year-old male, had the repair of a hernia performed elsewhere 20 years prior to entering Henry Ford Hospital for gastrointestinal bleeding. Since the cause was found to be peptic ulceration, treatment was by gastric resection.

While recovering in the hospital, the patient developed an incarceration of a small recurrent right indirect inguinal hernia. At operation, a portion of the cecum was found caught in a right internal ring. The bowel was viable and returned to the peritoneal cavity. The hernia was successfully repaired and remained so throughout a seven-year follow-up.

## Intestinal Obstruction Due to Richter's Hernia: Case Report

Besides appearance of a painful mass at the site of herniation, symptoms of intestinal obstruction should also alert the surgeon to the possible presence of a Richter s hernia. In the following case report, the surgeon was concerned about mechanical obstruction and entered the abdomen through a midline infraumbilical incision. At the time of operation, an indirect inguinal hernia accounted for the clinical symptoms

The patient was a 78 year-old male who appeared in the emergency room with an illness of over 24 hours. He complained of cramping abdominal pain, nausea, and vomiting. He had never undergone abdominal surgery. The abdomen was distended with hyperactive bowel sounds The temperature and leukocyte readings were slightly elevated. Abdominal films revealed dilated loops of small bowel compatible with mechanical small bowel obstruction. A small left indirect inguinal hernia was demonstrated

After proper preparation, the patient was operated on, with intestinal obstruction as the indication. His abdomen was opened infraumbilically in the midline. Exploration revealed dilated loops of viable small intestine. There was a round area (1.5 centimeters) of dark hemorrhage discoloration and edema in an antimesenteric portion of ileum. About the margin was a small identation, beyond which was normal bowel This was typical of the appearance of the bowel caught in a Richter s type of hernia. The only defect found was a small, tight fibrous ring at the site of the left internal abdominal ring. After a period of observation, it was found that the bowel was viable, and resection was unnecessary. The peritoneal sac was reduced excised. and the transversalis fascia repaired at the internal ring by the Henry-Cheatle-Nyhus approach The peritoneum and the abdominal incision were then closed

The patient had a period of ileus postoperatively but gradually improved and was discharged on the seventeenth postoperative day.

### Comment

Diverticulitis and appendicitis, as well as carcinoma of the colon, had been considered in the differential diagnosis of this 78-year-old patient.

The patient, when seen, had been at rest; and the hernia had reduced spontaneously. The acuity of the illness demanded prompt treatment; and the midline infraumbilical incision was chosen, since there was some doubt as to the precise diagnosis Exploration clearly revealed the cause of illness. Richter's hernias are most often seen in the femoral ring. They may occur at the um bilicus or in incisional hernias where the aperture in the fascia is small. I have only seen two Richter's hernias, both indirect, occurring in the inguinal region.

## Reduction En Masse

One danger that must be clearly understood in regard to Richter's hernia is reduction "en masse." In such a situation, the hernial mass may be completely replaced into the abdominal cavity without release of the strangulating hernial ring. Pearse (1931) presented this type of problem as a possible outcome of attempts at reduction of certain incarcerated hernias. The consequence is that the portion of the bowel incarcerated in the tight ring becomes gangrenous with eventual death from obstruction and infection in the absence of treatment. Treves (1887), remarkably enough, reported such a case in which operative treatment was life saving. Such cases must be extremely rare. Querna (1969) reported two cases of reduction en masse of femoral hernias; in one of these, a Richter's type of hernia was present.

## OPERATIVE TREATMENT

Before surgical treatment is attempted, the patient's condition and needs must be evaluated Nasogastric decompression is indicated in patients with prolonged incarceration and strangulation. Fluid replacement is needed to restore water and mineral levels to normal

A variety of procedures must be available to the surgeon. The technique for repair of a Richter's hernia that develops at the site of an incisional hernia is different from that for repair of a femoral hernia.

I favor the inguinal approach for repair of Richter's hernias that protrude through

either the inguinal or femoral ring. Pualwan (1958) preferred a preperitoneal approach, which is also effective The floor of
the inguinal canal can be opened sufficiently to permit proper inspection of the
bowel and, if necessary, resection. I place a
fine suture into the serosa of the bowel
prior to release of the bowel into the peritoneal cavity. The ends of the suture are
kept long, allowing retrieval of the bowel
for inspection after the peritoneal sac has
been freed. After the tension on the bowel
has been released, the color of the incarcerated bowel progresses toward normal. A decision as to the need for resection
can then be made. If the bowel is considered to be viable, the identifying suture is
cut at the knot, the bowel is replaced into
the peritoneal cavity, and the hernia appropriately repaired. If the bowel is gangrenous or if its viability appears questionable after a period of observation, then
resection and end-to-end anastomosis are
recommended. I have found that several
minutes must be allowed for return of
circulation to the injured area. The practice
of permitting the marked bowel to return to
the peritoneal cavity for a certain amount of
time has been found helpful.

The preperitoneal approach may be utilized in repair of a Richter's hernia developing in indirect or femoral hernias.

The repair of Richter's hernias developing at the umbilicus or at the epigastrium or
in incisional hernias has been described in
detail in the chapters dealing with those
specific problems.

## MORTALITY

The reported survival statistics for patients treated for Richter's hernias are
generally poor. Patients with Richter's
hernias are likely to be elderly and, too
frequently, neglected before receiving
medical care. Because the hernia is small, it
can easily be overlooked, so that treatment
is delayed; incarceration thus proceeds to
strangulation. Greater awareness of the
nature of Richter's hernia by members of
the nursing and medical professions will
eventually lead to better results.

To support the opinion that patients with
Richter's hernias are often neglected, we
can look at the statistics of Gillespie and
colleagues (1956). Among 20 patients, 6
died; but 2 of these patients were identified

as having Richter's hernias at postmortem
examination. In two other patients, gangrene of the bowel progressed to fecal
fistulae. Two patients died following resection of gangrenous bowel The mortality
figures reported in the literature range
between 20 and 56 percent following
surgical treatment of Richter's hernia.

## SUMMARY

Richter's hernia is deceptive because of
its small size and serious consequences.
Gangrene of the bowel can occur without
appearance of significant distention or
demonstration of air-fluid levels on x-ray
studies of the abdomen. Delay in diagnosis
has serious consequences, especially in
elderly patients.

Richter's hernias occur most often at the
femoral ring; but inguinal, umbilical, and
incisional hernias may also be sites of such
hernias.

Prompt surgical treatment is the only
approach to reduce the mortality.

## REFERENCES

Alexander, B.: Translation of Morgagni's *Book on the
Seats and Causes of Diseases,* Vol II. New York,
Hafner Publishing Co., 1960, pp. 136–147.
Botsford, T. W.: Richter's hernia in a sacral foramen:
New site for Richter's hernia. Arch. Surg. *112*:304,
1977
Bourke, J. B.: Small intestinal obstruction from a
Richter's hernia at the site of insertion of a
laparoscope. Br Med. J. 2:1393, 1977.
Burton, C. C.: Hernias of the supravesical inguinal
and lateral pelvic fossae. Int. Abstr Surg. *91*(1):1–
16, 1950
Burton, C. C.: Interligamentous inguinal hernia:
Classification and statistical study of 117 hernias.
Ann. Surg. *134*(1):119, 1951.
Cattell, R. B.: Richter's hernia. Surg. Gynecol. Obstet.
*56*:700, 1933
Cook, M. D., and Yarington, C. T., Jr.: Strangulated
Richter's hernia of the obturator canal: Report of two
cases. Am Pract. *13*:115, 1962.
Governale, S. L., Markiewicz, S. S., and Rotondi, A. J.:
Strangulated Richter's femoral hernia with report of
a case. J. Int. Coll Surg. *4*:160, 1941.
Cullen, T. H.: Herniation of acutely inflamed
Meckel's diverticulum through foramen of Winslow.
Arch. Middlesex Hosp. London *4*:278, 1954.
Foltz, E. L.: Richter's hernia. U. Mich. Hosp. Bull.
Ann Arbor *13*:105, 1947.
Fowler, R. S.: Partial enterocele. Ann. Surg. *29*:533,
1899.
Frankau, C.: Strangulated hernia: A review of 1487
cases Br J. Surg. *19*:176, 1931.
Gillespie, R. W., Glas, W. W., Mertz, G. H., and
Musselman, M. M.: Richter's hernia. Arch Surg.
*73*:550, 1956.

Keeley, J. L.: Meckel's diverticulum in a sac of ventral incisional hernia. Report of a case. Wis. Med. J. *36*:733, 1937.

Keynes, W. M.: Richter's hernia. Surg. Gynecol. Obstet. *103*:496, 1956.

Littre, A.: Observation sur une nouvelle espece de hernie. Mem. Acad. R. Soc. Paris p. 300, 1700.

Lyall, D., and Loumanen, R.: Richter's hernia. Am. J. Surg. *75*:828, 1948.

Meckel, J. F.: Uber die Divertikel am Darmkanal. Arch. Physiol. Rev. Autenrieth *9*:421, 1809.

Millard, D. G.: Richter's hernia through the inferior lumbar triangle of Petit A radiographic demonstration. Br J. Radiol. *32*:693, 1959.

Morgagni, J. B.: The Seats and Causes of Disease, Vol. II (translated by Benjamin Alexander). New York, Hafner Publishing Co., 1960, pp. 136–147.

Naylor, J.: Combination of Spigelian and Richter's Hernias: A case report. Am. Surg. *44*:750–752, 1978.

Orr, T. G.: Richter's hernia. Surg. Gynecol Obstet. *91*:705, 1950.

Pearse, H. E.: Strangulated hernia reduced "en masse". Surg. Gynecol. Obstet. *53*:822–828, 1931.

Pualwan, F.: Operative aspects of Richter's hernia. Surg. Gynecol Obstet. *106*:358, 1958.

Querna, M. H.: Reduction of hernia "en masse". Am. J. Surg. *118*:539–540, 1969.

Rhodes, R. L.: Partial enterocele; Richter's Littre's herniae. Trans. R. Soc. S. Afr. *61*:175, 1929.

Richter, A. G.: Abhandlung von den Bruchen. Gottingen, J. C., Dieterich, 1785, pp. 597–624.

Roser, W.: Ueber Darmwandbrüche. Arch f Klin. Chir *34*:435, 1886–1887.

Scarpa, A.: Sull'Ernie Memorie (Part 4). Milan, Anatomico-Chirurgische, 1809, p. 50.

Treves, F.: Richter's hernia or partial enterocele. Med Chir Trans. London *52*:149–167, 1887.

Watson, L. F.: Partial enterocele. Surg. Clin. North Am *2*:761–765, 1922.

White, C. S.: Richter's hernia. Surg. Gynecol. Obstet. *14*:45, 1914.

Wilson, G. E.: Richter's hernia. J.A.M.A. *102*:1938, 1934.

## Supplemental Reading

Bissell, A. H.: Richter's hernia. Am. J. Surg. *7*:864, 1929.

Brantigan, C. O.: Chicken bone hernia: An unusual presentation of a Richter's hernia. Am Surg. *41*:584–586, 1975.

Gray, H. K.: Meckel's diverticulum in hernia: Report of a case. Minn. Med *17*:68, 1934.

# LUMBAR HERNIAS

It is important to recognize that lumbar hernias may differ in their physical characteristics as well as in their etiology. They can present as a variety of anatomic defects, having a site of protrusion in the lumbar area. Lumbar hernias vary greatly in size and content of hernial sacs, and they may be congenital or acquired in origin. They can occur spontaneously, or they may be traumatic in origin—the trauma resulting either from physical factors or as a consequence of operative treatment.

The lumbar area is a broad anatomic area bounded below by the iliac crest, above by the twelfth rib, anteriorly by the external oblique muscle, and posteriorly by the erector spinae muscles (Fig. 24–4). Any protrusion in this rather large area is considered to be a lumbar hernia.

Specific anatomic areas of weakness have been identified by Petit (1774), Grynfeltt (1866), and Lesshaft (1870). Lumbar hernias may protrude through the superior lumbar triangle or the inferior lumbar triangle, or a large diffuse weakness may be evident in the lumbar area.

## DEFINITION

Any acceptable definition of lumbar hernia should include the variety of protrusions appearing in a well-defined anatomic area. Accordingly, a lumbar hernia is one that protrudes through some part of an area bounded by the twelfth rib above, the iliac crest below, the erector spinae muscles posteriorly, and the external oblique anteriorly. Superior and inferior lumbar hernias, of course, occur in this area.

## HISTORICAL BACKGROUND

Mastin in 1890 noted that Barbette in 1672, Garangoet in 1731, Ravaton in 1750, and LaChausse in 1759 all described hernias through the triangle of Petit. However, according to Mastin, it was not until 1783 that Petit published his paper describing a specific anatomic triangle.

Goodman and Speese reviewed the historical aspects of lumbar hernia in detail in 1916. The recorded historical facts were challenged by Jeannel (1902 to 1903), who failed to understand why the region was designated as "Petit's triangle"; Jeannel felt that description of the area by Dolee, Garangoet, Ravaton, and Bulin equaled that of Petit.

Grynfeltt in 1866 described the space with boundaries of the twelfth rib, the quadratus lumborum, and the external

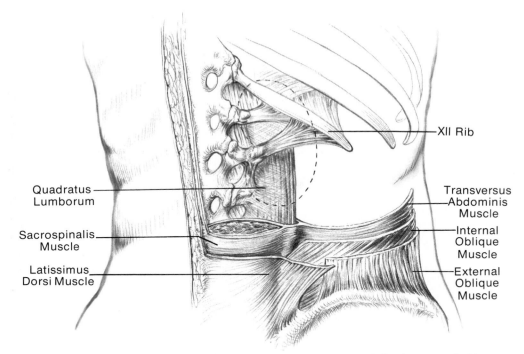

**Figure 24-4.** The lumbar area is limited above by the twelfth rib, anteriorly by the external oblique muscle, posteriorly by the erector spinae muscles, and below by the iliac crest.

oblique muscle. This space—although somewhat varied in its geometric form, depending upon anatomic arrangement—is generally known as the superior lumbar triangle of Grynfeltt-Lesshaft. Goodman and Speese stated that the form could be rhomboid, deltoid, trapezoid, or polyhedral. Lesshaft made his contribution in 1870, calling the space "the superior lumbar triangle." He was apparently unaware of the works of Grynfeltt at the time.

Larrey in 1869 referred to the superior lumbar triangle hernia as a costoiliac hernia.

Watson (1948) stated that de Huguier designated lumbar hernias as suprailiac hernias.

Once lumbar hernias were recognized as a specific entity, collective series began to appear in the literature. MacReady identified 25 cases of lumbar hernias and published his report in Lancet in 1890. His interesting paper referred to the cases of Garangoet (1731), Ravaton (1738), and Petit (1790). Mastin (1890) published a collected series in which he also referred to the cases of Garangoet and Ravaton. By 1923, Watson (1948) had accumulated 115 lumbar her-

nias, and in 1950 Thorek was able to locate 126 such cases.

Orcutt states that as of 1971, approximately 220 cases of lumbar hernia had been reported.

Dowd in 1907 and Rishmiller in 1917 presented effective methods of lumbar hernia repair. In 1963 Hafner, Wylie, and Brush utilized Marlex mesh in the repair of lumbar hernias. This is a noteworthy contribution, particularly in the repair of large incisional hernias in the lumbar area.

## ANATOMIC CONSIDERATIONS

In the broad sense, any protrusion in the lumbar region is a lumbar hernia (Fig. 24-4). Such hernias may be congenital, acquired, traumatic, or iatrogenic in origin. The boundaries include: twelfth rib, above; crest of the ileum, below; erector spinae muscles and vertebral column, posteriorly; and a vertical line from the tip of the twelfth rib to the iliac crest represents the anterior boundary.

Large congenital hernias and certain traumatic or postoperative lumbar hernias may occupy most of the area just outlined.

Other smaller lumbar hernias may protrude through the inferior lumbar triangle or the superior lumbar triangle.

## Inferior Lumbar Triangle

The anatomic boundaries of the triangle of Petit are rather easily identified and should be simply described  The inferior margin or base of the triangle is rigid and consists of the crest of the ilium (Fig. 24–5, A). The posterior margin of the external oblique forms the anterior boundary, while the posterior margin is the anterior edge of the latissimus dorsi muscle.

## Superior Lumbar Triangle

The superior lumbar triangle, which is covered by the latissimus dorsi muscle, was recognized initially by Grynfeltt in 1866; and, four years later, it was independently described by Lesshaft.

The superior lumbar triangle is bounded above by the twelfth rib (base of the triangle), and the posterior inferior spinae muscles form the posterior boundary. The posterior border of the internal oblique makes up the anterior-inferior boundary of this triangle. The latissimus dorsi covers this area, and the serratus posterior inferior must be retracted to gain access to this

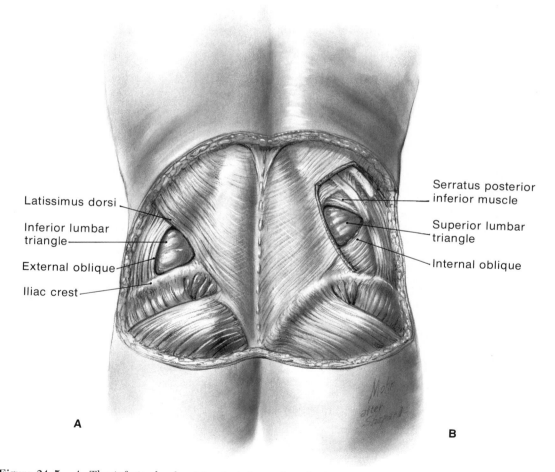

Latissimus dorsi

Inferior lumbar triangle

External oblique

Iliac crest

Serratus posterior inferior muscle

Superior lumbar triangle

Internal oblique

A

B

**Figure 24–5.** *A*, The inferior lumbar triangle is located in the lumbar area. It is bounded anteriorly by the posterior margin of the external oblique, posteriorly by the anterior margin of the latissimus dorsi, while the crest of the ilium forms the base. *B*, The superior lumbar triangle is bounded by the internal oblique muscle anterio-medially. The erector spinae muscles form the medial-most boundary, and the twelfth rib and serratus posterior inferior muscle form the base of the triangle.

small defect (Fig. 24–5, *B*). Thus, the sides of the "lumbo-costo-abdominal" triangles are made up of the internal oblique and the anterior border of the sacrospinalis, while the boundary above is the twelfth rib. The transversus abdominis muscle and its fascia form the floor of the superior lumbar triangle. The anatomic description just stated is an oversimplification; the space may indeed be quadrilateral, trapezoidal, or polyhedral in shape.

### Diffuse Lumbar Hernias

Diffuse lumbar hernias are among the largest protrusions that I have seen. They are usually iatrogenic or traumatic in origin, but, occasionally, large congenital lumbar hernias fit into this category.

Such hernias occupy the region from the costal margin to the iliac crest, and as far medially as the rectus abdominis muscle and sheath  The indexing of these hernias is poor  since most medical records departments categorize them as incisional hernias (which, of course, many of them are). These hernias often appear following operations on the kidney or after other procedures performed through a flank incision. Some of these large hernias are the consequence of operations on the iliac crest—the larger-sized lumbar hernias give the patient a grotesque appearance.

### Anatomic Relationships

It is useful to visualize the anatomic structures concerned in lumbar hernias in cross-sectional views  These relationships are well illustrated by Thorek (1950) in his book, *Modern Surgical Techniques* (Fig. 24–6, *A* to *D*). The relationship of the colon to these hernias is variable. Care must be taken in the dissection of every lumbar hernial sac because of possible injury to the viscera.

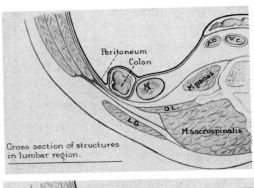

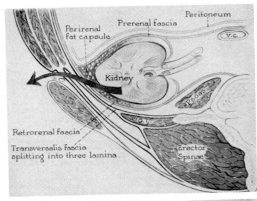

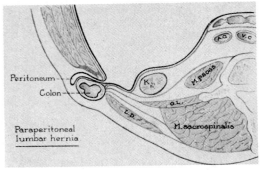

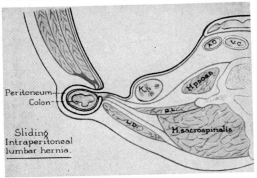

**Figure 24–6.** *A*, Normal visceral relationships viewed in cross section at the lumbar level. *B*, Pathway for herniation of kidney through the lumbar area. *C*, The colon may be a part of the herniated mass but in a location outside the sac. *D*, The colon in this illustration is part of a sliding hernia. (Reproduced by permission of author and publisher. From Thorek, Max: *Modern Surgical Technique.* Philadelphia, J. B. Lippincott Co., 1950).

**Table 24–3. CLASSIFICATION OF LUMBAR HERNIAS***

| Hernia | Site of Protrusion | Synonyms |
|---|---|---|
| Inferior Lumbar Hernia | Inferior Lumbar triangle of Petit | Inferior lumbar hernia<br>Hernia of Petit's triangle<br>Supra-iliac hernia of Huguier |
| Superior Lumbar Hernia | Superior lumbar Triangle of Grynfeltt-Lesshaft | Superior lumbar hernia<br>Grynfeltt's hernia<br>Lesshaft's hernia<br>Costo-iliac hernia of Larrey<br>Lumbo-costo-abdominal hernia |
| Diffuse Lumbar Hernia | Extensive in the lumbar area | Lumbar<br>Postoperative hernia<br>Traumatic lumbar hernia |

*Each type of hernia may be congenital or acquired.

In Figure 24–6, A, normal anatomic relationships are shown. The possible pathway for herniation of a kidney is shown in Figure 24–6, B. In Figure 24–6, C and D, the variable relationships of the colon to the hernial sac are clearly depicted.

## CLASSIFICATION OF LUMBAR HERNIAS

It is not possible to offer a simple classification of lumbar hernias that would include all anatomic variations and would reflect all the numerous and complex etiologic factors. From a practical point of view, however, an attempt at classification is desirable; and such an effort is presented in Table 24–3.

Some attempt at classification of lumbar hernias on an etiologic basis produces useful information that can lead to improved management of the problem (Table 24–4).

## Congenital Lumbar Hernias

Congenital lumbar hernias, which are thought to be due to arrested or abnormal development of the musculoskeletal system, have been described by Adamson (1958), Dowd (1907), Mastin (1890), Goodman and Speese (1916), Lee and Mattheis (1957), and Parkh and colleagues (1977) Muscles, aponeuroses, and bony structures show abnormalities.

It has been estimated that congenital lumbar hernias compose approximately 20 percent of all lumbar hernias.

### Acquired Lumbar Hernias

Acquired lumbar hernias consist of two varieties: spontaneous and traumatic.

**SPONTANEOUS LUMBAR HERNIAS** are seen in geriatric patients, patients with excessive weight loss, and occasionally in obese patients. Pulmonary diseases such as bronchitis and emphysema often occur in these elderly patients and may be contributing factors. I am not convinced that strenuous labor is an important factor.

Coley (1921), Goodman and Speese (1916), Menaker and Kulman (1971), and Musick and Schubert (1970) all reported examples of acquired lumbar hernias. Approximately 50 percent of lumbar hernias are of the spontaneous variety.

**TRAUMATIC LUMBAR HERNIAS** compose 26 percent of reported lumbar hernias with two varieties emerging in this classification. Physical trauma, such as occurs in accidents, is recognized as a cause of lumbar hernia. Everett (1974) reported a lumbar hernia case in which a five-year-old boy had been run over by the rear wheel of a lorry. Frazer (1968) reported such a hernia in a patient injured in an auto accident. Hancock's (1920) patient fell off a railroad car, while the patient reported by Hafner and colleagues (1963) fell from a height of

**Table 24–4. ETIOLOGIC FACTORS IN LUMBAR HERNIA**

I. Congenital Lumbar Hernias
   Arrest or defective development of abdominal musculature, ribs, vertebrae, and pelvis.

II. Acquired Lumbar Hernias
   A. Spontaneous
      Contributing factors include aging, weight loss; aggravated by chronic pulmonary disease.

   B. Traumatic—Nonoperative
      Contributing factors include: severe injury sustained in falls, gunshot, or crushing injuries.

   C. Traumatic—Postoperative
      Operative procedures on the kidney or adjacent structures resulting in large incisional hernias in the lumbar area.

      Operative procedures on the iliac crest, including bone-grafting technique and excision of tumors.

15 feet. Kretschmer (1951) reported a lumbar hernia in a patient who had the misfortune to be gored by a bull. Lewin and Bradley (1949) reported a lumbar hernia occurring in a soldier injured by a shell fragment. In all these cases, a common etiologic factor is present — namely, violent trauma. Thus, it can be seen that traumatic lumbar hernias are caused by severe direct injuries. Crushing injuries and injuries sustained in falls can lead to the development of lumbar hernias in some patients.

POSTOPERATIVE LUMBAR HERNIAS. It was with some reluctance that I included traumatic postoperative hernias among the etiologic factors of lumbar hernias. I have repaired four large postoperative incisional hernias in the lumbar area following operations upon the kidney. Kretschmer (1951) reported that 11 patients developed hernias following various renal operations. Such hernias are usually large and rather difficult to repair.

Operative procedures about the iliac crest occasionally result in lumbar hernias. Lotem and colleagues (1971) and Pyrtek and Kelly (1960) have reported instances in which lumbar hernias developed after bone grafts were taken from the crest of the ileum. Oldfield (1945) reported an iliac hernia following harvesting of iliac bone for grafting purposes Bosworth (1955) described a hernia that occurred through a defect created by resection of a portion of the ileum because of osteomyelitis.

## SYMPTOMS AND SIGNS

The most common symptom of lumbar hernia is the discovery of a protrusion by the patient, or by the parents if the patient is an infant. I have seen an acquired lumbar hernia the size of a hen's egg. At the other end of the spectrum, I recently repaired a recurrent postnephrectomy incisional hernia, approximately $25 \times 20$ centimeters in size, in an obese patient.

Patients often complain of discomfort and a dragging sensation; when the hernia is large, the deformity can prove embarrassing. In rare cases, the urinary tract or gastrointestinal tract may be involved; in these situations, urinary tract symptoms or bowel dysfunction may result. In the average patient with a lumbar hernia, the mass recedes or disappears on recumbency.

Incarceration of intestine with obstruction has been reported in 24 percent of 33 patients by Goodman and Speese (1916). Menaker and Kulman (1971) also reported such a case.

Most severe symptoms result from cases in which intestinal obstruction occurs. Cramping abdominal pain, vomiting, and distention vary in severity. Watson (1948) found strangulation to be present in 15, or 8 percent, of 186 cases of lumbar hernia due to all causes. He found strangulation to be present in 18 percent of 70 cases with spontaneous variety of lumbar hernias.

Some surgeons emphasize back pain as a prominent symptom of lumbar hernia; however, my experience has not confirmed this. If backache is a prominent symptom, then the musculoskeletal system should be evaluated through x-ray studies and consultation with an orthopedist. Herz (1945) and Ficarra (1955) attributed low back pain to herniation of adipose tissue. The explanation of back pain on a basis of panniculitis and pannicular hernia must be accepted with great caution, and only after all other causes for such pain have been excluded.

## DIFFERENTIAL DIAGNOSIS OF LUMBAR HERNIA

I suspect that many types of swelling in the lumbar area are considered to be lumbar hernias; but, in fact, comparatively few prove to be such hernias In my experience, a swelling (such as a lipoma in the lumbar area) is apt to be diagnosed as a hernia. The large hernias with obvious protrusion are comparatively easily diagnosed. A number of possibilities may account for tumefaction in the lumbar areas.

LIPOMA. A moderate-sized lipoma may be difficult to distinguish from a hernia. The tumor due to lipoma is firm and more or less circumscribed and, when located in Petit's triangle, can cause a problem in differential diagnosis. If the patient is asked to contract his musculature by lateral flexion of the trunk, it will be noted that the lipoma is superficial to the musculature. Although the presence of lipomas may lead to patient anxiety, there are usually no other complaints

**FIBROMA.** Tumors such as fibromas are painless and usually asymptomatic except for the presence of a worrisome protrusion. They are firm in consistency but may be confused with lipomas. Fibromas are not reducible and do not decrease in size upon recumbency.

**HEMATOMA.** Hematomas appear after a history of trauma, hence, pain of some magnitude will be present upon motion or palpation. Ecchymosis in the area should increase the suspicion that a hematoma is present. Athletes (such as football and hockey players or wrestlers) receive trauma to the iliac crest and can develop hematomas at the site. Repeated examinations over a period of time may be necessary to establish the diagnosis.

**ABSCESS.** In the past, when tuberculosis was a more common disease than it is today, it was not at all rare for an abscess to appear in the weakened area that is Petit's triangle. Such patients might present with pain and fever in addition to the chronic illness that is due to Pott's disease. Chest roentgenograms and x-ray films of the spine could prove helpful in the diagnosis. It should be recalled that the "cold abscess" of tuberculosis is not especially painful, and the degree of rubor may be minimal. Nonspecific abscesses due to a variety of causes are usually more acute in progression and, hence, cause greater discomfort. Fluctuation will develop in time if the abscess is left untreated. Infections may also arise from the kidney or the colon and present in the lumbar area.

**NEOPLASMS.** A number of neoplasms may appear in the lumbar area. Lipomas and fibromas have already been mentioned. Malignant tumors, although rare, do occur in the area. They originate from muscle, connective tissue, or bone. The diagnosis of rhabdomyosarcoma, sarcoma, or osteogenic sarcoma can only be made upon histologic examination of the removed tissue.

**MUSCLE HERNIAS.** Muscle hernias have been described by Watson (1948). Apparently, muscle fibers protrude through a disruption in the fascia of the involved muscle. In these cases, a defect is not palpable in the abdominal wall.

**POSTOPERATIVE AND POST-TRAUMATIC HERNIAS.** Postoperative and post-traumatic hernias in the lumbar area usually do not present a problem in diagnosis. The protrusion is usually large, soft, and reducible.

## TREATMENT

All symptomatic lumbar hernias should be repaired Lumbar hernias in infants should also be repaired, for the deformity will only result in emotional trauma to a growing child and embarrassment to the parents. There is some justification for use of a support in aged patients with serious cardiac, pulmonary, renal, or metabolic diseases. Even in those patients with obstructive symptoms, repair can be performed under local anesthesia.

In all patients with large hernias, the gastrointestinal and urinary tracts should be investigated with contrast studies prior to repair. It is important to know the position of the colon in relation to the hernial sac.

Patients with bronchitis and emphysema should discontinue smoking. Physical therapy and respiratory therapy should be commenced prior to surgery and continued in the postoperative period.

Since many patients with lumbar hernias—and, particularly, those with incisional hernias—are obese, weight reduction is a commendable goal.

### Operative Treatment

**POSITION OF PATIENT AND SKIN PREPARATION.** Some thought must be given to the position of the patient on the operating table. If a small Petit's triangular hernia is present, an oblique position will be adequate. If a large hernia is present, then the lateral position is needed. The affected side is up and the thigh extended; the opposite extremity is flexed at the knee. Use of a kidney elevator may be helpful in securing accessibility by separating the lower ribs from the ileum.

Painstaking efforts must be taken toward achieving asepsis. The skin is prepared with Povidone-iodine (Betadine) solution and alcohol.

If fascia lata is to be utilized in the repair, then the entire thigh must be prepared.

## Technique of Repair

Operative treatment might be deferred in certain patients with serious systemic disease; however, as with other hernias, the only possibility of cure lies in surgical repair. The skin incision may be made vertically over the hernia in Petit's triangle; another approach is obliquely from the area below the twelfth rib, over the hernial protrusion, toward the lower anterior abdomen. The incision thus lies above the iliac crest. The incision is developed through the skin and subcutaneous fat to the hernial sac. The protrusion may be quite small (one inch in diameter), or it may be enormous — measuring several inches in width and length. It is covered by an attenuated layer of lumbodorsal fascia, which is contiguous with transversalis fascia.

It is uncommon to find a hernial sac of the type seen in inguinal hernias. If such a sac is found, it must be opened with caution, since the colon and its mesentery may form a portion of the herniated mass. The peritoneal sac (if present) is dissected free, and high ligation carried out as a rule. Silk, catgut, or one of the synthetic sutures may be used. I prefer number 0 silk for the larger sac and finer sutures for smaller peritoneal sacs.

If the defect is large without an identifiable peritoneal sac, the mass may be inverted and plicating sutures carefully placed superficially to avoid visceral injury. The possible presence of a sliding viscus, such as colon, must be considered if injury to the bowel or its blood supply is to be avoided.

It is worthwhile to note contents of the lumbar hernial sac or protrusion as listed by Watson (1948). Omentum, fat, large and small intestine, mesentery, appendix, cecum, and stomach — and, more rarely, kidney — have been found in such sacs. Thorek (1950) found intestine (either large or small) in 41 of his patients, while fat was present in another 26 patients.

## Techniques for Reconstruction of the Abdominal Wall in Lumbar Hernia

A number of techniques have been utilized in the repair of lumbar hernias. The procedure chosen for a given patient obviously depends on the size and nature of the defect. Since the techniques are relatively simple, they will be described briefly with suggestions as to their application.

Owen (1888) felt that excision of the hernial sac was important. He was the first to close the operative wound with buried sutures

1. *Simple Closure of the Lumbodorsal Fascia*
   In instances where the hernia is small with protrusion of fat through the fascia, this simple method is adequate. The protruding fat is excised, with care taken to ligate the pedicle. Zimmerman and Anson (1967) advised a selective approach to repair of lumbar hernias. Opening of the peritoneal sac could be considered an elective matter, but closure of the fascia is essential. The defect in the transversus abdominis layer is easily seen and can be repaired with nonabsorbable sutures.
2. *Closure with Fascial Strips* (Swartz, 1954)
   In larger defects, most surgeons feel that some reinforcing structure is needed. Swartz described a technique in which he utilized strips of fascia lata, 1.0 to 1.5 centimeters in width, taken from the thigh. The strips of fascia were woven between the latissimus dorsi and the external oblique muscles. Transversalis fascia is included in the placement of fascial strips. Gallie and Le Mesurier described this principle in 1923.
3. *Closure with Fascial Sheets* (Ravdin, 1923)
   After disposition of the hernial sac as described earlier in this section, repair may be achieved with a sheet of fascia lata. This technique was beautifully described and illustrated by Ravdin in 1923 following repair of a post-traumatic lumbar hernia. First, he oversewed the inverted hernial sac, using chromic catgut (I prefer nonabsorbable sutures in these cases). He then placed a sheet of fascia lata deep to the musculature and closed the latissimus dorsi muscle over the implanted fascia. Finally, he placed another sheet of fascia lata over the repaired area. This is a useful method of repair; however, I recommend Marlex mesh in place of fascia lata.

4. *Closure with Musculofascial Pedicle or Flap Grafts* (Dowd, 1907; Rishmiller, 1917)

A number of surgeons have described effective and more complicated procedures appropriate for repair of large lumbar hernias. Such procedures are not often indicated, but occasionally they are useful. Dowd's technique, which is a classic method of repair, has been repeatedly referred to in the literature. The method is one in which major reconstruction is achieved through the use of musculofascial flaps. The essential features of the repair were clearly illustrated by Shepard in Watson's book on hernia (Fig. 24–7). Dowd developed a generous flap of fascia and aponeurosis largely from the gluteus maximus — which was elevated and sutured to the lumbar fascia above, the latissimus dorsi posteriorly, and the external oblique anteriorly (Fig. 24–7). In the upper portion of the defect, the latissimus dorsi and external oblique may be approximated. Finally, Dowd sutured a musculoaponeurotic flap from the latissimus dorsi over the area just described above. This is a method of proven value in repair of many lumbar hernias. Variations of the method are numerous.

Rishmiller in 1917 utilized a different application of the principles advocated by Dowd, forming a flap by splitting the aponeurosis of the latissimus dorsi.

Lewin and Bradley (1949) utilized more complicated and ingenious methods in repair of a traumatic unusual hernia. They utilized the iliopsoas muscle as a pedicle graft to partially replace loss of soft tissue and the iliac bone.

5. *Closure with Implants and Synthetic Meshes*

Fascia lata was employed by Ravdin in 1923 to add strength to the repair of a lumbar hernia. He actually utilized two sheets of fascia lata, placing one sheet deep to the musculature and the second over the previously approximated muscles.

Thorek in 1950 used tantalum in the repair of large lumbar hernias. Koontz in 1955 reported that he had used cutis grafts in the repair of two massive incisional lumbar hernias. In the repair of another large hernia, tantalum mesh was implanted. Pyrtek and Kelly in 1960 described their method of managing large iliac bone defects with herniation. They utilized tantalum prostheses to gain strength in the repair of two such defects.

Marlex mesh was successfully used by Hafner, Wylie, and Brush in 1963 in the repair of a post-traumatic lumbar hernia in Petit's triangle. The sac was imbricated; an aponeurotic flap was elevated from the gluteal area and sutured into the lower portion of the defect, utilizing Dowd's principle. At the apex of the defect, the latissimus dorsi and external oblique muscular layers were approximated. Marlex mesh was then sutured over the entire area.

The repair of many lumbar hernias may be a simple matter; but in unusual circumstances, reconstruction may be quite difficult. Careful evaluation of the problem at hand should then be followed by selection of an appropriate technique. I prefer the use of Marlex mesh as a prosthesis to that of cutis grafts and tantalum. Cutis grafts can become infected; they can develop retention cysts or even squamous cell carcinoma (as reported by Gomez and colleagues).[1] Tantalum gauze loses its strength because of fragmentation.

## Technique Preferred Today

Techniques that I have found useful for large lumbar hernias embody features recommended by Dowd, Ravdin, and Hafner and colleagues.

In large lumbar hernias (Fig. 24–8), I prefer identification of the peritoneal cavity, with entry into the peritoneal cavity. Exploration and high ligation of the peritoneal sac are performed. Excess of peritoneum as well as the attenuated and redundant trasversalis fascia and lumbodorsal fascia are excised. This layer is closed with number 2–0 nonabsorbable sutures.

I prefer placement of Marlex mesh at this level in those cases requiring reinforcement. The latissimus dorsi and external oblique musculoaponeurotic layers are closed at the apex over the mesh. Inferiorly, a flap of fascia from the gluteus maximus is turned upward to complete coverage of the deeply implanted mesh.

If necessary, a second layer of Marlex mesh may be sutured over the entire area. Sutures of number 2–0 nonabsorbable material should be placed to encompass the

fascia in the area. The connective tissue layer in the lumbar region does not resemble the aponeurosis of the external oblique in the groin. One suction catheter is

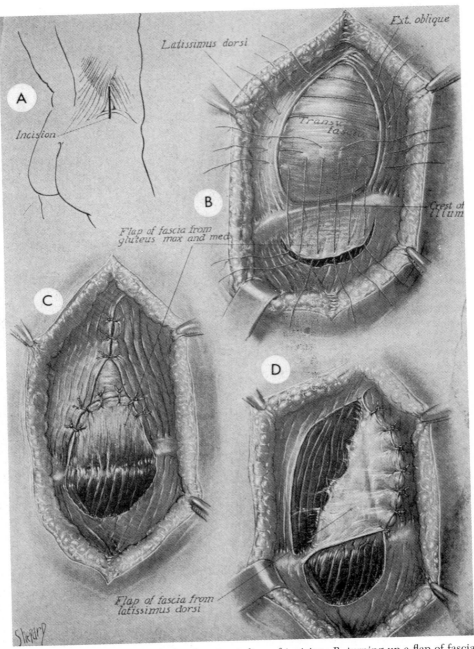

**Figure 24–7.** Dowd's operation for lumbar hernia: *A*, line of incision; *B*, turning up a flap of fascia lata and aponeurosis of gluteus maximus and medius muscles and suturing it to the lumbar fascia external oblique and latissimus dorsi muscles; *C*, the flap sutured; and *D*, closing of remaining gap with a flap of fascia from the latissimus dorsi. (Reproduced with permission of C. V. Mosby Co. From Watson, L. F.: *Hernia.* 3rd ed. St. Louis, C. V. Mosby Co., 1948.)

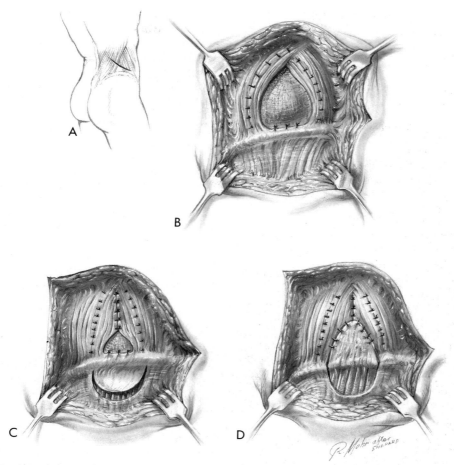

**Figure 24–8.**   Personal technique for repair of large lumbar hernia. *A*, An oblique skin incision is preferred. *B*, After the peritoneal sac has been entered and digital exploration performed, the Marlex mesh is placed over the defect and sutured to the external oblique and latissimus dorsi. *C*, The muscular layers as described above are partially closed over the implant. *D*, The fascial flap from the gluteal muscles is elevated and sutured over the remaining defect.

placed deeply over the lumbodorsal fascia and a second is placed superficially in the subcutaneous space.

## CLINICAL CASES

Hafner and colleagues in 1963 reported nine cases of lumbar hernias seen at Henry Ford Hospital. Two were located in the superior lumbar triangle; two, in the inferior lumbar triangle; five were diffuse—occupying a large portion of the lumbar area. All of the hernias in that report occurred in adults.

Since that time, 14 additional cases of lumbar hernia have been seen. One oc-

curred in a newborn female infant with multiple congenital anomalies—i.e., club-foot, spina bifida, meningocele, diaphragmatic weakness, and cystic fibrosis of the pancreas. No operative procedure was recommended, and the infant died six months later of her pancreatic disease.

Eleven of the lumbar hernias occurred in males and only two in females. With the exception of the one infant, all were adults ranging in age from 44 to 72 years.

Etiologic factors are summarized in Table 24–5.

In an institution involved in the caring of infants and children, the incidence of congenital lumbar hernias would be large. Since Henry Ford Hospital has an active

Table 24–5. ETIOLOGIC FACTORS—
14 PATIENTS WITH LUMBAR HERNIA

| | | |
|---|---|---|
| Congenital | | 1 |
| Acquired | | 13 |
| Spontaneous | 4 | |
| (Superior lumbar triangle, 2) | | |
| (Inferior lumbar triangle, 2) | | |
| Traumatic (nonoperative) | 5 | |
| Traumatic (postoperative) | 4 | |

emergency service, it is not surprising to find that post-traumatic lumbar hernias are fairly common.

## Acquired Lumbar Hernias

These tend to be large, occupying a generous portion of the lumbar area. Trauma, which results in lumbar hernias, is always of a severe degree and is sometimes bizarre in nature (such as being gored by a bull). In the cases seen at Henry Ford Hospital, a number of types of trauma had preceded the appearance of the lumbar hernia. Crushing injury at work (1 case), auto accidents (3), and falling from a height (1) accounted for the nonoperative trauma.

Three of the postoperative hernias in the lumbar area followed operations upon the kidney, and one developed secondary to removal of an iliac bone graft.

In four patients with spontaneous acquired hernias, obesity and severe chronic pulmonary disease were considered important etiologic factors. Two individuals were quite obese, and two had respiratory tract disease. Asthma, emphysema, chronic bronchitis, and bronchiectasis are underlying disorders that may occur prior to the appearance of lumbar hernias in some patients.

## Techniques of Repair

In general, the surgeons preferred to repair lumbar hernias without implants. In

Table 24–6. TECHNIQUES OF REPAIR—
13 LUMBAR HERNIAS

| | |
|---|---|
| Closure of lumbodorsal and transversalis fasciae | 2 |
| Closure in layers without implants | 6 |
| Repair with marlex mesh | 4 |
| Repair with Tantalum Mesh | 1 |

large lumbar hernias, however, implants were considered necessary (Table 24–6). Of our 14 cases, only one was not repaired because the infant had severe and multiple congenital anomalies.

In small lumbar hernias, the pedicle is clamped, ligated, and the lipomatous mass excised.

In the repair of moderate-sized lumbar hernias, the principles and technique of Dowd are useful. Six of 13 repairs were performed without implants.

For repair of the largest lumbar hernias, I prefer to use a Marlex mesh implant. Essentially, the hernial sac is dissected for identification of the weakness. I prefer to open the peritoneal sac and perform high ligation of the sac. In some lumbar hernias, the area of weakness is diffuse; and a sac (such as that seen in groin hernias) is not to be identified. Care must be taken to avoid injury to incarcerated contents or to sliding components.

The lumbodorsal and transversalis fascial layer is closed, or imbricated, to reduce the bulge. It is upon this layer and deep to the internal oblique and latissimus dorsi that I prefer to place the Marlex mesh.

The muscular layers are then closed over the mesh as completely as possible within the confines of sound technique. Excessive tension is avoided. If desired, an onlay implant of Marlex mesh may be added to the repair; however, this is rarely needed.

I do not use tantalum mesh in my current practice, nor do I recommend its use.

## Results

In general, I feel that excellent results are obtained with the small hernias and those repaired without implants. Follow-up studies are incomplete, and the patients with repaired lumbar hernias seemed to have disappeared into the general population. There was one recurrence in a patient who had had his hernia repaired with tantalum mesh. The metallic mesh was removed following a wound infection, and the lumbar hernia recurred.

Two patients developed seromas requiring aspiration; however, in both cases, the wounds healed satisfactorily Two other patients developed atelectasis and pneumonitis, but both responded to antibiotics and respiratory therapy. There were no deaths among the 13 surgical patients.

## SUMMARY

Lumbar hernias are protrusions of variable size, which develop in a well-defined anatomic area that is bounded above by the twelfth rib, below by the iliac crest, posteriorly by the erector spinae muscles and vertebral column, and anteriorly by a vertical line from the tip of the twelfth rib to the iliac crest. Within these confines are two potential areas of weakness; when protrusions occur, they are known as hernias of the superior triangle (Grynfeltt-Lesshaft) or inferior lumbar triangle (Petit).

Lumbar hernias may be classified, based on etiology, as congenital or acquired. Congenital lumbar hernias are relatively rare and are often accompanied by multiple congenital defects. Acquired lumbar hernias are the most common in our experience. Physical trauma—such as crushing injuries, falls, and auto accidents—account for many lumbar hernias. Operative trauma is another important cause of lumbar hernias. Operations on the kidney as well as bone grafting techniques in which the iliac crest is exposed account for a respectable number of lumbar hernias I feel that Marlex mesh should be implanted in cases requiring excision of generous quantities of iliac bone. Deep implantation of the prosthesis is an important principle to be followed.

Most lumbar hernias can and should be repaired without implants. The general principles and technique described by Dowd continue to be useful. Closure of the lumbodorsal fascia–transversalis fascia layer is an essential and important detail in successful repair.

Synthetic mesh if required should be deeply implanted over the lumbodorsal fascial layer, which is an excellent site for placement.

Fascia lata is infrequently used in repair of lumbar hernias, and tantalum mesh is obsolete.

## REFERENCES

Adamson, R. J.: A case of bilateral hernia through Petit's triangle with two associated abnormalities. Br. J. Surg. 46:88, 1958.

Bosworth, D. M.: Repair of hernia through iliac crest. J. Bone Joint Surg. 37(A):1969, 1955

Coley, W. B.: Lumbar hernia. Ann. Surg. 74:650, 1921.

Dowd, C. N.: Congenital lumbar hernia at the triangle of Petit. Ann. Surg. 45:245, 1907.

Everett, W. G.: Traumatic lumbar hernia. Injury 4:354, 1974.

Ficarra, B. J.: Pannicular lumbosacroiliac hernia. Arch. Surg. 70:229, 1955.

Frazer, E. H.: A case of lumbo-dorsal hernia with some unusual features. Med. J. Aust. 1:60, 1968.

Gallie, W. E., and MeMesurier, A. B.: Living sutures in the treatment of hernia. Can. Med. Assoc. J. 13:469, 1923.

Gomez, J., Wylie, J. E., and Ponka, J. L.: Epidermoid carcinoma in a cutis graft after repair of an incisional hernia. Rev. Surg. 29:381, 1972.

Goodman, E. H., and Speese, J.: Lumbar hernia. Ann. Surg. 63:548, 1916.

Grynfeltt, J.: Quleque mots sur la hernie lombaire. Montpellier Med. 16:323, 1866

Hafner, C. D., Wylie, J. H., and Brush, B. E.: Petit's lumbar hernia: Repair with Marlex mesh. Arch. Surg. 86:180, 1963.

Hancock, T. H.: Report of a case of traumatic hernia in Petit's triangle. South. Med. J. 13:521, 1920.

Herz, R.: Herniation of fascial fat and low back pain. J.A.M.A. 128:921, 1945.

Jeannel, M.: La hernie lombaire. Arch. Prov. Chir. Paris 11:389–418, 521–538, 649–665, 713, and 1279, 1902; 12:91–115, 159–174, 281–296, 1903.

Koontz, A. R.: An operation for massive incisional lumbar hernia. Surg. Gynecol. Obstet. 101:119, 1955.

Kretschmer, H. L.: Lumbar hernia of the kidney. J. Urol. 65:944, 1951.

Lee, C. M., Jr., and Mattheis, H.: Congenital lumbar hernia. Arch. Dis. Child. 32:42, 1957.

Larrey, L. D.: Recherches et observations sur la hernie lombaire. Bull. l'Academie Imperiale de Medicine, 1869.

Lesshaft, P.: Lumbalgegren in anatomisch–Chirurgischer Himsicht. Anat. Physiol. Wissensch. Med. 264, 1870.

Lewin, M. L., and Bradley, E. T.: Traumatic iliac hernia with extensive soft tissue loss Surgery 26:601, 1949.

Lotem, M., Maor, P., Haimoff, H., and Woloch, Y.: Lumbar hernia at an iliac bone graft donor site. Clin. Orthop. 80:130, 1971.

Macready, J.: Rarer forms of ventral hernia. Lancet Nov. 8, 1890.

Mastin, C. H.: On lumbar hernia. Ann. Surg. 12:20, 1890.

Menaker, G. J., and Kulman, H.: The intestinal complications of hernia and a case of lumbar hernia. Surg. Clin. North Am. 51:1337, 1971.

Musick, R. H., and Schubert, S. E.: Lumbar hernia: An instance reported. Ill. Med. J. 138:585, 1970.

Oldfield, M. C.: Iliac hernia after bone grafting. Lancet 1:810, 1945.

Orcutt, T. W.: Hernia of the superior lumbar triangle. Ann. Surg. 173:294, 1971.

Owen, E.: Lumbar hernia: Radical operation; recovery. Br. Med. J. 1:957, 1888.

Parekh, P., Parekh, B. R., and Singh, S. D.: Congenital lumbar hernia. Ind. Pediatr. 14:577, 1977.

Petit, J. L.: Traite des maladies chirurgicales et des

opérations qui leur conviennent. T. F. Didot, 2: 256–258, 1974.

Pyrtek, L. H., and Kelley, C. C.: Management of hernia through large iliac bone defects Ann. Surg. 152:988, 1960.

Radwin, I. S.: Lumbar hernia through Grynfeltt and Lesshaft's triangle. Surg. Clin. North Am. 3:267, 1923.

Rishmiller, J. H.: Hernia through triangle of Petit. Surg. Gynecol. Obstet. 24:589, 1917.

Swartz, W. T.: Lumbar hernia. J. Ken. Med. Assoc. 52:673, 1954.

Thorek, M.: Lumbar hernia. J. Int. Coll. Surg. 14:367, 1950.

Thorek, M.: *Modern Surgical Technic*. Philadelphia, J. B. Lippincott Co., 1950.

Watson, L. E.: *Hernia* (3rd ed.). St. Louis, C. V. Mosby Co., 1948, pp. 443–455.

## Supplemental Reading

Vannozzi, I.: Lumbar hernia, anatomo-clinical contribution. Minerva Chir. 16:511, 1961.

# SPIGELIAN HERNIAS

The precise identification of Spigelian hernia is made difficult by its location, uncommon occurrence, and unpredictable symptomatology. Although a mass does appear at the site of defect, the hernia is located in the linea semilunaris and beneath the external oblique aponeurosis where — unless the patient has lost significant amounts of subcutaneous adipose tissue — the mass is obscured. Furthermore, the various locations of the Spigelian hernia in the semilunar line create additional confusion. Pain of varying degrees of severity together with vague gastrointestinal symptoms also contributes to the difficulty in making a differential diagnosis. Even though Spigelian hernias are uncommon, they do occur often enough to confuse surgeons and other physicians as well.

## DEFINITION

A Spigelian hernia is one that protrudes through the linea semilunaris at any point in its extent. The most common location is at the junctional site of the linea semilunaris and the linea semicircularis of Douglas.

Although this description has practical merit, it may cause some confusion in that the semilunar line itself is not simply defined. In a review containing 149 references, Spangen (1976) pointed out four definitions for this important landmark, as follows:

1. The line created by the transition of the transversus abdominis muscle from muscle to aponeurosis.
2. The line created by the division of the internal oblique aponeurosis into anterior and posterior lamellae of the rectus sheath.
3. The indentation seen just lateral to the rectus abdominis muscle.
4. The line in the rectus abdominis sheath just lateral to the rectus muscle.

Each definition places the linea semilunaris at practically the same anatomic location.

It should be noted that the semilunar line extends from the costal cartilage of the ninth rib to the spine of the pubis. The anatomic details of the rectus sheath are of importance in any consideration of Spigelian hernias and have been described in Chapter 2.

The use of the eponymic designation Spigelian hernia to identify a lateral ventral hernia is questioned by some surgeons and is considered unacceptable by others. They make the valid point that Spigelius never saw such a hernia — although he was the first to describe the fascia through which such hernias protrude, a contribution that was of fundamental importance to all surgeons. Through usage, however, the term gained deep roots in the surgical literature; and even those surgeons who have a professed aversion to eponyms do recognize that Spigelian hernia does identify, with brevity, a particular type of hernia.

### Synonyms

A number of designations that have been applied to Spigelian hernia share a common undesirable feature — namely, the necessity of using several words in order to identify the protrusion. Some of the terms applied include: "hernia in the linea semilunaris" and "spontaneous lateral ventral hernia." Spigelian hernias have been called "masked hernias"; this is because, in some cases, the hernia protrudes deep to the aponeurosis of the external oblique and may be difficult to identify.

## HISTORICAL BACKGROUND

The credit for being the first to describe the semilunar line belongs to Adrian van der Spieghel (1578–1625). According to Spangen (1976), this anatomist studied in Padua and later held the Chair of Anatomy and Surgery at the university of that city.

The next significant contribution was made by Klinkosch, who, in 1764, first described a hernia that may well have been a spontaneous lateral ventral hernia. Burke (1975) researched the reference by contacting Professor Lensky at the Institute for History of Medicine at the University of Vienna. It is to be noted that Klinkosch's name is erroneously spelled "Klinklosch" in a number of references In order to provide the proper reference, I have cited that spelling identified by Burke.

Watson (1948) credits La Chausse with being the first to recognize a hernia in the linea semilunaris in 1721. It is clear that Sir Astley Cooper also recognized such hernias in 1804.

Spigelian hernias appeared to have been recognized much earlier in Europe than in this country By 1942, River had discovered only four cases in the American literature, while 112 were reported in foreign literature. By 1960, Read stated that over 200 cases had been reported in the literature.

Olson and Davis (1968) reported on six patients with Spigelian hernias seen in a period of two years. One of the six patients had an earlier repair elsewhere of what was described as a Spigelian hernia. Thus, Olson and Davis considered the defect to be a recurrent Spigelian hernia. A second patient had undergone an appendectomy and hysterectomy, on separate occasions, prior to the Spigelian repair. As a result of their findings, Olson and Davis felt that Spigelian hernias were more obscure than rare. I would add that other cases may be misdiagnosed and unreported.

## INCIDENCE

The male-to-female incidence of Spigelian hernias is approximately equal. Weiss and colleagues (1974) found the ratio to be 1:1.05 of males to females, based on cumulative data from cases in the literature.

Spigelian hernias occur most often in patients in the fourth, fifth, sixth, and seventh decades of life. Bailey (1957) found the greatest incidence to occur in patients in the fifth and sixth decades of life. Alsted (1973) noted that the youngest patient with spontaneous lateral ventral hernia was a neonate of six days, while the oldest was 94 years of age.

Graivier and colleagues (1970) were able to identify only six cases of Spigelian hernia occurring in children, and three other such hernias were of traumatic origin. Hurlbut and Moseley (1967) also treated a child with a lateral ventral hernia.

The bilateral occurrence of Spigelian hernias in infants was recognized by Hurwitt and colleagues (1955) and by Graivier and Alfieri (1978). Holloway (1922) noted that Berger reported bilateral spontaneous lateral ventral hernias occurring in a patient in 1918.

## ANATOMIC CONSIDERATIONS

In discussing the practical anatomic considerations, it is worthwhile to review the anatomy of the rectus sheath as described in Chapter 2.

Important anatomic details that have a bearing on the formation of the Spigelian fascia are well illustrated by Spangen (Fig. 24–9); the location of the semilunar line is clearly shown.

As can be seen in Figure 24–9, the semilunar line is located just lateral to the rectus sheath and extends from the ninth costal cartilage to the pubic spine. The external oblique is aponeurotic throughout the length of the rectus abdominis and provides the anteriormost lamella of the rectus sheath. The internal oblique divides into two lamellae to enclose the rectus muscle, and the aponeurosis of the external oblique, which lies over the linea semilunaris, makes up the anterior portion of the rectus sheath. The transversus abdominis aponeurosis contributes to the posterior lamina rectus sheath above the linea semicircularis of Douglas. Below the linea semicircularis of Douglas and approximately 5 to 8 centimeters below the um-

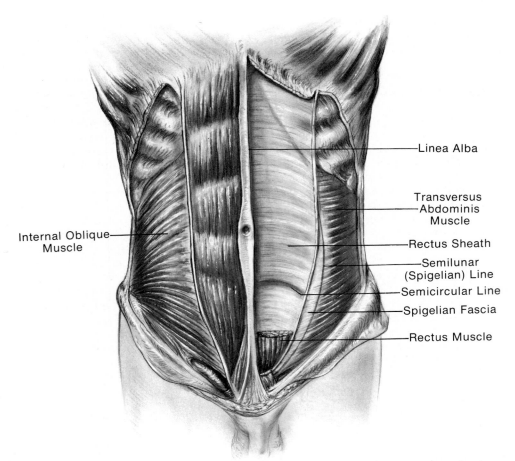

Internal Oblique
Muscle

Linea Alba

Transversus
Abdominis
Muscle

Rectus Sheath

Semilunar
(Spigelian) Line

Semicircular Line

Spigelian Fascia

Rectus Muscle

**Figure 24–9.** A ventral view of the abdominal wall showing the anatomical details. To the right, the external oblique muscle and ventral lamella of the rectus are cut away. To the left, the internal oblique and rectus abdominis muscle are removed. (Reproduced with permission of author and *Acta Chirurgica Scandinavica*. From Spangen, Leif: Spigelian hernia. Acta Chir. Scand. Suppl. *462*:7, 1976.)

bilicus, the fibers of the transversus abdominis join to form the anterior rectus sheath. Below this level, the posterior sheath of the rectus is quite thin. Furthermore, it is at this site of transition that the branches of the deep inferior epigastric artery enter the rectus abdominis muscle, disappearing under the posterior rectus sheath. Most of the Spigelian hernias I have operated on were found at this site. Thus, many Spigelian hernias appear at approximately the midpoint between the umbilicus and the pubic spine, in the linea semilunaris (Fig. 24–10). Such hernias are covered by the aponeurosis of the external oblique; hence, they may be considered a type of interparietal hernia.

Other terms that are encountered in the literature are the line of Spigel and Spigelian fascia. Actually, the linea semilunaris includes Spigel's line. A definition of Spigelian fascia is more difficult. It extends laterally to the internal oblique muscle and medially to the site of attachment of the external oblique aponeurosis to the sheath of the rectus. The width, depending on location, varies from a few millimeters to over three centimeters and tends to be widest in the vicinity of the linea semicircularis of Douglas

The location of Spigelian hernias in relationship to the layers of the abdominal wall is well indicated by Spangen (Fig. 24–11).

## ETIOLOGIC FACTORS

Numerous factors such as age, obesity, multiple pregnancies, straining (as due to cough), increased intra-abdominal pressure, and paralysis have been cited as predisposing to the formation of hernias of the linea semilunaris. Atrophy of tissues and loss of weight allow protrusion through weakened areas to occur as the result of increased intra-abdominal pressure due to coughing or heavy physical activity.

Watson (1948) identified a point of weakness at the junction of the linea semilunaris and linea semicircularis Cooper attributed the areas of weakness to the perforation sites by blood vessels, and River noted that branches of the deep inferior epigastric artery appear at this location.

## CLINICAL FEATURES

It is evident that most surgeons will see few Spigelian hernias in a productive surgical career, with only the exceptional case presenting a picture that the clinician will recognize. The symptoms tend to be confusing, and the physical manifestations

are often occult. A small Spigelian hernia in a well-nourished patient is well concealed under the aponeurosis of the external oblique muscle.

The following clinical picture is the result of a review of cases at Henry Ford Hospital, plus a review of the literature as shown in the reference list.

Pain, varying in type and severity, is present in nearly every patient with a hernia in the semilunar line; and occasionally it is suspected to be functional in nature. The pain may be dull, burning, or "dragging" in nature; it may be inconstant at times and can be aggravated by strenuous physical activity. Rest often relieves the discomfort. In a carefully taken history, it may be noted that coughing and straining aggravate the discomfort.

More severe pain indicates clearly the need for surgical intervention. Incarceration was rare, in my experience, as was intestinal obstruction. But when obstruction is present, the pain is cramping in nature; and nausea and vomiting, as well as distention, are all present. Constantino and Rocca (1974) reported an instance of strangulation occurring in a Spigelian hernia.

The identification of a protrusion or mass

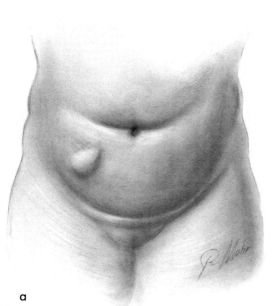

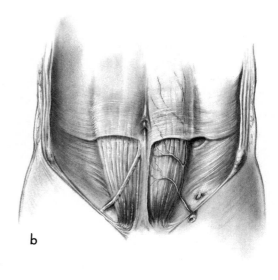

b

a

**Figure 24-10.** The general contour of a Spigelian hernia is shown in the illustration. The mass is ill-defined and located in the lower abdomen (*a*).

On viewing the site of the defect from within the abdomen, one may see it to be usually located where the semicircular and semilunar lines meet (*b*).

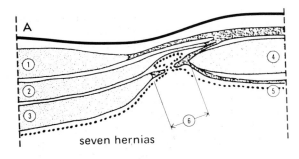

seven hernias

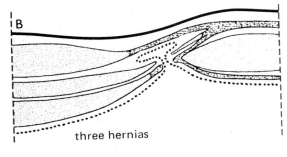

three hernias

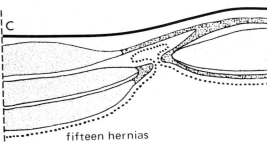

fifteen hernias

Figure 24–11.  In this illustration from Spangen, the locations of 25 Spigelian hernias are shown. These were located proximal or cephalad to the semicircular line. Significantly, the external oblique aponeurosis was intact in every case.
1. External oblique 2. Internal oblique 3. Transversus abdominis. 4. Rectus abdominis 5. Transversalis fascia 6. Spigelian fascia. (Reproduced with permission of author and journal publisher. From Spangen, Leif: Spigelian hernia. Acta Chir. Scand. Suppl. 462:15, 1976.)

is a great diagnostic aid. But unfortunately, a small hernia lying under the aponeurosis of the external oblique aponeurosis may not be evident; and, in such cases, diagnosis is quite difficult. On the other hand, a large reducible hernia simplifies the problem of diagnosis.

Examination for mass must be thorough and, in obscure cases, repeated. The patient should be examined standing and lying down, permitting observation of the abdominal musculature in tension and in relaxation. Localized tenderness and suggestion of a mass at the site may be substantial diagnostic contributions

In a patient with a low pain threshold, a palpable irreducible mass may represent a lipoma.

One other important point should be recalled—that in the lower one-third of the abdomen, the aponeurosis of the external oblique is firmly attached to the rectus sheath. The usual direction for expansion, according to Isaacson (1956), is downward and outward. Thus, the enlargement may be evident in the lower abdominal quadrants lateral to the rectus abdominis sheath.

Although Bryant (1947) found that most Spigelian hernias measure from one to two centimeters in diameter, Larson (1951) noted that some are much larger, measuring up to 14 centimeters in diameter.

## DIFFERENTIAL DIAGNOSIS

Spigelian hernias can be confused with a variety of disorders, and several conditions should be considered as important possibilities:

1. Lipomas of the abdominal wall. Since preperitoneal adipose tissue makes up most of the protruding mass in a Spigelian hernia, it is understandable that a clinical diagnosis of lipoma is often considered.

2. Disorders of the gastrointestinal tract must be differentiated from hernias in the linea semilunaris. Traction on incarcerated omentum may cause epigastric distress and gaseousness. Cholecystitis, intermittent small bowel obstruction, appendicitis, and diverticulitis must all be considered in arriving at the proper diagnosis in obscure cases.

3. Other hernias must be differentiated from Spigelian hernias. For example, a direct inguinal hernia might lead to confusion. In such cases, the Spigelian hernia presents in a low position or inferior to the common location. Careful examination of the groin with digital examination will help identify the defect in the floor of Hesselbach's triangle. Ventral, lumbar, and umbilical hernias

should be considered in the differential diagnosis.

4. Tumors of the abdominal wall and inflammatory lesions are uncommon as differential diagnostic possibilities. In obscure cases of abdominal pain and a phantom mass, complete gastrointestinal studies, as well as urologic investigations, are indicated, and in some patients, repeated physical examinations are advisable.

### Aids to Diagnosis

The key to the diagnosis of Spigelian hernia is consideration of that possibility. Reid (1949) stressed this point in describing a case in which appendicitis was considered in the differential diagnosis.

The clinical appraisal of a patient with careful attention to the history and physical examination is of the greatest importance. Direct inguinal hernias must be considered in the differential diagnosis.

Flat films of the abdomen may reveal abnormal gas patterns, or air-fluid levels in the occasional case where obstruction is present.

Barium enema examination may show a loop of colon within the sac as demonstrated by Read (1960) and by Owen (1971); Som and colleagues (1976) also pointed out the usefulness of contrast studies in identifying Spigelian hernias.

In obscure cases, it is important to obtain complete gastrointestinal studies and to investigate the genitourinary system.

Spangen (1976) recommended the use of ultrasonic scanning as a diagnostic aid. He was able to obtain a correct diagnosis in 19 out of 24 patients with spontaneous lateral ventral hernia.

### TREATMENT

The treatment of Spigelian hernia, once it is identified, is comparatively simple.

I prefer a transverse incision over the prominence of the mass. The skin incision measures from 8 to 10 centimeters (Fig. 24–12).

The protrusion becomes apparent upon opening of the aponeurosis of the external oblique. I prefer to open or incise the anterior rectus sheath and then retract the rectus muscle itself to the opposite side. By this approach, the defect can be better visualized.

The contents of the sac should be identified and replaced within the peritoneal cavity. The sac itself varies greatly, and the larger sacs are excised. I prefer to close the peritoneal sac, then repair the defect in the transversus abdominis layer with synthetic nonabsorbable sutures. Occasionally it is possible to close the internal oblique as a separate layer. The anterior rectus sheath is closed separately, followed by closure of the aponeurosis of the external oblique. Closure of skin and subcutaneous tissue is similar to that used in inguinal hernias.

### CLINICAL EXPERIENCE

In collecting a total of 19 operations for Spigelian hernias, it was necessary to review not only those records indexed as Spigelian but also those indexed as ventral and incisional hernias. This was due to poor indexing methods, and I suspect that many Spigelian hernias have become lost in medical record files for the same reason.

There were 11 females and 8 males among the 19 patients with hernias in the semilunar line.

The ages ranged from 20 to 77 years with the greatest number occurring in the sixth and seventh decades (Table 24–7).

Obesity was noted to be present in some degree, in 11 of 19 patients.

In this study, 12 Spigelian hernias were located on the right side and 7 on the left.

It is interesting that all of the Spigelian hernias in this study were located below the level of the umbilicus in the linea semilunaris; two of them were located in a low position, leading to the erroneous preoperative diagnosis of inguinal hernia.

The magnitude of the defect was characterized as small, moderate, or large. In 10 of the 19 hernias, a small defect was noted in the fascia. In a few of these patients, defects up to five centimeters were described. The size of the defect was considered moderate in seven patients and large in two individuals. One of the two patients was found to have a loop of sigmoid colon in the hernial sac.

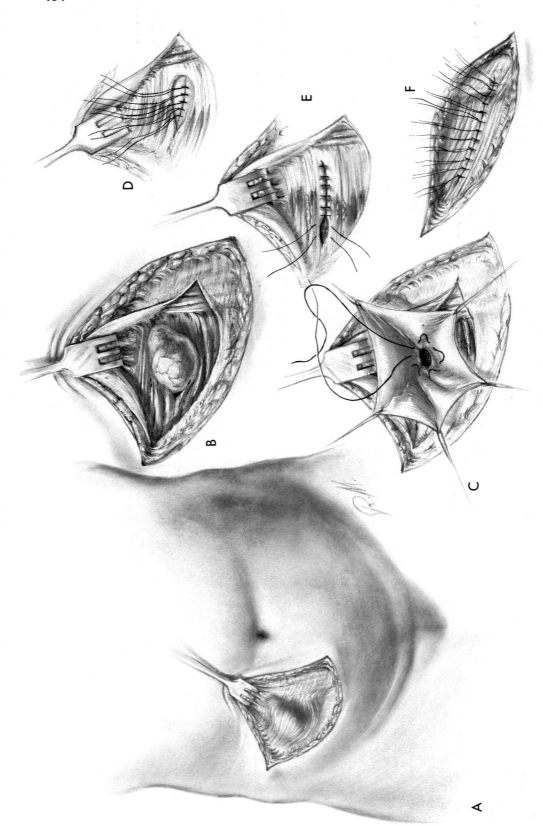

**Figure 24–12.** The skin incision is made obliquely over the protruding mass (*a*). The aponeurosis of the external oblique is opened, revealing the protrusion (*b*). In some cases, it is desirable to open the rectus sheath and refract the muscle medially. The globular mass is dissected free (*c*). I prefer to open the peritoneum, permitting digital exploration. Here the peritoneal sac is being closed. The transversalis fascia is closed (*d*). The internal oblique is closed (*d*). Steps (*d*) and (*e*) may be accomplished as a single-layer closure. The aponeurosis of the external oblique is approximated (*f*). Number 2–0 nonabsorbable sutures are preferred for

Table 24-7. AGE DISTRIBUTION—
19 PATIENTS WITH SPIGELIAN HERNIAS

| Age | No. of Patients |
|---|---|
| 0 to 20 yrs | 1 |
| 21 to 30 yrs. | 0 |
| 31 to 40 yrs. | 1 |
| 41 to 50 yrs. | 3 |
| 51 to 60 yrs. | 7 |
| 61 to 70 yrs. | 6 |
| 71 yrs. and older | 1 |

There were no instances of strangulation obstruction among the 19 patients.

Ten of the 19 patients were followed for five years or longer. There were no known recurrences among these patients.

The study of those patients was disappointing, since the information in several cases was incomplete. These patients were operated on by a number of surgeons, most of them repairing a single Spigelian hernia. I had occasion to repair 3 of the 19 hernias in the linea semilunaris. In each case, the peritoneal sac was surrounded by prolapsing preperitoneal fat. Each hernia measured less than five centimeters, and none of them contained viscera.

## SUMMARY

Spigelian hernias are uncommon. Many surgeons will complete a career in surgery repairing only one or two of them.

The diagnosis depends on a high index of suspicion accompanied with a detailed history and a searching physical examination. The patient should be examined in the standing and supine positions.

In the more obscure cases, a small protrusion of preperitoneal fat may cause rather severe pain. The protrusion, concealed by the aponeurosis of the external oblique, is difficult to demonstrate. Localized pain in the region of the linea semilunaris below the level of the umbilicus should arouse the clinician to the possible presence of a Spigelian hernia.

Such hernias tend to be of small size (less than 5 centimeters) and to occur in obese individuals in the fifth through seventh decades of life. Although Spigelian hernias tend to be unilateral and more common on the right side (as Graivier and colleagues have shown), they occur as bilateral defects in infants and children.

Surgical repair of Spigelian hernias is highly successful, with infrequent recurrence. Olson and Davis reported the only case of recurrent Spigelian hernia I have been able to locate.

## REFERENCES

Alsted, Uffe: Spontaneous lateral ventral or Spigelian hernia. Acta Chir. Scand. *139*:677, 1973.

Bailey, D.: Spigelian hernia: Report of five cases and review of the literature. Br. J. Surg. *44*:503, 1957.

Bryant, A. L.: Spigelian hernia. Am. J. Surg. 73:396, 1947.

Burke, J.: Spigelian and/or lateral ventral hernias. Rev. Surg. 32(5):310, 1975.

Cooper, A. P.: *The Anatomy and Surgical Treatment of Inguinal Hernia*, Vol. I. London, Longman & Co., 1804.

Constantino, L. C., and Rocca, E.: Strangulated Spigelian hernia in a child. Rev. Chir. Pediatr. *16*:236 (July–Sept), 1974.

Graivier, L., and Alfieri, A. L.: Bilateral Spigelian hernias in infancy. Am. J. Surg. *120*:817, 1970.

Graivier, L., Bernstein, D., and Rubane, C. F.: Lateral ventral (Spigelian) hernias in infants and children. Surgery *83*:288, 1978.

Holloway, J. K.: Spontaneous lateral ventral hernia. Ann. Surg. *75*:677, 1922.

Hurlbut, H. J., and Moseley, T.: Spigelian hernia in a child. S. Med. J. *60*:602, 1967.

Hurwitt, E., and Borow, M.: Bilateral Spigelian hernia in childhood. Surgery 37:683, 1955.

Isaacson, N. H.: Spigelian hernia: Report of four cases. Med. Annals D.C. *25*:23, 1956.

Klinkosch, J. T.: Programma quo divisionem herniarum novumque herniae ventralis speciem propouit. Pragae 1964. *In* Sandefort, Eduward: Thesaurus dissertationum Roterodami, Vol. 2. 383–402, 1769.

Larson, E. E.: Spigelian hernia. Am. J. Surg. 82:103, 1951.

Oen, E. Y.: Spigelian hernia and a "redundant" sigmoid colon. Med. J. Aust. 1(6):329, 1971.

Olson, R. O., and Davis, W. C.: Spigelian hernia: Rare or obscure? Am. J. Surg. 82:103, 1951.

Read, R. C.: Observations on the etiology of Spigelian hernia. Ann. Surg. 152:1004, 1960.

Reid, D. K.: Spigelian hernia simulating appendicitis. Br. J. Surg. 36:433, 1949.

River, L. P.: Spigelian hernia. Ann. Surg. *116*:405, 1942.

Som, P. M., Khilnani, M. T., Wolf, B. S., and Beranbaum, S. L.: Spigelian hernia. Acta Rad. Diag. 17:305, 1976.

Spangen, L.: Spigelian hernia. Acta Chirurg. Scand. Suppl. *462*:1–47 (Stockholm), 1976.

Watson, L. A.: *Hernia* (3rd ed.). St. Louis, C. V. Mosby Co., 1948, pp. 368–378.

Weiss, Y., Lernau, O. Z., and Nissan, S.: Spigelian hernia. *180*(6):836, 1974.

## Supplemental Reading

Aisenstein, I.: Hernia in the linea semilunaris Spigelii. Vrac delo, *ii*:116, 1928.

Arida, E. J., Shin, Keun Joh, and Cucolo, Gabrief, F.: Case Reports: The Spigelian hernia: Radiographic manifestations. Br. J. Radiol. *43*:903, 1970.

Beard, M., and Velander, A.: Lateral abdominal tenderness: Spigelian hernia. Mich. Med. *67*:857–860 (July), 1968.

Bertelsen, S.: The surgical treatment of Spigelian hernia. Surg. Gynecol. Obstet. *122*:567, 1966.

Charlesworth, D.: Spigelian hernia. Br. J. Clin. Pract. *23*:169, 1969.

Harless, M., and Hirsch, J. E.: Spigelian or spontaneous lateral ventral hernia. Am. J. Surg. *100*:515, 1960.

Hodges, P. J., and Pliskin, M.: Spigelian hernia. Penn. Med. *71*:51, 1968.

Holder, L. E., and Schneider, H. J.: Spigelian Hernias: Anatomy and roentgenographic manifestations. Radiology *112*(2):309, 1974.

Houlihan, T. J.: A review of Spigelian hernias. Am. J. Surg. *131*:734, 1976.

Ignatius, J. A.: Spigelian hernia. Am. J. Surg. *90*:388, 1955.

Jain, K. M., Hastings, O. M., Kunz, V. P., and Lazaro, E. J.: Spigelian hernia. Am. Surg. *43*(9):596–600, 1977.

Jarvis, P. A., and Seltzer, M. H.: Pediatric Spigelian hernia: A case report. J. Pediatr. Surg. *12*(4):609, 1977.

Koontz, A. R.: Hernia in the linea semilunaris. Ann. Surg. *135*:975, 1952.

Lawler, M. R., Jr., and Carlisle, B. B.: Giant Spigelian hernia. Am. J. Surg. *111*:562, 1966.

Leis, H. P., Jr., Mersheimer, W. L., and Winfield, J. M.: Spontaneous lateral ventral hernia. Surgery *43*(2):328, 1958.

Lovell, S. H.: Spigelian hernia and a "redundant" sigmoid colon. Med. J. Aust. *1*:499, 1971.

Masih, B., Swamy, S., and Altman, B.: Bilateral interstitial hernia in the newborn infant. Surgery *69*:577, 1971.

Matthews, F. S.: Hernia through the conjoined tendon or hernia of the linea semilunaris. Ann. Surg. *78*:300, 1923.

McAdam, W. A. F., and MacGregor, A. M.: Rupture of intestine in patients with herniae: A clinical study with a review of the literature. Br. J. Surg. *56*:657, 1969.

McVay, C. B., and Anson, J. B.: Composition of the rectus sheath. Anat. Rec. *77*:213, 1940.

McVay, C. B.: In *Davis–Christopher's Textbook of Surgery.* Philadelphia, W. B. Saunders Co., 1968. From Anson, B. J., and McVay, C. B.: *Surgical Anatomy,* Vol. I (5th ed.). Philadelphia, W. B. Saunders Co., 1971, p. 537.

Mersheimer, W. L., Winfield, J. M., and Ruggiero, W. F.: Spontaneous lateral ventral hernia. Arch. Surg. *63*:39, 1951.

Perrigard, G. E.: Superior linea semilunaris hernia subjacent to arcuate line. Can. Med. Assoc. J. *57*:575, 1947.

Porter, S. D.: Spigelian hernia, a cause of abdominal pain in young adults. J. Iowa Med. Soc. *59*:115, 1969.

Robinson, H. B.: Hernia through the semilunar line. Br. J. Surg. *2*:336, 1914.

Sarot, I. A.: Hernia in the linea semilunaris. J. Mt. Sinai. Hosp. *8*:164, 1941.

Strode, J. E.: Spigelian hernia. Surg. Clin. North Am. *43*:1379, 1968.

Tuononen, M. I., et al.: Spigelian Hernia. Ann. Chir. Gynaecol. (Helsinski) *65*(4):253, 1976.

Wakeley, C., and Childs, P.: Spigelian hernia through the linea semilunaris. Lancet *1*:1290, 1951.

Wassiljewskaja, Skijanskaja: Hernia in the linea semilunaris Spigelii. Int. Abstr. Surg. *49*:210, 1929.

Watson, D., and Scotter, B.: Strangulated Spigelian hernia (in Medical Memoranda). Br. Med. J. *1*:74, 1951.

Zimmerman, L. M., Anson, B. J., Morgan, E. H., and McVay, C. B.: Ventral hernia due to normal banding of the abdominal muscles. Surg. Gynecol. Obstet. *78*:535, 1944.

# SUPRAVESICAL HERNIAS

*Too often supravesical fossa and other collateral hernias are considered etiologically, diagnostically and therapeutically as being unrelated to external inguinal hernia which obviously is an erroneous assumption.*

*Burton, 1950*

There are certain hernias of the lower abdomen, directly or indirectly involving the bladder, that are extremely difficult to classify. Warvi and Orr (1940) noted that 27 different names have been applied to such hernias and the term supravesical hernia should be included in the list. Zimmerman and Anson (1967) pointed out that many hernias about the bladder are not recognized for what they are by the surgeon who encounters such defects. Since these her-

nias are not often seen, no individual surgeon is able to gain an extensive experience as to their characteristics. Many of these hernias form visible and identifiable protrusions in the groin; others appear within the peritoneal cavity, being a variety of internal hernia.

It is indeed impossible to apply a single term that will specifically identify the various types of hernia that appear in the supravesical and paravesical areas. Those who have studied this problem most seriously have experienced great frustration.

Since there is no present classification that is acceptable to all surgeons, the entire subject of hernias about the bladder deserves reconsideration. Rather than offer yet another classification, I prefer to develop a better application of the designations already available.

## DEFINITION OF TERMS

It might be useful to cite some of the synonyms that have been applied to internal supravesical hernias. The following terms—prevesical hernia, suprapubic hernia, paravesical hernia, intravesical hernia, vesicopubic hernia, and anterior retroperitoneal hernia—have all been used to designate hernias about the bladder. Other examples include: properitoneal supravesical hernia, hernia into the fovea or fossa supravesicalis, hernia juxtavesicalis, internal inguinal hernia, vesicoinguinal hernia, and retroperitoneal hypogastric hernia. All of these terms indicate that such hernias are positioned about the bladder.

In trying to identify types of supravesical hernias, Keynes (1964) proposed that they be classified as *external supravesical hernias* and *internal supravesical hernias*.

An external supravesical hernia originates in the supravesical fossa. It then may pass, in a lateral direction, to the lateral umbilical ligament (obliterated umbilical artery); however, more commonly, it will continue in an anterior direction to present as a femoral or direct inguinal hernia on abdominal examination. Although the direct inguinal and femoral hernia types are relatively common, I feel that most are not recognized by the surgeon as what they actually are. Keynes (1964) further noted that external supravesical hernias may appear in locations as follows:

1. Median, just lateral to the rectus abdominis muscle or tendon.
2. Trans-rectal, through the rectus abdominis.
3. Pararectal, lower portion of semilunar zone.
4. Lateral to the conjoined tendon; such hernias may appear as direct or femoral protrusions.

Such a classification system identifies the site of presentation of the hernia; thus, type 2 must be extremely rare, whereas types 3 and 4 probably occur much more frequently.

Keynes (1964) noted that external supravesical hernias may enlarge in a variety of directions. Foward, lateral, and downward enlargement may occur in different hernias. When forward or lateral enlargement occurs, demonstrable abdominal swelling is seen. When such hernias take a downward path into the pelvis, they assume various positions about the bladder and are not seen externally.

An internal supravesical hernia is one that arises in the supravesical space and may pass into the prevesical, paravesical, retrovesical, or supravesical position.

Warvi and Orr (1940) observed that internal supravesical hernias can be found in the prevesical, intravesical, paravesical, or lateral vesical positions.

Burton in 1950 presented an extensive, collective review on the subject of supravesical hernias. He divided them into prevesical, supravesical, paravesical, and lateral types (depending on their relationships to the bladder).

Skandalakis and colleagues (1976) have applied different terminology to define the course of internal supravesical hernias. They essentially divided these hernias into anterior supravesical, lateral supravesical, or posterior supravesical hernias. They identified retropubic and invaginating varieties of anterior supravesical hernias. Stated simply, external supravesical hernias will present with signs and symptoms ordinarily associated with inguinal hernias. The hernia is demonstrable on physical examination, and repair is performed according to established principles described in Chapter 13 and Chapter 15.

Internal hernias about the bladder lead to both obstructive symptoms and symptoms referred to the genitourinary tract.

## HISTORICAL BACKGROUND

Cooper in 1804 described supravesical fossae and illustrated external supravesical hernia at that time. Watson (1948) gives credit to Ring for reporting what was probably supravesical hernia in 1814. He considered that Linhart described the first authentic case in 1814.

Walker (1933) cited the various titles given to hernias of the prevesical space as follows: Wilms (1869), prevesical hernia; Lesser and Linhart (1866), inner inguinal hernia; Krönlein (1876), properitoneal hernia; Waldeyer (1889), supravesical hernia; and Wilms (1906), prevesical hernia. In scrutinizing the references quoted by Walker, it is evident that German surgeons were well aware of the unusual hernias of the supravesical space.

Warvi and Orr (1940) stated that in 1874 Waldeyer applied the term supravesical fossa to the prevesical area that we are discussing here. They indicated that other designations included fossa vesicomedialis, fossa interligamentosa, internal inguinal fossa, medial fovea, paravesical fossa, and fovea inguinalis intima. The papers of Chandler (1946), Warvi and Orr (1940), and Burton (1950) provide additional interesting historical and anatomical information.

The approach to surgical treatment of external supravesical hernias has been reasonably well developed. The usual preoperative diagnosis of external supravesical hernia is that of direct inguinal or femoral hernia.

Internal supravesical hernias present greater difficulties in diagnosis than in therapy. Symptoms may suggest gastrointestinal disease or genitourinary tract disease. The clinician is likely to suspect intestinal obstruction. The urologist will be aware of urinary frequency and symptoms due to pressure upon the bladder.

By 1976, Skandalakis and colleagues had identified only 59 instances of internal supravesical hernias.

## ANATOMY

The supravesical fossa is a triangular area in the lower anterior abdominal wall. The boundaries include the bladder inferiorly and the obliterated umbilical artery laterally. Thus, the urachal fold in the midline subdivides the area into compartments on the right and left (Fig. 24–13).

The lower boundary of the supravesical fossa, as defined by Keynes (1954), is the transverse fold of the bladder.

The middle inguinal fossa lies between the obliterated umbilical artery and the inferior epigastric artery, while the external inguinal fossa lies lateral to the inferior epigastric artery. Indirect inguinal hernias egress through the internal abdominal ring, which is lateral to the deep inferior epigas-

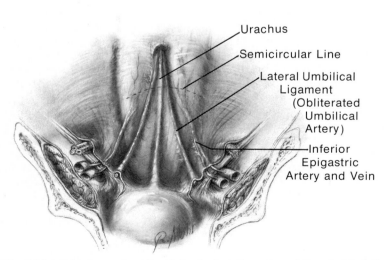

**Figure 24–13.** The folds of the lower anterior abdominal wall as viewed from behind. In the midline the urachal fold subdivides the area into right and left compartments. The transverse fold of the bladder is a lower boundary. The middle inguinal fossa lies between the obliterated umbilical artery and the deep inferior epigastric artery. The supravesical fossa lies between the urachus and the obliterated umbilical artery. Hernias originating in this fossa may appear as direct or femoral, or rarely as interparietal hernias.

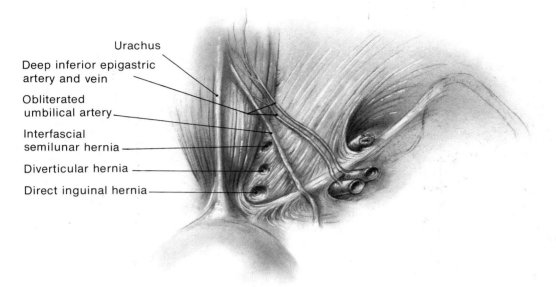

Urachus

Deep inferior epigastric
artery and vein

Obliterated
umbilical artery

Interfascial
semilunar hernia

Diverticular hernia

Direct inguinal hernia

**Figure 24–14.** Posterior view of the lower anterior abdominal wall. This diagrammatic presentation is designed to point out three defects that are diagnosed as direct inguinal hernias. They are located between the obliterated umbilical artery and the margin of the rectus sheath, but above the inguinal ligament. (Reproduced and modified from Burton, Claud: Supravesical inguinal and lateral pelvic fossae. Int. Abstr. Surg. *91*:5, 1950. By permission of *Surgery, Gynecology & Obstetrics.*)

tric artery. Direct inguinal hernias protrude medial to the deep inferior epigastric artery.

## PATHOLOGY

One finds that when attempting to describe external supravesical hernias, in effect, direct inguinal hernias and femoral hernias are being described. Such hernias protrude through the floor of Hesselbach's triangle. Femoral hernias should be included as well. It is extremely important to visualize the triangular area medial to the deep inferior epigastric artery and the midline. Cooper's ligament can be considered, for practical reasons, the base of this triangle. Furthermore, the rectus abdominis muscle and sheath play a powerful role in prevention of hernias in this anatomic area. On the other hand, lateral to the sheath of the rectus abdominis and medial to the obliterated umbilical artery occur a variety of defects that most surgeons identify as direct inguinal hernias (Fig. 24–14). These surgeons are not overburdened with semantic exercises that are of comparatively little substantive value. Nevertheless, I feel that a broad understanding of the

nature of hernia generally leads to somewhat better results in the management aspect.

Internal supravesical hernias are rare and may occur anterior to the bladder, posterior to the bladder, or to the right or left of the bladder. The anterior supravesical hernias are located in the retropubic space of Retzius (Fig. 24–15, *A*).

Certain supravesical hernias encroach on the area normally occupied by the bladder, resulting in urinary tract symptoms (Fig. 24–15, *B*). The protrusions may extend anteriorly, posteriorly, or laterally to the bladder.

## CLINICAL FEATURES

It is practical to consider the signs and symptoms of supravesical hernias on the basis of their anatomic location.

The external supravesical hernia may well appear as a more or less painful protrusion, which occurs at the lateral margin of the rectus abdominis sheath (Fig. 24–14). Such a hernia might appear as a femoral protrusion. External supravesical hernias are far more common than reported in various statistics, simply because most

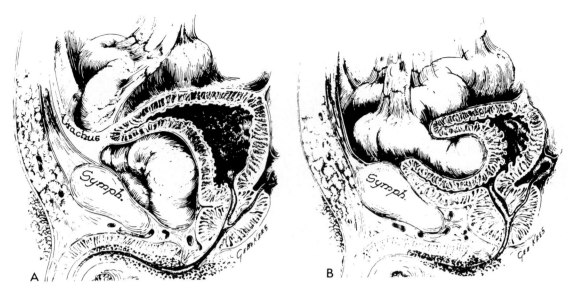

**Figure 24–15.** Supravesical hernias are extremely rare, but they occasionally encroach on the bladder. *A,* Prevesical hernia with a loop of bowel wedged into the space of Retzius. *B,* Supravesical hernia with pressure on the bladder. It is easy to understand why such hernias cause urinary tract symptoms. (Reproduced from Burton, Claud: Supravesical inguinal and lateral pelvic fossae. Int. Abstr. Surg. *91*:1–16, 1950. By permission of *Surgery, Gynecology & Obstetrics.*)

surgeons consider differentiation to be of little value. External supravesical hernias often appear as direct or femoral hernias in most medical record library statistics.

While it is not the intent of this volume to deal with internal supravesical hernias, it is appropriate to point out that such hernias can cause urinary tract symptoms where deformity of the bladder is the result of pressure exerted by loops of intestine. Should mechanical obstruction of the bowel occur, the results would be abdominal pain, nausea, vomiting, and distention. Cystoscopic examination may show deformity of the bladder. Cystograms might reveal indentation of a portion of the bladder due to pressure of the overlying mass. When obstruction has occurred, flat abdominal films will show dilated loops of small intestine with air-fluid levels. Tretbar and Gustafson (1968) used a water-soluble dye to identify obstruction in a patient with an internal supravesical hernia.

### TREATMENT

The treatment for both internal and external supravesical hernias is surgical.

Treatment of the external variety has been more successful, since such hernias tend to be visible upon physical examination. Any of the effective methods of repair of direct and femoral hernias may be used with a high degree of success.

The danger when dealing with internal supravesical hernia is to delay treatment. Prompt recognition of intestinal obstruction will lead to early exploration—before gangrene of the intestine can supervene. A lower abdominal midline or paramedian incision will permit location of the site of obstruction. The constricted neck of the sac is incised at its superior margin and the contents released. Gangrenous bowel (usually ileum), if present, is resected. The small defect is closed with monofilament nonabsorbable sutures, and the peritonneum closed after excision of any redundant peritoneum.

Mortality for external supravesical hernia following surgical correction should approach zero. Keynes (1964) has pointed out that since 1910, there have been 4 deaths among 41 patients undergoing surgical treatment for internal supravesical hernias, for a mortality of 10 percent.

## SUMMARY

A variety of groin hernias may originate in the supravesical fossa. These may present as external or internal hernias.

The external supravesical hernia is the more easily identified, though it may be classified as a direct or femoral hernia. Such hernias are visible through external examination.

Internal supravesical hernias present in a variety of locations about the bladder. They cause urinary tract symptoms or symptoms of intestinal obstruction. The key to diagnosis of such hernias is a high index of suspicion, which leads to x-ray studies of the abdomen and cystoscopy.

Surgical correction of external supravesical hernias is usually prompt, since they can be recognized on physical examination. Internal supravesical hernias are more dangerous because of a possible delay in diagnosis, since the defect cannot be seen on physical examination. Appropriate studies include flat films of the abdomen, cystoscopy, and cystograms. Prompt surgical correction is the proper treatment.

## REFERENCES

Barnes, D. R., and Dreyer, B. J.: Internal supravesical hernia. Br. J. Surg. 40:508, 1953.

Beck, W. C.: Internal supravesical hernia. Guthrie Clin. Bull. 23:133, 1953.

Berson, H. L.: Prevesical hernia. Am. J. Surg. 59:123, 1943.

Burton, C. C.: Hernias of the supravesical inguinal and lateral pelvic fossae: Their diagnosis, classification and relationship. Int. Abstr. Surg. 91(1):1, 1950.

Chandler, S. B.: Studies on the inguinal region. II. Anatomy of the inguinal (Hesselbach) triangle. Ann. Surg. 124:156, 1946.

Cooper, A.: The Anatomy and Surgical Treatment of Inguinal and Congenital Hernia. (1st ed.). London, Longman & Co., 1804.

Keynes, W.: The anatomy and surgery of the supravesical fossa (M.D. Thesis). University of Cambridge, 1954a.

Keynes, W.: Supravesical hernias. In Nyhus, L. M., and Harkins, H. N. (eds.): Hernia. Philadelphia, J. B. Lippincott Co., 1964, pp. 625–636.

Skandalakis, J. E., Gray, S. W., and Akin, J. T., Jr.: The surgical anatomy of hernial rings. Surg. Clin. North Am. 54:1227, 1964.

Skandalakis, J. E., Gray, S. W., Burns, W. B., Sangmalee, U., and Sorg, J. L.: Internal and external supravesical hernia. Ann. Surg. 42:142, 1976.

Tretbar, L. L., and Gustafson, G. E.: Internal supravesical hernia. A rare hernia causing small bowel obstruction. Am. J. Surg. 116:907, 1968.

Walker, I. J.: Hernia into the prevesical space. Ann. Surg. 97:706–712, 1933.

Warvi, W. N., and Orr, T. G.: Internal supravesical hernias. Surgery 8:312, 1940.

Watson, L. F.: Hernia (3rd ed.). St. Louis, C. V. Mosby Co., 1948.

Zimmerman, L. M., and Anson, B. J.: Anatomy and Surgery of Hernia (2nd ed.). Baltimore, Williams & Wilkins Co., 1967.

## Supplemental Reading

Cooper, A.: The Anatomy and Surgical Treatment of Abdominal Hernia (2nd ed.). London, Longman & Co., 1827.

Dixon, A. F., and Birmingham, A.: The peritoneum of the pelvic cavity. J. Anat. 36:127, 1902.

Downing, W.: Supravesical internal hernia. Am. J. Surg. 69:260, 1945.

Moynihan, B. G. A.: The anatomy and pathology of the rarer forms of hernia. Arris and Gale Lectures; Lecture 3: Hernia of the bladder. Lancet 1:596, 1900.

Pearce, A. E., and LaBove, N.: Internal supravesical hernia. Arch. Surg. 69:623, 1954.

Rowe, J. S., Jr., Skandalakis, J. E., and Gray, S. W.: Multiple bilateral inguinal hernias. Ann. Surg. 39:269, 1973.

Sawyers, J. L., and Stephenson, S. E.: Internal supravesical hernia. Surgery 42:368, 1957.

Wakeley, C. P. G.: Hernia of the bladder; its etiology and treatment: Report of 40 cases. Br. J. Urol. 2:1, 1930.

# INTERPARIETAL HERNIAS

## INTRODUCTION

From time to time, the surgeon encounters certain hernias where the sac finds its way into an unusual and unexpected location. In the case of the indirect inguinal hernia, the surgeon can expect to find the sac under the external oblique aponeurosis and within the cremasteric sheath. In the larger hernias, the sac will extend further along the spermatic cord through the external abdominal ring and toward the scrotum.

The sac of an ordinary direct inguinal hernia is found to be essentially free of the cord and under the external oblique aponeurosis. On the other hand, not all hernial sacs occur as expected. In the exceptional case the peritoneal protrusion is located between the various layers of the abdominal wall (Fig. 24–16).

## DEFINITION

An interparietal hernia can be defined as one in which the sac fails to take an expected direction through the abdominal wall, but protrudes between the various laminae of the abdominal wall.

As I have suggested, interparietal hernias, though uncommon, can present in a variety of forms and locations. In my opinion, little will be gained from attempts at complicated and exhaustive classifications of such hernias (Fuld, 1921).

Some of the synonyms for interparietal hernias include intraperitoneal hernia, intermuscular hernia, properitoneal hernia, interstitial hernia, and subcutaneous inguinal hernia.

## HISTORICAL BACKGROUND

Although interstitial hernias have been recognized for over 300 years, full appreciation of such defects is relatively recent. The association of intermuscular hernias with maldescent of the testes has become recognized during the present century.

Watson (1948) gives credit for recognition of interstitial hernias to Bartholin in 1661 and also notes that Petit described an interstitial hernia in 1790. Birkett, according to Watson, recommended in 1861 that the term "interstitial hernia" be applied to these hernias. Kronlein in 1875 and Le-Fort and Kuster in 1886, according to Watson, described anatomic features of inguino-superficial hernias.

Important contributions were made in 1900 by Göbell, who clearly illustrated the various types of interstitial hernias. The next significant contribution was that of Lower and Hicken (1931) who identified 590 cases in the literature. Their illustrations have been used extensively to depict the various types of interparietal hernia. These figures are utilized in a modified form in this chapter.

## VARIOUS TYPES OF INTERPARIETAL HERNIAS

The surgeon who would expect to treat hernias with a substantial degree of suc-

cess must be aware of the variety of interparietal hernias that can be encountered. In this particular section, I wish to direct attention to the position of the peritoneal sac in relation to the layers of the abdominal wall. Such an approach may be criticized as being oversimplistic, but it does lead to ease of understanding. I feel that interstitial hernias can be effectively divided into groups. Such a classification was appreciated by Göbell (1900) and by Lower and Hicken (1931):

1. Preperitoneal (properitoneal), Figure 24–17, A.
2. Interstitial (intermuscular), Figure 24–19, p. 494.
3. Extra-aponeurotic (superficial), Figure 24–20, p. 495.

Lower and Hicken (1931) studied the literature and found the incidence of the various types to be as follows:

| Type | Number | Percent |
|---|---|---|
| Preperitoneal (Properitoneal) | 119 | 19 |
| Interstitial (Intermuscular) | 384 | 61 |
| Extra-aponeurotic (Superficial) | 123 | 20 |

Statistics relative to the incidence of interparietal hernia are scanty. Bull and Coley (1893) reported an incidence of 0.02 percent for the preperitoneal variety. Langton (1900) found the incidence of interstitial hernias to be 0.084 percent, but Noonan (1950) reported the incidence to be 1.2 percent. These statistics probably represent an error on the low side, since surgeons are conditioned by training to recognize direct and indirect inguinal hernias with little anatomic attention given to the pathologic complexity of hernias. Reporting of various types of hernias should be more complete and detailed than it is currently.

## PREPERITONEAL HERNIA

This particular type of interstitial hernia—the preperitoneal hernia—has also been called properitoneal interstitial hernia (Fig. 24–18, A and B). Such hernias are located between the peritoneal layer and transversalis fascia. In some instances, a bilocular sac may be present, with a portion of the sac being interstitial in location. The preperitoneal sac may pass superolat-

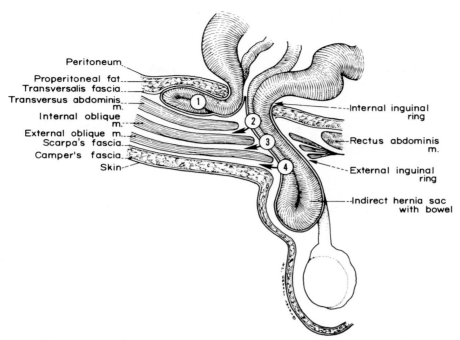

Peritoneum
Properitoneal fat
Transversalis fascia
Transversus abdominis m.
Internal oblique m.
External oblique m.
Scarpa's fascia
Camper's fascia
Skin

Internal inguinal ring
Rectus abdominis m.
External inguinal ring
Indirect hernia sac with bowel

**Figure 24–16.** This composite drawing summarizes the possible paths of protrusion of interparietal hernias. (Reproduced by permission of J. E. Skandalakis and *Surgical Clinics of North America*. From Skandalakis, John E., Gray, S. H., and Akin, J. T., Jr.: The surgical anatomy of hernial rings. Surg. Clin. North Am. *54*:1229, 1974.)

erally toward the anterior superior iliac spine; it may pass posterolaterally toward the iliac fossa; or, less often, it may take a course inferiorly and medially toward the bladder.

Usage has established the preperitoneal type of hernia as an "interstitial" hernia, but actually this portion of the sac has not penetrated the layers of the abdominal wall. It is important to recall that the sac may find its way into the iliac fossa, the inguinal area, the regions of the bladder and pelvis, and even into the femoral region. At the present time, separate classification for the above varieties of preperitoneal hernias hardly seems justified.

**Figure 24–17.** *A* is a preperitoneal interparietal hernia. *B* is a bilocular interstitial hernia. (*A* and *B* reproduced with permission from Anson, B. J., and Maddock, W. G.: *Callendar's Surgical Anatomy*, Philadelphia, W. B. Saunders Co., p. 209.)

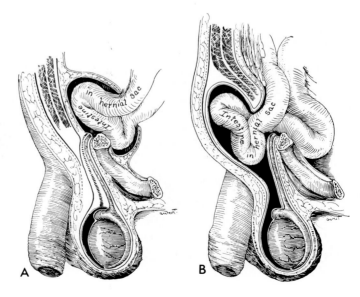

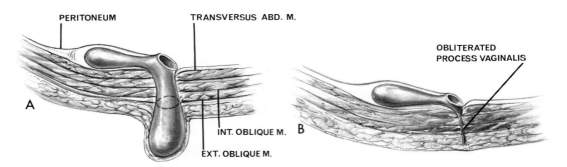

**Figure 24–18.** Preperitoneal types of interparietal hernia: *A*, bilocular; *B*, monolocular. (Reproduced and modified Ann. Surg. *94*:1070, 1931. By permission of J. B. Lippincott Company. Lower, W. E., and Hicken, N. F.: Interparietal hernias.)

## INTERSTITIAL HERNIA

Interstitial hernias compose the largest group of "interparietal" hernias. These hernias are among the most complicated hernias because the sac may find its way into a number of locations between the musculoaponeurotic layers of the abdominal wall. Thus, the sac may be located in a variety of positions between layers of the abdominal wall (Fig. 24–19, *A* and *B*).

The interstitial type of hernia accounts for approximately 60 percent of all interparietal hernias. In approximately three-fourths of the cases, there is some abnormality in either the testis or its descent.

## EXTRA-APONEUROTIC HERNIA

The extra-aponeurotic type of interstitial hernia has been called the inguinosuperficial hernia by Watson (1948). The sac passes through the external abdominal ring and projects toward the anterior superior iliac spine; thus it comes to lie upon the external oblique aponeurosis (Fig. 24–20, *A* and *B*).

## CLINICAL FEATURES

Although most interstitial hernias are described as protrusions occurring in the groin, I have seen a number of hernias where the sac is located under the aponeurosis of the external oblique in incisional hernias. Fisher (1946) encountered such a case in a postappendectomy patient. Macready (1893) recognized, however, that not all interparietal hernias present as obvious protrusions. In properitoneal hernias, the symptoms and signs will be those of intestinal obstruction and its consequences. In the interstitial type, an extra-aponeurotic mass can be palpated. Tenderness at the site of protrusion and intestinal obstruction logically lead to the generally correct diagnosis of incarcerated or strangulated hernia. The experienced surgeon will be prepared for an unusual presentation of the hernia in selected cases. He will entertain the possibility of an interparietal hernia when there is associated malposition of the testis. Interstitial hernias have presented as Spigelian hernias (Altman, 1960).

It is unfortunate that there are no pathognomonic signs and symptoms leading

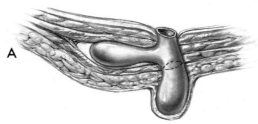
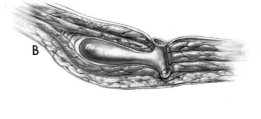

**Figure 24–19.** Interstitial types of interparietal hernia: *A*, Bilocular sac. *B*, monolocular sac. (Reproduced and modified from Lower, W. E., and Hicken, H. F. Interparietal hernias. Ann. Surg. *94*:1070, 1931. By permission of J. B. Lippincott Company.)

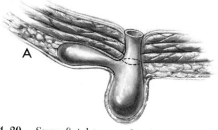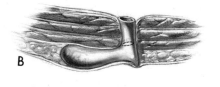

**Figure 24–20.** Superficial types of interparietal hernia: *A*, bilocular sac; *B*, monolocular sac. (Reproduced and modified from Hicken, N. F.: Interparietal hernias. Ann. Surg. 94:1070, 1931. By permission of J. B. Lippincott.)

to the diagnosis of interparietal hernia. Cramping, abdominal pain, distention, vomiting and impaired bowel function—together with a lower abdominal mass—should at least alert the clinician to the possibility. Such a presentation is common among patients with interparietal hernias. In a patient with malposition of the testis, the possibility of an interparietal hernia being present is increased.

The extra-aponeurotic or superficial type of interparietal hernia should be palpable unless the patient is obese.

Masih and colleagues (1971) treated bilateral interstitial hernia in a newborn infant (most unusual).

## TREATMENT

The treatment for interparietal hernias is surgical. The urgent indication for operative intervention is the presence of intestinal obstruction.

In those cases presenting as a mass in the groin, an inguinal incision should be made. Care in making the incision is extremely important if a subcutaneous mass is present. Unusual location of the sac and an abnormally located testis should alert the surgeon to the possible presence of an interstitial hernia.

In a substantial number of cases, the surgeon will enter the abdomen through an incision in the lower abdomen for intestinal obstruction. Upon entry into the abdomen, the surgeon should inspect the entire length of gut. In the preperitoneal variety of interstitial hernia, a portion of bowel will protrude into the sac as an incarcerated loop. The constricting ring is released, and inspection of the bowel will lead to resection if necrosis of the bowel wall is present. At laparotomy, the entire peritoneal surface should be carefully inspected, and any locules or defects repaired.

## SUMMARY

Perhaps the greatest benefit derived from recognition of interstitial or interparietal hernias as special entities is more effective surgical treatment. Identification of these unusual hernias will lead to proper anatomic dissection and effective repair of the defect encountered. The diagnosis is generally made by the operating surgeon. However, the possibility of encountering such hernias is greatest when intestinal obstruction is present along with the hernia.

The surgeon must thoroughly explore and dissect the peritoneal sac until the peritoneal lining of the abdomen has been identified. Such hernias point out the need for opening the hernial sac, which permits identification of unusual locules or configuration of the sac.

The high incidence of intestinal obstruction in patients with interstitial hernias dictates the need for appropriate surgical treatment. Strangulation obstruction, when present, requires resection.

## REFERENCES

Altman, B.: Interstitial hernia presenting as Spigelian hernia. Br. J. Surg. 48:60, 1960.
Bull, W. T., and Coley, W. B.: Observations on the mechanical and operative treatment of hernia at the hospital for ruptured and crippled of New York. Ann. Surg. 17:527, 1933.
Fisher, H. C.: Post-appendectomy interstitial inguinal hernia. Ann. Surg. 123:419, 1946.
Fuld, J. E.: Interparietal inguinal hernia. Int. J. Surg. 34:132, 1921.
Göbell, R.: Ueber interparietale Leistenbrüche. Deutsch. Ztschr. Chirc. 56:1, 1900.

Langton, J.: The association of inguinal hernia with descent of the testis. Lancet 2:1857, 1900.

Lower, W. E., and Hicken, N. F.: Interparietal hernias. Ann. Surg. 94:1070, 1931.

MacReady, J. F. C. H.: A Treatise on Ruptures (1st ed.). London, Blakiston & Co., 1893, p. 147.

Masih, B., Swamy, S., and Altman, B.: Bilateral interstitial hernia in the newborn infant. Surgery 69: 577, 1971.

Noonan, T. J.: Interstitial inguinal hernia. Lancet 2:849, 1950.

Watson, L. F.: Hernia (3rd ed.), St. Louis, C. V. Mosby Co., 1948, pp. 145–160.

## Supplemental Reading

Barling, E. V.: Interparietal hernia. Aust. N. Z., J. Surg. 26:32, 1956.

Beigler, S. K., and O'Brien, H.: Interstitial hernia. Wis. Med. J. 27:407, 1928.

Biasini, A.: Contribution to the study of strangulated inguinoproperitoneal hernia. Int. Abstr. Surg. 88: 338, 1949.

Cattell, R. B., and Aronoff, B. L.: An unusual hernia producing abdominal pain. Surg. Clin. North Am. 24:731, 1944.

DeGarmo, W. B.: Abdominal Hernia: Its Diagnosis and Treatment. Philadelphia, J. B. Lippincott, 1907.

Dickson, A. M.: Interstitial hernia. Am. J. Surg. 72: 186, 1946.

Dunphy, J. E.: Strangulated hernia. A report of two cases in which the sac was found in an unusual position. N. Engl. J. Med. 220:819, 1939.

Godfrey, N. G.: Strangulated interstitial hernia in females. Br. J. Surg. 31:413, 1944.

Golding-Bird, C. H.: Two cases of "hernie-en-bissac" in women, one being also "intraparietal." Trans. Clin. Soc. (London) 17:210, 1884.

Gray, W., and Horwitz, M.: Interstitial ventral hernia involving the small intestine. Am. J. Surg., 66:134, 1944.

Halstead, A. E.: Inguino-properitoneal hernia: Inguino-interstitial hernia: Report of cases. Ann. Surg. 43:704, 1906.

Koontz, A. R., and Stafford, E. S.: Unusual types of interparietal hernia. A.M.A. Arch. Surg. 71:723, 1955.

Koontz, A. R.: Interstitial hernia: A problem in diagnosis. Postgrad. Med. 19:45, 1956.

Russell, R. H.: Inguinal herniae: Their varieties, mode of origin and classification. Br. J. Surg. 9:502, 1922.

Thunig, L. A.: Recurrent incarceration of the left interstitial inguinal hernia. Am. J. Surg. 62:105, 1943.

Wilensky, A. O., and Gordon, J. A.: A case of interstitial hernia. Am. J. Surg. 45:330, 1939.

# REDUCTION OF HERNIA "EN MASSE"

There is a rare and unusually deceptive type of hernia, the clinical presentation of which is of an incarcerated hernia that, upon manipulation, appears to have been reduced. Actually, the incarcerated bowel and hernial sac are displaced into the abdominal cavity, and a loop of bowel remains incarcerated in the peritoneal sac. This entity results from what has been designated as "en masse" reduction. Some surgeons question this explanation of displacement, feeling that it is a variant of interparietal hernia. Lower and Hicken (1931) concurred in this opinion.

## DEFINITION

Reduction of hernia "en masse" refers to reduction of the external herniation with continued incarceration or strangulation of the initially prolapsed intestine. The most commonly reported instances of such complicated consequences following hernial reduction involve inguinal and femoral hernias. Querna (1969) reported two cases of reduction "en masse" occurring at femoral hernial sites.

## HISTORICAL BACKGROUND

Pearse (1962) reviewed the early history of hernias complicated by "en masse" reduction, noting that Saviard in 1702 reported a case in which a postmortem examination of the patient revealed that reduction of a strangulated femoral hernia had failed to achieve relief of the obstruction—despite what appeared to be a successful, although difficult, reduction of the hernia.

Pearse also noted that one case was subsequently reported by Le Dran in 1727, and in 1765 DeLafage added two more cases of "en masse" reduction to the literature.

Even as recently as 1859, Birkett was able to collect only 37 cases. He described a case in which posterior rupture of the sac occurred with displacement of the strangulated bowel posterior to the symphysis.

By 1941 Casten and Bodenheimer found that 205 cases of this entity had been reported. Barker and Smiddy (1970) noted that few additional cases were reported since that time—citing those of Coles (1941), Cooley (1942), Crowe (1943),

Chapple (1951), Bailie (1953), Millard (1955), Murdoch (1958), and Renton (1962). Also, Mings and Olson reported four successfully treated cases in 1965, and Wright and colleagues reported a single case, which was well documented, in 1977.

## INCIDENCE

In spite of the rare occurrence of reduction of a hernia "en masse," too many cases have been recorded to doubt their existence. I have personally seen two cases; one was associated with an inguinal hernia and the other with a femoral hernia. Pearse estimated the incidence to be approximately one in over 13,000 hernias, for a percent rate of .0077. It is easy to understand why most surgeons may not see a single case in their professional lifetime.

## PATHOLOGY

Differences of opinion as to the precise circumstances and events that result in "reductio-en-masse" following certain incarcerated hernias are recorded in the literature. According to Moynihan (1906), what really happened in such cases was that the incarcerated mass was reduced by taxis into the properitoneal sac of a bilocular hernial sac. Pearse held a similar view.

Casten and Bodenheimer (1941) felt that in the presence of both a weak internal ring and a small, scarred, firm, and unyielding sac, any incarcerated mass could be forced into the preperitoneal space. Nason and Mixter (1935) pointed out that the opening of the hernial sac must be large enough to permit entry of the viscera. The viscera are then trapped in a narrowed and firm ring, which prevents reduction of the contents.

Pearse illustrated a type of "reductio-en-masse" of hernia in which there was actual avulsion of the sac with displacement of the incarcerated mass into the peritoneal cavity. Such reduction must be extremely rare and would require more force than most of us would be willing to exert upon an incarcerated mass.

It is important to be aware that a hernial mass can be reduced into the preperitoneal space without eliminating the actual obstruction. Such hernial sacs may be found posterior to the pubis, in the abdominal cavity, or in the preperitoneal space. It might be well to think of such incarcerated hernias as "relocated" rather than as "reduced."

Barker and Smiddy illustrated clearly the concepts of reduction "en masse." In Figure 24–21, A, such reduction of a bilocular hernia is illustrated. The incarcerated external hernial mass was reduced into the preperitoneal pouch and space (Fig. 24–21, B).

The type of "reductio-en-masse" that I encountered in two cases is shown in Figure 24–22. The hernial sac and contents were reduced "en masse" into the abdominal cavity. Casten and Bodenheimer in 1941 offered such an explanation for "en masse" reduction of hernias.

Moss and coworkers (1976) reported an extremely unusual case of a sliding colonic Maydl's hernia. A double loop of colon was entrapped in a hernial ring (Fig. 24–23, A). The colon remained in the abdomen, forming a closed loop. A descriptive term for such a hernia is "hernia en-W," so called because of its configuration (Fig. 24–23, B). Any one of the loops may undergo strangulation.

## CLINICAL FEATURES

It is true that hernias associated with "en masse" reduction are rare; however, they do occur. When these hernias are overlooked, the results can be disastrous.

The patient will initially present with evidence of an incarcerated inguinal or femoral hernia. Furthermore, the visible protrusion will have been reduced. This might occur prior to admission to the hospital through efforts at reduction by the patient. Pearse, however, found that 60 percent of the hernial masses were reduced by the physician. Both hernia cases that I was involved in were reduced in the hospital.

Ordinarily, following successful reduction of an incarcerated hernia, improvement is prompt and continuous. However, with reduction "en masse," pain continues or recurs (as a colicky type of pain). Vomiting, constipation, and abdominal distention are symptoms caused by obstruction of the intestinal lumen.

Tenderness or palpable abdominal mass

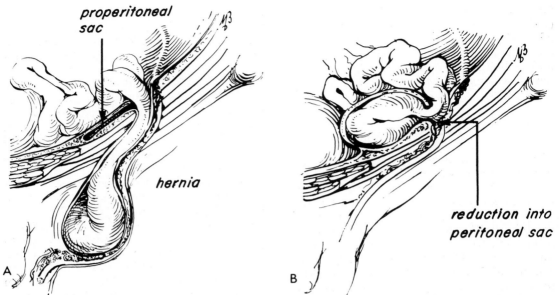

**Figure 24–21.** *A*, Bilocular hernia sac as illustrated by Barker and Smiddy. Such conditions permit reduction-en-masse. *B*, Location of hernias shown in *A*, into the preperitoneal site. (Reprinted from Barker, K., and Smiddy, F. G.: Mass reduction of inguinal hernia. Br. J. Surg. 57[4]:265 [April], 1974.)

or both may be present, depending on the type of hernia and on whether or not gangrene has developed. At this point, there is no evidence of an incarcerated external hernia. The presence of peritonitis suggests gangrene or perforation.

## X-RAY EXAMINATION

Any patient failing to improve following reduction of a hernia deserves x-ray studies of the abdomen. Dilated loops of small bowel with air-fluid levels will indicate the presence of an obstruction. The possibility of an "en masse" reduction of the hernia should then occur to the surgeon. In addition to the above evidences of obstruction, the surgeon should specifically look for a possible closed loop obstruction.

It is hardly necessary to perform barium studies in every case, but Parvey and coworkers found such studies helpful in an unusual case. In this case, although spontaneous reduction had occurred three years earlier, symptoms of obstruction led to roentgenographic studies, which revealed air-fluid levels. The authors sought additional information and performed barium studies of the small bowel, which demonstrated dilated small intestinal loops and

barium entering a small knuckle of ileum. Such information suggested the need for surgical intervention, and at operation a ring of thickened peritoneum was found to

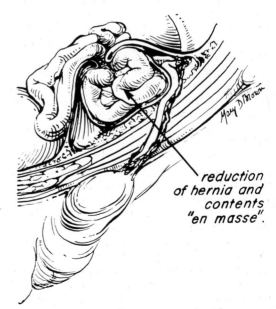

**Figure 24–22.** Another variety of reduction-en-masse of an inguinal hernia. Here the sac and contents are reduced into the abdominal cavity. (Reproduced from Barker, K., and Smiddy, F. G.: Mass reduction of inguinal hernia. Br. J. Surg. 57[4]:256 [April], 1974.)

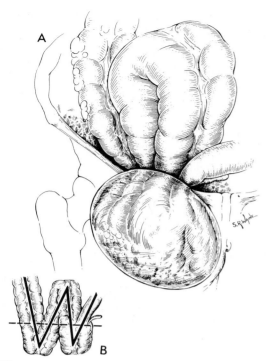

**Figure 24–23.** An unusual type of hernia in which a partial reduction is possible. *A*, Operative findings showing herniated cecum and colon. *B*, Maydl's hernia or "hernia en-W". (Reproduced by permission of author. From Moss, C. M., et al.: Sliding colonic Maydl's hernia. Dis. Colon Rectum *19*:637, 1976.)

be constricting an ischemic loop of ileum. The patient did well postoperatively. In my opinion, however, barium studies of the upper gastrointestinal tract could complicate the operative procedure in the presence of gangrene.

## TREATMENT

The treatment consists of prompt surgical reduction of the hernia and resection of gangrenous or seriously compromised bowel. The operative approach will vary depending on the circumstances faced by the surgeon. In two of my cases—one inguinal and one femoral hernia—the inguinal approach proved adequate. It was necessary to open the transversalis fascia in the floor of Hesselbach's triangle and incise the constricted ring in both cases. The incarcerated bowel was released, and re-

section was unnecessary. Both hernias were repaired by the Lotheissen-McVay technique.

Pearse noted that the inguinal incision was used in 76 percent, a rectus or midline incision in 18 percent; and in 6 percent, a combined inguinal and abdominal incision was necessary.

Wright and colleagues (1977) pointed out the advantages of a preperitoneal approach to hernias reduced "en masse." They observed that it was possible to visualize the hernial sac, resect the compromised bowel, and perform an anatomic repair.

## MORTALITY

There is currently no existing reason to justify a mortality of 70 percent in femoral hernias and 40 percent in inguinal hernias, as reported by Pearse. Surgeons are increasingly aware of the phenomenon of "reductio-en-masse." Prompt surgical intervention should result in survival for all but those cases involving neglected coexistent serious systemic diseases. In the cases being reported in current literature—such as those of Wright and colleagues (1977), Barker and Smiddy (1970), and Parvey and colleagues (1974)—survival is the rule. The key to improved results is prompt recognition, followed by expeditious surgical correction of the defect.

## SUMMARY

The reduction of hernia "en masse" occurs infrequently. It is dangerous to assume that once a hernial mass is reduced, it is no longer a problem. The reduced mass may continue as an obstructing hernia, or it may contain gangrenous bowel. It is most commonly located in the preperitoneal location.

Continued abdominal pain, vomiting, and distention should indicate the possibility of this rare type of hernia. A high index of suspicion that the problem might be due to "reductio-en-masse" will lead to further diagnostic efforts and prompt surgical correction of the defect.

Roentgen films of the abdomen are helpful when they show evidence of ileus or mechanical obstruction of the small bowel.

Prompt surgical correction of this rare type of hernia should result in a favorable outcome in nearly every case.

## REFERENCES

Barker, K., and Smiddy, F. G.: Mass reduction of inguinal hernia; description of a new physical sign of diagnostic value and aetiological significance. Br. J. Surg. 57(4):264, 1970.

Birkett, J.: Inquiry into the nature of those cases of strangulated oblique inguinal hernia termed "Reduction En Bloc Ou En Masse"; with special relation to the anatomy of the actual lesion and practical deductions derived from an examination of the cases. Med. Chir. Trans. 42:247, 1859.

Casten, P., and Bodenheimer, M.: Strangulated hernia reduced en masse. Surgery 9:561, 1941.

Lower, W. E., and Hicken, N. F.: Interparietal hernias. Ann. Surg. 94:1070, 1931.

Mings, H., and Olson, J. D.: Reduction "en masse" of groin hernia. Arch. Surg. 90:764–769, 1965.

Moss, C. M., Levine, R., Messenger, N., and Dardik, I.: Sliding colonic Maydl's hernia: Report of a case. Dis. Col. Rect. 19:636, 1976.

Moynihan, B. G. A.: Reduction of hernia en masse. Br. Med. J. 1:435, 1906.

Nason, L. H., and Mixter, C. C.: Hernia reduced en masse. J.A.M.A. 105:1675, 1935.

Parvey, L. S., Himmelfarb, E., and Rabinowitz, J.: Spontaneous reduction of hernia "en masse." Am. J. Roent. Radium Ther. Nucl. Med. 20(1):28, 1974.

Pearse, J. E.: Strangulated hernia en masse. Surg. Gynecol. Obstet. 1:1671, 1962.

Querna, M. H.: Reduction of hernia "en masse" Am. J. Surg. 118:539, 1969.

Wright, R. N., Arensman, R. M., Coughlin, T. F., and Nyhus, L. M.: Hernia reduction en masse. Am. Surg. 43(9):627, 1977.

## Supplemental Reading

Blackman, G. C.: On the reduction of strangulated hernia "en masse" or "en bloc". Am. J. Med. Sc. 12:336, 1846.

Levack, J. H.: En masse reduction of strangulated hernia. Br. J. Surg. 50:582, 1962.

Renton, C. J. C.: Reduction en masse of direct inguinal hernia. Br. Med. J. 1:1671, 1962.

# LITTRE'S HERNIA

*It is to rupture that contains a Meckel's process that the term Littre's hernia should alone be applied.*

*Treves, 1887*

Littre's hernia (1700) merits some discussion here because of its historical interest and specificity. The finding of a single case of this type of hernia is distinction enough to warrant publication, and surgeons regularly succumb to the urge to do so. I, too, am anxious to add one more case to the literature (Fig. 24–24).

## DEFINITION

In Littre's hernia, a Meckel's diverticulum—including the contiguous ileum—is the only viscus within the hernial sac. The term "hernia of Meckel's diverticulum" is cumbersome; hence, Littre's hernia is the preferred designation.

## HISTORICAL BACKGROUND

Although there was some early confusion as to what constituted a Littre's hernia,

Treves in 1887 clearly identified this entity. According to Treves, Littre described what he called a new form of hernia in 1700. He presented two instances in which Meckel's diverticula found their way into hernial sacs (Fig. 24–25).

Stahl (1897) located an unusual illustration of Littre's first case (1699) of hernia and Meckel's diverticulum (Fig. 24–25). This drawing is of such interest that I have reproduced it here. Littre referred to the diverticulum itself as "appendice de l'intestin ileon."

It is important to recognize that the congenital diverticulum bearing the name of Meckel was not described by him until 1809. According to Treves, the diverticulum was discovered in hernial sacs by Mery in 1701, Wrisburg in 1797, Gunz in 1744, Ruysch in 1707, and Morgagni in 1741. To further clarify the differentiation between a Littre's hernia and a partial enterocele, Richter described a specific type of hernia in 1785 in which a portion

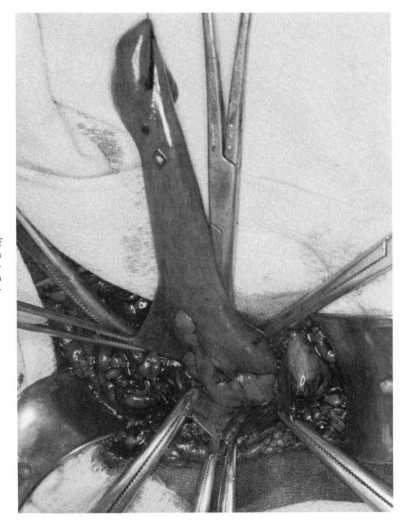

**Figure 24-24.** Photograph of Meckel's diverticulum which presented at an indirect inguinal hernial sac. Note location of diverticulum on antimesenteric side of the ileum.

the bowel wall was either incarcerated or strangulated or both. Thus, by 1809, the pathologic anatomy of Littre's and Richter's hernias was appreciated by the surgical cognoscenti.

Mason (1933) gave an interesting account of the life of Littre (also known as de Litre). Littre was an excellent teacher and studied anatomy when "sentimental and legal barriers to dissecting abounded." Police permits were necessary for dissection. Littre made the appropriate acquaintances, and he and a friend dissected over 200 subjects during the long and cold winter of 1684.

Watson reviewed the history in considerable detail. By 1946 he had collected 259 cases reported in the literature.

## INCIDENCE

The appearance of a Meckel's diverticulum is an unusual experience for both the patient and the surgeon. The incidence of Meckel's diverticula has been reported to range from 1.1 to 4.5 percent. Gray and Skandalakis (1972) noted that in a collected autopsy series, Meckel's diverticula were found in 1.1 to 2.5 percent; but during appendectomy, the incidence increased, ranging from 2.0 to 4.5 percent. Zimmerman and Anson (1967) estimated that the incidence of all types of hernias ranged from 3 to 8 percent. The likelihood of a hernia and a Meckel's diverticulum occurring in the same individual is small; the

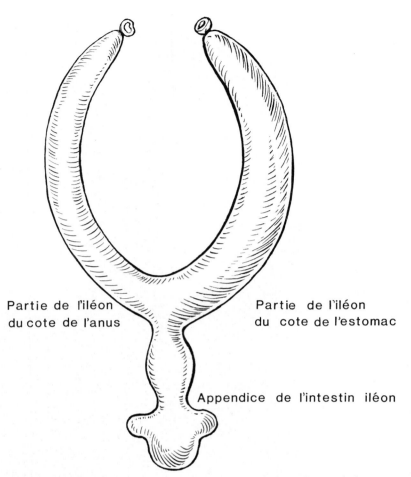

Partie de l'iléon
du cote de l'anus

Partie de l'iléon
du cote de l'estomac

Appendice de l'intestin iléon

**Figure 24–25.** This illustration of Littre's first case in 1699 is taken from the article by F. A. Stahl. Note the interesting terminology used to describe the components. (Reproduced and modified by permission of J.A.M.A. From Stahl, F. A.: Acute partial enterocele. J.A.M.A. 2:687, 1897.)

possibility of a Meckel's process finding its way into a hernial sac is remote.

The combination of hernia and Meckel's diverticulum has been reported in infants, adults, and geriatric patients. The inci-

#### Table 24–8. LITTRE'S HERNIAS— INCIDENCE IN VARIOUS TYPES OF HERNIAS*

| Author | Site | Percent |
|--------|------|---------|
| Watson (1948) | Inguinal | 50 |
| Davis (1954) | Inguinal | 50 |
| Watson (1948) | Umbilical | 25 to 30 |
| Gray (1934) | Femoral | 25 to 30 |

*Other sites include: incisional hernia, Keeley (1937); femoral hernia, Weinstein et al. (1938); umbilical, Kremer and Morton (1938), Goni-Moreno (1941); sciatic, Brodnax (1924).

dence in infants is quite low. Watson found only four cases in infants up to one week following birth. The majority of reported Littre's hernias were seen in adults and older individuals.

Frankau (1931) identified 5 Littre's hernias among 1487 strangulated hernias, for an incidence of 0.3 percent. This was based on a highly selected group of patients who had not only incarceration but strangulation as well.

### ANATOMIC AND PATHOLOGICAL FEATURES

A Meckel's diverticulum is the result of incomplete obliteration of the omphalo-mesenteric duct. It is due specifically to persistence of the abdominal part of the vitelline duct and is named after Johann Frederick Meckel, who described it in 1809. This congenital diverticulum is located on the antimesenteric portion of the ileum and is situated between 30 and 130 centimeters from the ileocecal valve. The outpouching varies in size and shape. It may appear as a shallow, wide-mouthed diverticulum; or it may be long, narrow, and fingerlike, measuring up to ten centimeters in length. A true diverticulum, it is made up of mucosal, submucosal, muscularis, and serosal layers.

It is important to recall that a Meckel's diverticulum may contain ectopic pancreatic tissue and gastric or duodenal mucosa. Bleeding, perforation, and ulceration of the diverticulum are complications that arise due to the presence of such aberrantly located epithelium.

Other complications that might occur as a result of the Meckel's diverticulum include intestinal obstruction and inflammation of the diverticulum.

Gray and Skandalakis (1972) state that 15 percent of obstructions attributable to Meckel's diverticulum are the result of incarceration of such diverticula in hernial sacs.

The significant occurrence of Littre's hernia in women has been recognized by Zuniga and Zupanec (1977). This observation is consistent with the prevalence of femoral hernias in females. Zuniga and Zupanec felt that over 50 percent of recently reported Littre's hernias are located at the femoral hernial site.

Gray (1934) found that approximately one-third of such hernias appeared at the femoral ring. Sweet (1930), Strohl and McArthur (1939), and Kanazawa and co-workers (1972) also reported similar cases.

The unusual occurrence of a Littre's hernia at the site of an incisional hernia was reported by Keeley (1937) and by Payson and colleagues (1956).

## TREATMENT

The urgent problems in the treatment of Littre's hernia are intestinal obstruction and peritonitis, when present. Management of obstruction by nasogastric intubation and fluid replacement are the first steps to take. Administration of antibiotics is indicated by the presence of infection.

It is important to identify the type of hernia present. When the diverticulum is encountered, resection is in order. A long narrow diverticulum may be excised with closure of the base. I approximate the mucosal layer with number 3–0 chromic catgut placed as a continuous interlocking suture. Then, serosa to serosal closure is completed with interrupted Lembert sutures of number 4–0 silk. Inspection of the problem might demand resection of a portion of the ileum along with the diverticulum if simple excision is contraindicated by the presence of gangrene and inflammation at the diverticular site.

In the patient whom I operated on for Littre's hernia, the presenting problem appeared to be an incarcerated inguinal hernia. The long Meckel's diverticulum was excised, and transverse closure was possible. The indirect inguinal hernia was repaired successfully by the modified Bassini technique.

## Results

In my opinion the results obtained following repair of Littre's hernias should approximate those obtained generally in repair of comparable hernias.

Watson, in a collected series of 124 cases, reported 13 deaths, for a mortality of 10 percent. In my opinion, the significant number of deaths can no longer be justified. This high mortality, however, can be explained. Three cases were treated prior to 1948—when antibiotic therapy was not yet available—for complications resulting from intestinal strangulation.

## SUMMARY

There are no pathognomonic signs and symptoms leading to the diagnosis of Littre's hernia. The presence of an incarcerated hernia, which is also accompanied by evidence of local inflammation, should alert the surgeon to the presence of an unusual hernia. In the differential diagnosis, a Richter's hernia or the presence of the appendix in the sac must be considered. At the time of the operation, it is important to recognize the problem and resect the diverticulum.

## REFERENCES

Brodnax, J. W.: Hernia of Meckel's diverticulum through the greater sciatic foramen. J.A.M.A. 82: 440, 1924.

Davis, C. E., Jr.: Littre's hernia. Ann. Surg. 139:370, 1954.

Frankau, C.: Strangulated hernia: a review of 1487 cases. Br. J. Surg. 19:176, 1931.

Goni-Moreno, L.: Prolapso umbilical del diverticulo de Meckel. Arch. Argent. Enferm. Apar. Dig. Nutr. 17:72, 1941.

Gray, H. K.: Meckel's diverticulum in hernia: Report of a case. Minn. Med. 17:68, 1934.

Gray, S. W., and Skandalakis, J. E.: Embryology for Surgeons. Philadelphia, W. B. Saunders Co., 1972, pp. 156–167.

Kanazawa, K., Ishikawa, K., Shoji, R., and Okamoto, A.: Littre's femoral hernia causing intestinal fistula. Jap. J. Surg. 2(1):37, 1972.

Keeley, J. L.: Meckel's diverticulum in sac of ventral incisional hernia. Wisc. Med. J., 36:733, 876, 1937.

Kremer, R. M., and Morton, J. H.: Strangulated Littre's umbilical hernia. Am. Surg. 34(6):432, 1968.

Littre, A.: Observation sur une nouvelle espèce de hernie. Mem. Acad. R. Sc. Paris, pp. 300–310, 1700.

Mason, G.: Note on association of Meckel's diverticulum with hernia. Newcastle Med. J. 13:73, 1933.

Meckel, J. F.: Uber die divertikel am darmkanal. Arch. Physiol. Riel. Autenreith 9:421, 1809.

Payson, B. A., Schneider, K. M., and Victor, M. B.: Strangulation of a Meckel's diverticulum in a femoral hernia (Littre's). Ann. Surg. 144:277, 1956.

Richter, A. G.: Abhandlung von den Brüchen Göttingen. J. C. Dieterich, 1785.

Stahl, F. A.: Acute partial enterocele. J.A.M.A. 2:683, 1897.

Strohl, E. L., and McArthur, S. W.: Incarcerated Meckel's diverticulum in femoral hernia. Arch. Surg. 38:783, 1939.

Sweet, R. H.: Incarceration of a Meckel's diverticulum in a femoral hernia. N. Engl. J. Med. 202:997, 1930.

Traves, F.: Richter's hernia or partial enterocele. Med. Chir. Trans. 52:149, 1887.

Watson, L. F.: Hernia (3rd ed.). St. Louis, C. V. Mosby Co., 1948, pp. 547–554.

Weinstein, B. M.: Strangulated Littre's femoral hernia with spontaneous fecal fistula. Ann. Surg. 108:1076, 1938.

Zimmerman, L. M., and Anson, B. J.: Anatomy and Surgery of Hernia. (2nd ed.). Baltimore, Williams and Wilkins Co., 1967, pp. 15–21.

Zuniga, D., and Zupanec, R.: Littre hernia. J.A.M.A. 237:1599, 1977.

### Supplemental Reading

Dent, C. T.: A case of strangulated hernia (Littre's) or partial enterocele. Trans. Clin. Soc. London 15:16, 1882.

Dunn, T. M., and Markgraf, W. H.: Littre hernia—incarcerated Meckel's diverticulum. Am. J. Surg. 103:144, 1962.

Goodman, B. A.: Meckel's diverticulum. Arch. Surg. 36:144, 1938.

Haber, J. J.: Meckel's diverticulum. Review of literature and analytical study of twenty-three cases with particular emphasis on bowel obstruction. Am. J. Surg. 73:480, 1947.

Krausz, M., Rubin, S., and Schiller, M.: Infantile strangulated Littre's hernia with a gangrenous homolateral testis: Report of a case. Aust. N. Z. J. Surg. 44:45, 1974.

Lind, S. W.: A Meckel's diverticulum in a hernia sac. Ohio State Med. J. 29:549, 1933.

Lium, R., and Ladd, S. T.: Left inguinal hernia with acute Meckel's diverticulitis and peritonitis. New Engl. J. Med. 226:15, 1942.

Matt, J. G., and Timpane, P. J.: Peptic ulcer of Meckel's diverticulum: Case report and review of the literature. Am. J. Surg. 47:612, 1940.

Meyerowitz, B. R.: Littre's hernia. Br. Med. J. 1:1154, 1958.

Moses, W. B.: Meckel's diverticulum: Report of two unusual cases. New Engl. J. Med. 237:118, 1947.

Wollgast, G. F., and Hilz, J. M.: Littre's hernia: strangulation of Meckel's diverticulum in a femoral and inguinal hernia. Am. Surg. 28:841, 1962.

# GASTROSCHISIS

A controversy exists even to the present time as to the precise nature and genesis of gastroschisis as an entity. It is to be noted that the term "gastroschisis" was formerly an all-inclusive one—being applied in the early part of this century to all types of developmental wall defects (with the exception of hernia into the umbilical cord). A careful search of the Cumulative Index Medicus, covering a 40-year period, revealed that recognition of gastroschisis as an entity is a comparatively recent development.

According to Shaw (1975), Ballantyne in 1904 collected so many cases of "gastroschisis" that the task of compiling them was a difficult one. However, once the term was redefined by Moore and Stokes (1953), somewhat fewer cases appeared to meet the specifications recorded. Also, another facet of the problem stemmed from a misunderstanding, or erroneous interpretation, of the development of the abdominal wall.

To be noted is the scarcity of early published reports, suggesting an ambiguous conception of the defect. Cullen in his exhaustive volume, Diseases of the Umbilicus (1916), does not even mention gastroschisis in the index. And, although Iason (1941) does refer to "gastroschisis completa"—using the word once in his massive volume—he does not describe the entity that is currently accepted as gastroschisis. In an early publication on gastroschisis, Phineas Berstein in 1940 referred to the defect as a rare teratologic condition in the newborn. He found reference to the word *gastroschisis* in only 6 of the 34 references he used. In 1946, Johns called attention to the defect and other anomalies in a paper entitled "Congenital Defects of the Abdominal Wall in the Newborn"; in parenthesis after the title, he added the term "gastroschisis." He compiled 97 assorted articles on the subject. Gross, in his volumes on surgery of infancy and childhood, did not include the word "gastroschisis" in the index. Watson (1948) also failed to include the word "gastroschisis" in the index of his works. In 1964, Nyhus and Harkins included in their book a chapter by Thomas C. Moore on the subject of gastroschisis.

## DEFINITION

There is no doubt in my mind that defects such as gastroschisis were recognized for many years, but the terminology required refinement. As pointed out by Johns, such terms as "abdominal fissure," "agenesis of the abdominal wall," "eventration," "amniotic hernia," and "ectopia intestinalis" were all applied to gastroschisis, and, of course, the relationship of gastroschisis to omphalocele is still unresolved.

In view of the fact that the term "gastroschisis" is now firmly established in surgical literature, some attempt at definition is in order. As previously stated, Schuster felt that some of the confusion resulted from an incomplete understanding or erroneous interpretation of the development of the abdominal wall.

Gastroschisis can be defined as a developmental defect of the periumbilical abdominal wall, characterized by prolapse of viscera (usually small intestine) through a defect to the right of the umbilical cord, which is separated from the cord by a bridge of skin. Significantly, there is no sac present, but the foreshortened intestines are covered with a thickened, adherent gelatinous material.

The gross features of hernia into the umbilical cord, omphalocele, and gastroschisis are illustrated in Figure 24–26, A–C.

In hernia into the umbilical cord (Fig. 24–26, A), the intestine remains prolapsed through a small midline defect, usually under 4 centimeters in diameter. The intestine is covered by amniotic membrane. Skin of the abdominal wall is normal and adequate and extends up to the margin of the defect where it is contiguous with the amniotic membrane. These features were pointed out by Benson and coworkers in 1949.

In omphalocele, the defect in the abdominal wall is usually larger than 4 centimeters; and prolapsed viscera, including intestine and other abdominal organs, are covered by a transparent membrane (Fig. 24–26, B). The covering consists of peritoneum and amniotic membrane. The umbilical cord is attached to the apical part of the protruded mass. In hernia into the umbilical cord, the peritoneal cavity is well developed, but in omphalocele it is frequently too small to allow replacement of the viscera without creating greatly increased pressure on the major abdominal vessels and elevation of the diaphragm.

Gastroschisis must be differentiated from ruptured hernia into the umbilical cord or omphalocele (Fig. 24–26, C). The defect in the abdominal wall appears to be independent of the umbilical cord and lies to the right of it. The defect is separated from the umbilical cord by a bridge of epithelium. There is no hernial sac or amniotic membrane over the viscera, usually intestine. The thickened, apparently foreshortened, bowel is covered by a thick, gelatinous material. This causes adherence of the intestinal loops, one to the other. The peritoneal cavity is somewhat better developed than that seen in omphalocele, but it may still be too small to permit visceral replacement and closure of the abdominal wall defect. Infarction of the prolapsed bowel occurs in the occasional case.

## HISTORICAL BACKGROUND

It is practical to divide the historical developments dealing with gastroschisis into two periods—early and current. Unfortunately, the early history is one

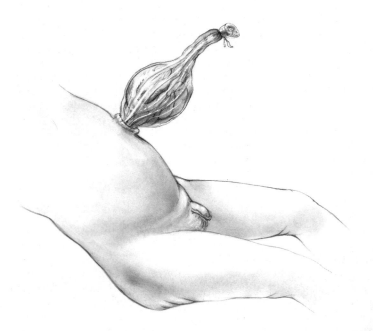

**Figure 24–26.** *A,* The important features of hernia into the umbilical cord; *B,* large omphalocele with intact membrane. *C,* In gastroschisis, the extruded mass is covered with a gelatinous material, and the umbilicus is usually located to the left of the defect.

**A.** Hernia into the Umbilical Cord

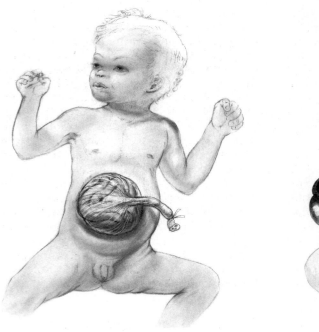

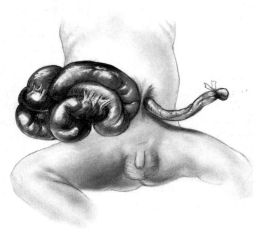

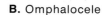

**B.** Omphalocele                                                    **C.** Gastroschisis

clouded by incomplete descriptions of infants with numerous anomalies. Bernstein (1940) stated that Lycostenes described such a case in Chronicon in 1557 in which the infant was severely deformed with numerous defects. By 1946, Johns had identified 96 case reports dealing with the subject of gastroschisis. He divided the infants being studied into three groups. Sixty-eight cases were considered in Group 1, consisting of stillborn monstrosities. In Group 2, 19 infants were alive and normal at birth except for abdominal wall defects, and surgical repair was not attempted. All of these infants, according to Johns, died of peritonitis, gangrene, pneumonia, dehydration, and "exhaustion." I would like to emphasize that in modern practice, these individual and collective complications can be treated successfully. Also, because of the ability to provide effective preoperative and operative treatment, increasing numbers of cases are being reported. In Group 3, Johns included those cases in whom attempts at repair were undertaken; six of nine infants survived operation. In this group, he identified cases treated successfully by Hogue (1882), Benedect (1892), Caffer (1929), Gamble (1930), Watkins (1943), and his own case, reported in 1946.

The current or modern period of understanding of gastroschisis began in 1953, when Moore and Stokes identified only five cases in the literature. They called attention to an entity that simply had not yet been clearly defined prior to their observations. It is also appropriate to emphasize that modern advances in the science of medicine have made effective surgical treatment of gastroschisis a possibility.

Important developments that preceded progress in the surgical treatment of gastroschisis are:

1. Improved physiologic knowledge of prematurity in infants and neonates. Definition of fluid and electrolyte needs in such infants was accomplished through the efforts of innumerable pediatricians, pediatric surgeons, and neonatologists. Definition of unstable thermoregulatory mechanisms in those infants, with emphasis on the importance of proper environmental temperature and moisture.

2. Effective methods of ventilatory support developing from an awareness of the fact that forced replacement of viscera into a small peritoneal cavity seriously interfered with circulatory and respiratory function.
3. Effective methods of intravenous feeding, sustaining the infant until ileus abated.
4. Effective antibiotic therapy.
5. Manufacture of inert materials for protection of the viscera during that period of time required to permit enlargement of the peritoneal cavity through growth.
6. Need for immediate postpartum protection of infant's viscera by a protective covering over sterile saline-soaked gauze.
7. Isolettes to provide ideal environments during transport to specialized treatment centers prepared to manage such precarious problems.
8. Recognition of need for individualization of surgical correction of gastroschisis: primary repair, closure after manual stretching of the abdominal wall, closure with widely fashioned skin flaps, and use of silos or pouches of plastic materials have all been employed.

## EMBRYOLOGY

Complete satisfaction with the explanation of developmental events resulting in gastroschisis has not been achieved, since some uncertainty still exists as to whether or not omphalocele and gastroschisis are caused by the same developmental aberration. Margulies (1945) and Duhamel (1963) explained a small omphalocele or hernia into the umbilical cord as being due to incomplete return of the intestine into the peritoneal cavity after its normal earlier sojourn into the extra-embryonic celom. The abdominal wall develops normally in these cases; and the defect, usually less than four centimeters, lies between the rectus abdominis muscles, which are normal. The failure of closure of the umbilical ring is secondary to the herniation. Hernia into the umbilical cord is described in detail and illustrated in Figure 22–14, page 420. Gross and Blodgett (1940) felt that omphalocele resulted from arrested development of the abdominal cavity during the third month of gestation. Ladd and Gross, however, in 1941 concluded that omphalocele was a consequence of maldevelopment of the abdominal wall itself.

Margulies in 1945 pointed out that development of the abdominal wall is nearly complete during the third week of fetal life. It is generally appreciated that after ten weeks, the growth of the abdominal cavity is rapid, permitting the abdominal viscera to return into the peritoneal cavity. On the other hand, should some event lead to interference with normal development of the abdominal wall before the third week, the subsequent return of the midgut is modified. The well-known fact that omphaloceles are accompanied by numerous associated anomalies suggests that interference with development of the embryo occurs early in fetal life. Fewer such associated abnormalities occur with gastroschisis than with omphalocele, suggesting gastroschisis occurs later in the period of embryogenesis.

Irving and Rickham (1978) compiled an impressive list of anomalies associated with omphalocele. In 145 cases they found 323 abnormalities: gastrointestinal abnormalities in 115 (79 percent), craniofacial abnormalities in 75 (45 percent), genitourinary abnormalities in 56 (39 percent), and cardiovascular abnormalities in 43 (30 percent). Such evidence strongly supports early and complicated disruption of developmental processes during embryonic growth.

From the embryologic point of view, gastroschisis has not lent itself to simple explanation even though the defect in the abdominal wall is not large. Hernia into the umbilical cord and omphalocele, in contrast, are more easily comprehensible and demonstrable as developmental abnormalities. There is agreement among embryologists, pediatricians, and pediatric surgeons on the embryogenesis of hernia into the umbilical cord and exomphalos; however, gastroschisis has not been explained to the satisfaction of all interested observers. In the case of gastroschisis, we seem to be trying to explain a final event by conjecture and speculation.

Duhamel in 1963 stated that exomphalos results in the embryo from a disturbance of the vital mechanism of body closure. He applied the term *celosomia* to defects arising from improper development of abdominal folds. Where there is failure of development of the cephalic fold with its splanchnic layer, complicated anomalies (such as that reported by Cantrell, Haller, and Ravitch in 1968) result in the absence of the thoracoabdominal wall, leading to ectopia cordis. Sternal defects, diaphragmatic defects, and omphalocele are present in such cases. Failure in caudal fold development and its splanchnic layer results in a variety of abnormalities that can involve the hindgut, bladder, and lower abdominal wall. Failure of lateral folds to develop results in exomphalos.

Duhamel (1963) stated that in gastroschisis there is a teratogenic action that prevents differentiation of the embryonic mesenchyme. He further stated that once the ectoblastic layer is deprived of its mesenchymal support, it is resorbed. He noted that when the ectoblastic layer of the somatopleure is thus resorbed gastroschisis results.

Moore and Stokes (1953) postulated that it is possible for the defect of gastroschisis to result from a distortion or interference with ventral extension of the myotomes in this area. The views on embryogenesis of gastroschisis noted by Duhamel (1963) and by Lewis and colleagues (1973) are most widely quoted in the literature. Izant (1966), Lewis and colleagues (1973), Colombani (1973), Cunningham (1977), and Noordijk and Bloemsma-Jockman (1979) all indicated that there are developmental differences between gastroschisis and antenatal rupture of a hernia into the umbilical cord.

Shaw (1975) felt that while there are clinical differences between gastroschisis and omphalocele, they can easily be explained by differences in fetal age at the time of the noxious influence of the teratogenic agent or event. Shaw holds the view that gastroschisis, similar to hernia of the umbilical cord and small omphaloceles, is an anomaly of the umbilical ring and not a form of independent maldevelopment of the abdominal wall. Thomas and Atwell (1976) agree with those views, noting that they have never been able to identify muscle fibers between the defect in gastroschisis and the umbilical cord. They felt that evidence suggests that gastroschisis is the result of intrauterine rupture of a hernia into the umbilical cord.

The matter of apparent separation of the cord from the defect was explained by Shaw (1975), who pointed out that it was possible for an ingrowth of epithelium to result in separation of the defect from the umbilical cord. While such an event would result in an apparently "normal" insertion of the cord, the defect is nevertheless medial to the rectus abdominis muscles.

Some attempt is needed to apply a uniform terminology to congenital defects of the abdominal wall. The classification, a brief description proposed by Schuster (1979), is reproduced in Table 24–9.

## CLINICAL FEATURES

In gastroschisis the intestines protrude through a defect that is usually located to the right of what is described as a normally located umbilical cord. In any event, the prolapsed bowel is separated from the cord by an epithelial bridge. The absence of a sac over the protruded viscera is striking. Typically, it is the small intestine that prolapses through the defect. Colon and stomach may also comprise a portion of the herniated contents, but the bladder and internal genitalia are uncommonly encountered. A gelatinous layer over the viscera results in adherence of loops of intestine, one to the other. The bowel wall is thickened and appears to be foreshortened. In the occasional infant, the bowel may undergo strangulation obstruction. Atresia of the bowel is uncommonly seen.

One of the earliest descriptions of gastroschisis is that of Bernstein, who, in 1940, noted the absence of a sac and the enlarged, thickened cyanotic intestine that presents as a thickened, adherent mass. The leathery consistency of the mass was thought to be due to the fact that the extruded viscera were bathed in amniotic fluid.

Moore and Stokes (1953) described gastroschisis in detail, noting the extraumbilical location of the protruding mass, which was not covered by a sac but by a leathery, gelatinous mass. They pointed out the discrepancy in size of the protruded mass and the peritoneal cavity.

In 1963 Moore identified antenatal and perinatal types of gastrochisis. Infants with the antenatal variety had small peritoneal cavities, and the protruded bowel was covered with a thick, homogenous material. Such events were attributed to prolonged exposure of the viscera to amniotic fluid in utero. Less serosal reaction was seen in infants having perinatal occurrence of the abnormality, since the viscera were exposed to amniotic fluid for shorter periods of time.

## ASSOCIATED ANOMALIES IN GASTROSCHISIS

The significant incidence of associated anomalies occurring in exomphalos has been noted in Chapter 22 and also earlier in this chapter. Moore and Stokes (1953) noted that associated anomalies are unusual in gastroschisis and tend to involve the intestinal tract. Moore in 1977 noted that serious additional congenital abnormalities occurred in 37 percent of 236 cases of omphalocele, but in only 18 percent of 278 cases of gastroschisis. Moore noted that jejunoileal malformations were far more common in infants with gastroschisis.

**Table 24–9.  PROPOSED TERMINOLOGY FOR CONGENITAL ABDOMINAL WALL DEFECTS RELATED TO ETIOLOGY AND DEFINITIVE FEATURES**

| Terminology | Etiology | |
|---|---|---|
| Epigastric omphalocele | Cephalic fold abnormality | Diameter of |
| Omphalocele | Lateral fold abnormality | defect greater |
| Hypogastric omphalocele | Caudal fold abnormality | than 4 cm. |
| Ruptured omphalocele | Ante- or perinatal rupture of the above. | |
| Hernia of the umbilical cord | Incomplete closure of umbilical ring (diameter of defect less than 4 cm; contains small bowel only) | |
| Gastroschisis | Ante- or perinatal rupture of hernia of umbilical cord. | |

Moore and Stokes (1953), Touloukian and Spackman (1971), and Gilbert and colleagues (1972) all observed shortening and thickening of the bowel. This is considered to be a reversible condition once the intestines are returned to the peritoneal cavity.

Atresia due to constriction of the gastroschisis defect has been described by Gilbert and colleagues (1972) and by Grosfeld and Clatworthy in 1970. Irving and Rickham (1978) also identified two such cases.

Kiesewetter (1957), Denes and coworkers (1968), and Firor (1971) observed gangrenous intestine beyond the point of constriction at the abdominal wall defect.

## TREATMENT

Effective treatment of gastroschisis is truly a modern development, and most of those contributing toward a solution to this problem are still living. I have cited a number of important references (indicating dates) to emphasize that most of the advancements have occurred in the past two decades.

Prior to 1953, survival following any modality of treatment of gastroschisis was a rare event. Moore and Stokes reported two cases at that time, both of whom died. An early surviving case was that of Watkins in 1943. He was able to close the defect primarily after replacing the viscera into the peritoneal cavity.

Proper management of infants in the neonatal period is of great importance. The assistance of a pediatrician, and preferably a neonatologist, is highly desirable. The care of infants with such anomalies in a setting providing excellent pediatric intensive care is highly desirable.

Bennington and colleagues (1974) identified these factors as resulting in the exceedingly high mortality that occurred in the past:

1. Low body temperature and acidosis.
2. Postoperative ventilatory problems.
3. Sepsis.
4. Small size of the abdominal cavity.
5. Prolonged dysfunction of the bowel.
6. Malnutrition.

Recognition of the above factors has

resulted in implementation of corrective measures with increasing success.

## IMMEDIATE NONOPERATIVE TREATMENT

The initial nonoperative treatment of the infant is important if a favorable outcome is to be achieved. Unnecessarily prolonged exposure of the mass of prolapsed viscera to contamination, desiccation, and loss of body warmth will threaten the very survival of the infant.

Nasogastric decompression is necessary to empty the upper gastrointestinal tract of contents and to aspirate swallowed air.

The viscera are covered with sterile, saline-soaked dressings.

The infant is placed in an Isolette with controlled temperature and humidity.

Intravenous fluids and broad-spectrum antibiotic coverage is provided. Need for vitamin K therapy, oxygen administration, and correction of acidosis should be recognized in individual infants.

## SURGICAL REPAIR

Techniques available for repair of gastroschisis have been described by Irving and Rickham (1978). In some cases, repair can be comparatively simple; but in others multiple problems already alluded to are encountered. Girvan and colleagues (1974) indicated a need for individualization of surgical repair.

Three approaches to repair of gastroschisis are possible.

1. Primary closure (Fig. 22–16). This technique had been used successfully by Watkins (in 1943), Izant (in 1966), Mahour and Lee (in 1974), and Zwiren and Andrews (also in 1974). Closure may be performed either in layers or as a single-layer closure. A number of authors have added manual stretching of the abdominal wall to permit visceral replacement and primary closure. Such principles were employed by Izant (1966), Rangaratham and colleagues (1969), Gilbert and coworkers (1972), Lewis and coworkers (1973), Bennington and colleagues (1974), and Raffens-

berger and Jona (1974). Primary closure should only be utilized if it does not interfere with ventilation and circulation.

2. Closure of skin over the viscera. In this method a ventral hernia is deliberately created. It was performed for the first time by Gross and Blodgett (1940 and later by Gross (1948). The details of this method are illustrated in Figure 22–22, pp. 430–431. The technique is objectionable because it results in an incisional hernia, often associated with numerous adhesions. Nevertheless, this approach saved lives of infants when other methods of treatment had not yet been developed. Thomas and Atwell (1976) preferred this method for 12 of 13 infants with gastroschisis.

3. The use of prosthetics to create a temporary domicile for the viscera, allowing time for enlargement of the abdominal wall through growth—a comparatively

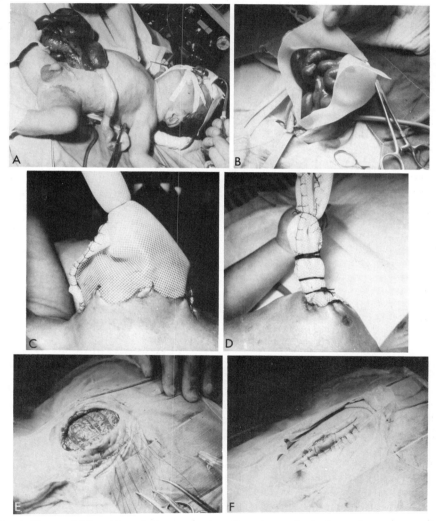

**Figure 24–27.** *A,* Gastroschisis with typical presentation. Note the marked edema, distention, and matting of the bowel. *B,* A silon pouch is being fashioned of sufficient size to contain the intestine. *C,* The silon pouch is completed. *D,* The silon pouch is being constricted from the top towards the abdomen. Notice the distention of the abdomen. *E,* The residual defect is being closed. *F,* Appearance after closure has been completed. (Reproduced by permission of author and journal. From Firor, H. V.: Technical improvements in the management of omphalocele and gastroschisis. Surg. Clin. North Am. 55(1):133, 1975.)

recent development (Fig. 24–27, A–F). Schuster (1967) beautifully illustrated the principles and techniques when he advocated a new method for staged repair of large omphaloceles. This type of treatment was utilized in gastroschisis by Allen and Wrenn (1969), Cordero and coworkers (1969), Bryant and coworkers (1970), Gilbert and colleagues (1968 and 1972), Mahour and colleagues (1974), Shermeta and Haller (1975), Firor (1975), Rubin and Ein (1976), Kim (1976), and Aaronson (1977). Hutchin and Goldenberg in 1965 utilized Teflon mesh to bridge large defects in omphaloceles. They later removed the mesh and closed the fascial defect.

The use of a temporary plastic pouch or silo allows time for growth and enlargement of the abdominal cavity. Rubin and Ein (1976) pointed out the hazard of infection and stressed the need for early removal of the pouch. Candida sepsis was a serious complication, often resulting in death. The hazard of pseudomonas infection has also been identified. Many authors have stressed the hazard of local infection and generalized sepsis incident to the use of pouches to accommodate the prolapsed bowel. From a survey of current literature, most surgeons favor earliest possible removal of the synthetic pouch. It is apparent that most pouches can achieve their purpose in 10 to 12 days. Closure of the abdominal wall defect then causes no major respiratory or circulatory embarrassment in most infants.

## MORTALITY

The earliest survival following repair of gastroschisis is that reported by Watkins in 1943. Moore and Stokes (1953) reported treatment of two patients, neither of whom survived. In 1964 Moore reported 17 (56 percent) surviving patients among 30 infants. Girvan and colleagues (1974) reported that mortality of omphalocele and gastroschisis range between 40 and 50 percent. Lewis and colleagues (1973) treated 31 patients with gastroschisis, with a survival rate of 68 percent. Zwiren and Andrews (1974) treated 18 patients with a remarkable rate of survival of 83 percent.

## SUMMARY

Gastroschisis is an anomaly of development of the abdominal wall that presents with recognizable clinical features. The protruding viscera (usually small intestine) present through an abdominal wall defect just to the right of the umbilical cord. The cord is separated from the defect by a bridge of epithelium. The viscera are covered by a gelatinous material, and no hernial sac is identified.

Preoperative care has been described here in general terms, as have the complications of gastroschisis.

Operative treatment should be individualized; primary closure, two-staged repair, and use of temporary plastic pouches are modalities of treatment.

Primary repair with visceral replacement carries the dangers of circulatory and respiratory embarrassment.

Staged procedures with closure of skin over the prolapsed viscera require later secondary repair of ventral herniation. Adhesions make dissection of the bowel tedious and somewhat dangerous.

When plastic pouches are fashioned, the risk of infection is great. Early, but appropriate, removal of the pouch is highly desirable.

Recently gained knowledge of the pathophysiology of gastroschisis, with particular attention to circulatory and respiratory functions, has resulted in improved management. With availability of effective antibiotic therapy and parenteral feeding, survival rates for infants with gastroschisis have steadily improved. Rates of less than 30 percent have been reported for mortality.

The matter of embryogenesis of gastroschisis has not yet been resolved.

## REFERENCES

Aaronson, I. A., and Eckstein, H. B.: The role of the silastic prosthesis in the management of gastroschisis. Arch. Surg. 112:297, 1977.

Allen, R. G., and Wrenn, E. L., Jr.: Silon as a sac in the treatment of omphalocele and gastroschisis. J. Pediatr. Surg. 4(1):3, 1969.

Benson, C. D., Penberthy, G. C., and Hill, E. J.: Hernia into the umbilical cord and omphalocele (aminocele) in the newborn. Arch Surg. 58:833, 1945.

Berman, E. J.: Gastroschisis, with comments on embryological development and surgical treatment. Arch. Surg. 75:788, 1957.

Bernstein, Phineas: Gastroschisis, a rare teratological condition of the newborn. Arch. Pediatr. 57:505, 1940.

Binnington, H. B., Keating, J. P., and Ternberg, J. L.: Gastroschisis. Arch. Surg. 108:455, 1974.

Bryant, L. R., Beargie, R. A., Segnitz, R. H., Trinkle, J. K., and Griffen, W. O., Jr.: Surgical management of gastroschisis. Trans. S. Surg. Assoc. 81:150, 1970.

Cantrell, J. R., Haller, J. A., and Ravitch, M. M.: A syndrome of congenital defects involving the abdominal wall, sternum, diaphragm, pericardium and heart. Surg. Gynecol. Obstet. 107:600, 1958.

Colombani, P. M., and Cunningham, D.: Perinatal aspects of omphalocele and gastroschisis. Am. J. Dis. Child. 131:1386, 1977.

Cordero, L., Touloukian, R. J., and Pickett, L. K.: Staged repair of gastroschisis with silastic sheeting. Surgery 65(4):676, 1969.

Cullen, T. S.: Embryology, Anatomy and Diseases of the Umbilicus. Philadelphia, W. B. Saunders Co., 1916.

Cunningham, A. A.: Exomphalos. Arch. Dis. Child. 31:144, 1955.

Dénes, J. Léb, J., and Lukács, F. V.: Gastroschisis. Surgery 63:701, 1968.

Duhamel, B.: Embryology of exomphalos and allied malformations. Arch. Dis. Child. 38:142, 1963.

Firor, H. V.: Technical improvements in the management of omphalocele and gastroschisis. Surg. Clin. North Am. 55(1):129, 1975.

Gilbert, M. G., Mencia, L. F., Brown, W. T., and Linn, B. S.: Staged surgical repair of large omphaloceles and gastroschisis. J. Pediatr. Surg. 3(6):702, 1968.

Gilbert, M. G., Mencia, L. F., Puranik, S. R., Litt, R. E., and Altman, D. H.: Management of gastroschisis and short bowel: report of 17 cases. J. Pediatr. Surg. 7(5):598, 1972.

Girvan, D. P., Webster, D. M., and Shandling, B.: The treatment of omphalocele and gastroschisis. Surg. Gynecol. Obstet. 139:222, 1974.

Grosfeld, J. L., and Clatworthy, H. W.: Intra-uterine midgut strangulation in a gastroschisis defect. Surgery 67:519, 1970.

Gross, R. E.: A new method for surgical treatment of large omphaloceles. Surgery 24:277, 1948.

Gross, R. E., and Blodgett, J. B.: Omphalocele in the newly born. Surg. Gynecol. Obstet. 71:520, 1940.

Hutchin, P., and Goldenberg, I. S.: Surgical therapy of omphalocele and gastroschisis. Arch. Surg. 90:22, 1965.

Iason, A. H.: Hernia. Philadelphia, Blakiston Co., 1941.

Irving, I. M., and Rickham, P. P.: In Rickham, P. P., Lister, J., and Irving, I.: Neonatal Surgery (2nd ed.). London, Butterworths, 1978, pp. 309–333.

Izant, R. J., Jr., Brown, F., and Rothmann, B. F.: Current embryology and treatment of gastroschisis and omphalocele. Arch. Surg. 93:49, 1966.

Johns, F. S.: Congenital defect of the abdominal wall in the newborn. Ann. Surg. 123:886, 1946.

Jones, P. G.: Exomphalos, a review of 45 cases. Arch. Dis. Child. 38:180, 1963.

Kieswetter, W. B.: Gastroschisis. Arch. Surg. 75:28, 1957.

Kim, S. H.: Omphalocele. Surg. Clin. North Am. 56(2):361, 1976.

Ladd, W. E., and Gross, R. E.: Abdominal Surgery of Infancy and Childhood. Philadelphia, W. B. Saunders Co., 1941.

Lewis, J. E., Jr., Kraeger, R. R., and Danis, R. K.: Gastroschisis. Ten-year review. Arch. Surg. 107:218, 1973.

Mahour, G. H., and Lee, F. A.: Gastroschisis: Mortalities and growth of survivors. Am. Surg. 40(7):425, 1974.

Margulies, L.: Omphalocele (Amniocele). Am. J. Obstet. Gynecol. 49:695, 1945.

Moore, T. C., and Stokes, G. E.: Gastroschisis. Surgery 33:112, 1953.

Moore, T. C.: Gastroschisis and omphalocele: Clinical differences. Surgery 82(5):561, 1977.

Moore, T. C.: In Nyhus, L. M., and Harkins, H. N.: Hernia. Philadelphia, J. B. Lippincott Co., 1964.

Noordijk, J. A., and Bloemsma-Jonkman, F.: Gastroschisis: No myth. J. Pediatr. Surg. 13(1):47, 1978.

Nyhus, L. M., and Harkins, H. N.: Hernia. Philadelphia, J. B. Lippincott Co., 1964.

Raffensperger, J., and Jona, J.: Gastroschisis. Surg. Gynecol. Obstet. 138:30, 1974.

Rangarathnam, C. S., Lal, R. B., and Swenson, O.: Gastroschisis. Arch. Surg. 98:742, 1969.

Rickham, P. P.: Rupture of exomphalos and gastroschisis. Arch. Dis. Child. 38:138, 1963.

Rubin, S. Z., and Ein, S. H.: Experience with 55 silon pouches. J. Pediatr. Surg. 11:803, 1976.

Schuster, S. R.: A new method for the staged repair of large omphaloceles. Surg. Gynecol. Obstet. 125:837, 1967.

Schuster, S. R.: In Ravitch, M. M., Welch, K. J., Benson, C. D., Aberdeen, E., and Randolph, T. G.: Pediatric Surgery (3rd ed.). Chicago, Year Book Medical Publishers, Inc., 1979, pp. 778–801.

Shaw, A.: The myth of gastroschisis. J. Pediatr. Surg. 10(2):235, 1975.

Shermeta, D. W., and Haller, J. A., Jr.: A new preformed transparent silo for the management of gastroschisis. J. Pediatr. Surg. 10(6):973, 1975.

Thomas, D. F. M., and Atwell, J. D.: The embryology and surgical management of gastroschisis. Br. J. Surg. 63:893, 1976.

Touloukian, R. J., and Spackman, T. J.: Gastrointestinal function and radiographic appearance following gastroschisis repair. J. Pediatr. Surg. 6:427, 1971.

Watkins, D. E.: Gastroschisis with case report. Va. Med. J. 70:42, 1943.

Watson, L. F.: Hernia (3rd ed.). St. Louis, C. V. Mosby Co., 1948.

Zwiren, G. T., and Andrews, G.: Progress in the management of gastroschisis. Am. Surg. 40:662, 1974.

## Supplemental Readings

Carlson, K. P., Campbell, G. D., and Hindle, R. C.: Gastroschisis: Case report and comment. N. Z. Med. J. 84:315, 1976.

Chato, L. M., Jr., Schairer, A. E., and Schmitz, R. L.: Staged repair of gastroschisis with an enteric fistula as a complication. Ill. Med. J. 148:467, 1975.

Collins, D. L., and Schumacher, A. E.: Omphalocele ruptured before birth. Proceedings of Pediatr. Surgery Congress, Roy. Child. Hosp. Melbourne, 21:71, 1970.

Croom, R. D., and Thomas, C. G.: Repair of gastroschisis. Surg. Gynecol. Obstet. *132*:689, 1971.

Eckstein, H. B.: Exomphalos. A review of 100 cases. Br. J. Surg. *50*:405, 1963.

Firor, H. V.: Omphalocele — An appraisal of therapeutic approaches. Surgery 69:208, 1971.

Graivier, L.: Changing concepts in treatment of ruptured omphalocele (Gastroschisis). Texas Med. 70:70, 1974.

Gray, S. W., and Skandalakis, J. E.: Embryology for Surgeons. Philadelphia, W. B. Saunders Co., 1972.

Grob, M.: *Lehrbuch der Kinderchirurgie.* Stuttgart, George Thieme Verlag, 1957, pp. 312–315.

Hollabaugh, R., and Boles, T.: The management of gastroschisis. J. Pediatr. Surg. 8:263, 1973.

Janoski, E. O., Jona, J. Z., and Belin, R. P.: Congenital anomalies of the umbilicus. Am. Surg. *43*(3):177, 1977.

Johnson, A. H.: Omphalocele and related defects. Am. J. Surg. *114*:297, 1967.

Judd, D. R., Wince, L., and Moore, T. C.: Gastroschisis: Report of two cases successfully treated. Surgery 58:1033, 1965.

Kling, S.: Massive omphalocele: A method of treatment employing skin allograft. Canad. J. Surg. *10*:445, 1967.

Lafer, D. J.: Rectus muscle transection for visceral replacement in gastroschisis. J. Surg. 63:988, 1968.

Lewis, J. E.: *Atlas of Infant Surgery.* St. Louis, C. V. Mosby Co., 1967.

Mahour, G. H., Weitzman, J. J., and Rosenkrantz, J. G.: Omphalocele and gastroschisis. Ann. Surg. *177*:478, 1973.

Moore, T. C.: Gastroschisis with antenatal evisceration of intestines and urinary bladder. Ann. Surg. *158*:263, 1963.

Othersen, H. Biemann, Jr., and Hargest, T. S.: A pneumatic reduction device for gastroschisis and omphalocele. Surg. Gynecol. Obstet. *144*:243, 1977.

Panovski, J.: Gastroschisis. Acta Chir. 7:263, 1960.

Seashore, J. H., MacNaughton, J. R., and Talbert, J. L.: Treatment of gastroschisis and omphalocele with biological dressings. J. Pediatr. Surg. *10*(1):9, 1975.

Shaw, A.: Differences between omphalocele and gastroschisis (letter). Am. J. Dis. Child. *132*(9):936, 1978.

Shaw, A.: Gastroschisis: Not omphalocele (letter). Surg. 83(6):752, 1978.

Shaw, A.: Gastroschisis: No myth (letter). J. Pediatr. Surg. *13*(6):560, 1978.

Shermeta, D. W.: Simplified treatment of large congenital ventral wall defects. Am. J. Surg. *133*:78, 1977.

Simpson, R. L., and Caylor, H. D.: Gastroschisis. Am. J. Surg. 96:675, 1958.

Thompson, J., and Fonkalsrud, E. W.: Reappraisal of skin flap closure for neonatal gastroschisis. Arch. Surg. *111*:684, 1976.

Thunig, L. Albert: Hernia into the umbilical cord and related anomalies. Arch. Surg. *1*:1021, 1936.

Venugopal, S., Zachard, R. B., and Spitz, L.: Exomphalos and gastroschisis: A 10 year review. Br. J. Surg. 63:523, 1976.

Wesselhoeft, C. W., Porter, A., and Deluca, F. G.: The treatment of omphalocele and gastroschisis. Ann. Chir. Infant. *13*:237, 1972.

# HERNIORRHAPHY AND APPENDECTOMY

*The free mobility and uncertain length of the cecum and the variations in its position due to developmental anomalies are such that the appendix may be found in any region of the abdomen and in close relations with the various abdominal rings, in which it may finally become engaged. As a matter of fact this little organ has been discovered in the inguinal and femoral canals on either the right or left side, also within the umbilicus, within the obturator foramen and in the various retrocolic and retrocecal fossae.*

*Kelly, 1905*

From time to time, the surgeon will encounter a hernia with an appendix presenting at the opened peritoneal sac — an invitation for the surgeon to perform an appendectomy; this circumstance is most likely to occur in the presence of indirect sliding inguinal and femoral hernias. It has been my policy to remove the appendix, if it can be done easily and without traction on the mesoappendix.

However, in today's medicolegal climate, it would be advisable to obtain the patient's approval prior to simultaneous appendectomy. Local anesthesia provides a distinct advantage in this regard, since the surgeon who is performing the herniorrhaphy can inform the patient of the situation and obtain his or her consent for simultaneous appendectomy during the operative procedure. A much more remote possibility is the need for appendectomy as dictated by the presence of an acutely inflamed appendix in association with a hernial sac.

## HISTORICAL BACKGROUND

There is little to be gained from a lengthy historical review regarding the relationship of the appendix to hernia. Watson, who reviewed the subject in some detail, noted that Berengerius Carpus in 1524 was the first to recognize the appendix. Vesalius in 1543 and Fallopius in 1560 described it further, and in 1561 Vidus Vidius named it "appendix vermiformis." Watson pointed out that it was not until 1731 that deGarengoet identified an appendix in a hernial sac.

It is interesting that the first recorded appendectomy is attributed to Cladius Amayand in 1735. The appendix in this interesting case was located in a hernial sac. In his exhaustive works on the ver-

miform appendix and its diseases (1905), Kelly gave credit to Morgagni for recognizing an appendix in a hernial sac in 1751. Kelly (1905) noted that the appendix had been found in inguinal, femoral, umbilical, and obturator hernias. The illustration of an appendix encountered in a hernial sac is taken from Kelly (Fig. 24–28).

Wakeley (1938) stated that hernias of the appendix constitute approximately one percent of all hernias. Furthermore, in 2000 personal cases, he found that 12 were associated with inguinal hernias, 3 with femoral hernias, and 1 with an umbilical hernia.

Watson (1946) made the observation that prior to the mid-nineteenth century, operative treatment of the diseased organ was undertaken only when abscesses formed at hernial sites. He found that it was in the latter part of the nineteenth century that the accessible appendix was being more frequently removed.

By 1946 Watson was able to accumulate 924 instances in which the appendix was

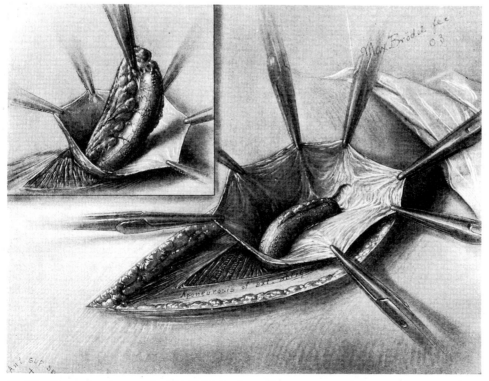

**Figure 24–28.**    These drawings are by Max Brödel, whose illustrations are classics. In the insert, the appendix is quite mobile. In the larger drawing, the appendix is adherent to the sac. Such conditions may be seen in sliding hernias of the appendix. (Reproduced by permission of W. B. Saunders Company. From Kelly, H. A., and Hurdon, E.: *The Vermiform Appendix and its Diseases.* W. B. Saunders Co., Philadelphia, 1905, p. 790.)

present in a hernial sac. Thus, it can be seen that the anatomic association of appendix to hernia is not rare. Every busy general surgeon will be faced with this combination from time to time. He must be prepared to make a decision regarding possible appendectomy in each case, based on the anatomic findings and the benefit-risk ratio. For example, appendectomy in an elderly patient with an atrophic appendix that cannot be reached easily might be ill conceived.

## HERNIAS CONTAINING THE APPENDIX—CLINICAL FEATURES

Kelly (1905) cited evidence that the appendix is more commonly located in hernial sacs of very young patients and of those in the advanced years of life. Young adults and middle-aged patients are afflicted with this combination much less frequently.

Quoting Rivet, Kelly noted that more males presented with appendices in hernial sacs than did females. The sex incidence was 70 percent in males and 30 percent in females.

As to the type of hernia, 70 to 80 percent of hernias containing the appendix were inguinal and 20 to 30 percent were femoral. In females, according to Kelly, there is a preponderance of femoral hernias containing the appendix.

Griffin (1968), Chatterjee (1966), Garland (1955), and Gerami and colleagues (1970) reported cases of incarcerated appendices in femoral hernial sacs. Griffin summarized the incidence of appendices found in femoral hernia sacs as reported by various authors.

Cutolo and coworkers (1978), Gualt and Bayles (1936), Griffin (1968), Gerami and colleagues (1970), Powell (1954), and Rose (1954) all reported acutely inflamed appendices in femoral hernial sacs.

Voitk and coworkers (1974) called attention to the infrequent occurrence of ruptured appendicitis in femoral hernias. In reviewing the English literature, they found only 59 cases of acute appendicitis occurring in femoral hernias. In only 7 patients was the appendix ruptured. They noted the condition was misdiagnosed as an abscess. Prompt incision and drainage initially may be life-saving. Later, definitive treatment may consist of fistulectomy, appendectomy, and herniorrhaphy.

It is rare to find the appendix in an obturator or umbilical hernia. Although the appendix is most often found in right indirect inguinal hernias, it can be located in remote areas, as in the case reported by Kelly (Fig. 24–29). The mobile cecum permitted the cecum and appendix to reach the left inguinal region. The presenting symptoms of patients with hernias containing the appendix are of two types. First, sliding indirect inguinal hernias containing the appendix and cecum will present as a mass, which is more or less reducible. Second, patients with hernias containing an acutely inflamed appendix—whether due to primary appendicitis or strangulation obstruction—will complain of localized pain and swelling. Depending on the state of progression, evidence of peritonitis may be present.

Carey (1967) noted that acute appendicitis may occur in a variety of hernias. He reported the occurrence of five such cases in right indirect inguinal hernias, three in femoral hernias, and one each in an incisional hernia and in a left indirect inguinal hernia. He recommended appendectomy and en bloc resection where appropriate. Patients in whom the appendix had not perforated did well. Carey felt that repair of the hernia was indicated.

Piersol in 1901 reported that 23 percent of hernias of the appendix occurred during childhood.

DeGormo reported in 1907 a sliding appendiceal hernia in an adult female.

Rose and Santulli (1978) reported that in rare examples, the mesoappendix forms the sliding component of an inguinal hernia. They found that such hernias occurred predominantly in male infants. They performed appendectomy plus herniorrhaphy in 16 patients without need for counterincisions. Antibiotics were not given, and there were no complications in this series.

Srouji and Buck (1978) studied acute appendicitis in infants up to 30 days following birth. From 1901 to 1975 they identified 106 cases, pointing out that incarceration leads to pressure with eventual strangulation. Variable degrees of infarction, perforation, gangrene, and even phlegmon may be the result. They suggested that the high mortality with acute intra-abdominal appendicitis can be attributed to a failure to make a proper diagnosis. In hernial appendicitis, earlier recognition is possible because of a visible inflammatory protrusion. The obstruction

at the hernial ring tends to protect the peritoneal cavity from generalized peritonitis and sepsis. The need for surgical intervention, and avoidance of soilage of the peritoneal cavity, is clear.

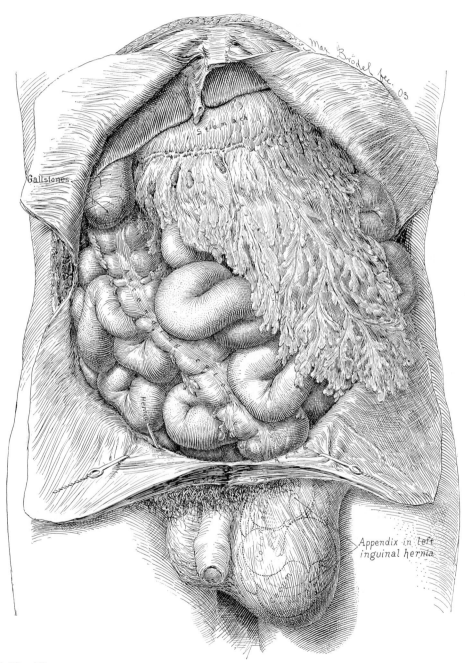

**Figure 24–29.** Illustration by Brödel showing that the appendix may find its way to a remote location. In this case, it is seen to be in the left inguinal region, relocating in the left scrotum. (Reproduced by permission of W. B. Saunders Company. From Kelly, H. A., and Hurdon, E.: *The Vermiform Appendix and its Diseases*, p. 788.)

**Table 24–10.  AGE INCIDENCE
–27 PATIENTS HAVING
APPENDECTOMY AND
HERNIORRHAPHY**

| Age | Number |
|---|---|
| 0 to 10 yrs. | 3 |
| 11 to 20 yrs | 0 |
| 21 to 30 yrs. | 1 |
| 31 to 40 yrs. | 2 |
| 41 to 50 yrs. | 3 |
| 51 to 60 yrs. | 4 |
| 61 to 70 yrs. | 9 |
| 71 yrs. and older | 5 |
| | 27 |

## CLINICAL STUDY

I tried to collect as many examples as I could find where the patient had had an appendectomy along with hernia repair. Such records are extremely difficult to locate, since there is no special indexing to permit easy retrieval.

Nevertheless, between 1942 and 1972 I was able to identify 27 records of patients having appendectomy plus herniorrhaphy.

### Age Incidence

The age incidence among our cases is similar to that reported by Kelly (Table 24–10). The youngest patient was 18 months old and presented with a sliding hernia; a second patient was two years old. The oldest patient was 86 years of age.

### Sex Incidence

As might be expected, access by the appendix into a hernial sac can most easily be accomplished in association with in-

**Table 24–11.  TYPE OF HERNIA
CONTAINING APPENDIX–
27 PATIENTS**

| Type of Hernia | No. of Patients |
|---|---|
| Indirect sliding, right | 13 |
| Indirect, right | 6 |
| Femoral | 6 |
| Indirect and femoral | 1 |
| Direct | 1 |
| | 27 |

direct sliding inguinal hernias (Table 24–11). In such cases, the cecum and terminal ileum are in proximity to the internal ring. A mobile cecum may permit entry into the femoral hernia in a female.

From this study it can be seen that the appendix can be most readily removed when an indirect sliding hernia is present. Such hernias are seen in older patients.

In six female patients, the appendix was present in femoral hernias. This is also consistent with the observation of Kelly that in females there is a preponderance of femoral hernias with appendices, whereas in males it is the indirect inguinal hernia that is more often found to contain the appendix.

Cutolo and colleagues (1978) reported an instance in which a patient had acute suppurative appendicitis occurring in a femoral hernial sac. Voitk and associates (1974) identified 59 cases of acute appendicitis within femoral hernias, then added two new cases.

### Operative Treatment

The principles of management of the appendix are comparatively simple. Appendectomy is performed only if the appendix can be delivered through the opened peritoneal sac without further disrupting or incising the abdominal wall. Good access to the cecum, mesoappendix, and the appendiceal base is essential if a safe appendectomy is to be performed.

A variety of techniques were utilized in the repair of hernias in the 27 patients in this study; the procedure was adapted to the needs of the particular case. Methods of repair are described and illustrated in appropriate chapters in this text.

Surgeons will often select monofilament wire sutures in the repair of hernias when there is a possibility of infection.

In our technique of appendectomy, the serosa of the appendix is incised; the stump is ligated with plain catgut and inverted into the cecum. A purse-string of number 4–0 silk, previously placed into the cecal wall about the appendix, is then tied. The vessels of the mesoappendix are secured with number 4–0 silk sutures.

Antibiotics are not administered routinely but are given to selected patients, such as those with acute appendicitis or with some degree of inflammation.

During appendectomy of acute appendicitis, if exposure of the ileocecal area is difficult and unsatisfactory, an abdominal incision should be made to insure clear visualization of the area.

## Operative Findings

In three patients, the operative findings were of unusual interest; two of these will be reported here in some detail.

One patient had an incarcerated femoral hernia, and the peritoneal cavity was entered through a right lower transverse abdominal incision. The patient had acute appendicitis; appendectomy was performed and the hernia repaired by the Henry-Cheattle-Nyhus technique. Recovery was uneventful.

The second patient presented a more complicated problem, as the following case indicates.

## Incarcerated Indirect Inguinal Hernia and Acute Appendicitis (Case in Point)

The following interesting case is presented from the service of Dr. Thomas Fox.

The patient was a 39-year-old Maltese male who had been ill for one week with severe abdominal pain, distention, and absence of bowel movements for two or three days. Enemas gave no relief. When seen in the emergency room, he was acutely ill with temperature elevation and a rapid pulse. The abdomen was tense, protuberant, and tender in the right lower quadrant. An incarcerated left indirect inguinal hernia was found.

The patient was taken to the operating room where after adequate preparation and spinal anesthesia a left inguinal hernia was repaired by Dr. Thomas Fox. An extraordinary amount of pus was encountered upon opening the peritoneal sac. As so often happens, the incarceration became reduced once the anesthetic was administered. When the peritoneal cavity was entered, the small intestine was found to be viable. Exploration revealed the presence of acute appendicitis with perforation, and appendectomy was performed through a McBurney incision. Postoperatively, the patient was acutely ill and developed a

subphrenic abscess, which required drainage later.

## Comment

It was reasonable to assume that this patient's illness was due to an incarcerated and possibly strangulated hernia. The surgeon was alert to the fact that profuse pus in the presence of relatively normal small intestine must be due to pathology other than the hernia; the appendiceal area was suspect, and acute perforated appendicitis discovered.

The performance of an appendectomy through a small McBurney incision was a simple matter. This incision healed without a hernia, but the lateral extension of the herniorrhaphy incision was the site of a recurrent hernia.

The protrusion and incarceration of a hernia following onset of acute intra-abdominal pathology are not rare. Carcinoma of the colon and rectum, diverticulitis, and other inflammatory diseases of the bowel can contribute to incarceration of an established hernia.

The following case report is unusual in that an appendix incarcerated in a direct inguinal hernia in a female showed inflammatory changes. The patient was operated on by Dr. Ahmad M. Hamzah.

## Incarcerated Appendix in a Direct Inguinal Hernia

The patient was an 80-year-old hypertensive female who was admitted to the hospital with a history of sudden onset of pain and a protruding tender mass in the right groin. The past history was unremarkable. There was no nausea or vomiting, but constipation was present. The patient was in good general health except for a grade II systolic murmur and hypertension. The abdomen was soft with active bowel sounds. Above the right inguinal ligament, a palpable, tender, and irreducible mass could be appreciated. Skin discoloration was present. Rectal examination revealed normal sphincter tone with no particular tenderness. Laboratory analyses of the blood and urine were within normal limits. The clinical diagnosis was incarcerated right inguinal hernia with possible strangulation; operative repair under local anesthesia was advised. At operation, performed by Dr. Ahmad Hamzah, a direct inguinal hernia was found with the hernial sac located medial to the deep inferior epigastric vessels. Upon opening the sac, an incarcerated inflamed appendix with definite demarcation at its base was found. An appendectomy was performed easily, and hernia repair accomplished. Broad-spectrum antibiotics were administered, and the patient made an uneventful recovery.

The pathologist reported that the hernial sac showed acute peritonitis. The inflammation involved the external layers of the appendix, being reported as periappendicitis.

The patient continued to do well for three months after discharge.

## Discussion

The presence of an appendix in a hernial sac is seldom diagnosed prior to surgery, since appendiceal incarceration in an inguinal hernia is extremely rare; the presence of an incarcerated appendix in a direct inguinal hernia must be extremely rare.

Our operative findings of appendiceal congestion, discoloration, and clear demarcation at the base of the appendix led us to conclude that the appendix was entrapped at some point by the direct fascial defect. The added process of inflammation and adhesion prevented its reducibility and explained its subsequent presentation as a groin mass with skin discoloration. The occurrence of an incarcerated appendix in a direct inguinal herniation in an elderly female makes this a unique case. Direct inguinal hernias are uncommon in females and, when they do occur, reducibility of prolapsing contents is the rule.

## Complications

The fear of postoperative complications tends to deter surgeons from performing elective appendectomy during herniorrhaphy. Those surgeons who have performed such operations do not report unusually high complication rates; this is, in my opinion, because the surgeon takes special precautions to prevent contamination.

Eisman and colleagues studied the problem of simultaneous appendectomy and herniorrhaphy in 1959 and 1962. They were able to perform both procedures in 44.4 percent of 1040 cases. They reported an infection rate of 4.7 percent, stating that this result was comparable to the control group within their study. They recommended that removal of the appendix is reasonable during herniorrhaphy if it does not entail prolonging operative time, if the appendix is easily delivered, and if the base is clearly visualized to permit accurate amputation and subsequent closure. Eisman and coworkers do not advise persistence in performing appendectomy at the risk of extending the incision laterally. I agree with the above concepts.

In the 27 cases that I reviewed, there were two postoperative hematomas, one major hemorrhage from an aberrant obturator artery, and one genitourinary tract infection. One patient with acute suppurative appendicitis developed a wound infection and a recurrent hernia. Our complication rate was respectable, but we do not persist in performing routine appendectomies during herniorrhaphy.

## SUMMARY

Hernias that most commonly contain the appendix are of the indirect variety, followed much less frequently by femoral hernias.

When acute appendicitis is present in a hernia, operative intervention is mandatory. The preferred treatment is appendectomy; however, if a groin abscess has formed (as in a femoral hernia), carefully performed drainage followed by definitive surgery is a reasonable course.

When an appendix prolapses into the opened peritoneal sac during herniorrhaphy, appendectomy is advisable if the organ can be easily removed without undue traction. Control of the mesoappendix and access to the base of the appendix as it joins the cecum are essential.

I do not recommend extension of the incision laterally to permit removal of a normal appendix.

Whenever a thick purulent exudate is encountered during herniorrhaphy, its source should be explained, even if a secondary abdominal incision is necessary.

If appendectomy is to be performed for removal of a normal appendix during herniorrhaphy, permission should be obtained prior to the procedure. If appendicitis is present, the indication for appendectomy is clear.

It is unreasonable to assume that it is possible to continue the practice of appendectomy plus herniorrhaphy with a complication rate no higher than that encountered with herniorrhaphy alone.

## REFERENCES

Amayand, C.: Of an inguinal rupture with a pin in the appendix cocci encrusted with stone: And some observations on wounds in the guts. Philosoph. Trans. Roy. Soc. 39:329, 1736.

Carey, L. C.: Acute appendicitis occurring in hernias. A report of 10 cases. Surgery 61:236, 1967.

Chatterjee, S. N.: The appendix in a femoral sac. J. Ind. Med. Assoc. 46:377, 1966.

Cutolo, L. C., Wasserman, I., Pinck, R. L., and Mainzer, R. A.: Acute suppurative appendicitis occurring in a femoral hernia. Dis. Col. Rect. 21(3):203, 1978.

DeGarmo, W. B.: Abdominal Hernia. Philadelphia, J. B. Lippincott Co., 1907, pp. 256–259.

Eisman, B., Fowler, W. G., and Robinson, J. M.: Appendectomy during right inguinal herniorrhaphy. Ann. Surg. 149:110, 1959.

Eisman, B., Robinson, R. M., and Brown, F. H.: Simultaneous appendectomy and herniorrhaphy without prophylactic antibiotic therapy. Surgery 51:578, 1962.

Fox, Thomas: (Personal communication).

Frankau, C.: Strangulated hernia: A review of 1487 cases. Br. J. Surg. 19:176, 1931.

Garland, E. A.: Femoral appendicitis. J. Ind. Med. Assoc. 48:1292, 1955.

Gault, E. W., and Baylis, E. I.: Appendicitis in a femoral hernia. Med. J. Aust. 1:789, 1936.

Gerami, S., Easley, G. W., and Mendoza, C. B., Jr.: Appendiceal abscess as contents of right femoral hernia. A case report. Int. Surg. 53:354, 1970.

Griffin, J. M.: Incarcerated inflamed appendix in a femoral hernia. Am. J. Surg. 115:364, 1968.

Hamzah, Ahmad M.: (Personal communication).

Kelly, H. A.: Appendicitis and Other Diseases of the Vermiform Appendix. Philadelphia, W. B. Saunders Co., 1905, pp. 786–793.

Piersol, G. A.: Early infantile hernia of the vermiform appendix. Univ. PA Dept. Med. Bull. Reprint 278–282, 1901.

Powell, H. D. W.: Gangrenous appendix in femoral hernial sac. Lancet 267:1211, 1954.

Rose, E., and Santulli, T. V.: Sliding appendiceal inguinal hernia. Surg. Gynecol. Obstet. 146:626, 1978.

Rose, T. F.: The acutely inflamed appendix in a hernial sac. Med. J. Aust. 2:216, 1954.

Srouji, M. H., and Buck, B. E.: Neonatal appendicitis; ischemic infarction in incarcerated inguinal hernia. J. Pediatr. Surg. 13(2):177–179, 1978.

Voitk, A. J., Macfarlane, J. K., and Estrada, R. L.: Ruptured appendicitis in femoral hernias: report of two cases and review of the literature. Ann. Surg. 179:24, 1974.

Wakeley, C. P.: Hernia of the vermiform appendix. A record of sixteen personal cases. Lancet 2:1282, 1938.

Waring, H. J., and McAdam Eccles, W.: Cases from Mr. Langton's Wards. St. Bart. Hosp. Rep. 27:179, 1891.

Watson, L. F.: Hernia (3rd ed.). St. Louis, C. V. Mosby Co., 1946, pp. 523–546.

## Supplemental Reading

DeGarengot, R. J. C. (Cited by Garland, E. A.): Femoral appendicitis. J. Ind. Med. Assoc. 48:1292, 1955.

Hamilton, A. T., and Wilson, W. H.: A femoral hernia containing a strangulated appendix preoperatively diagnosed as a metastatic lymph node. N. Car. Med. J. 2:295, 1950.

Harf, A.: Einklemmung des Meckelschen Divertikels in einer Schenkelhernie. Deutsche Med. Wochenschr. 45:881, 1919.

Hodgson, N.: Strangulated femoral hernia associated with an appendix abscess in the hernial sac. Br. J. Surg. 13:386, 1925.

Holliday, T. D. S., and White, J. R. A.: Inflamed appendices in femoral hernial sacs. Br. Med. J. 11:779, 1953.

Keeley, J. L., and Schairer, A. E.: Incidental appendectomy during repair of groin hernias. Surgery 52:421, 1962.

Kia-Nouri, M.: Isolated incarcerated appendix in a femoral hernia. J. Albert Einstein Med. Cen. 10:38, 1962.

Koontz, A. R.: Femoral hernia. Arch. Surg. 64:298, 1952.

Love, R. J. M.: Herniorrhaphy plus appendectomy. Br. Med. J. 2:746, 1948.

McClure, R. D., and Fallis, L. S.: Femoral hernia. Report of 90 operations. Ann. Surg. 109:987, 1939.

Mitchell, J. E.: Hernial appendicitis. Br. J. Clin. Pract. 18:419, 1964.

Morrison, J. T.: Hernio-appendectomy. Lancet 1:625, 1937.

Myers, W. H., and Rominger, R. F.: Combined appendectomy and inguinal herniotomy. Am. J. Surg. 74:441, 1947.

Oliveira, A. B.: Acute appendicitis presenting as a strangulated left femoral hernia. Br. J. Clin. Pract. 17:213, 1963.

Rogers, F. A.: Strangulated femoral hernia: Review of 170 cases. Ann. Surg. 149:9, 1959.

Ryan, W. J.: Hernia of the vermiform appendix. Ann. Surg. 106:135, 1937.

Schrager, V. L.: Routine appendectomy through right indirect inguinal hernia sac in afebrile cases. Surg. Clin. North Am. 3:387, 1919.

Shawan, H. K., and Altman, R.: Appendices found as contents of femoral herniae. Ann. Surg. 101:1270, 1935.

Taylor, K. P. A.: Routine removal of appendix in right inguinal herniorrhaphy: 96 Appendectomies in 100 consecutive operations for hernia. Ann. Surg. 90:266, 1929.

Torek, F.: Combined operation for removal of appendix and cure of inguinal hernia. Ann. Surg. 43:665, 1906.

Wakeley, C. P. G.: Hernia of the vermiform appendix. In Maingot, R.: Abdominal Operations. New York, Appleton-Century-Crofts, 1969, p. 1288.

Wise, L., and Tanner, N.: Strangulated femoral hernia appendix with perforated sigmoid diverticulitis. Proc. Roy. Soc. Med. 56:1105, 1963.

Wood, A. C.: Appendicular femoral hernia with notes of 100 cases. Ann. Surg. 43:668, 1906.

# INGUINAL HERNIA AND CARCINOMA

## INTRODUCTION

The possibility of uncovering a concomitant carcinoma along with an inguinal hernia prior to hernia repair has prompted some surgeons to recommend "routine" barium enema and/or sigmoidoscopic examination preoperatively. The importance of substantiating such a possibility is obvious, since surgeons would be understandably loath to have overlooked a neoplasm of the large bowel or rectum in a patient with a recent herniorrhaphy. Unfortunately, the yield of colorectal malignancies by this expedient has been disappointingly small.

## HISTORICAL BACKGROUND

Publications on the subject are of recent vintage, and the more informative articles have been written in the current decade.

Myers and Rominger (1947) were among the first to call attention to the need for thorough clinical evaluation of patients with hernia, recommending that special attention be given to gastrointestinal symptoms. However, of the 200 patients studied, only one eventually was found to have a gastric neoplasm and another carcinoma of the sigmoid. The suspected presence of malignancy following removal of a nodule with the hernial sac was subsequently proved by histologic examination. The carcinoma was located on postoperative barium enema. As a result of their studies, Myers and Rominger recommended that patients with gastrointestinal symptoms have appropriate studies prior to hernia repair.

In 1961 Zollinger and Kinsey indicated that elderly patients with direct hernias often have prostatic obstruction of some degree. They called attention to the occasional patient who will present with gastrointestinal neoplasm as well as hernia. They pointed out that incidence of hernias, as well as of carcinoma of the colon, increases with the age of the patient population. Of 107 male patients with proven carcinoma of the large bowel, 17 percent first presented with symptoms suggestive of hernia. Zollinger and Kinsey recommended sigmoidoscopy and barium enema examination on all patients over 40 years of age. They made this recommendation even though they noted that not one patient under the age of 54 years had both carcinoma of the large intestine and hernia.

Craighead and colleagues (1964) investigated the occurrence of associated disorders with acutely incarcerated groin hernias among 127 patients. They found that 11 percent of these patients had obstruction of the lower urinary tract and a similar number had pulmonary emphysema.

Nine of 127 patients returned in from 19 to 60 months with other disorders. Four patients, or 3 percent, re-entered because of far-advanced malignancies. The site was not specified.

In 1965 Maxwell and coworkers investigated the occurrence of colon carcinoma in patients with inguinal hernia. They found that 22.5 percent of all patients with cancer of the large bowel also had inguinal hernias or gave a history of having had hernia repairs within two years of treatment for the malignancy. As a consequence, they recommended sigmoidoscopy and barium enema for all patients over 55 years of age. They stated that all symptomatic patients should be appropriately studied.

In 1971 Brendel and Kirsch raised an important question. They were interested in the frequency of asymptomatic colonic carcinomas in patients with inguinal herniorrhaphy. They studied 312 patients with preoperative barium enema examinations. All of these patients were males ranging in age from 19 to 98 years of age. Not one case of carcinoma of the colon was identified by this approach. During this period, 106 patients were treated for carcinoma of the colon. In this group, 16 percent had a history of hernia. Only four patients in this group had their hernias for less than two years, and they presented with symptoms suggestive of colonic malignancy. Brendel and Kirsch noted that the average age of patients with large bowel malignancies was 65 years.

Brendel and Kirsch suggested that gonadal irradiation incident to barium enema studies could have long-term adverse effects on patients in the reproductive age group. However, the long-term somatic and genetic effects are not established at this time.

The authors concluded that routine barium enema examination in patients with inguinal hernia was a poor survey procedure in their practice.

Further contributions came from Juler and colleagues in 1972. These authors found that among 969 patients with hernia repairs, 201 barium enema examinations were performed. Furthermore, of patients so examined, 65 percent were over 50 years of age. Not one case of carcinoma of the large bowel was discovered.

In addition, Juler and coworkers (1972) studied 210 patients with large bowel malignancies, 18 of whom also had inguinal hernias. The patients in this group presented with symptoms attributable to the colonic malignancies rather than to hernia.

Sannella (1973) also studied the results obtained with routine barium enema examinations in 493 patients. There was no incidence of colonic malignancy. One patient with a lengthy history of inguinal hernia was admitted to the hospital for rectal bleeding and proved to have a carcinoma of the sigmoid colon. Sannella also recorded significant observations on the occurrence of prostatism in patients with hernia. He found that 7.3 percent of patients in the seventh decade of life, with a history of hernia less than 2 years, had prostatectomies during the admission. He pointed out the high incidence of prostatic disease in patients with hernia.

## DISCUSSION

Evidence is accumulating that routine barium enema examination in asymptomatic patients with hernia has limited value. This is particularly true in younger patients without symptoms — i.e., those under the age of 50 years. Such investigations become valuable in patients with symptoms referable to the gastrointestinal tract.

In an evaluation of the elderly patient with hernia, such symptoms as abdominal pain, even minimal changes in bowel habits, bloody stools, anemia, and weight loss should lead to thorough investigation of the gastrointestinal tract. Physical examination should include palpation of the entire abdomen.

Rectal tumors cause such symptoms as bleeding, loose stools, perineal pain, constipation, abdominal pain, and changes in caliber of the stool; these symptoms must be explained, and rectal and sigmoidoscopic examinations are indicated.

Ponka and colleagues (1960) have studied the problem of differential diagnosis between carcinoma and diverticulitis. The age incidence for both is cited in Figure 24–30. It is to be noted that the age incidence for these conditions is quite similar to that seen in indirect inguinal hernias in adults (Chapter 13). A significant incidence of symptoms in patients with carcinoma and diverticulitis was noted. Change in bowel habits — including constipation, diarrhea, and bleeding — occurred in over three-fourths of 100 patients with proven carcinoma.

I have attempted to evaluate the late results obtained following herniorrhaphy. In Chapter 11 on indirect inguinal hernias, in adults, late deaths occurred in 41 of 548 patients. Arteriosclerosis and arteriosclerotic heart disease accounted for most deaths (18), and malignancies ranked second with 11 late deaths. In two cases, carcinoma of the colon was the cause of death (0.36 percent), and three patients died of prostatic carcinoma.

Among 493 patients who had repair of direct inguinal hernias, there were 14 late deaths from malignancy. There were three late deaths (0.60 percent) from carcinoma of the colon and five late deaths from prostatic carcinoma (1.0 percent). These figures are cited to support the increasing evidence that routine screening of every patient with hernia will at best yield positive findings in a limited number of patients. Even in prolonged follow-up studies of post-herniorrhaphy patients, a limited number will develop carcinoma of the colon.

I cannot recall identifying a single case of colonic carcinoma in an asymptomatic patient as a result of preoperative sigmoidoscopy and barium enema examination. Two patients with hernias were discovered to have colonic cancers, but both were symptomatic. A third patient, 78 years old and anemic, bled from the rec-

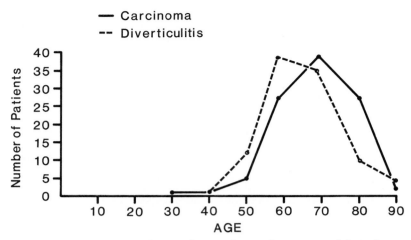

**Figure 24–30.** Age incidence — diverticulitis and carcinoma of the colon.

tum; a large lesion was discovered by proctoscopy.

In my experience it is the symptomatic patient who needs proctoscopic and barium enema examinations. I have not been impressed with the positive results of such examinations in younger patients with hernia — i.e., those under 55 years of age.

## CONCLUSION

The need for routine sigmoidoscopy and barium enema examination in patients under the age of 55 without gastrointestinal symptoms has not been established.

As patients increase in age, the incidence of colorectal malignancies increases (Fig. 24–31). In this group diverticular disease, prostatism, and pulmonary disease show a greater incidence than does colorectal neoplasia. In patients with hernia, but without gastrointestinal symptoms, the yield of positive findings with routine sigmoidoscopy and barium enema examination will be small. On the other hand, such investigations in symptomatic patients will be rewarding.

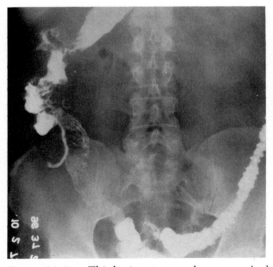

**Figure 24–31.** This barium enema shows a marked filling defect in the right colon. The patient was 60 years of age and presented for repair of a large right inguinal hernia. Although the patient denied bowel dysfunction, the mass in the right abdomen was palpable. Colectomy was performed before repair of the hernia.

## REFERENCES

Brendel, T. H., and Kirsh, I. E.: Lack of association between inguinal hernia and carcinoma of the colon. N. Engl. J. Med. *284*:369, 1971.

Craighead, C. C., Cotlar, Capt. A. M., and Moore, K.: Associated disorders with acute incarcerated groin hernia. Ann. Surg. *159*:987, 1964.

Juler, G. L., Stemmer, E. A., and Fullerman, R. W.: Inguinal hernia and colorectal carcinoma. Arch. Surg. *104*:778, 1972.

Maxwell, J. W., Jr., Davis, W. C., and Jackson, F. C.: Colon carcinoma and inguinal hernia. Surg. Clin. North Am. *45*:1165, 1965.

Myers, H. M., and Rominger, R. F.: Gastrointestinal symptoms and inguinal hernia. N. Engl. J. Med. *227*:660, 1942.

Ponka, J. L., Brush, B. E., and Fox, J. DeWitt: Differential diagnosis of carcinoma of the sigmoid and diverticulitis. J.A.M.A. 98:516, 1960.

Sannella, N. A.: Inguinal hernia and colon carcinoma: Presentation of a series and analysis. Surgery 73(3): 434, 1973.

Terezis, N. L., Davis, W. C., and Jackson, F. C.: Carcinoma of the colon associated with inguinal hernia. N. Engl. J. Med. *268*:774, 1963.

Zollinger, R. M., and Kinsey, D. L.: The management of hernia: all ages. Postgrad. Med. *30*:20, 1961.

# 25

# The Relaxing Incision

My experience with use of the relaxing incision now covers a period of 28 years. I was introduced to this technique in hernia repair by the late Dr. Laurence S. Fallis, former Chief of Surgery at the Henry Ford Hospital. The procedure is not new; however, for some unknown reason, many surgeons have been reluctant to take advantage of it. I have used it most often in repairing large direct inguinal hernias, but it also can be used in repairing femoral hernias, large indirect inguinal hernias, and many recurrent groin hernias. It is most applicable for those situations in which the distance from the transversus abdominis arch, or "conjoined tendon," to Cooper's ligament or to the inguinal ligament is too great to permit approximation with acceptable tension. The incision is made vertically in the anterior sheath of the rectus abdominis muscle and extends upward near to but not including the linea alba. It is thus possible to strengthen the floor of Hesselbach's triangle without creating undue tension on the suture line. The integrity of the abdominal wall is not violated by this incision. The relaxing incision should be utilized far more often than it is, in my opinion.

## HISTORICAL BACKGROUND

I have previously reviewed the history of the development of the relaxing incision in hernia repair in Chapter 1. The changes in technique of performance and the evolution of the relaxing incision are shown in Figure 25–1. Note how the incision has shifted toward but not beyond the midline; in addition, its length has somewhat increased. At one time, the incision had been used to gain access to the rectus abdominis muscle, which was sutured to the inguinal ligament. Some of the earlier publications appeared in the German and French literature; these will be referred to in this chapter because of their importance. Brief descriptions made by various authors of the incision and its applicability to hernia repair, will follow.

Anton Wölfler, a student of the great Billroth, had used a relaxing incision for four years prior to his publication in 1892. In his work, Wölfler stated, "Then the lateral border of the rectus muscle is approximated and sutured to Poupart's ligament which is sometimes very easily accomplished and at other times more difficult to achieve. In the latter case the fascia of the rectus muscle is incised." Fortunately, the relaxing incision made by Wölfler was clearly illustrated (Fig. 25–2). In his repair, Wölfler then sutured the "posterior fascia of the rectus muscle and the muscle belly" to the aponeurotic lateral leaflet of the external oblique muscle or to the inguinal ligament.

Bloodgood, in close collaboration with Halsted, studied the hernia problem. In 1899 he noted that in certain cases the "conjoined tendon was obliterated." I interpret this statement to mean that the internal oblique and transversus abdominis muscles were deficient in the floor

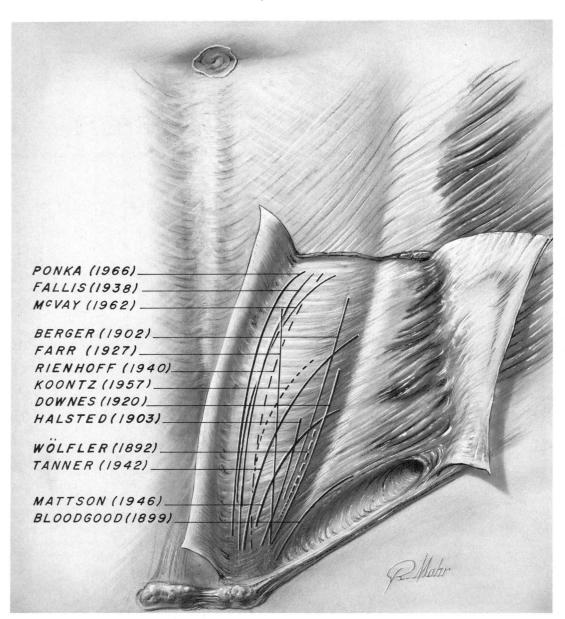

PONKA (1966)
FALLIS (1938)
McVAY (1962)

BERGER (1902)
FARR (1927)
RIENHOFF (1940)
KOONTZ (1957)
DOWNES (1920)
HALSTED (1903)

WÖLFLER (1892)
TANNER (1942)

MATTSON (1946)
BLOODGOOD (1899)

**Figure 25–1.**   This illustration includes the relaxing incision as performed by a number of surgeons. Note how the incision has moved toward the midline and increased somewhat in length.

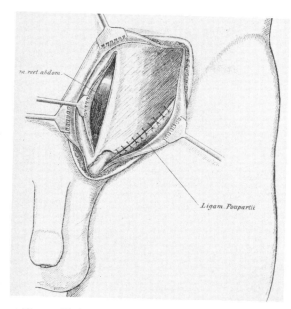

**Figure 25–2.** Reproduction of the original drawing of the incision into the rectus sheath as performed by Anton Wölfler. (From Wölfler, A.: Zur Radikaloperation des Freien Leistenbruches. Beitr. Chir. Festschr. Gewidmet Theodor Billroth, p. 573, Stuttgart, 1892, p. 573.)

of the inguinal canal. Bloodgood employed a maneuver that included suturing the rectus muscle to Poupart's ligament; time has shown this procedure to be unsatisfactory. He stated that the technique of performing the relaxing incision

was very simple. He divided the sheath of the rectus in the direction of the muscle bundles, from its insertion in the symphysis pubis, for a distance of 5 cm. This exposure gained access to the rectus abdominis muscle, which he employed in repair of the hernia. Bloodgood noted that by June 1898 Dr. Slajmer had repaired 150 hernias using Wölfler's method.

In 1902 Berger published a lengthy article on repair of hernia in the Revue de Chirurgie. Fortunately, his version of the relaxing incision was well illustrated (Fig. 25–3). Berger utilized an incision in the anterior sheath of the rectus, particularly in the treatment of direct inguinal hernias.

I then expose the anterior surface of the rectus abdominis sheath by elevating the superior border of the external oblique incision. I incise this anterior fascia parallel to and a fingerbreadth inward from the external border over a length of 8 to 10 cm until muscle fibers become visible throughout the entire length of the incision.

The technique of performance and the applicability of the relaxing incision were clear to Berger.

Halsted was a truly great student of the hernia problem. He continued his interest in the field throughout his career. He was

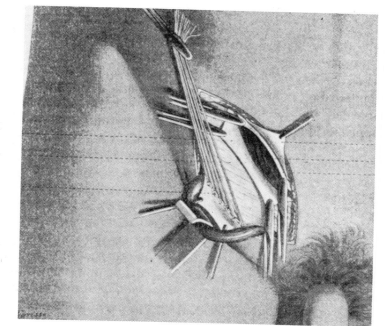

**Figure 25–3.** The original drawing of the incision into the rectus sheath as performed by Berger. (From Berger, P.: La hernie inguino-interstitielle et son traitment par la cure radicale. Rev. Chir. 25: 39, 1902.)

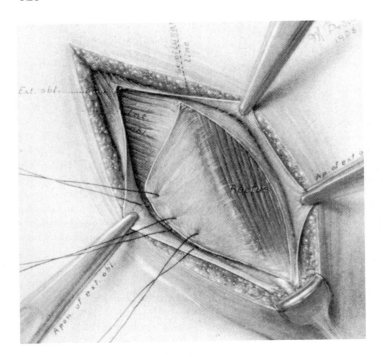

**Figure 25–4.** The relaxing incision as performed by Halsted. The lateral margin of the sheath of the rectus abdominis was utilized in the repair. (Reproduced with permission of The Johns Hopkins University Press, Baltimore, Maryland. From Halsted, W. C.: The cure of the more difficult as well as the more simple inguinal ruptures. Bull. Johns Hopkins Hosp. *14*:208, 1903.)

extraordinary in his ability to explore techniques and honest enough to reject those measures that proved ineffectual. In 1903 he performed his modification of the relaxing incision as follows: "The internal oblique muscle, mobilized and possibly further released by incising the anterior sheath of rectus muscle, is stitched (the conjoined tendon also) to Poupart's ligament in the Bassini-Halsted manner." It is through the availability of excellent illustrations that the evolution of the relaxing incision can be traced, and we are fortunate to have the drawing of Halsted's relaxing incision by Max Brödel (Fig. 25–4).

Both Halsted and Bloodgood appreciated the need for some method that permitted closure of the area of weakness between the conjoined tendon and the inguinal ligament.

Other surgeons have recognized the need for a maneuver that would permit repair of defects in the floor of the inguinal canal without undue tension. Among the interesting publications dealing with attempts to achieve relaxation of the conjoined tendon are the Transactions of the New York Surgical Society of 23 April, 1913. In this article, Lusk recommended that a vertical incision be made in the anterior sheath of the rectus and that the

sheath be divided transversely. In the same publication, Downes reported that he had employed rectus muscle transplantation in 165 patients. In 1920 Downes described his technique of opening the rectus sheath to gain access to the rectus abdominis muscle. Thus, he used a method that was similar to the one described earlier by Bloodgood.

Farr was a perceptive surgeon who pointed out in 1927 that although the Bassini repair gave excellent results in children with indirect inguinal hernias and in adults with good musculature, the results in repair of direct inguinal hernias were far from satisfactory. He observed that in direct inguinal hernias, the conjoined tendon could not be sutured to Poupart's ligament without excessive tension. To avoid this tension, in the aponeurotic layers of the middle of the belly of the rectus abdominis muscle, he made a vertical incision that extended from the symphysis upward for a distance ranging from 3 to 4 in. He observed that marked relaxation occurred, permitting the conjoined tendon and the edge of the rectus sheath to approximate Poupart's ligament without excessive tension.

Fallis in 1938 fully appreciated the importance of the relaxation incision in hernia repair (Fig. 25–5). Through his

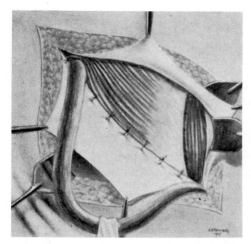

**Figure 25–5:** This illustration shows the relaxing incision as performed by Fallis in 1938. (Reproduced with permission of the J. B. Lippincott Company. From Fallis, L. S.: Direct inguinal hernia. Ann. Surg. *107*(4):579, 1938.)

efforts, many surgeons became aware of the importance of this technique. He made the relaxing incision as close as possible to the reflection of the aponeurosis of the external oblique muscle and extended it upward for approximately 2½ to 3 inches. Fallis used the relaxing incision in most direct inguinal hernias, but he also employed the technique in certain large indirect hernias and in a few femoral hernias.

Rienhoff in 1940 made an incision through the anterior sheath of the rectus, exposing the rectus abdominis muscle and the pyramidalis muscle. The incision in the rectus sheath was carried down to the superior ramus of the pubis and was made superiorly as far as permitted by the reflection of the aponeurosis of the external oblique muscle. He noted that such an incision released the anterior sheath and permitted bulging of the enclosed muscles.

Tanner in 1942 did much to call attention to the importance of the relaxation principle and advocated the use of what was to become known as the "Tanner slide." He made a curved incision through the aponeurosis of internal oblique and transversus abdominis muscles as they form the anterior sheath of the rectus abdominis muscle (Fig. 25–6). The incision commences approximately at the pubic crest and passes straight upward for a distance of 4 in. He advised a cautious

approach so as not to inflict injury on the iliohypogastric nerve. He noted that as soon as the incision is made, there is a tendency for the lateral margin of the incision to slide downward and laterally. Tanner suggested that if the insertion of the pyramidalis into the rectus sheath interfered with the "slide," the fascia between the pyramidalis and the sheath could be incised. He advocated use of his modification of the relaxing incision for direct inguinal hernias and for those indirect inguinal hernias with weakness in the floor of the inguinal canal.

Mattson in 1946 employed a relaxing incision in the repair of direct inguinal hernias, certain indirect inguinal hernias, femoral hernias, and recurrent hernias. From the anterior sheath, he fashioned a boomerang-shaped flap and sutured it to the pubic (Cooper's) ligament for a distance of 5 cm from the pubic spine.

Koontz in 1957 described his personal technique for performing a relaxing incision. He used it almost routinely in repair of inguinal hernias in adults. Koontz elevated the upper flap of the aponeurosis of the external oblique muscle. Blunt finger dissection is possible in initial operations, but in recurrent operations, the upper leaf of the external oblique muscle must be separated from the rectus sheath by sharp dissection. After the aponeurosis of the external oblique muscle is elevated with a retractor, an incision is made just lateral to

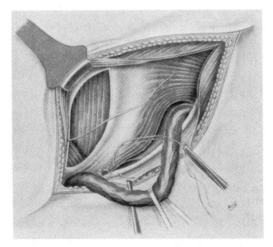

**Figure 25–6.** Tanner contributed to the popularization of the relaxing incision. (Reproduced with permission of *The British Journal of Surgery* and the author. From Tanner, N. C.: A slide operation for inguinal and femoral hernia. Br. J. Surg. 29:287 (January), 1942.)

the insertion of the external oblique apo-neurosis into the rectus sheath. Koontz extended the incision upward from the symphysis for a distance of about 3 in.

In 1960 Poth described his technique in which the rectus-pyramidalis sheath was used as a transplant or flap in the repair of groin hernias.

In 1962 McVay thoroughly studied the relaxing incision from the anatomic point of view, stating that "the relaxing incision begins just off center immediately above the pubic crest, and continues in a ce-phalic direction, following the line of fusion of the external oblique aponeurosis with the rectus sheath." The length of the incision ranged from 5 to 7 cm, in the average case.

Monasch of Rotterdam in 1966 pointed out that Dutch literature contained little on the subject of the relaxing incision. He advocated its use in the repair of inguinal hernias as a means of avoiding tension. He realized that not all inguinal hernias re-quired repair of the inguinal floor but felt that when repair of this area was indicated, a relaxing incision was a logical means of avoiding excessive tension on the suture line. His method of performing the relax-ing incision was very similar to McVay's.

Nielsen and his colleagues in 1972 recognized that in repair of direct inguinal hernias, the weak point is the most medial part of the posterior inguinal wall. They pointed out that the excessive tension in this area can be avoided by the use of a vertical relaxing incision in the rectus sheath. They plan to use this incision more frequently in the future.

## ANATOMY OF THE RELAXING INCISION

The surgeon who would employ the relaxing incision should be thoroughly familiar with the anatomy of the lower abdomen and the rectus sheath. Many general anatomic facts have already been discussed in Chapter 2. In this section, some of the important details will be con-sidered.

On careful examination, the line of fusion of the external oblique with the rectus sheath can be seen to approach the midline immediately above the pubic

crest. McVay states that occasionally this fusion fails to occur, making it possible for the surgeon to perform the relaxing inci-sion on the opposite side of the repair. It would be possible, in rare instances, to incise the linea alba. I have never seen such an anatomic arrangement. As the line of fusion of the external oblique with the rectus sheath is followed upward in a cephalad direction, it progresses laterally until it fuses inseparably with the anterior sheath of the rectus abdominis muscle (Fig. 25-7).

After a relaxing incision has been per-formed, the external oblique aponeurosis provides a strong protective layer over the gaping defect.

The relaxing incision is made through the anterior sheath of the rectus abdominis muscle. Its components are aponeurotic elements from the internal oblique and transversus abdominis as they pass an-terior to the rectus abdominis muscle to fuse in the midline with similar structures from the contralateral side (Fig. 25-8).

Koontz (1926) has shown experimentally that the incision in the sheath of the rectus does not produce an area of weakness. Furthermore, regeneration of connection tissue occurs. I can confirm these observa-tions based on operations in man. Al-though the defect produced as a result of the "slide" can be recognized, a connec-tive tissue develops over the once visible rectus muscle. The rectus muscle and the transversalis fascia combine to form an effective barrier against herniation.

When the relaxing incision is made, one additional structure is often recognizable. Anson and his coworkers, have found that the pyramidalis muscle is present in 90 per cent of individuals, but it varies consider-ably in size and form. The fascia of the anterior rectus sheath also encompasses the pyramidalis muscle. In a small number of patients, it may be necessary to incise the connective tissue sheath or septum, which passes posteriorly and somewhat obliquely to the pyramidalis muscle.

In addition to the external oblique aponeurosis and the rectus abdominis and pyramidalis muscles, there is another structure that contributes to the integrity of the abdominal wall following the relax-ing incision. The transversalis fascia, as well as the peritoneum, remains intact

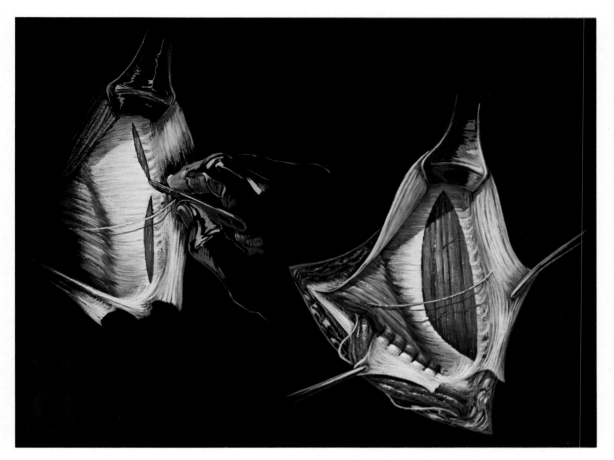

**Figure 25-7.**    This illustration shows an anterior view of important structures to be considered in performance of the relaxing incision. The incision must be made in the anterior sheath of the rectus abdominis muscle. The pyramidalis muscle is often seen. The incision curves laterally in the cephalad direction since the external oblique aponeurosis becomes tightly fused with the sheath.

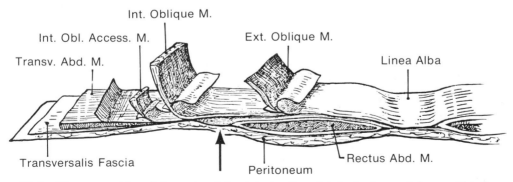

**Figure 25-8.**    The composition of the rectus abdominis sheath as it is in the lower abdomen. This figure also shows the rectus fascia — and how the rectus abdominis muscle and transversalis fascia (arrow) prevent a hernia through the relaxing incision. (Reproduced by permission of authors. From McVay, C. B., and Anson, B. J.: Composition of the rectus sheath. Anat. Rec. 77:217, 1940.)

posterior to the muscles of the rectus sheath (Fig. 25–8, p. 531).

I have alluded to the danger of erroneously incising the linea alba when fusion fails to occur between the external oblique aponeurosis and the anterior sheath of the rectus abdominis. Also, a problem arises if the relaxing incision is made just lateral to the rectus abdominis muscle where the aponeurotic lamina fuse before continuing onto the rectus abdominis muscle.

It is truly remarkable that I have never seen a hernia occur through a relaxing incision as described in this chapter. McVay has made precisely the same observations in his practice. It is a safe procedure and definitely increases the possibility of cure of hernias in which a shift of tissues is necessary to strengthen areas of weakness in the floor of the inguinal canal.

## TECHNIQUE OF PERFORMING THE RELAXING INCISION

The skin and subcutaneous tissues are first divided. Hemostasis is achieved, and an incision is made in the fascia of the external oblique at the level of the superior crus. The ilioinguinal nerve lies on the spermatic cord, along with the cremaster muscle. The upper leaflet of the external oblique aponeurosis is elevated as far superiorly and medially as possible. Blunt dissection will suffice as a means to separate the fascia from the anterior sheath of the rectus muscle. The iliohypogastric nerve may now be seen and protected. In patients who have recurrent inguinal hernias or have had previous lower abdominal surgery, sharp scalpel dissection may be necessary.

The anterior sheath of the rectus muscle is made up of aponeurotic contributions from the internal oblique and transversus abdominis muscles. The rectus abdominis and pyramidalis muscles are enclosed in the sheath. Care is taken to make the incision as near to the midline as possible, commencing at the pubic crest or slightly above and extending upward for a distance ranging from 5 to 8 cm, depending on the size of the individual patient.

Two structures must be recognized and spared during performance of a relaxing incision — the iliohypogastric nerve and a branch of the deep inferior epigastric artery. If the artery is divided, it must be ligated, lest a troublesome hematoma develops. If the incision is performed after the transversus arch or conjoined tendon is sutured to either the inguinal or Cooper's ligament, gaping of the incised sheath occurs, revealing the rectus abdominis muscle. It has occurred to me that this surprising distraction of the rectus sheath may cause some surgeons to doubt the advantage to using this in the repair of any hernia. If any fibrous attachments of the pyramidalis muscle interfere with relaxation, these may be divided. I am particularly careful to neither incise the linea alba nor cut through the fascial lamina just lateral to the rectus abdominis muscle. A properly made relaxing incision always results in a separation or gaping of the cut edges of the sheath, thus exposing the red rectus abdominis muscle (Fig. 25–7, p. 531).

## ADVANTAGES OF THE RELAXING INCISION

1. It permits approximation of the transversus arch (conjoined tendon or lateral margin of the rectus sheath) to Cooper's ligament or to the inguinal ligament without excessive tension.
2. Its use does not result in weakness of the abdominal wall.
3. The relaxation, or "slide," permits the lower fibers of the internal oblique to lie more nearly parallel to Poupart's ligament.
4. After the relaxing incision is made, sutures are less likely to cause tissue necrosis and more likely to remain intact.
5. Since the defect can be bridged with the patient's available tissues, synthetic meshes, grafts, and foreign materials are unnecessary.
6. Bilateral hernia repairs can be carried out as a simple operative procedure, since tension can be avoided through the use of the "slide."
7. Operative time is less when compared to more elaborate grafting techniques, whether fascia or synthetic meshes are used.

## SUMMARY

Surgeons who have had experience with the relaxing incision generally agree on its usefulness in the repair of direct inguinal and recurrent direct inguinal hernias. They use it frequently in repairing large indirect inguinal hernias, particuarly when there is a weakness in the floor of Hesselbach's triangle. McVay does not feel that the relaxing incision is needed in small or medium hernias or in most femoral hernias. I find that I am using the relaxing incision with increasing frequency in the repair of femoral hernias or when I consider the tension on the suture line to be excessive in the repair of direct inguinal hernias, including those of moderate size. Tanner used the "slide" in repair of direct inguinal hernias and certain indirect and femoral hernias. The relaxing incision, or "Tanner slide," is an extremely useful adjunct in repair of those hernias resulting from a weakness in the inguinal floor. It permits approximation of the fused portions of the transversalis fascia, the transversus abdominis, and the internal oblique (i.e., the transversus arch, or conjoined tendon) to Cooper's ligament or to the inguinal ligament without excessive tension.

## REFERENCES

Anson, B. J., Beaton, L. E., and McVay, C. B.: The pyramidalis muscle. Anat. Rec. 52:405–411, 1938.

Berger, P.: La hernie inguino-interstitielle et son traitment par la cure radicale. Rev. Chir. 25:1, 1902.

Bloodgood, J. C.: Operations on 459 cases of hernia in the Johns Hopkins Hospital from June, 1889 to January 1899. Rep. Johns Hopkins Hosp. 7:223, 1899.

Downes, W. A.: Management of direct inguinal hernia. Arch. Surg. 1:53, 1920.

Fallis, L. S.: Direct inguinal hernia. Ann. Surg. 107(4): 572, 1938.

Farr, C. E.: A modified technic for difficult inguinal hernias. Surg. Gynecol. Obstet. 44:261, 1927.

Halsted, W. C.: The cure of the more difficult as well as the simpler inguinal ruptures. Bull. Johns Hopkins Hosp. 14:208, 1903.

Koontz, A. R.: Personal technique and results in inguinal hernia repair. J. A. M. A. 164:29, 1957.

Koontz, A. R.: Muscle and fascia suture with relation to hernia repair. Surg. Gynecol. Obstet. 42:222, 1926.

Lusk, W. C.: Rectus transplantation by a special technique. Ann. Surg. 58:675, 1913.

Mattson, H.: Use of rectus sheath and superior pubic ligament in direct and recurrent inguinal hernia. Surgery 19:498, 1946.

McVay, C. B.: The anatomy of the relaxing incision in inguinal hernioplasty. Q. Bull. Northwestern University Med. Sch. 36:245, 1962.

McVay, C. B., and Anson, B. J.: Composition of the rectus sheath. Anat. Rec. 77:213–225, 1940.

Monasch, S.: The relaxing incision in the anterior rectus sheath in the operative treatment of inguinal hernia. Arch. Chir. Neerl. 17:13–21, 1966.

Nielsen, O. V., Jørgensen, S. P., and Ottsen, M.: Inguinal herniorrhaphy by anatomical transversalis fascia repair. Acta Chir. Scand. 138:701–704, 1972.

Ponka, J. L.: The relaxing incision in hernia repair. Am. J. Surg. 115:552–557, 1968.

Poth, E. J.: A basic concept in the use of the rectus-pyramidalis sheath and transplants in the repair of hernias. Surg. Gynecol. Obstet. 3:515–516, 1960.

Rienhoff, W. F.: The use of the rectus fascia for closure of the lower or critical angle of the wound in the repair of inguinal hernia. Surgery 8:326, 1940.

Tanner, N. C.: A slide operation for inguinal and femoral hernia. Br. J. Surg. 29:285, 1942.

Wölfler, A.: Zur Radikaloperation des Freien Leistenbruches. Beitr. Chir. (Festchr. Gewidmet Theodor Billroth), Stuttgart, 1892, p. 552.

# 26

# Prosthetics in Hernia Repair

*The choice of herniorrhaphy must have basis: sound knowledge of the anatomy and physiologic requirements of the region; a recognition of the fundamental factors concerned in wound healing and tissue repair; and a certain ingenuity which allows an occasional disregard of "routine procedures."*

*Dr. Tom Dercum Throckmorton, 1947*

## INTRODUCTION

The ingenious use of reinforcing materials to strengthen a weakened abdominal wall is a comparatively recent development that was initiated during the present century. Laparotomies were performed with increasing frequency, and intra-abdominal inflammatory and neoplastic diseases were treated with increasing success; however, the favorable results were not achieved without complications. Some patients were left with large disabling herniations; and, although many could be repaired successfully with the patient's own tissues, others recurred repeatedly. Surgeons searched diligently for a material to implant into the abdominal wall — something that would add strength while avoiding the excessive tension created when large defects, either inguinofemoral or abdominal incisional, were bridged by approximating the patient's own tissues.

### Definition of Terms

It is interesting that long before the need for tissue substitutes was identified, there already existed a suitable vocabulary for appropriate use by the surgeon. Furthermore, a definition of terms was essential, since a clear understanding of terminology is the key to implementation of known facts regarding implantation surgical techniques.

*Webster's New International Dictionary* was consulted for most of the definitions that follow:

**PROSTHESIS:** The addition to the human body of some artificial part.

**IMPLANT:** To set securely or deeply. Through usage, the term has also been more or less accepted as a noun; in this context an implant might consist of any material placed within the human body.

**FILIGREE:** The term originally referred to ornamental work in which fine wire of gold, silver, or copper was used in the decoration of art objects. It is used here to describe an open arrangement of fine wire.

**FABRIC:** A cloth that is woven or knit from fibers (vegetable, animal, or synthetic in origin).

**NETTING:** A piece of network; any fabric of crossing cords (threads, ropes, wires, or the like) with open spaces between them.

**CLOTH:** A woven, pliable fabric.

**MESH:** Pertains to a network or netting. Yarns might be monofilamentous or multifilamentous. The interval between the material used is usually much greater than the diameter of the yarn.

**SPONGE:** A flexible porous material. The term originally described natural sponges; currently, it refers to a synthetic, plastic, porous material that resembles the natural sponge physically but not chemically.

**TEXTILES:** This term includes fabrics that are woven, braided, or knitted. In textiles, the diameter of the interstices is less than the diameter of the yarn. According to Wesolowski and colleagues (1966), the most useful textile implants are fabricated from multifilament yarns.

## Desirable Qualities in a Prosthetic Material

The ideal prosthetic material has not yet been produced; nevertheless, many effective and useful materials are available. The need for prosthetic materials is universal in the practice of surgery. Surgeons who employ such materials should be aware of their desirable features as well as their limitations. Cumberland in 1952 and Scales in 1953 identified a number of desirable qualities in materials to be used as prosthetics. Since 1959, I have had an interest in materials that might be used to strengthen the abdominal wall. Wesolowski and coworkers have considered the use of artificial materials in surgery in an exhaustive report, which includes an impressive list of 424 references.

The demands placed on a material that is to serve as a replacement or reinforcement for some portion of the abdominal wall are enormous. The desirable qualities in an ideal prosthetic material, which are listed in Table 26–1, are briefly described as follows:

**STRENGTH:** This is an extremely important quality; a prosthetic material must be capable of holding the abdominal wall together in a relatively normal state.

Table 26–1. **DESIRABLE QUALITIES IN A PROSTHETIC MATERIAL**

Strength
Durability
Tissue tolerance
Flexibility
Ease of handling
Nonwandering
Tolerated in presence of infection — stability
Availability
Porosity
Easily sterilized
Nonallergenic
Does not undergo alterations: cyst formation
                                               malignant changes
Economic

**DURABILITY:** This is an essential quality if the implanted material is to remain effective over a long period of time. Permanent and unaltered strength is a highly desirable quality in any material implanted into the abdominal wall for retaining purposes.

**TISSUE ACCEPTANCE:** Implies that the material is incorporated into the abdominal wall without excessive or prolonged inflammatory response. It is well known to surgeons, especially those involved in organ transplantation, that the tissues of one individual will have no inclination whatsoever to accept those of another. Furthermore, synthetic materials are not really "accepted" by the tissues.

When tissues are exposed to a chemical, physical, or mechanical irritant, an inflammatory response follows. Foreign materials evoke a great variety of responses that can be summarized briefly as follows:

1. Destruction and lysis of the foreign material.
2. Incorporation and tolerance.
3. Rejection and extrusion.

Destruction takes place through the action of phagocytes and enzymatic degradation of foreign proteins. Catgut sutures, as well as those of silk, are removed from sutured wounds.

Certain implanted materials may be isolated or incarcerated in a dense fibrous capsule. Here, the foreign body interferes very little with the biologic integrity of the individual and, thus, is permitted to remain relatively isolated.

Other materials, such as meshes, possess open spaces that are invaded by fibrous tissue. Such circumstances result in minimal objections on the part of the host's biologic identity. We recognize the situation as a state of "tolerance" or "acceptance." On the other hand, certain closely woven materials evoke a severe cellular reaction, with prolonged exudation leading to infection and extrusion in an unacceptably high percentage of cases. Such a response is called "rejection" or extrusion. Arnaud and colleagues (1977) observed that cloth materials resulted in encystment or extrusion following implantation.

It is important to realize that implanted material is subject to biologic scrutiny on the part of the host. If the material can be incorporated into the tissues without evoking excessive reaction, then the result is acceptable. It is unlikely that any material that is completely nonreactive in the body will ever function as a prosthetic material for hernia repair, since such material would fail to gain attachment to the abdominal wall.

**FLEXIBILITY AND PLIABILITY:** These are obvious qualities that a material must have in order to assure comfort to the patient following implantation. Conversely, rigid materials lead to erosion, ulceration, and discomfort. Infection may well follow such events. The ideal material would approach the consistency of the normal abdominal wall after implantation.

**EASE OF HANDLING:** Consideration of ease in handling must be given by the surgeon in selecting a prosthetic. Materials that are soft, pliable, and can be cut into desirable shapes without unravelling are preferable. Rigid materials that lack conformity are generally avoided.

**NONFRAGMENTATION:** This is an essential quality in a prosthetic material, since it must retain its strength for a prolonged period of time. Fragmentation is a serious limitation inherent in certain metallic implants such as tantalum.

**NONWANDERING:** The ability of materials to provide continued strength in a previous area of weakness is a necessity. Metallic meshes have been found to wander considerable distances, causing complications.

**TOLERANCE:** The material must be able to withstand the effects of infection. Incisional hernias occasionally contain incarcerated and strangulated bowel; in such situations, the mesh must be used only on strong indication. When infection supervenes, certain meshes can interfere with healing, and occasionally it becomes necessary to remove the material.

**AVAILABILITY:** Consideration of this important aspect in implantation explains the popularity of synthetic prosthetic materials, since a second operative procedure is unnecessary (as is the case with fascia lata).

**POROSITY:** This characteristic is universally present in the prosthetic materials currently being used. It is this feature that permits ingrowth of fibrous tissue and capillaries. Such incorporation of the material adds strength and permanency to the implant (Fig. 26–1).

Surgeons who use implants should be familiar with the fundamentally important work of Vorhees and colleagues in 1951. Their research was done in the field of vascular surgery—employing tubes of fine mesh cloth to serve as a conduit. Vorhees and colleagues postulated that the interstices would become filled with fibrin plugs and that eventually fibroblasts would grow into the porous material. The area would subsequently become covered with an endothelial layer. Such, indeed, was the chain of events. On autopsy of the animals, Vorhees and coworkers found that fibroblasts grew into the interstices of the implanted Vinyon "N" cloth. The quality of porosity in a prosthetic material is as important for an abdominal wall implant as it is for a vascular prosthesis. The pores permit strong incorporation of the implanted material by virtue of fibrous tissue ingrowth and, hence, continuity with the body wall of the host.

**EASE OF STERILIZATION:** This must be considered, since avoidance of infection is of the greatest importance when implants are used. Furthermore, if the material can be resterilized without loss of strength, a saving will result from use of portions of mesh remaining from previous repairs.

**NONALLERGENICITY:** An essential quality if the implanted material is to function without causing a severe local reaction. Extrusion and infection are other

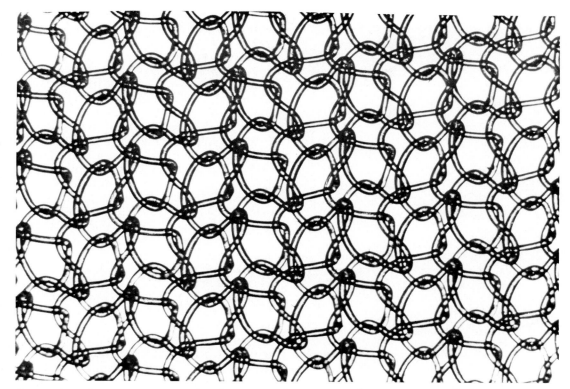

**Figure 26–1.** Porosity is an essential quality in a prosthetic material that permits ingrowth of connective tissue and, hence, incorporation of the implant into the abdominal wall. (Reproduced by permission of the author and *Archives of Surgery.* From Usher, F. C.: A new technique for the repair of inguinal and incisional hernias. Arch. Surg. *81*:847–854, 1960.)

sequelae that may occur if a sensitizing material is used in hernia repair.

ALTERATIONS FOLLOWING IMPLANTATION: This includes cyst formation and malignant degeneration. Inclusion cyst formation and malignant degeneration have been seen following repair of hernias with cutis graft for reconstruction of the abdominal wall.

ECONOMICAL: The cost of production of the material to be employed in a reconstruction of abdominal wall defects must be reasonable. It must be kept in mind that the patient's own tissues might serve the need without additional expenditure.

In Table 26–1, I have enumerated most of the qualities desirable in a material to be considered for use in repairing abdominal wall defects. As new materials are introduced, they are followed by a wave of enthusiastic acceptance. After a period of evaluation, too many of these materials fade into oblivion. Tantalum has suffered such a fate.

## CLASSIFICATION OF REINFORCING MATERIALS FOR USE IN HERNIA REPAIR

No single classification of implantable materials is completely satisfactory. A variety of tissues, metallic substances, and synthetic materials have been used to replace tissues destroyed by infection or excised by surgery (as in removal of malignant tumors). In some instances, the patient's own tissues were shifted or relocated as free grafts and, hence, cannot be considered prosthetic materials even though they do provide reinforcement of weakened abdominal wall areas.

In Table 26–2, I have listed several materials that have been used, or are currently employed, in the repair of abdominal wall defects. Some of these materials perished in the experimental laboratory and were never used in patients, while others enjoyed a short life-span.

Table 26–2.  A CLASSIFICATION OF
REINFORCING MATERIALS FOR
HERNIA REPAIR

I **Autografts**
  A. *Fascia Lata*
    1. Free
    2. Pedicle
  B. *Tendon*
  C. *Cutis Graft*
  D. *Whole Skin*
II **Homograft**
  A. *Fascia Lata*
  B. *Aorta*
III **Heterografts**
  A. *Fascia*
  B. *Tendon*
  C. *Pericardium*
IV **Metallic**
  A. *Stainless Steel*
  B *Tantalum*
  C. *Silver*
V **Synthetic-Plastic**
  A. *Marlex Mesh (High-density polyethylene)*
  B. *Mersilene (Dacron polyester)*
  C. *Nylon (Polyamide)*
  D. *Others*
    1. Teflon (Polytetra-fluoroethylene)
    2. Ivalon sponge (formalized polyvinyl)

The large variety of substances used experimentally and clinically as prosthetic materials suggests that the perfect substitute has yet to be developed.

## AUTOGRAFTS

### Fascia Lata

Autografts have been used extensively in repair of both incisional and recurrent inguinal hernias. Fascia lata was the most popular autologous tissue because of its strength, availability, and tissue acceptance.

McArthur was the first to use aponeurotic strands of the external oblique in repair of inguinal hernias in1901. In 1910 Kirschner utilized a rectangular piece of fascia lata to strengthen the inguinal area during herniorrhaphy, transplanting the fascia as a free graft. Gallie and LeMesurier in 1921 and 1923 demonstrated that when autologous fascial strips were used in hernia repair, the material did not stretch or contract when placed in a location similar to that from which it was removed. It is to be noted that Gallie and LeMesurier utilized strips of fascia lata in the repair of inguinal hernias. They observed that the incision from which

the fascia was obtained—in the lateral aspect of the thigh—healed without disability even when the remaining defect in the fascia of the thigh was not closed.

Others who utilized fascia lata grafts in hernia repair included: Joyce (1940), Cowell (1946), Singleton and Stehouwers (1945), and Hamilton (1956). The aponeurosis of the external oblique may also be used as a reflected flap for repair of defects in the abdominal wall. Austin and Damstra (1951) utilized fascial flaps, pedicle grafts of fascia lata, and free transplants of fascia lata in a variety of large, complicated, ventral hernia repairs. They found that the transplants became incorporated in the transplanted position without significant loss of strength.

Chaimoff and Dintsman utilized the anterior sheath of the rectus abdominis for repair of midline incisional hernias in 1973.

The advantages of autogenous fascia are numerous. First, the patient has his own supply in the form of fascia lata. Second, it causes no abnormal tissue reaction. Third, because of its width, autogenous fascia does not cut through tissues. Fourth, it will survive in the patient, retaining its strength for prolonged periods of time.

Why, then, is the use of autogenous fascia not more popular? The need for a second operative procedure is an inconvenience to both the patient and the surgeon, as well as an added expense. Also, patients do not appreciate a lengthy scar on the thigh, and surgeons are not enthusiastic at the prospect of harvesting a sheet of fascia. In addition, complications at the donor area do occur; Hamilton (1968) reported a significant incidence of complications (such as seromas and hematomas), occurring at the donor site in the thigh.

### Tendon

Pilcher (1939), in an effort to strengthen the floor of the inguinal canal, used the plantaris tendon—which was fixed in position in a zig-zag fashion. The method has not been a popular choice and probably will not become one, since the tendon is absent or inadequate in a substantial number of patients and a secondary procedure would be necessary to obtain the graft.

## Cutis Grafts and Whole Skin Grafts

In early attempts to discover a readily available and strong prosthetic material for repair of various bodily defects, cutis and whole skin grafts were explored as possible sources. Serious drawbacks to successful use of these materials included the presence of hair follicles and sebaceous glands.

Cutis grafts, which consist of the skin minus the epidermal covering, have been utilized since 1913 in repair of hernias and also in plastic surgery. The epidermis may be removed by scraping, shaving, or cutting it off with a dermatome (split-thickness layer) as reported by Swenson and Harkins. Microscopically, the cutis graft contains the normal layer and sebaceous sudoriferous glands, hair follicles and a thin layer of adipose tissue.

According to Cannaday (1942), Loewe first used cutis grafts in 1913. Rehn utilized cutis transplants in reconstructive surgery in 1914. By 1928, Uihlein had reviewed 104 cases operated on by Rehn, including 65 incisional hernias and 11 inguinal hernias. Cannaday in 1942 believed that cutis grafts were of value in repair of large incisional hernias.

Harkins in 1943 reported on the use of a cutis graft in the repair of a large incisional hernia. With his usual thoroughness, Harkins later studied the behavior of cutis grafts in more detail and reported on eleven additional operated cases in 1945. He specifically noted that it was impossible to remove all epithelial elements from a cutis graft and retain sufficient dermis in the tissue to be transplanted.

In 1937 Peer and Paddock carried out extensive experimental studies on the fate of deeply implanted dermal grafts. They noted that in obtaining a cutis graft there remained some epithelial elements. Closed cyst cavities, although of microscopic size, contained horny epithelial material and fragments of hair. Sebaceous glands, hair follicles, and sweat glands were seen at variable periods postimplantation. Granulation tissue surrounded the implant and consisted of lymphocytes, macrophages, and epithelioid cells as well as giant cells. The studies of Peer and Paddock provided carefully documented information as to the fate of dermal grafts.

Couris and Wylie (1964) reported a case in which a huge epidermal cyst developed 17 years and 9 months after it had been implanted by Harkins (Fig. 26–2). Not only did this patient develop a huge cyst, but it eventually developed into a squamous cell carcinoma; this case was reported by Gomez, Wylie, and Ponka (1972). This possible consequence of the use of skin is a

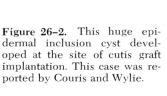

**Figure 26–2.** This huge epidermal inclusion cyst developed at the site of cutis graft implantation. This case was reported by Couris and Wylie.

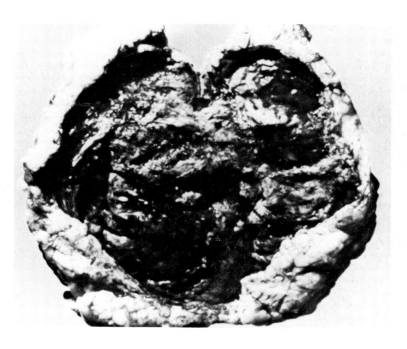

serious limitation of its use as a long-term prosthesis (Fig. 26–3).

The use of whole skin was used briefly as a prosthetic material in hernia repair. Mair utilized whole skin in hernia repair, and by 1944 he reported on 88 such repairs. He felt that atrophy of the epithelial elements occurred when the graft was sutured under tension. A lengthy follow-up study of these cases was not, to my knowledge, available. Marsden failed to identify cyst formation among 164 inguinal hernia patients in whom whole skin was used as a prosthesis.

Subsequent to the increased use of cutis and whole skin grafts for hernia repair during the late 1940's, a rash of postoperative cysts appeared in the 1950's; this complication is so significant that some of the early cases will be briefly discussed here (Table 26–3).

Chodoff in 1949 found that the incidence of wound complications was no greater following skin graft repair of hernias. But, in a significant study in 1951, Strahan found 9 cysts or wound sinuses among 413 patients who had a variety of hernias repaired with whole-skin grafts as a supporting material. In addition, sepsis was encountered in 4.3 percent of Strahan's patients. The recurrence rate was 6.8 percent in this group of hernias repaired with whole-skin grafts.

Rutter in 1955 reported formation of a large cyst seven years after cutis graft of a hernia. It measured 7 × 3 centimeters and contained waxy inspissated material and several hairs. Microscopically, the cyst was found to be lined with squamous epithelium. Fortunately, the hernia repair remained sound, although dense scar was present.

Powell and Ewing described a postimplantation dermoid cyst in 1952 following earlier whole-thickness skin repair of an incisional hernia in a female patient. Her postoperative course was complicated and prolonged, requiring several operations. Two large cysts, containing debris and opalescent fluid, were excised.

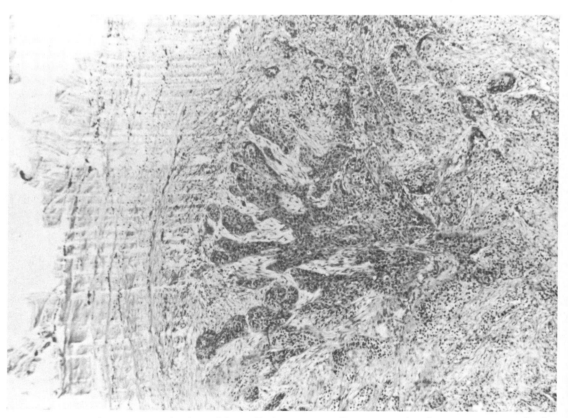

**Figure 26–3.**    A photomicrograph taken of the wall of squamous cell carcinoma developing in a cutis graft. This case was reported by Gomez, Wylie, and Ponka.

Table 26–3.   REPORTED CASES OF CYST FORMATION FOLLOWING CUTIS
OR SKIN GRAFTS

| Author | Cases | Material | Type of Hernia | Interval | Size (cm) |
|---|---|---|---|---|---|
| Strahan (1951) | 9 | Skin | Inguinal | 16 mos. | 6.5 × 3.0 (Average) |
| Powell (1952) | 1 | Skin | Incisional | 9 mos. | 6.5 × 3.5 |
| Clarke (1952) | 1 | Skin | Inguinal | 12 mos. | 1.5 × 0.5 |
| Rutter (1955) | 1 | Cutis | Inguinal | 84 mos. | 7.0 × 3.0 |
| Wylie (1964) | 1 | Cutis | Incisional | 113 mos. | 10.0 × 4.5 |

Piper in 1969 compared the repair of direct and indirect inguinal hernias in men by the whole thickness skin graft method and the Bassini method. He obtained significantly better results with whole-thickness skin grafts in the repair of direct hernias than he did with the Bassini method in the repair of indirect inguinal hernias. The problem of sepsis was significant—occurring in 7 percent of the cases, with wound discharge continuing for an average of 8.8 months. Piper found the rate of cyst formation to be 3.2 percent.

Because of the danger of infection, sinus formation, epidermoid cyst formation, and even epidermoid carcinomatous degeneration, I do not advise the use of cutis grafts or whole-thickness skin grafts in hernia repair. Furthermore, the easy availability of effective synthetic prosthetic materials or fascia lata should render the use of dermal grafts obsolete in hernia repair.

## HOMOGRAFTS

### Fascia Lata—Aorta

In 1954 Usher and colleagues began using homologous human fascia and heterologous ox fascia that had been preserved by a freeze-drying process, or lyophilization. Human fascia lata was removed from the thighs of suitable individuals, cut into strips, and threaded on needles. These strips were then treated with antibiotics, placed in Pyrex glass tubes, and frozen. At the completion of this procedure, the fascial strips were almost completely dehydrated; however, they could be reconstituted by their being placed in a saline solution for 15 minutes. They were then suitable for use in the repair of hernias. Usher and colleagues repaired 63 hernias with lyophilized fascia, with 3 recurrences. When two of these specimens were removed at autopsy, they showed no foreign body reaction on microscopic examination. The lyophilized fascia also retained its strength, as shown by tensiometer tests.

Fogelson and Jackson (1959) utilized lyophilized aortic homographs to repair what they described as tissue-deficient inguinal hernias. They found the tissue to be well tolerated in five patients and recommended further use of the material.

## HETEROGRAFTS

### Fascia—Tendons—Pericardium

Heterografts have been utilized in the past but never gained popularity as prosthetic materials for hernia repair. Ox fascial grafts and kangaroo tendons had been explored for possible use in humans.

Heterografts have been far more effective in the research laboratory animal than they have in man. Horsley (1931) found that alcohol-preserved fascia of the ox is quickly absorbed and rapidly loses its tensile strength.

Koontz reviewed the early history of tendon transplantation. He pointed out that Nageotte in 1917 was able to transplant pieces of alcohol-preserved tendon successfully. The changes incident to the successful incorporation of the tissue were described. Initially, Koontz performed animal experiments to determine the fate of dead fascial transplants. He preserved fascia derived from various sources in 70 percent alcohol and later implanted it into the connective tissue of these animals. He utilized fascia lata, sheath of the rectus, fascia lata and pericardial sac of the ox, and the submucous coat of pig's bladder. These materials were used to repair defects in abdominal walls of dogs and cats. He found that the grafted material was incorporated into the surrounding tissue of the host ingrowth of fibroblasts. The implanted tissue became vascularized, and dead cells were replaced by living cells within the graft.

Favorably impressed with his experiments on animals, Koontz then utilized strips of ox fascia lata that had been preserved in alcohol. The material was threaded onto needles and sutured into the defect.

Because of the general availability of animal tissues, this possible source of a strong fascial suture was explored by Koontz in 1927. The material proved unsatisfactory on clinical trial, because wound infection, fascial sloughs, and recurrence of hernias were all too common. For these reasons, he abandoned the use of this material.

The use of kangaroo tendon in hernia repair is of historical interest. Koontz cited the report of Hutchinson who employed kangaroo tendon in hernia repair.

Heterografts have largely been used experimentally to bridge defects in animals. Such materials ordinarily undergo dissolution and rejection. Chemical modification of heterografts alters the response but does not stop the rejection mechanisms. Heterografts cannot be recommended as desirable materials for hernia repair at this time.

## METALLIC PROSTHESES

### Stainless Steel

Based on a knowledge of the nature of stainless steel, it would theoretically seem likely that such a metallic prosthesis could well provide strength for a defective area. The material is durable and inert in living tissues.

Preston and Richards have found annealed steel mesh to possess great and permanent strength. They also found that it did not have a tendency to work-harden. They emphasized that stainless steel is well tolerated in infected wounds, and it need not be removed in the presence of wound infection or drainage.

Preston and Richards in 1973 reported their experiences with the use of wire-mesh prostheses in treatment of hernias in 2000 patients; extending over a period of 24 years. These surgeons emphasized the need for rigid adherence to aseptic principles. Strict hemostasis, gentleness, avoidance of undue trauma, and use of sharp dissection were identified as important technical details. They recognized that excessive tension interfered with healing because it compromised the blood supply to the area. The authors used annealed stainless steel — which is inert, has permanent strength, does not work-harden, and is malleable. Preston and Richards advised that wide coverage of the defect area was important if abdominal pressure was to be distributed over a wide area. In inguinal hernia repair, the mesh is attached under the conjoined tendon and under the edge of the rectus sheath. The authors reported the rate of infection to be 0.1 percent. They did not find it necessary to remove the mesh in any patient.

Abel and Hunt utilized stainless steel wire somewhat ingeniously in 1948 when they improvised a technique in which the wire was used as a suture for darning the defect.

Babcock popularized the use of stainless steel in 1952. Haas and Ritter utilized a specially prepared stainless steel net for repair of huge incisional hernias in 1958. Bapat and Patel found stainless steel mesh to be effective in repair of inguinal hernias.

Mathieson and James continue using stainless mesh and report only two recurrences among 93 operated cases in a follow-up of from one to five years.

It appears that stainless steel mesh has not yet been eliminated as a strong and well-tolerated prosthetic material. With currently improved methods of manufacture, it is apparent that in the hands of Preston and Richards the material is highly effective.

There is some prejudice against the material because it is a "metal." There is also the fear that the material will fragment, migrate, and cause pain. Richards and Preston have not been able to confirm the occurrence of such events.

### Tantalum Gauze

Tantalum gauze as a prosthetic material became popular after both Throckmorton and Koontz presented their experiences with this material. Throckmorton submitted his findings for publication in April, 1947, followed by Koontz in December of 1947. Douglas (1948) and Lam and colleagues (1948) reported their experiences with this metal. Tantalum is an element that chemically is capable of resisting acids and alkalis, much as glass does. It exhibits excellent tensile strength and is quite malleable. It may be manufactured into wire or woven into a gauze. The material is pliable and, hence, may be handled with comparative ease. When implanted into living tissues it serves as a network for ingrowth of fibrous tissue, which is sometimes excessive.

Koontz initially utilized tantalum in the repair of incisonal hernias; Throckmorton repaired groin hernias, incisional hernias, and one obturator hernia with the metallic mesh. There is no doubt that when tantalum was introduced, it was a reasonably good material for repair of abdominal wall defects. After 1948, the popularity of this metallic mesh increased as evidenced by a number of favorable reports, including that of Dunlop (1950). In 1951, Koontz utilized tantalum gauze to reinforce Hesselbach's triangle in the repair of large defects in the groin. He discovered only one recurrence out of 77 patients operated on and followed for 25 months. He did not discuss postoperative complications.

In 1951 Flynn and colleagues reported their experiences with 45 ventral hernias repaired with tantalum gauze and followed for 55 months. In this series, there was only one recurrence. The authors noted that, with the passage of time, fragmentation of the gauze occurred after a "work-hardening" process. In two cases, gross infection did not require removal of the tantalum. Flynn and coworkers observed that pain occurs when the mesh is implanted adjacent to bone.

Burton in 1959 and Adler in 1962 cited several disadvantages to the use of tantalum mesh; the relative inflexibility of the material, its tendency to undergo fragmentation, and the possibility of erosion and even occasional protrusion through the skin were noted. In some cases, the material would fragment and permit development of a small hernia.

My early experience with tantalum was generally favorable; however, discomfort, if not pain, was a common complaint among many patients. Collections of serum were not at all uncommon, many requiring aspiration. Tantalum, wherever it came in contact with bowel, became intimately attached to it—making subsequent dissection difficult, if not impossible. Migration following fragmentation became a problem in a few cases where the mesh had been utilized in repairing lower abdominal wall defects (Fig. 26–4).

In 1959, Burton summarized serious objections to the use of tantalum succinctly as follows: (a) fatigue fractures of the mesh were often seen; (b) tantalum is less pliable than autografts and, hence, is not as comfortable; (c) the contour of the abdominal wall may become irregular. If excision of the graft becomes necessary, it must be removed in its entirety with some sacrifice of the remaining abdominal wall. Subsequent repair of any residual hernia would thus be more difficult.

In spite of a brief period of popularity in the 1950s, tantalum gauze lost a great deal of its attractiveness to surgeons. Fragmentation and wandering of the material are serious objections to its use. If it is properly implanted, Koontz and Kimberly found that it is well accepted in the presence of infection. If the material is loosely sutured and does not come in contact with the tissues, removal of the foreign body may be necessary if infection supervenes. If silk, cotton, or other braided sutures are utilized, they can contribute to chronic draining sinuses.

In my opinion, tantalum—because of its relative inflexibility, its tendency to undergo fragmentation, and its propensity for wandering—has lost most of its appeal to surgeons. Early enthusiasm for this material as an implant for hernia repair has largely abated. At the present time, I do not employ it in any hernia repairs.

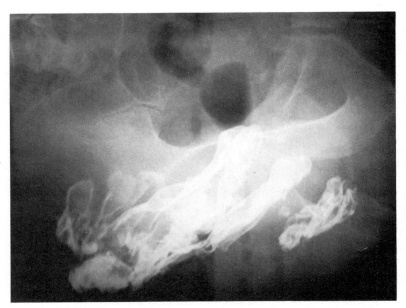

**Figure 26–4.**   X-ray film of abdomen following hernia repair with tantalum. The wrinkling, fragmentation, and wandering are strikingly demonstrated.

### Silver Wire

Metallic prosthetic materials such as filigrees, grids, plates, and meshes have been used in hernia repairs since 1894, according to Throckmorton (1948). He stated that Phelps utilized coiled silver wire in repair of inguinal hernias. Throckmorton noted that Witzel in 1900 had fashioned a network of crossed silver wires. Witzel further suggested the possibility of implanting ready-made filigree; however, it was Goepel who (in 1900) was the first to employ such material in a herniorrhaphy. Throckmorton also noted that Meyer in 1902 used a silver wire netting and that Bartlett in 1903 utilized a filigree of wire loops as prosthetic materials. McGavin in 1909 and Warren in 1921 both employed a silver wire filigree in hernia repair in 1909.

More recently, Cole (1941) reported his experiences in applying the filigree operation for hernia repair—placing the silver wire network in the floor of the inguinal canal. The results could not be accurately reported, since many of his patients were British seamen who, of necessity, traveled afar. Since that time, silver wire as mesh or filigree has been infrequently utilized.

Gradually, the use of silver wire and filigree fell into disrepute. Throckmorton noted the observations of McGavin and summarized the objections to use of silver wire. (1) Discomfort was experienced by a number of patients. Silver wire and filigree lack pliability, and the rigidity causes discomfort. (2) The material is not completely inert and becomes work-hardened. (3) There is an aversion on the part of patients to the idea of having foreign materials placed in their bodies.

## SYNTHETIC PLASTIC MATERIALS

### Marlex Mesh

The search for more desirable prosthetic implants continues, with a variety of synthetic materials being presented to surgeons for their acceptance and use. These plastic materials possess enduring strength. They are pliable but are not always well accepted by the recipient. The easy availability and reasonable cost of these materials are also desirable features. A number of investigators have contributed important information regarding the biologic reactions evoked by implantation of plastic materials into both man and animals. Some of the materials result in fibrous tissue ingrowth and tolerance by the host. Others provoke the foreign body reaction that necessitates extrusion of the material should implantation be followed by infection.

Usher deserves credit for his early and extensive researches on the use of prosthetic materials in hernia repair. His excellent techniques of implantation have been amply illustrated in his numerous publications. As early as 1958, Usher and Wallace investigated tissue reaction to the following plastics: nylon, orlon, Dacron, Teflon, and Marlex. They placed these materials into the peritoneal cavities of dogs. Upon sacrificing the animals seven days later, the two researchers found that Teflon and Marlex caused less foreign body reaction than did nylon, orlon, or Dacron. Usher and Wallace suggested that Marlex might be valuable in fabrication of surgical prostheses; and by 1958 Usher, Ochsner, and Tuttle had repaired 34 incisional hernias with Marlex mesh.

Usher and Wallace presented their observations on a new substance, "Marlex 50 polyethylene." The new material was described as possessing high tensile strength and pliability. This high-density polyethylene, as an implant, became infiltrated with connective tissue. It is impervious to water and is resistant to many chemicals. It has a softening temperature of 260° F and may be sterilized in boiling water without damage. The tensile strength of the monofilamentous material was found to vary from 50,000 to 150,000 lbs/sq. inch. It definitely possesses more strength than silk.

The use of high-density polyethylene (Marlex) increased rapidly. By 1962 Adler found that it was used by 20 percent of the surgeons whom he questioned; since that time, the material has continued to gain in popularity.

In 1959 Usher and colleagues reported their results with 78 patients with hernias (23 with inguinal hernias) and other tissue defects. Usher and coworkers observed the implanted material in three patients who developed abscesses and found it to be well tolerated. Incision and drainage plus antibiotic therapy resulted in eventual healing.

In January of 1959 Usher reported further experimental studies with Marlex mesh. In these experiments, the surgical repairs were performed on dogs. Usher found that the material was well tolerated when utilized in the repair of defects of the abdominal wall, chest wall, and diaphragm. The mesh was found to be infiltrated with fibrous tissue, and granulation tissue grew into the interstices. Marlex was well tolerated even in the presence of infection.

At the Henry Ford Hospital, we have been interested in Marlex mesh since it first became available to us in 1959 (Ponka, et al.). At that time, we found that the material was well tolerated following implantation in experimental animals. The connective tissue ingrowth into the meshes of the Marlex was striking. We subsequently implanted it into patients with excellent results. I have since been impressed that the material is well tolerated and retains its strength for indefinite periods of time.

By November of 1960, Usher and colleagues described techniques for implantation of Marlex into patients with inguinal and incisional hernias. They pointed out that tension could be avoided in the repair of large hernias with the implantation of a prosthesis.

Usher continued his interest in the use of Marlex mesh in the repair of large incisional hernias and complicated inguinal hernias. By 1962 (according to Usher), 541 hernias had been repaired by various surgeons in the United States, utilizing this material.

Drainer and Reid (1972) found that Marlex mesh was an effective substance for implantation, but they reported an infection rate of 22.2 percent and a mortality of 7.5 percent. These results are not as good as those reported by other authors (e.g., Usher).

Gilsdorf and Shea (1975) used Marlex mesh in the repair of massive ventral abdominal wall defects. Of the six patients involved, four survived. It should be pointed out that Gilsdorf and Shea used the mesh as a protective covering for the exposed intestine and permitted early ambulation by the patient.

Jacobs and colleagues (1965) found knitted Marlex mesh to be useful in the repair of difficult incisional hernias and clearly illustrated the variety of techniques for implantation of the material. They reported the incidence of seroma to be 45 percent. This is higher than the 6.3 percent reported by Usher in 1963.

Walker and Langer (1976) repaired large ventral hernias in 14 patients. Three other patients required excision of the adjacent abdominal wall along with their tumors. There were only two recurrences among those patients who underwent surgery for hernia repair. Walker and Langer found Marlex mesh to be the best synthetic material available. In three patients, it was well tolerated in the presence of infection.

Schmitt and Grinnan (1967) found that Marlex mesh was well suited for use in infected abdominal war wounds.

Of all the synthetic materials currently available, Marlex is probably the most useful, possessing most of the qualities listed in Table 26-1. It has been used liberally for two decades, with an established record of excellence as a prosthesis. Findings have shown it to be both well incorporated into and well tolerated by adjacent tissues. Its strength, flexibility, and durability have been established through clinical use.

Marlex is well tolerated in infected areas, provided that monofilament sutures are used. Heavy braided sutures serve as foci of residual infection and prolonged drainage from sinuses. Double thicknesses of Marlex mesh might also complicate healing in the occasional case. Of all materials in the surgeon's armamentarium, Marlex has an established record of excellence as a prosthesis.

## Mersilene (Dacron) Mesh

Mersilene is a synthetic mesh of polyester fibers. This material was used in the repair of 23 hernias by Abdul-Husn (1974). The author stressed the need for rigid adherence to aseptic principles in the repair of hernias with this material.

Calne (1974) utilized Mersilene mesh in the repair of bilateral inguinal hernias, placing the mesh behind the rectus abdominis muscles. The material was well tolerated in the patients studied.

Cerise and coworkers (1975) carried out experimental and clinical studies to evaluate the worth of Mersilene mesh in repair of abdominal wall defects. They found the material to be effective, with both a complication rate and recurrence rate of only one percent.

Durden and Pemberton (1974) used Dacron in the repair of ventral and inguinal hernias. They stressed the need for adequate dissection, careful hemostasis, and asepsis. They recommended that a single layer of mesh be used as an extraperitoneal implant. They sutured the Dacron implant in place with number 2–0 synthetic nonabsorbable sutures placed 6 mm apart.

Adler (1962) found Dacron to be an effective prosthetic material. Wolstenholme (1956) also found Dacron mesh to provide strength in the repair of both inguinal and femoral hernias. Haskey and Bigler (1975) repaired ventral herniations in 20 patients without major complications.

Linn and Vargas (1973) utilized Silastic-encased Dacron to generate a fibrous tissue reaction at the site of hernia repair. The material was removed after a growth of connective tissue developed at the hernia site.

Casebolt (1975) utilized both Marlex mesh and Mersilene and concluded that there was little to choose between the materials—both were effective for hernia repair.

Mimms and Tinckler (1976) utilized Mersilene mesh to provide support for a weakened transversalis fascia, which they demonstrated on special studies utilizing a scanning electron microscope. The mesh provided a trellis for fibrous tissue ingrowth.

## Nylon

Nylon initially gained acceptance among surgeons through its use as a strong and durable suture material, which caused minimal tissue reaction. Nylon has been used somewhat more often in England than in the United States. Doran and colleagues (1961) used thin nylon net in the repair of 86 inguinal hernias. They reported 19 recurrences in 67 operations. They tried using a thick or heavier netting with very poor results—of the 15 patients in whom this material was tried, chronic sinuses occurred in over 50 percent. Doran and colleagues also used a medium nylon netting in 212 inguinal hernia repairs. With this material, the results were more acceptable; they reported 4 recurrences in 189 repair cases followed for two years. In six septic cases, removal of the mesh was necessary.

Moloney has been using nylon since 1958 and has described a nylon-darn method for the repair of hernias. He does not advocate use of braided sutures but has found that the monofilamentous material withstands sepsis.

Adler and Firme (1962) pointed out that nylon tended to lose its tensile strength and to fall apart when used as an implant.

Ludington and Woodward (1959) observed that nylon loses 80 percent of its strength due to hydrolysis and chemical deterioration.

At present, nylon cannot be recommended as a desirable prosthetic material for repair of abdominal wall defects.

### Teflon—Ivalon

TEFLON. LeVeen and Barberio (1949) studied the tissue reaction evoked by Teflon. They called attention to the fact that Teflon cannot be rendered "wet" when exposed to water. Nothing will adhere to it, and it is remarkably inert. When Teflon was placed in the peritoneal cavity, finely divided chips were seen to lie free with no gross evidence of tissue reaction. Without an inflammatory response, connective tissue proliferation does not occur under conditions just described.

Gibson and Stafford (1964) attempted to repair large ventral hernias with Teflon mesh in 25 patients but found it necessary to remove the mesh in five patients in order to achieve complete healing. They reported wound complications in 50 percent of their patients.

Ludington and Woodward (1959) utilized Teflon (polytetrafluoroethylene) mesh in repair of abdominal wall defects in 26 patients. They felt that the results justified further use, as indicated by a 6- to 12-month follow-up of their patients. Copello (1968) found Teflon mesh useful in repair of complicated recurrent groin hernias.

Teflon, in its current state of manufacture, cannot be recommended for repair of hernias. The material is not incorporated into body tissues, and an unacceptably high rate of wound complications has been reported (Gibson and Stafford, 1964).

IVALON (Polyvinyl) sponge was implanted in dogs to repair diaphragmatic defects. In studies up to 12 months, Pesek and Keeley (1958) found that the sponge underwent fragmentation and that there was a dense fibrous tissue ingrowth. Numerous foreign body giant cells were seen on microscopic examination.

Adler and Darby (1960) found that Ivalon (Polyvinyl formal) sponge possessed poor tensile strength following implantation. Ivalon has not been identified as a suitable prosthetic material for repair of abdominal wall defects.

### SUMMARY

Of all the synthetic materials advocated for repair of hernias, Marlex and Mersilene meshes are currently the most useful.

My personal experience with Marlex mesh dates back to 1959. I have found it to be an effective material for hernia repair. It is durable, pliable, and well tolerated by the tissues; and it performs well in the presence of infection, provided that a single layer of mesh is used and nonbraided sutures are employed for fixation.

### CLINICAL STUDY

In order to evaluate our experience with fascial and prosthetic implants, I reviewed available records of 266 patients who had incisional hernias repaired at the Henry Ford Hospital from 1946 through 1976.

### Sex Distribution

In this particular study, the use of some adjunct in incisional hernia repair was required somewhat more often in males than in females. It is to be noted that, generally, incisional hernias are reported to be more common in females. Prosthetic material was used in the repair of 142 hernias (or 53.4 percent) in males and 124 (or 46.6 percent) in females.

### Age Incidence

The need for prosthetic implants arises infrequently in young patients. Only 12, or

4.5 percent, of the patients were under 36 years of age. In these patients, infection was a complicating factor in wound healing following initial surgery. Adult and geriatric patients were found to be appropriate candidates for hernia repair with prosthetic materials (Fig. 26–5).

### History and Physical Examination

The clinical histories of the patients with incisional hernias were very much alike. Protrusion with discomfort was the most common complaint. Furthermore, often numerous unsuccessful operations had been performed in an attempt to correct the protrusion.

Incarceration of omentum and bowel was common, but symptoms of intestinal obstruction were infrequent. Even in cases of large and long-standing herniation, intestinal obstruction was unusual. Surgeons were reluctant to use implants when gangrenous intestine was present. The danger of infection was obviously a deterring factor. Only 13 of the 266 patients included

in this study had symptoms suggestive of intestinal obstruction.

Obesity was a factor in 132 of the 266 patients. The adverse effect of obesity on the postoperative patient is well known to surgeons. It is unfortunate that so many fat people would rather switch doctors than lose weight! Use of implants has proved to be useful in repair of hernias in many obese individuals.

Most of the incisional hernias, on physical examination, were found to be large — generally over 10 centimeters in diameter. One hundred forty-nine hernias were large; 87 were of medium size; and only 30 patients had hernias measuring less than 6 centimeters in diameter.

Incarceration of viscera was common in these hernias; however, obstruction was encountered in four patients, and strangulation occurred in only two patients.

### Initial Surgical Procedures

It is useful to note the initial operative procedures that led to herniations ulti-

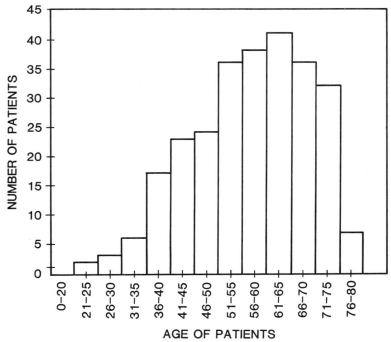

Figure 26–5.   Age incidence of 266 patients with incisional hernias repaired with implants.

## Table 26–4. INITIAL OPERATIVE PROCEDURE

| Type | Number |
|---|---|
| Cholecystectomy and biliary tract surgery | 58 |
| Hysterectomy | 38 |
| Gastric surgery | 34 |
| Appendectomy | 31 |
| Umbilical and epigastric hernia repair | 18 |
| Colectomy | 10 |
| Trauma | 10 |
| C-section and other pelvic operations | 10 |
| Small bowel resection | 8 |
| Vascular operations | 5 |
| Miscellaneous | 44 |
| Total | 266 |

mately requiring some type of prosthesis (Table 26–4).

Well over half of the initial operations required incisions in the upper abdomen. It was difficult to gather details; however, it can be stated that most of the patients who required implants had some type of postoperative complication.

Little will be gained from a further discussion of Table 26–4; however, since the miscellaneous group is so large, it may be helpful to identify some of the cases included in this category. Operations on the spleen, kidneys, adrenals, and pancreas were occasionally followed by the occurrence of hernias, which were repaired with implants. Specific operative procedures included in this group were sympathectomies, urethropexy, transabdominal repairs of rectal prolapse, excision of pubic ramus, and secondary operations upon the gastrointestinal tract. Some of the procedures could not be well identified, either after the patient's history had been taken or at the time of the repair.

## Postoperative Complications

The complications that occurred following initial operative procedures were difficult to establish in every case, since many patients had their first operative procedure (or procedures) performed at other institutions. Despite this fact, some useful information can be gained from the experience. The complications that were most often recognized are summarized in Table 26–5.

The adverse effects of wound infection, wound disruption, pulmonary complications, ileus, and hematomas on the healing wound have been discussed at length in Chapter 20 on wound disruption.

Placement of a drain through an operative incision predisposes the area to infection and interferes with wound healing at the drain site. We had ample opportunities to observe the deleterious effects of drains placed through appendectomy incisions in the right lower quadrant or through the middle portion of subcostal incisions utilized for cholecystectomy. We have discontinued this practice with a great reduction of hernias at these locations. Drains should be placed through specially placed stab wounds in the flank, not through operative incisions.

Surgeons of experience recognize that patients who have had radiotherapy to the abdomen heal with difficulty. Postoperative hernias are not at all uncommon in patients who have undergone pelvic irradiation. Such therapy was identified in only 4 of 266 patients included in this study. Tissues become atrophic, and blood supply to the irradiated area is definitely decreased. Connective tissue in such areas is of poor quality and, in the presence of herniation, poorly suited for use in hernia repair. The skin in such cases is also atrophic and heals slowly.

The destructive effects of repeated operative procedures on the abdominal wall are obvious when one considers that 104 patients out of 266 in this study required 2 or

## Table 26–5. POSTOPERATIVE COMPLICATIONS FOLLOWING INITIAL PROCEDURE IN 266 PATIENTS

| Type | Number |
|---|---|
| Wound infection | 58 |
| Wound disruption | 33 |
| Pulmonary complications | 30 |
| Ileus | 20 |
| Hematoma | 12 |
| Other factors: | |
|     Drain through wound | 48 |
|     Irradiation | 6 |
|     Multiple operations | 104 |
| Total° | 311 |

°Total is greater than number of operations because some patients had more than one complication.

Table 26–6.  NUMBER OF PREVIOUS
REPAIRS – 266 PATIENTS WITH
INCISIONAL HERNIAS

| Number of Previous Repairs | No. Patients |
|---|---|
| 1 | 162 |
| 2 | 51 |
| 3 | 30 |
| 4 | 23 |
| 5 | 5 |
| 6 | 4 |
| 7 | 2 |
| 8 | 1 |
| 9 | 3 |

more operative procedures (Table 26–5). The history of multiple previous abdominal operations should alert the surgeon to the possible need of some prosthetic material in the repair of a hernia.

### Number of Previous Operations

While it is true that 162 patients (or 61 percent) had one operative procedure prior to undergoing repair with a prosthesis, it is noteworthy that another 104 (or 39 percent) had two or more abdominal operations (Table 26–6).

For 104 patients requiring numerous repairs, 317 attempts were made at reconstruction before implants were considered to be indicated. These statistics point out the repeated morbidity and enormous cost associated with every incisional hernia. Every helpful device must be utilized in repair of difficult recurrent hernias.

### Time of Appearance of Incisional Hernias

Incisional hernias usually appear promptly after unsuccessful repair. Furthermore, patients become surprisingly skillful at recognizing a recurrence, indicating this event by the simple and distressingly accurate observation: "It came back." Even obese patients develop a tactile sense that permits identification of a small or moderate defect hidden in the depths of a heavy panniculus (Table 26–7).

Most of the hernias ultimately repaired with prosthetic materials appeared within

the first year following some type of operative procedure or repair of an incisional hernia. As I have noted, patients become remarkably skillful at identifying recurrences.

### Site of Hernias Repaired with Implants

In some cases, it was most difficult to identify the actual location or site of certain defects. Such hernias were large and involved a considerable portion of the abdominal wall. Many of them were the result of numerous attempts at repair through a variety of incisions into the abdominal wall (Table 26–8).

### Indications for Use of Prosthetic Materials in Repair of Hernias

Indications for the use of prosthetic materials in hernia repair must be more clearly defined. As more desirable synthetic materials become available, implants will be used more frequently. It appears to me that the significant recurrence rate following incisional and inguinal hernia repairs provides a strong argument for greater use of a prosthetic material to repair defects without generation of excessive tension.

In this series of 266 patients undergoing repair of incisional hernias, I could identify a number of indications for use of implants; these are listed in Table 26–9.

The presence of a large defect with loss of substance of the abdominal wall is a picture altogether too familiar to surgeons. In the occasional patient, generous amounts of tissue must be excised because of malignancy. In such situations, bringing the edges of the defect together creates such

Table 26–7.  TIME OF APPEARANCE OF
INCISIONAL HERNIAS

| Time of Appearance | Number of Patients |
|---|---|
| 0 to 1 mo. | 56 |
| 2 to 6 mos. | 108 |
| 7 to 12 mos. | 56 |
| 13 to 24 mos. | 12 |
| 3 to 5 yrs. | 12 |
| 6 yrs. and longer | 22 |
| Total | 266 |

Table 26–8. SITE OF DEFECTS
REPAIRED WITH IMPLANTS IN
266 PATIENTS

| Area | Number of Patients |
|---|---|
| Right upper quadrant | 67 |
| Upper abdominal midline | 61 |
| Lower abdominal midline | 58 |
| Right lower quadrant | 53 |
| Left lower quadrant | 17 |
| Left flank | 5 |
| Left subcostal | 5 |
| Total | 266 |

excessive tension that failure is all too
common.

Multiple repairs result in heavy scar
formation at the site of repair. It is becoming recognized that the fibrous tissue of a
large cicatrix is, at best, a poor substitute for
normal tissues.

Loss of substance is somewhat difficult to
describe, but the experienced surgeon
recognizes the situation as one in which
there has been destruction of tissue.
Wound infection was recognized as a factor
contributing to incisional hernias in 58, or
21 percent, of the cases included in this
study.

Obesity, per se, can hardly be considered
as an indication for prosthetic implants, but
when this factor is present in a patient with
a moderate or large defect the use of
additional supporting material to the repair
is reasonable.

Pulmonary disease — such as severe emphysema, chronic bronchitis, and severe

Table 26–9. INDICATIONS FOR USE OF
PROSTHETICS IN 266 PATIENTS

| Indication | Number of Patients |
|---|---|
| Large defect | 149 |
| Loss of substance | 108 |
| Multiple operations | 104 |
| Obesity | 132 |
| Pulmonary disease | 24 |
| Irradiation | 6 |
| Strenuous work | 3 |
| Patient on steroid therapy | 1 |
| Total* | 527 |

*Some patients had more than one indication for
use of implants; hence, the total number of indications will be greater than the number of patients.

cough — places additional stress on the site
of repair. Again, the use of an implant is
often indicated.

The adverse effect of irradiation on
healing wounds is well known. Atrophic
tissues receive an impaired blood supply
and, consequently, heal poorly.

Some patients must perform heavy labor
and place great pressure upon any abdominal incision. This also is true of weight
lifters and those who perform strenuous
muscular exercises. Some thought should
be given to the use of prosthetic materials
in such individuals if incisional hernias are
a problem.

Clinical experience with patients on
prolonged steroid therapy has shown that
hernias tend to recur in such individuals.
The use of a prosthetic material is indicated
in the occasional patient who has an
incisional hernia but must continue steroid
medication for prolonged periods of time.

## Techniques of Placement of Prosthetic Materials for Hernia Repair

During the past 50 years, surgeons have
gained much useful information regarding
the use of prosthetic implants as a means of
adding strength to a more or less compromised abdominal wall. (Most of the
significant contributors are cited in the
references.) Surgeons have increasingly
recognized that excessive tension produced by injudicious attempts at closure of
all hernias without implants results in an
unacceptably high number of recurrences.
Strong synthetic materials that provide
strength while being tolerated by the
tissues are available. These implants are
ultimately incorporated into an infiltrating
connective tissue network.

In this section I will discuss the techniques now available and the general
principles for implantation of prosthetic
materials.

Koontz was a pioneer in search of a
suitable prosthetic material, beginning in
1927 with his utilization of preserved
fascial grafts. He reported his experiences
with tantalum in 1951 and in 1959 (as a
coauthor with Kimberly). Koontz later
summarized many of his ideas in a book
published in 1963. In that publication, he
illustrated use of a prosthetic material as an
onlay graft.

Usher recognized the need for a prosthetic material that could be used to repair abdominal wall defects in 1954. He published many articles alone and with colleagues. I have cited 12 of his references in which he describes a number of techniques for implantation of prosthetic materials. Usher illustrated a number of methods for implantation of Marlex mesh in his publications in 1970 (Fig. 26–6). He showed that

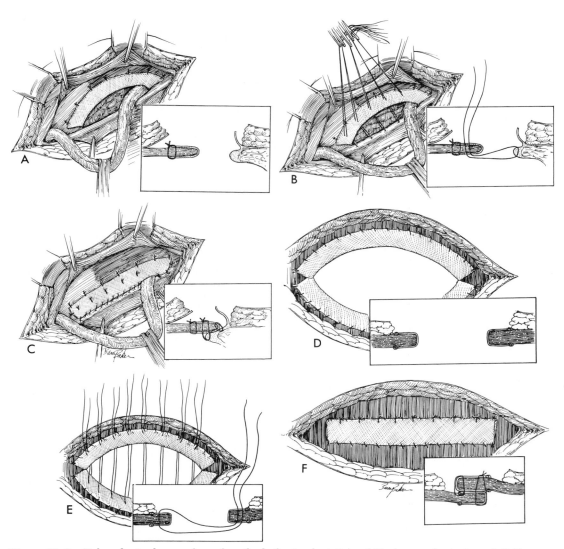

**Figure 26–6.** Usher devised a number of methods for implantation of Marlex mesh. *A*, *B*, and *C* illustrate Usher's techniques for repair of inguinal hernias; *D*, *E*, and *F* show Usher's techniques for repair of incisional hernias.

*A*—A strip of Marlex mesh, 1 inch width, is sutured as a cuff over the free edge of the conjoined tendon; the transversalis fascia has been incised. *B*—Imbricating sutures of number 0 polypropylene are placed ½ inch apart; these sutures must pass through the mesh anteriorly and posteriorly. *C*—The imbricating sutures are pulled up and tied, and a second row (continuous number 0 polypropylene) is placed to complete the overlap; additional interrupted sutures are placed lateral to the cord. *D*—Two 2-inch strips of Marlex mesh are sutured as a cuff over the opposing edges of the hernial ring, using a continuous suture of number 0 polypropylene monofilament. *E*—Imbricating sutures of number 0 polypropylene monofilament are placed ¾ inch apart; these sutures must pass through the mesh anteriorly and posteriorly. *F*—The imbricating sutures are pulled up and tied, and a second row of continuous number 0 polypropylene (reinforced with a few interrupted sutures) is placed to complete the overlap. (*A-F*, Reproduced by permission of author and publisher. From Usher, F. C.: The repair of incisional and inguinal hernias. Surg. Gynecol. Obstet. *131*:325, 1970. Copyright 1970 by *Journal of Surgery, Gynecology, and Obstetrics.*)

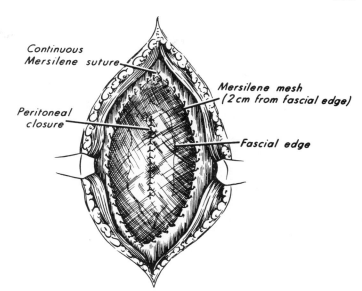

**Figure 26–7.** Cerise and coworkers applied the prosthetic material as an onlay graft after closure of the peritoneum. In this instance, the material implanted bridged the defect to provide strength in the repair. (Reproduced by permission of the author and J. B. Lippincott Company. From Cerise, E. J., et al.: The use of Mersilene mesh in repair of abdominal wall hernias. Ann. Surg. *181*(5):731, 1975. Copyright 1975, J. B. Lippincott Company.)

the implanted material could be implanted deeply within the abdominal wall or more superficially as an onlay graft. He also utilized the mesh in repair of difficult inguinal hernias.

In 1965 Jacobs, Blaisdell, and Hall identified a number of methods for implantation of Marlex mesh. More recently (1975), Casebolt summarized the various methods available for implantation of prosthetic materials.

Cerise and coworkers (1975) utilized Mersilene mesh in repair of incisional hernias and inguinal hernias. They pointed out the need for closure of the transversalis fascial layer (Fig. 26–7).

Copello (1968) illustrated important details in the attachment and placement of prosthetic materials in repair of difficult hernias in the lower abdomen and groin (Fig. 26–8).

Surgeons have accepted the premise that prosthetic implants do, in fact, increase the strength of repair. Cerise and coworkers and Arnaud and coworkers demonstrated that implanted materials increased the strength of healing wounds in rats. The determined bursting pressures in animals with and without implants demonstrated the effectiveness of prosthetics in providing additional support to the operative area.

### Placement of Prostheses

I have utilized a variety of locations for implantation of prosthetic materials (Fig.

26–9). In general, I favor the preperitoneal position for implantation. Positioning of the mesh posterior to the rectus abdominis muscle is also effective (Fig. 26–9). Synthetic meshes may be placed in these common locations:

1. Intra-abdominal (inlay graft)
2. Preperitoneal
3. Subaponeurotic
4. Subcutaneous (onlay graft)

The mesh may be implanted in two layers, or it may serve to bridge a defect in the abdominal wall.

In 266 patients included in this clinical study, I found that the synthetic material was implanted as indicated in Table 26–10.

It can be seen that, as a general principle, implantation of the prosthesis into the depths of the repair is desirable. The subcutaneous location for implantation of a prosthetic material was not frequently chosen and was employed in only 2.6 percent of the repairs.

### REPAIR OF INCISIONAL HERNIAS IN 266 PATIENTS IN WHOM PROSTHETIC IMPLANTS WERE USED

#### Anesthesia

In the early years of this study (during the 1950s), spinal anesthesia was popular. This modality of anesthesia provided excellent relaxation. The undesirable sequelae of spinal anesthesia included backache,

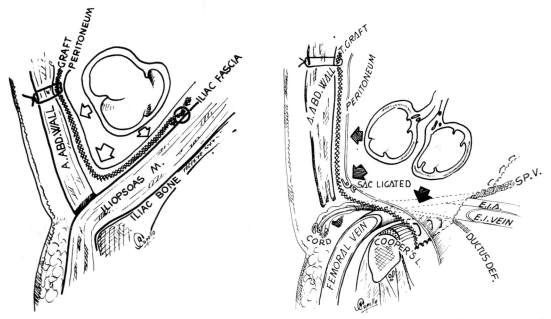

**Figure 26–8.** Copello illustrated a number of methods for attachment of mesh in the repair of lower abdominal and groin hernias. His methods of implantation and fixation are sound. *A* shows a sagittal view lateral to the femoral vessels. The mesh is attached to the iliac fascia. Note the generous piece of mesh used. In *B*, the sagittal view is in the region of the iliac and femoral vessels. Note attachment of the mesh to Cooper's ligament. (Reproduced by permission of the author and J. B. Lippincott Company. From Copello, A. J.: Technic and results of Teflon mesh repair of complicated re-recurrent groin hernias. Rev. Surg. 25(2):98–100, 1968. Copyright 1968. J. B. Lippincott Company.)

headache, and urinary retention (Table 26–11). Although these complications were uncommon, they were annoying and occasionally led to prolonged periods of morbidity.

Gradually, endotracheal general anesthesia gained in popularity, so that now it is a preferred method of anesthesia for repair of complicated incisional hernias.

Local anesthesia was used in only 27 patients who either were considered increased surgical risks or had comparatively small hernias. At the present time, I prefer endotracheal general anesthesia for repair of incisional hernias.

### Suture Material

During the 1950s, silk and catgut were the most popular suture materials. Wire was used infrequently; however, with the improved quality of this material, its use has gained in popularity. Wire retains its strength and is well tolerated in the presence of infection.

Currently, synthetic nonabsorbable monofilamentous sutures are popular. Number 2–0 Dacron is commonly selected when strength is important.

### Implants Used in Repair of 266 Incisional Hernias

In an experience with incisional hernias at Henry Ford Hospital from 1948 to 1973, implants were utilized in 34 percent (as noted in Chapter 21).

During the 1950s and early 1960s, fascia lata and tantalum metallic mesh were the materials most often used. Since Marlex mesh became available, it has been used almost exclusively (Table 26–12).

Although Harkins (1943) employed cutis grafts in repair of incisional hernias at Henry Ford Hospital in 1943, this material has since fallen into disfavor because of cyst formation and malignant degeneration. Couris and Wylie (1964) documented the case in which a large epidermoid cyst developed in the grafted area (Fig. 26–2). Later, Gomez, Wylie, and Ponka (1972) reported growth of epidermoid carci-

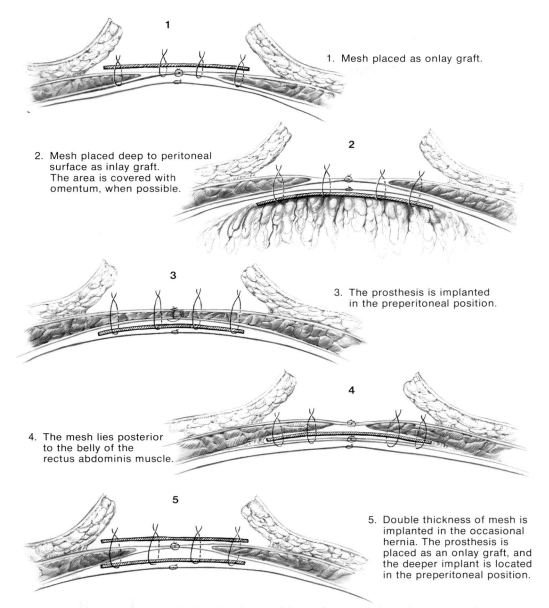

1. Mesh placed as onlay graft.

2. Mesh placed deep to peritoneal surface as inlay graft. The area is covered with omentum, when possible.

3. The prosthesis is implanted in the preperitoneal position.

4. The mesh lies posterior to the belly of the rectus abdominis muscle.

5. Double thickness of mesh is implanted in the occasional hernia. The prosthesis is placed as an onlay graft, and the deeper implant is located in the preperitoneal position.

**Figure 26–9.** Methods which author has used for implantation of prosthetic materials.

**Table 26–10. PLACEMENT OF IMPLANT IN 266 PATIENTS WITH INCISIONAL HERNIAS**

| Site of Implant | Number of Patients |
|---|---|
| Preperitoneal | 109 |
| Posterior to rectus abdominal muscle | 73 |
| Intraperitoneal (Inlay) | 65 |
| Subaponeurotic | 12 |
| Subcutaneous (Onlay) | 7 |
| Total | 266 |

noma at the site of the cutis graft implantation (Fig. 26–3). The chain of events described above is undoubtedly rare, but the fact that it can occur is a strong deterrent

**Table 26–11. ANESTHESIA USED IN 266 PATIENTS WITH INCISIONAL HERNIAS**

| Anesthesia | No. Patients | Percent |
|---|---|---|
| Spinal | 134 | 50.4 |
| General | 105 | 39.5 |
| Local | 27 | 10.1 |

**Table 26–12.    TYPE OF PROSTHETIC MATERIAL USED IN REPAIR OF 266 INCISIONAL HERNIAS**

| Material | No. Patients | Percent |
|---|---|---|
| Marlex mesh | 219 | 82.3 |
| Tantalum mesh | 31 | 11.7 |
| Fascia lata | 16 | 6.0 |

to the use of either cutis grafts or skin grafts in repair of hernias.

In our practice, tantalum mesh has also been found unacceptable as a prosthetic material for hernia repair. We found that in many cases it proved useful, but in other cases it tended to migrate and fragment (Fig. 26–4). Furthermore, if it came in direct contact with viscera, the resultant fusion defied even the most patient efforts at separation. Enterotomies were embarrassingly frequent. Dense adhesions were too often encountered in the vicinity of the implanted tantalum. In its day, tantalum mesh served a useful purpose but still fell short of meeting the important qualities of implants described earlier in this chapter.

Fascia lata is an effective material for reinforcing areas of weakness in the abdominal wall or groin. The need for both a lengthy incision in the thigh and a second operative procedure is a significant drawback to the use of this adjunct.

Marlex mesh remains the prosthetic material of choice in our practice, currently being used in over 90 percent of the instances in which an implant is used. In an experience of 20 years, Marlex mesh has been found to be strong and durable. It is pliable and becomes incorporated into a connective tissue network. It can tolerate infection if heavy braided sutures are not used for fixation.

### Operative Findings in Repair of 266 Incisional Hernias with Mesh

Hernias that required some type of implant for secure repair had often been operated upon several times previously. Furthermore, large hernias easily accommodate the wandering abdominal viscera (Table 26–13).

It is understandable that the omentum, hanging apronlike over the viscera, finds its way into any protrusion. The small intestine is encountered most often in hernias of the lower abdomen. The colon, being relatively fixed to the posterior abdominal wall on the right and left, is less commonly encountered in incisional hernias than is the small intestine. The transverse colon and the sigmoid colon can easily enter large hernial sacs. It is seen that over 80 percent of incisional hernias in this study had viscera in them. The surgeon must always be alert to the possibility that the thin cicatrix covers protruding intestine. Keeping this in mind, the surgeon will perform fewer inadvertent enterotomies.

### Deaths

There was only one postoperative death, occurring in a 72-year-old male. Death occurred 18 days postoperatively and was caused by pneumonia and congestive heart failure. The patient had advanced arteriosclerotic heart disease. There is always the possibility, no matter how remote, that an occasional patient might not survive repair of a complicated hernia—especially if the patient is elderly and has advanced cardiovascular, pulmonary, or renal disease.

### Postoperative Complications Following Repair of 266 Incisional Hernias

There is no doubt in my mind that the incidence of complications is greater when implants are used in repair of incisional hernias than when they are omitted. The advantages to the patient in additional strength at the site of repair, however, outweigh the disadvantages that might arise should complications develop. Besides,

**Table 26–13.    OPERATIVE FINDINGS IN 266 PATIENTS WITH INCISIONAL HERNIAS**

| Viscus | No. Instances | Percent |
|---|---|---|
| Omentum | 131 | 49.3 |
| Omentum and small bowel | 57 | 21.4 |
| Omentum and colon | 27 | 10.2 |
| Small intestine | 3 | 1.1 |
| Not described | 48 | 18.0 |

Table 26–14. POSTOPERATIVE
COMPLICATIONS IN 266 PATIENTS
WITH INCISIONAL HERNIAS
REPAIRED WITH IMPLANTS

| Complication | No. Patients | Percent |
|---|---|---|
| Seroma° | 27 | 10.2 |
| Hematoma° | 13 | 4.9 |
| Infection° | 11 | 4.1 |
| Sinuses° | 7 | 2.6 |
| Mesh—Foreign body | 6 | 2.3 |
| Tenderness | 16 | 6.0 |
| Induration | 32 | 12.0 |
| Skin necrosis° | 2 | 0.8 |
| Wound disruption° | 1 | 0.4 |
| Pulmonary | | |
| Atelectasis, bronchitis | 12 | 4.5 |
| Pulmonary embolism | 2 | 0.8 |
| Urinary tract | | |
| Retention | 12 | 4.5 |
| Infection | 4 | 1.5 |
| Gastrointestinal | | |
| Ileus | 7 | 2.6 |
| Thrombophlebitis | 3 | 1.1 |

°These are considered to be serious wound complications, whereas tenderness and induration are of minor significance.

most of the complications are of a minor nature and self limiting.

Since postoperative complications are discussed in detail in Chapter 28, I will confine my remarks here to those complications peculiar to hernias repaired with implants. The more common complications are summarized in Table 26–14.

There are comparatively few studies alluding to postoperative complications following implantation of prosthetic materials. Surgeons who have experience with various materials realize that wound complications do arise. Most of our complications occurred during the early years of this study. Tantalum mesh was accompanied by disturbingly high rates of complications. Rigid adherence to aseptic principles and careful surgical technique has decreased the rate of infection.

Wound induration and tenderness following implantation of prosthetic material are annoying to some patients. The tenderness is somewhat greater when the implant is placed in the subcutaneous position. Induration may result as a response to trauma of the procedure, but it should be recalled that fibroplasia is an expected response to implantation of various materials.

Seromas and hematomas could be reduced in frequency through sharp dissection and meticulous hemostasis. In three patients, seromas developed in the thigh where the fascia lata graft was obtained. The use of currently available suction devices permits continuous evacuation of serum and blood (Fig. 21–10, p. 388).

In a few patients, sinuses develop and continue to drain for months or even years. In order to remedy this situation it is necessary to remove heavy braided suture material, or both. Before I advise removal of the mesh, wide drainage and a search for suture material is performed under anesthesia. The wound is subsequently irrigated with an antiseptic solution periodically. If healing does not occur within 6 weeks to 2 months, I advise removal of the implant. This was not a rare eventuality when tantalum mesh was used. It was necessary to remove mesh in 6, or 2.3 percent, of the patients in whom implants were used.

Even though nasogastric suction is used in almost every patient with complicated and recurrent incisional hernias, ileus was a significant complication in 2.6 percent of the patients in this study. In the largest and most complicated incisional hernias, I advise the use of the Miller-Abbott tube as well as more effective decompression of the small bowel.

The other complications noted in Table 26–14 are those seen occasionally in patients undergoing major operative procedures.

## Recurrence Rates Following Repair of Incisional Hernias with Implants

The results following repair of incisional hernias with implants are reasonably good but still fall short of perfection. There were 13 recurrences recognized during a period when 68 percent of the patients were followed longer than one year.

It is impossible to draw a sweeping conclusion from this small number of recurrent hernias, but a few observations can be recorded.

Tantalum gauze was used as the implant in four patients with recurrences. One of these individuals developed a large seroma; the second developed a wound infection; the third suffered a wound dehiscence; and only one of the four appeared to heal satisfactorily.

Two patients with fascia lata implants ultimately developed recurrent hernias.

In seven patients, Marlex mesh was implanted but failed to prevent reappearance of the hernia. In one patient it was later obvious that the implant was too small. In three others the mesh was implanted as an intraperitoneal implant. The recurrence was small in two of the three patients. Reduction in the size of an incisional hernia through a surgical effort, while not an ideal to be pursued, can be a progressive step towards eventual complete repair.

A recurrence rate of 4.9 percent in the repair of complicated hernias is acceptable. Given a longer follow-up period, other recurrences would undoubtedly appear.

### Repair of Large Supraumbilical Hernias with Mesh

Certain large midline incisional hernias above the umbilicus can best be repaired with placement of a synthetic mesh. Patients with incisional hernias that developed following wound infection often show significant weakness in the epigastrium. Those patients with severe pulmonary disease — including emphysema, bronchitis, and asthma — are good candidates for hernia repairs with mesh. Other individuals who have diastasis recti with a large midline defect, make approximation of available tissues possible at the price of increased tension. Severe obesity with resultant increase in intra-abdominal pressure is another possible indication for use of prosthetics in selected patients.

The previous cicatrix in the midline is excised from the xiphoid process to the umbilicus (Fig. 26–10). The incision is developed laterally to the margin of the rectus sheath on each side. The sac protrudes through the linea alba, which has been forced or spread more or less laterally. Often the epigastric hernial sac contains a wide attachment of omentum. The dissection is carried out around the entire sac at the level of the anterior sheath of the rectus and the external oblique aponeurosis. Exposure of normal tissue for repair is essential.

The hernial sac is carefully opened to avoid visceral injury and any adherent omentum, small intestine, or colon is detached.

The posterior rectus sheath is now identified on each side. If the rectus abdominis muscle is freed from the sheath to the linea semilunaris, greater mobility of this structure is obtained.

If nylon retention sutures are to be used, they should be placed at this point in the procedure. They should be spaced at intervals of approximately three centimeters and inserted through the abdominal wall where normal tissues remain.

The posterior rectus sheath is approximated with interrupted figure of eight sutures of number one chromic catgut (Fig. 26–11). I do not use continuous sutures in hernia repair.

After the posterior rectus sheath and peritoneum are closed, the mesh is placed deep to the rectus abdominis muscle (Fig. 26–11). The mesh must be of adequate size, extending from the lateral margin of one rectus sheath to the opposite side and from the costal margin above to the umbilical area below. Nonabsorbable sutures, such as number 2–0-coated Dacron, are useful and dependable; however, stainless steel wire may be used as well. These are inserted so that some lateral tension is placed on the mesh; this maneuver relieves some of the tension on the suture line (Fig. 26–11).

Placement of the prosthesis deep to the belly of the rectus abdominis, but anterior to the posterior rectus sheath, is highly desirable. In this position it cannot become adherent to the intestine, and it is well incorporated into the abdominal wall at this depth. Placement of the mesh in this location results in excellent strength following healing (Fig. 26–12).

The anterior sheath of the rectus is closed with interrupted figure-of-eight sutures of nonabsorbable material.

If excessive tension is encountered, relaxing incisions may be made in the anterior sheath of the rectus. A single lengthy incision is desirable in some cases. In others numerous small incisions are made. Suction catheters are placed deep to the mesh and at the subcutaneous level (Fig. 21–10, p. 388).

The skin and subcutaneous tissues are

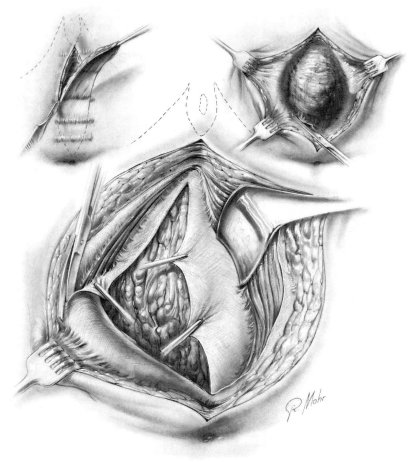

**Figure 26–10.** In the repair of large recurrent incisional hernias, certain principles must be followed. The previous cicatrix is usually best excised (insert); the margins of the defect must be clearly identified, as must the peritoneal layer or posterior rectus sheath.

approximated with interrupted sutures of number 3–0 nylon.

If nylon retention sutures were placed earlier, then they are tied over segments of rubber catheters at this point. Dressings are then applied. With use of suction catheters, pressure dressings are unnecessary and may cause respiratory embarrassment.

## Repair of Large Complicated Incisional Hernias of the Lower Abdomen with Mesh

One may see the occasional patient with huge abdominal wall defects in the lower abdomen. In some patients, appendectomy is followed by infection and later multiple attempts at repair. A few patients had earlier operations through a poorly placed pararectus incision with destruction of nerve and blood supply to the abdomen. Large hernias are the result. Inguinal hernias later follow these events in several individuals as well. Because of loss of substance of the abdominal wall, the implantation of mesh is necessary (Fig. 26–13, *A* and *B*).

After excision of the cicatrix and excess skin is performed, the incision is developed about the hernial sac to the external oblique aponeurosis. The sac is opened and adhesions are freed from the sac. Care must be taken to avoid accidental enterotomy. Viscera are freed and replaced in the peritoneal cavity. The peritoneal sac of any coexisting inguinal or femoral hernia is reduced at this time.

The peritoneal sac and transversalis fascia are closed as a separate first layer. The

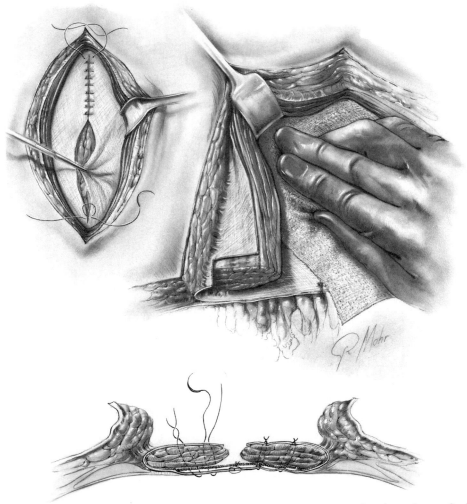

**Figure 26–11.** It is preferable to close the peritoneum and posterior rectus sheath as shown. Such closure protects viscera from the implant. The prosthetic material is placed, so that it lies posterior to the rectus abdominis muscle. The implant is cut and sutured so that it extends beyond the defect and is attached to musculoaponeurotic structures.

transversus abdominis and internal oblique muscles are usually atrophic or nonexistent in these cases; therefore, implantation of a prosthesis becomes necessary at this level.

The dissection is carried out at the preperitoneal level in the same manner as it is performed during a preperitoneal inguinal or femoral herniorrhaphy.

Cooper's ligament and the femoral vessels are visualized in selected cases.

The mesh is sutured to the pubic tubercle and Cooper's ligament medially and to the anterior superior iliac spine laterally.

Number two nonabsorbable monofilamentous sutures are recommended. Wire sutures may be used if desired (Fig. 26–14).

With firm attachment achieved inferiorly, the mesh is then placed beneath the rectus muscle medially, and sutures are placed between the mesh and the anterior sheath of the rectus.

Superiorly, the mesh may be placed just anterior to the internal oblique muscle and aponeurosis. In some cases, the prosthesis may be located in the preperitoneal position just anterior to the closed peritoneal layer. It should be noted that the muscles and aponeurosis referred to may be more or less destroyed due to infection or trauma of repeated surgical procedures in the area (Fig. 26–15).

The portion of mesh implanted must be of generous size, extending from the midline to the region of the inguinal ligament and Cooper's ligament below, to the level of the umbilicus above, and as far laterally as the anterior superior iliac spine (Fig. 26–15, p. 563). An error is made occasionally when a piece of mesh of insufficient size is used in an attempt to cover a large defect.

If it is possible, the transversus abdominis arch may be approximated to Cooper's ligament independently prior to attaching the mesh to the abdominal wall superiorly and medially. This technique will eliminate direct or femoral hernias.

It is desirable to cover the mesh with remaining musculoaponeurotic structures. Practically, it is usually possible to cover a great deal of the mesh with the transversus abdominis and internal oblique muscles lateral to the rectus muscle. Medially, the mesh may be under the belly of the rectus abdominis muscle. The external oblique aponeurosis is approximated with interrupted sutures, usually number 2–0 nonabsorbable.

Suction catheters are placed deep to the prosthesis and in the subcutaneous space. The skin is closed with fine nylon sutures, or subepidermal sutures of synthetic ab-

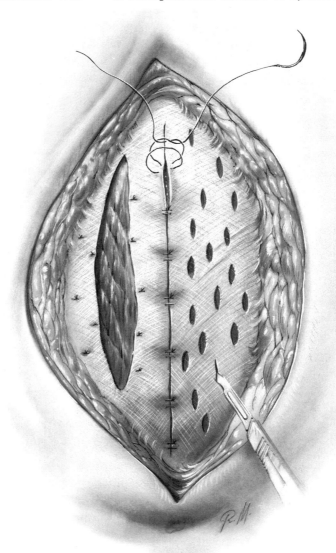

**Figure 26–12.** The anterior sheath of the rectus abdominis muscle is closed over the prosthetic material whenever possible. This objective must not be gained at the cost of excessive tension on the suture line. A relaxing incision may be made as illustrated; a long vertical incision is shown on the left, and numerous smaller incisions accomplish a similar result on the right.

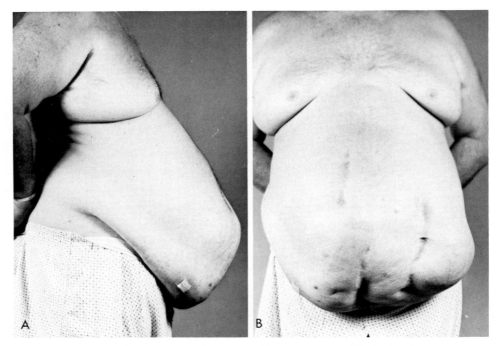

**Figure 26–13.** AP and lateral views of a huge incisional hernia in a man who had eight previous attempts at repair.

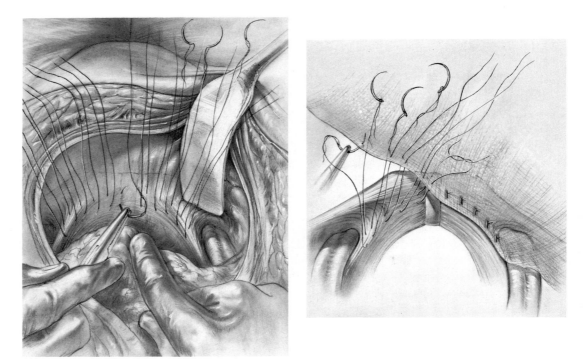

**Figure 26–14.** In certain large and often recurring hernias, it is necessary to attach the prosthetic material deeply. Cooper's ligament is exposed bilaterally through the preperitoneal approach. Sutures are individually placed into the ligament under direct vision. After these have all been properly placed, the sutures are delivered through the mesh as indicated and individually ligated. The illustration shows the location of the mesh in relation to the peritoneum and repaired abdominal wall.

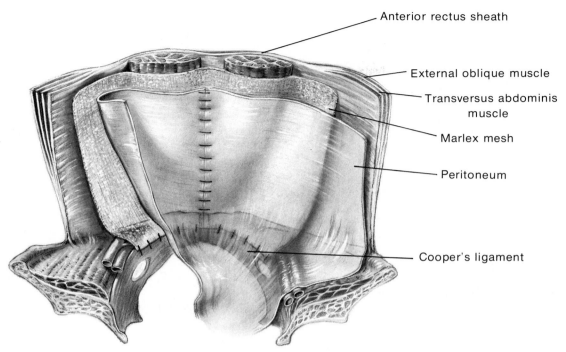

Figure 26–15. The illustration shows the attached mesh in place and depicts the extent of reinforcement needed in certain uncommon but large hernias.

sorbable material plus strips of nonallergenic adhesive tape placed transversely across the incision.

The postoperative result of the patient shown in Figure 26–13, A and B, is shown in Figure 26–16. A panniculectomy was performed in which 9.5 pounds of skin and subcutaneous fat were removed. The skin removed measured 32 inches in length. It is not necessary to attempt to fashion a completely flat abdominal wall. Domicile must be allowed for the viscera and omentum. Patients with incisional hernias have been accustomed to great protuberances and a significant reduction in size of the abdomen is gratefully appreciated by the patient, but, more importantly, the compromise is physiologically and anatomically sound.

## REPAIR OF INGUINAL AND FEMORAL HERNIAS WITH IMPLANTS—CLINICAL EXPERIENCE

It has been difficult to obtain the medical records of patients repaired with implants.

I have been able to identify records of 68 patients having had inguinal and femoral defects repaired with implants. Few cases were identified in the 1940s, but most of them were repaired since 1950. Change in the prosthetic preferred as a reinforcing material is apparent. The general indications for use of implants are being identified more clearly.

### Age

It can be seen from Table 26–15 that young infants, children, and young adults rarely, if ever, require implants for inguinal or femoral hernia repair. Over two-thirds of the patients fell into the age group between 50 and 70 years.

### Sex

This study points out that females with inguinal or femoral hernias seldom require implants to achieve strong repairs. Only two (or nearly 3 percent) of the patients

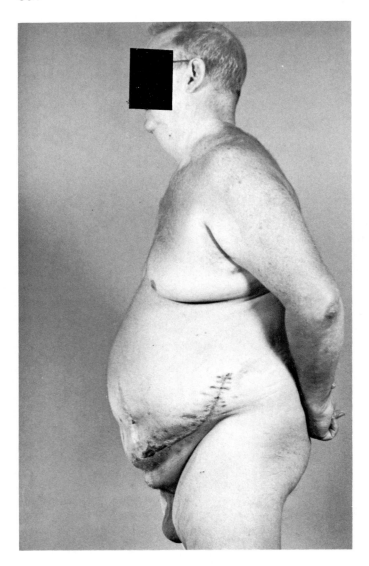

**Figure 26–16.** This lateral view shows the postoperative result obtained in repair of the hernia shown in Figure 26–13. Panniculectomy was performed in which 9.5 pounds of skin and subcutaneous fat were removed. The ellipse of skin excised measured 32 inches in length. It is neither necessary nor advisable to attempt to create a scaphoid abdomen in patients with generously protuberant bellies.

were females. The structures normally available in the lower abdomen of the female permit repair of hernias in the groin area with remarkable success.

### Clinical Features

Over 70 percent of the recurrent hernias included in this study appeared within six years.

Twenty-six percent of the patients had previously undergone repair of bilateral inguinal hernias, either simultaneously or separately.

The common indication for use of prosthetic materials was recurrence of in-

guinal or femoral hernias or both. Forty-four patients had undergone one repair previously and 24 had required numerous repairs. Sixteen individuals had two earlier attempts at repair. Clearly previous failures at hernia repairs should suggest the possible need of an implant.

### Initial Repairs

It is unfortunate that accurate information concerning the initial hernia is so often wanting. It is difficult to determine the nature of the original defect or precisely how it was repaired. Even with these constraints, some worthwhile observations

**Table 26–15. AGE INCIDENCE OF 68 PATIENTS HAVING INGUINAL OR FEMORAL HERNIAS REPAIRED WITH MESH**

| Age | No. Patients | Percent |
|---|---|---|
| Birth to 30 yrs. | 0 | 0.0 |
| 31 to 40 yrs. | 5 | 7.4 |
| 41 to 50 yrs. | 14 | 20.6 |
| 51 to 60 yrs. | 26 | 38.2 |
| 61 to 70 yrs. | 18 | 26.5 |
| 71 to 80 yrs. | 3 | 4.4 |
| 81 to 90 yrs. | 2 | 2.9 |
| | 68 | 100.0 |

emerge. Direct inguinal hernias were the most common type initially repaired, and the recurrence presented as a direct protrusion. Femoral hernias were second in frequency to direct inguinal hernias as the initial defect. Indirect inguinal hernias presented much less frequently.

## Type of Groin Hernias Repaired with Mesh

Even though I was able to collect only a small number of groin hernias repaired with prosthetic materials, a few pertinent observations can be made (Table 26–16). Sixty-eight patients had 70 repairs (2 patients had bilateral repairs). It can be seen from Table 26–16 that recurrent direct inguinal and recurrent femoral hernias are common indications for use of prosthetic implants. Furthermore, combinations of

**Table 26–16. TYPE OF INGUINAL AND FEMORAL HERNIAS REPAIRED WITH MESH**

| Type of Hernia | No. Patients | Percent |
|---|---|---|
| Direct-recurrent | 35 | 50.0 |
| Femoral-recurrent | 9 | 12.9 |
| Inguinofemoral-recurrent | 8 | 11.4 |
| Direct and femoral-recurrent | 6 | 8.6 |
| Indirect-recurrent | 5 | 7.1 |
| Direct and indirect-recurrent | 4 | 5.7 |
| Direct-indirect-femoral-recurrent | 2 | 2.9 |
| Indirect-femoral-recurrent | 1 | 1.4 |
| | 70 | 100.0 |

defects (such as inguinofemoral recurrent hernias) are repaired with implants.

On the other hand, less than 10 percent of the recurrent hernias were of the indirect variety. Such indirect hernias had often undergone a number of previous repairs with recurrence. Indirect inguinal hernias even if recurrent, seldom require insertion of prosthetic materials.

## Methods of Repair of Recurrent Groin Hernias with Implants

A number of possible locations can be found for implantation of prosthetic materials into the groin; however, the two areas that cause the greatest difficulty are the floor of Hesselbach's triangle and the femoral ring. At times, both these areas require strengthening with an implant.

The onlay graft, in which the mesh is placed over the external oblique aponeurosis, is not a preferred method of implantation.

The method for inserting mesh that I prefer requires complete exposure of Cooper's ligament. The mesh is attached to this strong ligament from the pubic tubercle to the femoral vein. Number 2–0 monofilamentous synthetic nonabsorbable sutures are placed at right angles to Cooper's ligament (Fig. 26–17); such attachment will prevent development of a recurrent femoral hernia as well. It should be noted that the transversalis fascia is closed separately at the internal ring. After attachment of the mesh to Cooper's ligament, the transversus arch is sutured to this same structure with interrupted sutures as performed in the Lotheissen-McVay repair (Fig. 26–17). In a few cases, this is not possible; and the implanted mesh must provide the needed strength of repair. In some cases, the sheath of the rectus may be incised and the mesh attached to the posterior sheath of the rectus abdominis muscle. In this situation, it may be useful to implant the mesh under some portion of the internal oblique as well. It should be recalled that many hernias requiring implants for repair present with destruction of tissues and loss of normal landmarks due to innumerable previous attempts at repair.

After the mesh has been attached to Cooper's ligament and the transversus arch

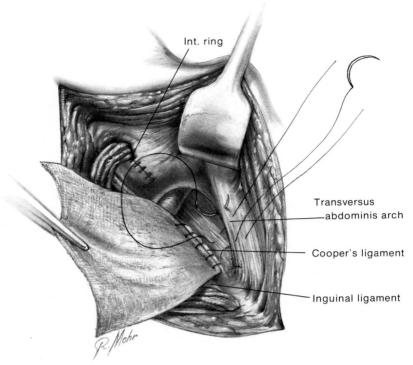

**Figure 26–17.** In the repair of difficult recurrent inguinal or femoral hernias, it is often advisable to attach the mesh to Cooper's ligament. Such attachment will preclude recurrence of femoral hernias. The transversus arch is usually sutured to Cooper's ligament, when possible.

sutured to this same structure, the mesh is sutured to the anterior sheath of the rectus and aponeurosis of the internal oblique (Fig. 26–18).

In another method of insertion of the mesh, the prosthetic material is implanted deep to the aponeurosis of the external oblique muscle and attached to the inguinal ligament and to the aponeurosis of the internal oblique muscle. Such placement is suitable for direct and indirect recurrent inguinal hernias, but obviously is of no value in repairing femoral hernias.

## PROSTHETIC MATERIAL USED FOR GROIN HERNIAS

It is interesting that as a result of the influence of Gallie and LeMesurier (1923) strips of fascia lata were used in repair of two early cases included in this study. Later, sheets of fascia lata were used to repair 10 recurrent inguinal hernias. Following the influence of Koontz in 1948, tantalum gauze was utilized as an implant in the 1950s. The material was utilized in only five patients.

Marlex mesh was used in 53 or 75 percent of the operations included in this study. Currently, Marlex mesh is used as the prosthetic material of choice in hernia repair.

## Recurrences

Only 52 percent of the patients were followed up to 10 years. During this time, 2 recurrences were identified for a recurrence rate of 2.9 percent. I am convinced that excellent results can be obtained with effective use of prosthetic materials. Attachment of the mesh to such strong structures as Cooper's ligament, the inguinal ligament, and such aponeuroses as are available provides excellent strength. Tension must be avoided in repair of hernias and implantation of mesh makes this possible.

## Complications

In any study of recurrent inguinal hernias, the incidence of hematomas and seromas will be significant; this is especially true if implants must be used during the repair.

Seromas occurred in 6 (or 8.8 percent) of the patients, while 4 (or 5.9 percent) developed hematomas. Two patients had wound infections, and in one of the early cases, it was necessary to remove the tantalum mesh. One of these patients suffered a recurrence.

Urinary retention was reported in three patients with significant infection developing in one.

Postoperative ileus was annoying to two patients, eventually requiring nasogastric suction.

Three patients, or 4.4 percent, had atrophic testicles prior to repair of their recurrent inguinal and femoral hernias, and one additional individual was found to have developed atrophy postoperatively. These observations confirm my opinion that testicular atrophy following hernia repair is a significant problem. In this group of cases, nearly 6 percent had atrophic testicles.

## INDICATIONS FOR IMPLANTATION OF PROSTHETIC MATERIALS IN REPAIR OF RECURRENT INGUINAL AND FEMORAL HERNIAS

To the best of my knowledge, little effort has been made to identify patients whose hernias might best be repaired with implants. It is clear that infants, children, and young adults with indirect inguinal hernias do not require prostheses. In this group, the patent processus vaginalis must be eliminated and little, if anything, needs to be done to the internal abdominal ring.

It has become apparent to me that groin

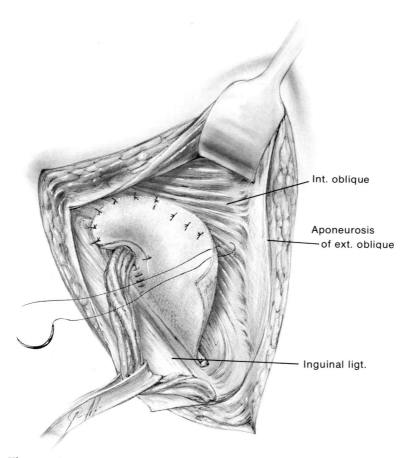

Int. oblique

Aponeurosis of ext. oblique

Inguinal ligt.

**Figure 26–18.** The prosthetic material is then attached to the anterior sheath of the rectus and to the aponeurosis of the internal oblique. A relaxing incision may be utilized before final fixation of the mesh to decrease tension. In such cases, the mesh is sutured over the incision site.

hernias in females can also be repaired with a high rate of success without resorting to implants.

On the other hand, certain recurrent inguinal and femoral hernias require extraordinary measures to insure strong repairs. At this time, I cannot assign a numerical value to each indication, but significant reasons for prosthetic implantation are identified in Table 26–17.

In the Henry Ford Hospital experience, the most common indication for use of prosthetic materials is recurrence of herniation. With repeated operative procedures, scar tissue replaces normal tissue; and experience teaches that fibrous tissue is inferior to normal tissue in strength.

Bilateral repair of inguinal hernias places an additional burden on the suture line, even with relaxing incisions. The use of prosthetic reinforcement of the inguinal floor should be employed more frequently than it is currently. As a result of my studies of femoral hernias, I am using implants with increasing frequency in repair of recurrent femoral hernias. Even though the defect in such hernias is small, the structures available for repair are rigid (such as Cooper's ligament) or inflexible (such as the inguinal ligament). Furthermore, a small prosthetic implant provides great strength at the site of repair.

During repair of certain recurrent inguinal hernias, it is evident that considerable tension is the result. This is better seen when repair is performed under local anesthesia, since the abdominal wall generally retains its tone. If there is undue tension on the line of repair even after a relaxing incision is made, a prosthetic implant is indicated.

A few patients will be seen whose inguinal ligament had been sacrificed during a previous repair. The Lotheissen-McVay repair of direct hernias in such patients is often successful, but a few will require a prosthetic implant.

Patients who perform heavy work or indulge in strenuous exercises are reasonable candidates for prosthetic implants, particularly when recurrent direct inguinal hernias are being repaired.

An occasional patient is seen with tissues of poor quality. Patients on large doses of steroids for prolonged periods of time show deterioration of their connective tissue strata. Use of prosthetics in repair of recurrent inguinal or femoral hernias is reasonable in such cases.

## APHORISMS APPLICABLE TO PROSTHETIC IMPLANTS

Thirty-three years of experience with implants produced a considerable amount of useful knowledge from which a number of general principles can be identified. Some of these I have found to be applicable to the use of prosthetic implants for hernia repair. Although the degree of usefulness varied with the type of hernia encountered, I made no attempt to place them in order of importance and simply listed them numerically.

1. Use a piece of mesh or implant of sufficiently large size. It should extend at least 1.5 to 3 centimeters beyond the margins of the defect.
2. Implant the prosthesis as deeply into the abdominal wall as is reasonable for the hernia being repaired.
3. Attach the prosthesis widely—well beyond the margins of the defect.
4. Suture the implant into position with synthetic monofilament nonabsorbable sutures placed at intervals of 4 to 6 millimeters.
5. Cover the mesh with a musculoaponeurotic layer but not when this objective would result in excessive tension.

**Table 26–17. INDICATIONS FOR USE OF PROSTHETIC MATERIALS IN REPAIR OF RECURRENT INGUINAL AND FEMORAL HERNIAS**

**Attenuated tissues**
   Heavy cicatrix
   Postoperative infection
   Loss of some portion of abdominal wall
**Repeated attempts at repair**
**Bilateral inguinal or femoral hernias**
**Excessive tension with conventional repairs**
**Patient with severe pulmonary disease**
   Emphysema
   Bronchitis
   Asthma
**Patient performing strenuous work**
   Heavy labor
   Athletics
**Patients with abnormal tissues**
   Prolonged steroid therapy
   Marfan's syndrome
   Hypothyroidism

6. Place the prosthesis anterior to the peritoneum and transversalis fascia when possible, thus achieving deep implantation.
7. Intraperitoneal placement of the implant is necessary in some cases. In such situations, a layer of omentum should cover the viscera.
8. Anchor the prosthesis to strong supporting structures such as Cooper's ligament, the inguinal ligament, and musculoaponeurotic layers as dictated by the individual case.
9. Placement of mesh anterior to the peritoneum-transversalis fascia-posterior sheath of the rectus abdominis muscles provides excellent reinforcement.
10. Placement of the implant under the aponeurosis of the external oblique is acceptable when the deeper layers have been properly closed.
11. Use of a prosthetic material as an onlay graft may be of value in relieving tension on the site of repair in selected cases.
12. Meshes should be implanted as smoothly as possible and under slight tension. Wrinkles and folds in the material should be avoided.
13. When more than one layer of prosthetic material is used, it is advisable that some portion of the abdominal wall be interposed between them.
14. Double thicknesses of mesh with surfaces in immediate apposition are not always well tolerated. The need for such an approach is not great.
15. Heavy braided sutures, such as silk, should be avoided.
16. Drainage tubes should be placed between the layers of the abdominal wall and suction applied thereto. Blood and serum collections will be an infrequent complication as a result.
17. Prostheses should be used on good indication to add strength to the abdominal wall or inguinal region whenever loss of tissue has occurred, when ordinary repairs would create excessive tension on the site of repair, or when the patient is likely to inflict great stress upon the suture line.
18. If infection should supervene, it may not be necessary to remove the material if a nonbraided suture material was used during the repair. Wide drainage is essential, together with use of appropriate antibiotics and irrigation of the wound.

## SUMMARY

The important qualities required of a prosthetic material for implantation have been identified in detail. Strength, durability, tissue tolerance, ease of handling, and porosity are the desirable qualities that have been identified. Such materials must be tolerated in the presence of infection; they must be nonallergenic; and they must not lead to cyst formation or neoplasia.

Autologous fascia lata is a desirable material for implantation biologically, but it requires an incision into the thigh. This requires a secondary operative procedure and heals with a bulging defect, which is objectionable in some patients.

Of the plastic materials, Marlex mesh is currently most popular in this country. It is an excellent material in my experience and currently preferred over other materials.

Mersilene mesh has been used with significant success, but its final role in prosthetic repair of hernias is yet to be determined. Stainless steel mesh is used comparatively infrequently, but some surgeons have reported good results following implantation.

The principles to be followed in placement of prosthetic materials have been discussed. Implantation of the material into the depths of the defect is important. Covering of the implanted material with aponeurosis is highly desirable. The prosthetic implant must be large enough to extend well beyond the defect. I cut the prosthesis so that it extends two to four centimeters beyond the defect. It is sutured in place with numerous number 2–0 synthetic nonabsorbable suture materials. Technical details for implantation are well illustrated.

The indications for implantation are numerous and are steadily being better recognized. The presence of a large defect, loss of substance of the abdominal wall, and numerous previous repairs are among the most important indications for implantation of reinforcing materials. Obesity is an important factor when added to the above indications for use of implants.

Certain significant complications occur following use of various materials in hernia repair. Seromas, hematomas, and wound infections occur more frequently when implants are used. Sinuses occur less often, but can be an annoying complication requiring months for eradication. Occasionally in such wounds, braided suture material and the implant itself must be removed.

The recurrence rate following repair of incisional hernias with implants was 4.9 percent; this seems excessive, but many of the hernias had been subjected to repeated efforts at repair. Furthermore, even when recurrences were seen, they were frequently of smaller size than the original defect.

The recurrence rate following repair of inguinal and femoral hernias was 2.9 percent. This is considered to be a reasonable incidence of recurrence, since the hernias encountered were considered to be difficult problems.

It is felt that there should be less reluctance to utilize prosthetic materials in hernia repair. Large defects and bilateral recurrent inguinal hernias are often best repaired with implants. Such materials provide strength to the abdominal wall without generating excessive tension at the site of repair.

## REFERENCES

Abel, A. L., and Hunt, A. H.: Stainless steel wire for closing abdominal incisions and for the repair of herniae. Br. Med. J. 2:379, 1948.

Abul-Husn, S.: The use of polyester mesh in hernia repair. J. Med. Liban. 27:437, 1974.

Adler, R. H.: An evaluation of surgical mesh in the repair of hernias and tissue defects. J. Arch. Surg. 85:836, 1962.

Adler, R. H., and Darby, C.: Use of a porous synthetic sponge (Ivalon) in surgery: I. Tissue responses after implantation: II. Studies of tensile strength. U. S. Armed Forces Med. J. 11:1349, 1466, 1960.

Adler, R. H., and Firme, C.: The use of nylon prostheses for diaphragmatic defects. J. Surg. Gynecol. Obstet. 104:669, 1957.

Arnaud, J. P., Eloy, R., Adloff, M., and Grenier, J. F.: Critical evaluation of prosthetic materials in repair of abdominal wall hernias. Am. J. Surg. 133:338, 1977.

Austin, R. C., and Damstra, E. F.: Fascia lata repair of massive ventral hernias. Am. J. Surg. 82:466, 1951.

Babcock, W. W.: The range of usefulness of commercial stainless steel cloths in general and special forms of surgical practice. Ann. W. Med. Surg. 6:15, 1952.

Bapat, R. D., and Patel, R. A.: Stainless steel mesh, A neglected implant for inguinal hernia repair. J. Postgrad. Med. 20:94, 1975.

Bartlett, W. F.: An improved filigree for the repair of large defects in the abdominal wall. Ann. Surg. 38:47, 1903.

Burton, C. C.: Classification and techniques of fascial grafts in repair of inguinal hernia. Surg. Gynecol. Obstet. 105:521, 1957.

Burton, Claud: Fascia lata, cutis and tantalum grafts in repair of massive abdominal incisional hernias. Surg. Gynecol. Obstet. 109:621, 1959.

Calne, Roy Y.: Repair of bilateral hernia with mersilene mesh behind rectus abdominis. Arch. Surg. 109:532, 1974.

Cannaday, John E.: The use of the cutis graft in the repair of certain types of incisional herniae and other conditions. Am. Surg. 115:775, 1942.

Casebolt, Buford T.: Use of fabric mesh in abdominal wall defects. Mo. Med. 72:71, 1975.

Cerise, Elmo J., Busuttil, Ronald W., Craighead, Claude C, and Ogden, William W. II: The use of mersilene mesh in repair of abdominal wall hernias. Ann. Surg. 181:728, 1975.

Chaimoff, C., and Dintsman, M.: Repair of huge midline hernias in scar tissue. Am. J. Surg. 125:767, 1973.

Chodoff, R. J.: Use of full-thickness skin grafts in repair of large hernias. Ann. Surg. 129:119, 1949.

Clarke, S. H. C.: The formation of inclusion dermal cysts following whole thickness graft for repair of hernia. Br. J. Surg. 39:346, 1952.

Cole, Percival P.: The filigree operation for inguinal hernia. Br. J. Surg. 29:168, 1941.

Copello, A. J.: Technic and results of Teflon mesh repair of complicated groin hernias. Rev. Surg. 25(2):95, 1968.

Couris, G., and Wylie, J.: Epidermoid cyst formation following cutis graft repair of incisional hernia. H. F. H. Med. Bull. 12:141, 1964.

Cowell, Ernest: Recurrent inguinal hernia. Br. Med. J. 2:330, 1946.

Cumberland, V. H.: A preliminary report on the use of prefabricated nylon weave in the repair of ventral hernia. Med. J. Aust. 1:143–144, 1952.

Dales, H. C., and Kyle, J.: Late results of using tantalum gauze in the repair of large hernias. Surgery 43:294, 1958.

Doran, F. S. A., Gibbins, R. E., and Whitehead, R.: A report on 313 inguinal herniae repaired with nylon net. Br. J. Surg. 48:430, 1961.

Douglas, D. M.: Repair of large herniae with tantalum gauze. Lancet 1:936, 1948.

Drainer, Ian K., and Reid, D. K.: Recurrence-free ventral herniorrhaphy using a propylene mesh prosthesis. J. Roy. Surg. 17:253, 1972.

Dunlop, George R.: The use of tantalum gauze in the repair of hernias with tissue deficiencies. New Eng. J. Med. 242:542, 1950.

Durden, John G., and Pemberton, L.: Dacron mesh in ventral and inguinal hernias. Am. Surg. 40:662, 1974.

Flynn, W. J., Brant, A. E., and Nelson, G. G.: A four and one-half year analysis of tantalum gauze used in the repair of ventral hernia. Ann. Surg. 134:1027, 1951.

Fogelson, J., and Jackson, C. R.: The repair of tissue deficient hernias by aortic implants. Surg. Gynecol. Obstet. 109:245, 1959.

Gallie, W. E., and LeMesurier, A. B.: Living sutures in the treatment of hernia. Can. Med. Assoc. J. *13*:469, 1923.

Gibson, L. Dean, and Stafford, Clarence E.: Synthetic mesh repair of abdominal wall defects. Am. Surg. *30*:481, 1964.

Gilsdorf, R. B., and Shea, M. M.: Repair of massive septic abdominal wall defects with Marlex mesh. Am. J. Surg. *130*:634, 1975.

Gomez, J., Wylie, J. H., and Ponka, J. L.: Epidermoid carcinoma in a cutis graft after repair of an incisional hernia. Rev. Surg. *29*:381, 1972.

Gove, P. B. (ed.): *Webster's New International Dictionary* (3rd ed.). Springfield, Mass., G. & C. Merriam Company, Publ., 1960.

Haas, A., and Ritter, S. A.: Use of stainless steel ring chain net for reinforcement in repair of large and recurrent hernias of the anterior abdominal wall. Am. J. Surg. *95*:87, 1958.

Hamilton, Joseph E.: The repair of large or difficult hernias with mattressed onlay grafts of fascia lata. Ann. Surg. *167*:85, 1968.

Harkins, Henry N.: A new type of relaxing incision—The dermatome-flap method. Am. J. Surg. *59*:79, 1943.

Harkins, Henry N.: Cutis grafts. Ann. Surg. *122*:996, 1945.

Haskey, Robert S., and Bigler, F. Calvin: Difficult hernias—Mersilene mesh in the repair of hernias. J. Kans. Med. Soc. *76*:239, 1975.

Horsley, Guy W.: The behavior of alcohol preserved fascia lata of the ox, autogenous fascia and chromicized kangaroo tendon in dog and in man. Ann. Surg. *94*:410, 1931.

Jacobs, Elias, Blaisdell, F. William, and Hall, Albert D.: Use of knitted Marlex mesh in the repair of ventral hernias. Am. J. Surg. *110*:897, 1965.

Joyce, T. M.: Fascial repair of inguinal hernias. J.A.M.A. *115*:971, 1940.

Kimberly, R. C.: *Problems of Recurrent Hernia*. Springfield, Ill., Charles C Thomas, 1975.

Kirschner, M.: Die praktischen Ergebnisse der freien Fascien-Transplantation. Arch. Klin. Chir. *92*:888, 1910.

Koontz, Amos R.: Dead (preserved) fascia grafts for hernia repair. J.A.M.A. *89*:1230, 1927.

Koontz, Amos R.: Preliminary report on the use of Tantalum mesh in the repair of ventral hernias. Ann. Surg. *127*:1079, 1948.

Koontz, Amos R.: Preserved fascia in hernia repair with special reference to large postoperative hernias. Arch. Surg. *26*:500, 1933.

Koontz, A. R.: *Hernia*. New York, Appleton-Century-Crofts, 1963.

Koontz, Amos R.: The use of Tantalum mesh in inguinal hernia repair. Surg. Gynecol. Obstet. *92*:101, 1951.

Koontz, Amos R.: Tantalum mesh in the repair of large ventral hernias. Surg. Gynecol. Obstet. *93*: 112, 1951.

Koontz, Amos, R., and Kimberly, Robert C.: Further experimental work on prostheses for hernia repair. Surg. Gynecol. Obstet. *1*:321, 1959.

Lam, Conrad R., Szilagyi, D. Emerick, and Puppendahl, Magda: Tantalum gauze in the repair of large postoperative ventral hernias. Arch. Surg. *57*:234, 1948.

Lattimore, T. J., and Koontz, A. R.: Suction drainage after implantation of Tantalum gauze sheets. J.A.M.A. *155*:1333, 1954.

LeVeen, H. H., and Barberio, J. R.: Tissue reaction to plastics used in surgery with special reference to Teflon. Ann. Surg. *129*:74, 1949.

Linn, Bernard S., and Vargas, Abelardo: Use of temporary prostheses to repair difficult hernias. South. Med. J. *66*:925, 1973.

Ludington, L. G., and Woodward, E. R.: Use of Teflon mesh in repair of musculofascial defects. Surgery *46*:364, 1959.

Mair, George B.: Analysis of a series of 454 inguinal herniae with special reference to morbidity and recurrence after the whole skin-graft method. Br. J. Surg. *33*:42, 1946.

Mair, George B.: Preliminary report on the use of whole skin-grafts as a substitute for fascial sutures in the treatment of herniae. Br. J. Surg. *32*:381, 1944.

Marsden, C. M.: Whole skin graft repair of hernias with report of 163 operations with follow-up of 136 operations of 12 months. Br. J. Surg. *35*:390, 1948.

Mathieson, A. J. M., and James, J. H.: A review of inguinal hernia repair using stainless steel mesh. J. R. Coll. Surg. Edinb. *20*:58, 1975.

McArthur, D. L.: Autoplastic suture in hernia and other diseases: Preliminary report. J.A.M.A. *37*: 1162, 1901.

McGavin, Lawrie: The use of filigrees of silver wire in the cure of herniae usually considered inoperable. Br. Med. J. *2*:1395, 1907.

Minns, R. J., and Tinckler, L. F.: Structural and mechanical aspects of prosthetic herniorrhaphy. J. Biomech. *9*:435, 1976.

Moloney, G. E.: Results of nylon-darn repairs of herniae. Lancet *2*:273, 1958.

Peer, Lyndon A., and Paddock, Royce: Histologic studies on the fate of deeply implanted dermal grafts. Arch. Surg. *34*:268, 1937.

Pesek, I. George, and and Keeley, John L.: Polyvinyl forma (Ivalon) sponge in repair of diaphragmatic hernia. A.M.A. Arch. Surg. *77*:18, 1958.

Pilcher, Robin: Repair of hernia with plantaris tendon grafts. Arch Surg. *38*:16, 1939.

Piper, J. V.: A comparison between whole-thickness skin-graft and Bassini methods of repair of inguinal hernia in men. Br. Surg. *56*:345, 1969.

Ponka, J. L., and Brush, B. E.: Problem of femoral hernia. Arch. Surg. *102*:417, 1971.

Ponka, J. L., Wylie, J. H., Chaikof, L., Sergeant, C., and Brush, B. E.: Marlex mesh—A new plastic mesh for the repair of hernias. H. F. H. Med. Bull. *7*:278, 1959.

Powell, T., and Ewing, M. R.: Postoperative implantation dermoid cysts. Br. Surg. *39*:366, 1952.

Preston, Daniel J., and Richards, Charles: Use of wire mesh prostheses in the treatment of hernia. Surg. Clin. North Am. *53*:549, 1973.

Rutter, A. G.: Cyst formation seven years after a cutis graft repair of hernia. Br. Med. J. *1*:951, 1955.

Scales, F. T.: Discussion on metals and synthetic materials in relation to soft tissues: Tissue reaction to synthetic materials. Proc. R. Soc. Med. *46*:647, 1953.

Schmitt, Henry J., Jr., and Grinna, George L. B.: Use of Marlex mesh in infected abdominal war wound. Am. Surg. *113*:825, 1967.

Singleton, A. O., and Stehouwers, O. W.: The

fascia-patch transplant in the repair of hernia. Surg. Gynecol. Obstet. *80*:243, 1945.

Strahan, A. W. B.: Hernial repair by whole-skin graft with report on 413 cases. Br. J. Surg. *38*:276, 1951.

Swenson, S. A., and Harkins, H. N.: Cutis grafts: Application of the dermatome-flap method. Arch. Surg. *47*:564, 1943.

Throckmorton, Tom Dercum: Tantalum gauze in the repair of hernias complicated by tissue deficiency. Surgery *23*:32, 1948.

Usher, Francis C.: A new plastic prosthesis for repairing tissue defects of the chest and abdominal wall. Am. J. Surg. *97*:629, 1959.

Usher, Francis C.: A new technique for repairing large abdominal wall defects. Arch. Surg. *82*:870, 1961.

Usher, Francis C.: Hernia repair with knitted polypropylene mesh. Surg. Gynecol. Obstet. *117*:239, 1963.

Usher, Francis C.: Hernia repair with Marlex mesh. Arch. Surg. *84*:325, 1962.

Usher, F. C.: Use of a mesh prosthesis. In Mulholland, J. H., et al.: Current Surgical Management III. Philadelphia, W. B. Saunders Co., 1965, pp. 469–474.

Usher, Francis C.: Use of freeze dried human fascia lata in the repair of incisional hernias. Am. Surg. *21*:364, 1955.

Usher, F. C.: The repair of incisional and inguinal hernias. Surg. Gynecol. Obstet. *131*:525, 1970.

Usher, Francis C., et al.: Polypropylene monofilament. A.M.A. *179*:780, 1962.

Usher, Francis C., et al.: A new technique for the repair of inguinal and incisional hernias. Arch. Surg. *81*:847, 1960.

Usher, Francis C., et al.: Marlex mesh: A new plastic mesh for replacing tissue defects. Arch. Surg. *78*:138, 1959.

Usher, Francis C., et al.: Lyophilized human and ox fascia in the repair of hernias. Surgery *36*:117, 1954.

Usher, Francis C., Ochsner, John, and Tuttle, L. L. D., Jr.: Use of Marlex mesh in the repair of incisional hernias. Am. Surg. *24*:969, 1958.

Usher, Francis C., and Wallace, Stuart A.: Tissue reaction to plastics. Arch. Surg. *76*:997, 1958.

Vorhees, A. B., Jaretzki, A., and Blakemore, A. H.: The use of tubes constructed from Vinyon "N" cloth in bridging arterial defects. Ann. Surg. *135*:332, 1952.

Walker, P. M., and Langer, B.: Marlex mesh for repair of abdominal wall defects. Can. J. Surg. *19*:211, 1976.

Warren, Richard: Surgery of ventral hernia. Cli. J. *1*:481, 1921.

Wesolowski, Sigmund A., Martinez, Alfred, and McMahon, James D.: Use of artificial materials in surgery. In Current Problems in Surgery. Year Book Medical Publ., December, 1966.

Wolstenholme, J. T.: Use of commercial Dacron fabric in the repair of inguinal hernias and abdominal wall defects. Arch. Surg. *73*:1004, 1956.

## Additional Readings

Ali, Munawar: Cutis strip and patch repair of large inguinal hernias. New Engl. J. Med. *251*:932, 1954.

Dunphy, J. Englebert: The cut gut. Am. J. Surg. *119*:1, 1970.

Ein, Sigmund H., Fallis, James C., and Simpson, James S.: Silon sheeting in the staged repair of massive ventral hernias in children. Can. J. Surg. *13*:127, 1970.

Jefferson, Nelson C., and Dailey, U. G.: Incisional hernia repaired with tantalum gauze. Am. J. Surg. *75*:575, 1948.

Linder, F., and Linder, M.: Krebsige Entartung in Hautschlauch einer Ösophagoplastik. Thoraxchir. *16*:48, 1968.

Mahorner, Howard: Umbilical and midline ventral herniae. Ann. Surg. *111*:979, 1940.

Narat, J. K., and Khedrous, L. G.: Repair of abdominal wall defects with Fortisan fabric. Ann. Surg. *136*:272, 1952.

Nataras, M. J.: Experience with Mersilene mesh in abdominal wall repair. Proc. R. Soc. Med. *67*:1187, 1974.

Peacock, Erle E., Jr.: Some aspects of fibrogenesis during the healing of primary and secondary wounds. Surg. Gynecol. Obstet. *115*:408, 1962.

Peacock, E. E.: Subcutaneous extraperitoneal repair of ventral hernias. Ann. Surg. *181*(5):722–727 (May), 1975.

Porell, William J., and Parsons, Langdon: Perineal hernia repair with nylon mesh. Surgery *43*:447, 1958.

Smith, R. S.: The use of prosthetic materials in the repair of hernias. Surg. Clin. North Am. *51*:(6)1387, 1971.

Walke, Lacey: Treatment of large ventral herniations with fascia lata, Tantalum mesh and other foreign bodies. House Staff Lectures, Henry Ford Hospital, Gen. Surg. Rev. *81*:1–17, 1966.

Wilkinson, Tolbert S., Rybka, F. James, and Paletta, F. X.: Studies in nonsuture immobilization of skin. South. Med. J. *65*:25–28, 1972.

# 27

# Intraoperative Complications During Hernia Repair

*Preoperative preparation for the surgeon involves a mental survey of the anatomy and physiology of the part to be surgically disturbed. For an operation performed repeatedly by the fully experienced surgeon, the flash of a mental anatomical image may suffice, but for the initiate a review of the pertinent anatomy is essential. The type of hernial pathology that is anticipated and the potential problems that might be encountered must be mentally reviewed. The proposed operative steps to be performed should be organized and clearly in mind. Technical deviations that might be indicated by possible alterations in the anticipated findings should also be mentally catalogued.*

*Longmire, 1978*

## INTRODUCTION

It is clear that unusual pathologic and anatomic conditions present at the time of repair contribute to the development of complications; however, the inescapable fact that the surgeon might have had something to do with a particular complication often creates an understandable attitude of denial insofar as occurrence of intraoperative complications is concerned. Such involvement produces an additional burden on the surgeon. And, in the light of these statements, the wisdom of Longmire's quotation is evident.

It is extremely easy to produce an inadvertent enterotomy when dealing with gangrenous intestine, since the bowel is delicate and easily entered. The presence of bladder in an oft-recurrent hernia makes injury to these structures a frequent possi-

bility. An anomalous anatomic situation sometimes contributes to an intraoperative complication; for example, an abnormal accessory obturator artery might be injured in a Cooper's ligament repair of a hernia.

Despite the surgeon's extreme vulnerability to possible error, there are but a few reports dealing systematically with intraoperative complications. Yet in today's era of informed consent, it is increasingly important for the surgeon to identify the formidable list of potential complications and problems (Table 27-1).

The surgeon should inform the patient of the relative risk involved in herniorrhaphy—for instance, in aged patients with strangulation, the risk is significant; however, in young healthy patients, the risk of a fatality is remote.

Of great importance to some patients is the matter of testicular function. After

**Table 27–1.   INTRAOPERATIVE
COMPLICATIONS**

I **Fatalities**

II **Hemorrhage**

A. *Minor*
   1. Superficial and deep circumflex iliac arteries
   2. Superficial epigastric artery
   3. Superficial external pudendal artery
   4. Deep inferior epigastric artery
   5. External spermatic artery
   6. Pampiniform plexus
   7. Veins of Retzius

B. *Major*
   1. Femoral artery
   2. Femoral vein — hemorrhage — constriction
   3. Accessory obturator artery

III **Injury to Testicular Blood Supply**

A. *Injury to Internal Spermatic Artery*
B. *Injury to External Spermatic Artery*

IV **Injury to Intestine**

A. *Large Intestine*
   1. Sigmoid colon
   2. Cecum

B. *Small Intestine*

V **Injury to Bladder**

VI **Injury to Nerves**

A. *Ilioinguinal*
B. *Iliohypogastric*
C. *Genitofemoral*
D. *Lateral Femoral Cutaneous*
E. *Femoral*

VII **Injury to Vas Deferens**

VIII **Injury to Fallopian Tubes and Ovaries**

explaining the problem to the patient, the sacrifice of a testicle during the repair of a recurrent inguinal hernia in a 70-year-old male might be undertaken without great concern; however, the sacrifice of the sole remaining viable testicle in a young patient undergoing recurrent inguinal hernia repair is an entirely different situation — and a much more serious one. In such situations, the risks should be discussed with the patient, his wife, and his employer. There is a direct relationship between the incidence of atrophic testicles and the number of previous repairs to which the patient has been exposed. Both the patient and his wife should be aware of the available options and should be consulted in the decision making on the course of action to be taken.

Since serious operative accidents are rare, the surgeon, when queried about any of the complications listed in Table 27–1, is apt to reply that he either has never seen such complications or is aware of only minor ones. But realistically, these problems do occur from time to time; and recognition of the intraoperative complication, together with its proper management, will result in eventual recovery in most cases. Relegation of major responsibility to anyone who is not well acquainted with anatomic relationships in the groin and who is inexperienced in the potential complexity of strangulated hernias should be avoided.

Previous books on the subject of hernia discuss briefly the problem of intraoperative complications. Iason (1941) describes

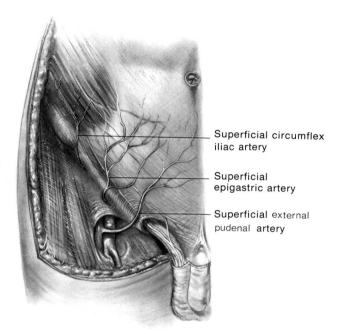

**Figure 27-1.** The superficial vessels encountered in performing the incision for herniorrhaphy include the superficial external pudendal, the superficial epigastric, and the superficial circumflex iliac arteries.

Superficial circumflex iliac artery

Superficial epigastric artery

Superficial external pudenal artery

surgical accidents and complications in one page — listing injuries to the bladder, intestine, spermatic cord, internal spermatic artery, deep inferior epigastric arteries, and the external iliac arteries. Watson (1948) describes operative complications, briefly mentioning injuries to the bowel and bladder. Zimmerman and Anson (1967) discuss operative injuries and accidents at some length. Nyhus and Condon (1978) recognize the importance of identifying postoperative complications by devoting a chapter in their book to this important matter.

## INTRAOPERATIVE DEATHS

Deaths during operations for hernia are extremely rare. Cardiac arrests, strokes, and "anesthetic accidents" account for a few fatalities. Deaths occurring in the early postoperative period are more common and will be discussed at length in Chapter 28.

## HEMORRHAGE

Bleeding from the subcutaneous vessels — including superficial circumflex iliac, superficial epigastric, and the superficial external pudendal — is seldom pro-

fuse (Fig. 27-1). If these vessels are not recognized and ligated, hematomas of some size often occur, especially in hypertensive patients. Residents seldom know these vessels by name or location and must be introduced to them repeatedly. Active bleeding from these vessels is rarely a

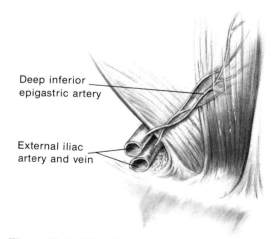

Deep inferior epigastric artery

External iliac artery and vein

**Figure 27-2.** The deep inferior epigastric artery arises from the external iliac artery, and lies deep to the transversalis fascia, where it forms a portion of the medial boundary of the internal abdominal ring. The inferior epigastric artery supplies the cremaster muscle through a cremasteric branch. It should be recalled that in large indirect inguinal hernias, the deep inferior epigastric artery may be dislocated far medially.

problem that requires reoperation for hemostasis, but postoperative hematomas are seen in significant numbers in studies of postoperative complications.

Unrecognized bleeding from the deep inferior epigastric artery is more troublesome. If this artery is not seen in its position at the internal ring, the needle may be easily placed through it, with resulting blood loss. The location and identification of the external spermatic artery at the internal ring will largely eliminate the problem of bleeding from this source. The deep inferior artery and vein are located just under the transversalis fascia, medial to the internal abdominal rings, and constant awareness of their locations is necessary if they are to be spared injury (Fig. 27–2). Ligation of the deep inferior epigastric vessels causes little interference with healing, although some wound edema and induration may follow.

## BLEEDING FROM THE PAMPINIFORM PLEXUS

Although bleeding from the venous plexus in the spermatic cord is seldom great, it can be troublesome and result in hematomas of substantial size. Rough dissection, including the use of sponges in separating cord structures from the peritoneal sac, is likely to injure the delicate veins of the pampiniform plexus. Accurate sharp dissection of the peritoneal sac is possible by inserting a finger into the sac in order to determine its thickness and to locate the cord at the internal ring. Avulsion of the cord structures from the sac is unnecessarily traumatic. Any bleeding venules must be individually clamped and ligated with fine silk.

In dissecting a lengthy hernial sac from the cord, it is always important to avoid excessive traction on the cord and to ligate every bleeding vessel, carefully and individually. Interference with the venous blood flow from the testicle may result in significant testicular swelling.

In some patients, it might be prudent to avoid dissecting out the entire peritoneal sac. The peritoneal sac might best be transected at the internal abdominal ring and dissection of the proximal portion completed to permit high ligation of the sac. The distal sac rarely results in a

hydrocele. If desired, the anterior portion of the sac might be opened. The cord structures are thus spared injury.

In recurrent direct hernias, care must be taken to avoid injury to the veins of Retzius in any dissection at the preperitoneal level.

## VASCULAR INJURIES

It is unusual for surgeons to report complications such as major vascular injuries. The reluctance on the part of surgeons to identify such surgical errors is easily understandable; yet, as previously stated, it would be totally unrealistic to take the position that such accidents never occur. Accidents such as vascular injuries should be discussed and faced realistically. Once identified, vascular injuries should be treated promptly and properly. With such an attitude on the part of surgeons, serious and permanent complications will be quite rare.

In 1913 Kahnan reported an instance in which ligature of the femoral artery following injury during herniorrhaphy led to amputation (Fig. 27–3).

Anatomy of the femoral vessels must be taught enthusiastically to residents. It is difficult to grasp the anatomic fact that as

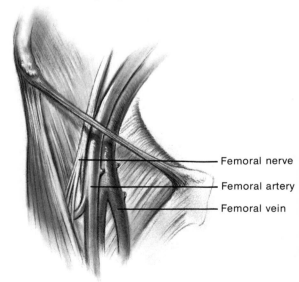

**Figure 27–3.** The femoral vein and femoral artery are always in some danger of injury because they lie just under the inguinal ligament and the iliopubic tract in the groin. The femoral nerve, which lies laterally and more deeply than the vein or artery, is in less danger than the vessels.

the iliac vessels come up out of the depths of the pelvis, they lie in dangerous proximity to the iliopubic tract and inguinal ligament where they are identified as femoral vessels (Fig. 27–3). In my experience, it is just under the inguinal ligament that injury to the femoral vessels might occur. At other times, the iliac vessels may be injured in the floor of the inguinal triangle, deep to the transversalis fascia.

The surgeon should suspect a surgical misadventure when blood appears promptly at the site of suture placement; the blood is of a bluish color if the femoral vein is injured and bright red if the femoral artery is perforated with the needle. The action taken by the surgeon at this point is of enormous importance. There are two approaches that some surgeons tend to use at this point, both of which are less than desirable. First, there is the tendency to complete the suture placement with ligature. Obviously, the suture so placed must have a site of entry as well as a point of exit, and ligation of this suture may well result in a larger defect by tearing the segment of vessel between perforations of entry and exit of the suture (Fig. 27–4). Second, when bleeding is a problem, the urge is always present to grasp the bleeding site with a clamp of some size; this, too, is a maneuver that is not recommended. What, then,

should be done? Simple fundamentals of technique are effective in solving the problem. It should be recalled that with the first insertion of the needle, we have what amounts to a vascular puncture. The needle should be withdrawn without completion of suture placement and digital pressure applied over the area for several minutes. Bleeding will stop in almost every instance. In an occasional patient with hypertension, bleeding from a perforated femoral artery may continue in spite of the above maneuvers. Application of damaging clamps should be avoided. Pressure with one digit over the bleeding site will control hemorrhage while the transversalis fascia is divided, permitting dissection of areolar tissue and identification of the bleeding site. The tiny perforation can usually be closed with a single number 6–0 vascular suture.

It is important to recall that in certain geriatric patients the circulation to the lower extremities may be marginal, and the need to preserve all collaterals is obvious. I am aware of one patient who lost a lower extremity because of vascular injury during herniorrhaphy. A second patient had a highly complicated course, eventually requiring ligation of the femoral artery in the groin. After a prolonged period of disability, he fortunately made an acceptable

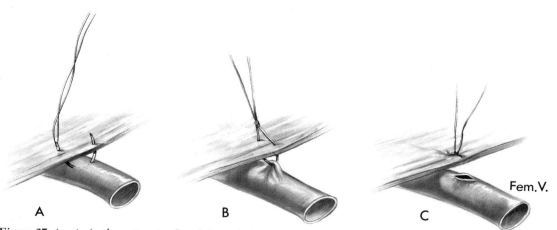

**Figure 27–4.** *A,* As the suture is placed through the inguinal ligament, the femoral vessel, which lies in close proximity to the ligament, is penetrated. *B,* As the ligature is tied tightly, the vessel is injured. *C,* The defect in the damaged vessel is variable. Most such injuries are minor, but, in the occasional case, a large hematoma or profuse hemorrhage is the result.

recovery. Such complications are rare; but, given a number of unfortunate circumstances, disaster can occur.

## INJURY TO THE FEMORAL VEIN

The femoral vein can be damaged through blind improper placement of sutures or traumatized through improper placement of retractors during repair of direct or femoral hernias.

Pulmonary embolism remains a significant threat to the health, and even the life, of the occasional patient undergoing hernia repair. Surgeons who must expose the region of the femoral artery and vein during hernia repair recognize that in occluding the femoral ring or in repairing the inguinal floor, it is possible to constrict the lumen of the femoral vein by placing sutures too far laterally—that is, sutures placed between the inguinal ligament and Cooper's ligament or between the transversus abdominis lamina might encroach on the lumen of the vein.

Surgeons with experience in the field recognize the possibility of venous constriction during herniorrhaphy. They can, when approached on the matter, recall cases in which swollen extremities or pulmonary emboli, or both, occurred. Such cases are rarely reported; cases reported by Nissen (1975) are of interest in this regard.

## ACCESSORY OBTURATOR ARTERY

Another source of major operative hemorrhage might be the accessory obturator artery. This artery may be encountered in dissections performed to expose Cooper's ligament (Fig. 27–5). Fortunately, even if injured, this vessel may be ligated with safety. Direct visualization and identification of such vessels will minimize the risk of injury.

Obviously, those vessels are most likely to be encountered in a Lotheissen-McVay repair.

I have seen one instance of major hemorrhage from an accessory obturator artery. In this case, reoperation was necessary following hernia repair because of continued

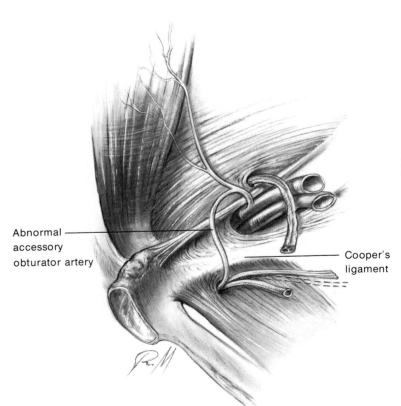

Abnormal accessory obturator artery

Cooper's ligament

**Figure 27–5.** An abnormal accessory obturator artery may communicate with the inferior epigastric artery and course over the iliopectineal eminence. This vessel is occasionally large and may be injured during dissection over Cooper's ligament. Sutures should not be placed blindly in this area.

bleeding and hypotension. This patient required six blood transfusions to replace his blood loss.

When faced with a large hematoma or continued bleeding, the surgeon must be prepared to take the occasional patient back to the operating room. If the blood clotting mechanism is normal and if simple measures such as pressure fail to stop the bleeding in a reasonable time, then it is recommended to proceed with exploration of the wound in the operating room under aseptic conditions. I have been forced to re-explore two patients in whom bleeding was a problem. In one patient, the bleeding came from an accessory obturator artery; in the second patient, the bleeding came from the pampiniform plexus. This second patient had a large indirect scrotal recurrent hernia. His spermatic cord was large, and the internal ring was closed too tightly for this particular patient. As a result, the pressure on the venous plexus was great, and bleeding continued. Removal of one suture at the internal abdominal ring and ligature of a few small venules corrected the problem.

# INJURY TO THE TESTICULAR BLOOD SUPPLY

The surgeon must be aware that the testicle derives its major blood supply from the internal spermatic artery, the deferential artery, and the external spermatic artery (Fig. 27–6). The possibility of injuring one or more of these vessels is always present.

The internal spermatic artery arises from the aorta and then courses over the psoas muscle in the retroperitoneal plane toward the internal abdominal ring. It becomes vulnerable to injury at the internal abdominal ring during hernia repair. Even with constant awareness of the artery and minimal manipulation of the cord, there is some danger of compromise of the blood supply to the testicle. This danger is increased significantly when recurrent hernias are repaired. In such situations, the position of the remaining spermatic cord is uncertain. If the spermatic cord had been transplanted and the cremaster previously removed, the difficulty of identifying the cord structures is sometimes enormous.

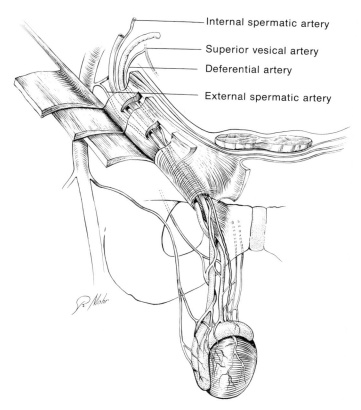

- Internal spermatic artery
- Superior vesical artery
- Deferential artery
- External spermatic artery

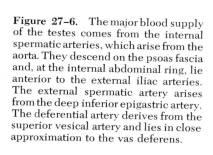

**Figure 27–6.** The major blood supply of the testes comes from the internal spermatic arteries, which arise from the aorta. They descend on the psoas fascia and, at the internal abdominal ring, lie anterior to the external iliac arteries. The external spermatic artery arises from the deep inferior epigastric artery. The deferential artery derives from the superior vesical artery and lies in close approximation to the vas deferens.

The deferential artery originates from the superior vesical artery. It lies in close proximity to the vas throughout its course to the globus major of the testicle where it divides into branches supplying the body and tail of the epididymis.

The external spermatic, or cremasteric, artery arises from the deep inferior epigastric artery and becomes a portion of the cord at the internal abdominal ring.

The location of the vessels just described must always be kept in mind during dissection. Careful surgical technique is essential in attempting to preserve the testicular blood supply. Sharp dissection and careful hemostasis are necessary. Only fine-pointed hemostats should be used and ligatures should be no larger than number 4–0. Even with strict operative precautions, every surgeon will encounter an occasional case in which there has been compromise of the blood supply to the testicle.

## INJURY TO THE BLADDER

*It is said that on several occasions the urinary bladder has been mistaken for the hernia sac and has been tied off and amputated, resulting in a urinary fistula.*

*Kahnan, 1913*

Bladder injuries are uncommonly reported. Davis (1916) found only 2 such injuries among 1500 operations. He pointed out the need for recognition of the defect, closure of the cystotomy, and catheter drainage.

Injury to the bladder is also possible in the repair of direct sliding hernias (Fig. 27–7). It should also be recalled that the bladder may find its way into a sliding femoral hernia.

Kahnan (1913) cited an instance in which a patient developed lower abdominal pain, chills, fever, and pyuria postoperatively. The patient later voided a large chromic catgut suture per urethra and subsequently recovered. He felt that a portion of the bladder was tied off with the ligature.

The distended bladder may appear in the inguinal region as a direct, indirect, or femoral hernia. It should be recalled that the bladder is a distensible organ; and as it distends, it becomes thinner. An enormously distended bladder may be easily confused with the peritoneal sac. The surgeon must be aware that a huge bladder may reach the umbilicus or the external abdominal ring. Under these conditions, the erroneous identification of the bladder as a hernial sac is quite possible. It is, therefore, of great importance that the bladder be emptied prior to herniorrhaphy.

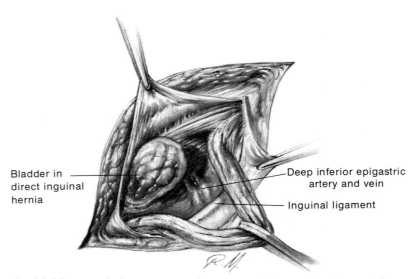

Bladder in direct inguinal hernia

Deep inferior epigastric artery and vein

Inguinal ligament

**Figure 27–7.**   The bladder may find its way into the occasional hernia as a direct sliding component. On palpation, the sac is firm, irregular, and can be reduced with difficulty. Greatest caution is essential whenever the surgeon wishes to open a direct hernial sac.

The greatest danger to the urinary bladder arises in repair of direct inguinal or femoral hernias and recurrent hernias of both these varieties. The injuries that I myself have seen occurred in two patients with recurrent direct inguinal hernias. In both instances, we were prepared for the possibility, having made cystograms indicating the location of the bladder. A Foley catheter had been inserted preoperatively in both cases in which the bladder was inadvertently entered. It is most important to recognize injury to the bladder. Closure of the defect in two layers with continuous number 4–0 chromic catgut and interrupted fine silk sutures will solve the problem. Foley catheter drainage continues for several days. Prompt improvement can usually be expected if the bladder injury is recognized and repaired. In the repair of such hernias, I use catgut and monofilament wire rather than silk. Drains are used in selected cases.

## INJURY TO THE BOWEL

While not common, injuries to the intestine do occur. Levy and coworkers (1951) reported 2 inadvertent enterotomies among 1001 operations, while Davis (1916) found only 1 operative intestinal injury in 1500 operations.

Intestinal injuries may occur when small intestine becomes incarcerated in an indirect or femoral inguinal hernia. Direct inguinal hernias almost never result in incarceration because of the wide opening into the sac. When either small intestine or a femoral hernia becomes incarcerated and possibly strangulated, the serious symptoms of nausea, vomiting, pain, and the presence of a tender, palpable, irreducible mass make the problem of diagnosis a comparatively simple one. A Richter's type of hernia (considered in much more detail in Chapter 24) may be quite small and difficult to recognize. In complicated cases, the bowel may be tightly incarcerated and inadvertent enterotomy performed.

Such accidents may be avoided by utilizing a generous but careful incision on either side of the protruding mass. With release of tension, disruption is less likely to occur. If the problem is a Richter's femoral hernia, it must be approached from a position above the inguinal ligament. Incision into Gimbernat's ligament me-

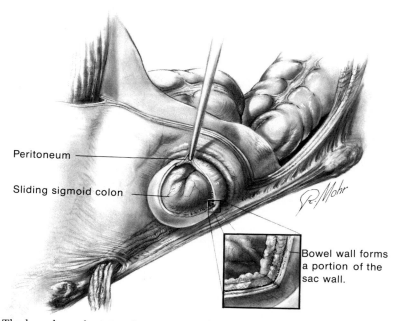

Peritoneum

Sliding sigmoid colon

Bowel wall forms a portion of the sac wall.

**Figure 27–8.**   The bowel may be injured in incisional hernias where it lies just under the epidermis. At other times, a sliding inguinal hernia may contain sigmoid on the left or some part of the iliocecal segment on the right. Such hernias occur in older, obese patients; following reduction, they reappear promptly. The peritoneum may be identified at the upper or superior portion of the sac.

dially will often free the incarcerated bowel. Should resection be necessary, it can be performed from this vantage point. In the event that exposure of the area is unusually difficult, it may be prudent to gain control of the proximal and distal limbs of the bowel through a transabdominal incision. With application of rubber bands or atraumatic Pott's type clamps, the incarcerated hernial mass may be managed without danger of spillage.

In the event of gross contamination, I recommend repair of the hernia with monofilament wire and catgut sutures. Drains are recommended and broad-spectrum antibiotics should be administered.

Injury to the colon may occur when dealing with sliding components of the sigmoid colon on the left and the cecum on the right (Fig. 27–8). At least five errors may

occur in dealing with sliding hernias containing bowel; they are:

1. Failure to recognize the colon in the sac.
2. Dissection in an incorrect, or nonanatomic, plane while trying to free the sliding hernia from the spermatic cord.
3. Suture, or injury, to vessels that supply the colon.
4. Poor placement of sutures in an ill-advised attempt to cover "raw areas", as when dealing with cecal sliding hernias.
5. Performing inadvertent colotomies — erroneously identifying the colon as a hernial sac.

It is most important to recognize the sliding hernia preoperatively, or to at least suspect the possibility at operation. If

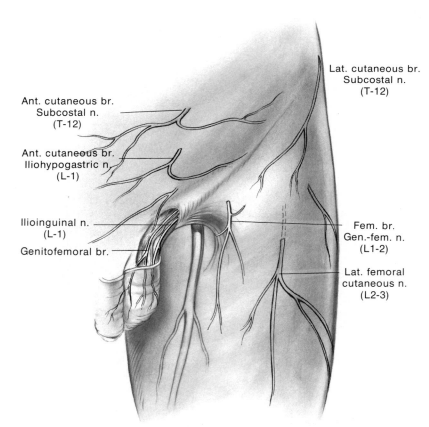

**Figure 27–9.** The iliohypogastric and ilioinguinal nerves can be seen to lie in a dangerous position just under the external oblique aponeurosis. The ilioinguinal nerve often presents at the superior crus of the external abdominal ring. It is at this site where it might be injured in opening the external oblique aponeurosis. The postoperative anesthesia which follows sacrificing of these nerves is temporary because of overlapping nerve supply to the area.

erroneous entry into a clean colon occurs, it must be repaired with two layers—using chromic catgut for mucosal closure and number 4–0 silk, interrupted, for serosal closure. The wound must be drained and the repair accomplished with catgut and single-strand wire sutures. Broad-spectrum antibiotics are given at the time of injury rather than at the point when complications occur. The problem of the sliding hernia is discussed at length in Chapter 28. Experiences with colonic injuries are also discussed.

## INJURY TO THE ILIOINGUINAL, ILIOHYPOGASTRIC, AND LATERAL FEMORAL CUTANEOUS NERVES

The ilioinguinal and iliohypogastric nerves are particularly exposed to injury during herniorrhaphy (Fig. 27–9) since they are located directly in the paths of surgical effort at repair. The lateral femoral cutaneous nerve comes under consideration during more extensive, but uncommon, dissections involving the posterolateral aspects of the abdominal wall and upper thigh.

Andrews in 1926 noted that the ilioinguinal and iliohypogastric nerves were particularly prone to injury. This is explained in part by the fact that these nerves show great variation in anatomic arrangement (Fig. 27–9).

The ilioinguinal and iliohypogastric nerves arise from the first lumbar but often receive fibers from the twelfth thoracic nerve as well. These nerves then penetrate the internal oblique muscle lateral and superior to the internal abdominal ring. The ilioinguinal nerve commonly lies upon the cremasteric muscle of the cord and is most easily injured when the external oblique aponeurosis is incised. According to Andrews (1926), at this point it functions purely as a sensory nerve. He found that while the iliohypogastric nerve provides fibers to the lower fibers of the internal oblique muscle, it does so before it appears at the herniorrhaphy site. Therefore, muscular paralysis is not a consequence of section of the iliohypogastric nerve.

More recently, Moosman and Oerlich (1977) pointed out that while injury to the ilioinguinal nerve does not endanger life of the patient, the consequence of hypesthesia, paresthesia, or numbness in the inguinoscrotal area is annoying to some patients. They emphasized that in 35 percent of 424 dissections, the ilioinguinal nerve was located in an aberrant location within the cremasteric sheath or its counterpart in the round ligament. At this site, the nerve is more vulnerable to injury.

Careful incision of the external oblique aponeurosis at a distance three or four centimeters from the margin of the external abdominal ring will permit direct visualization of the nerve and its preservation. Constant awareness of possible injury to the iliohypogastric and ilioinguinal nerves while in the operative field will lead to preservation of these nerves.

The lateral femoral cutaneous nerve may be injured in extensive dissections which include the lower abdomen. Such injuries are rare and result in anesthesia of the anterolateral portion of the thigh. The numbness subsides over a period of several months.

The annoying problem of nerve entrapment and postoperative pain will be discussed in Chapter 29 on late complications.

## INJURIES TO THE VAS DEFERENS

Injuries to the vas deferens are uncommon. Fortunately, the vas is comparatively easily located by palpation and by sight. Its cordlike consistency is a quality that makes it stand out among other structures of the spermatic cord. The vas is most vulnerable to injury in operations for recurrent hernias and especially when numerous operative procedures have been performed previously.

The vas deferens is fairly easily repaired at the time of initial injury (Fig. 27–10). I place a plain catgut suture through the lumen to serve as a splint. The catgut is placed on a straight needle, inserted obliquely through the wall of the vas deferens, then into the lumen of the proximal vas; and then, it is again passed obliquely through the wall. With this suture serving as a splint, the areolar tissue about the wall of the proximal and distal vas deferens is incorporated in interrupted sutures to achieve accurate approximation.

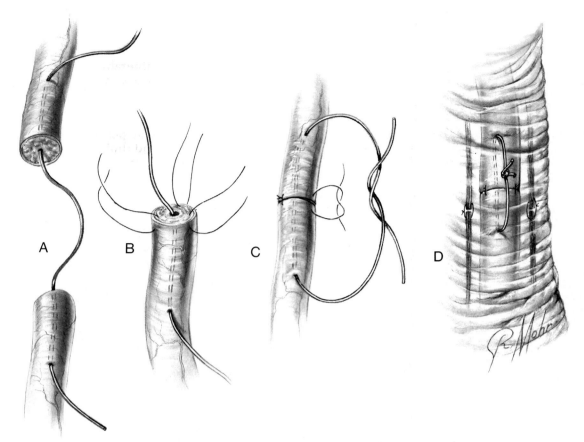

**Figure 27–10.** The vas deferens might be severed during repair of recurrent inguinal hernias. Reconstruction should be attempted at the time. A simple technique is illustrated.

*A*, The lumen may be preserved with a removable number 2–0 nylon suture stent. *B*, The wall of the vas is then approximated with interrupted number 6–0 absorbable sutures. *C*, The cut ends of the vas deferens are approximated with number 6–0 absorbable sutures. *D*, The nylon stent suture is tied in order to maintain the ends of the vas in approximation.

After healing is complete the nylon stent is removed. This method is recommended by Dr. Riad Farah of the Department of Urology of Henry Ford Hospital.

## INJURY TO FALLOPIAN TUBES AND OVARIES

*The discovery of a sliding hernia involving internal genitalia in a female infant evokes both surprise and confusion in a general surgeon of average experience.*

*Richardson, 1963*

The relative infrequency of inguinal hernias in female infants may account for a lack of appreciation of the magnitude of the problem as it affects these individuals when they become adults.

Goldstein and Potts (1958) observed that the incidence of sliding hernias in female infants is 20 percent, but Stevenson and Johnson (1964) felt that this figure is probably nearer to 50 percent. Only during the past quarter-century have surgeons recognized the importance of the problem of sliding hernias in female infants (Fig. 27–11).

Operative complications are not always manifest at once. The tragic consequences of operative injury to the Fallopian tubes may not be evident until the infant reaches

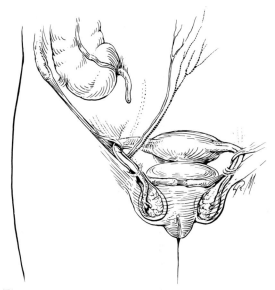

**Figure 27–11.** The need for surgeons to recognize the tremendous importance of sliding hernias in female infants is now being recognized. Tubes and ovaries damaged during surgical repair in infancy may not be recognized as a cause of sterility until the reproductive age is reached. Too often the surgeon who performed the initial operation is unaware of the long-term result of his effort.

sexual maturity—when it is found sterility is a problem.

Swanson and Chapler (1977) have recently called attention to infertility in females following bilateral inguinal herniorrhaphies in infancy. This particular type of operative injury has been only recently recognized.

It is important that during the operative procedure in female infants, the presence of a sliding hernia be recognized and properly managed. The fimbriae of the tube must not be roughly handled with large crushing instruments. It is important that all structures be identified; hence, I recommend that the peritoneal sac be carefully opened at its upper margin at the internal ring. There are two methods for management of the peritoneal sac; it may be inverted after a purse-string suture has been placed at the internal ring, or it may be managed as illustrated in Figure 18–23, A; page 311. Gentle handling of the fragile tube and replacement of both the tube and ovary into the peritoneal cavity are essential.

## SUMMARY

It is an impossible feat to conduct a large surgical practice without ever encountering an operative complication of major proportions or a postoperative fatality. The surgeon who studies the problem of hernia in all its aspects and devotes a great deal of time to this area will have fewer such complications than will the surgeon who performs the occasional herniorrhaphy. Since intraoperative complications are not always recorded, it would be difficult to offer an accurate estimate as to their frequency. Fortunately, most minor problems are promptly and effectively managed without incident. Some of the significant operative complications have been presented along with suggestions for prevention and management. I believe that an awareness of all the possible complications is the key to their avoidance or, at least, a factor in reduction of their numbers. Most of these complications referred to in Table 27–1 have occurred at some time on my division and in my surgical practice. Some of the problems occurred elsewhere and were referred to me for resolution. Fortunately, most of the complications listed are easily managed if recognized! The important lesson to be learned is that herniorrhaphy should command the respect of the surgeon who undertakes to perform the operation. He should be aware of the dangers that await him at each step of the repair. The fatality rate must approach zero, and complications must be kept to a minimum. The outline of intraoperative complications might be useful to those who must seek "informed consent" from the patient and his relatives.

Intraoperative complications are not always avoidable, but they should be recognized as they occur and promptly corrected. I feel that many postoperative complications have their origins in surgical misadventure of some degree. This statement is not intended to be an accusation but rather a recognition of certain events. In the repair of complicated hernias or recurrent hernias, injury may occur to the testicular blood supply. When the surgeon is dealing with gangrenous bowel, inadvertent enterotomy is not rare. The bowel wall is delicate and easily ruptured. The surgeon, in dealing with sliding inguinal hernias, may easily injure the bowel or bladder.

Management of sliding inguinal hernias in female infants requires great respect for the particular problem at hand. The ovaries and tubes with delicate fimbriae must be handled with the lightest touch. Consideration must be given to the blood supply of these structures if they are to be functional when the patient reaches sexual maturity.

This chapter emphasizes the need for accurate anatomic knowledge on the part of surgeons who wish to repair hernias with a measure of success. The relationship of one anatomic structure to another must be clearly understood, and these structures must be appreciated in a three-dimensional perspective.

## REFERENCES

Andrews, E.: The ilio-hypogastric nerve in relation to herniotomy. Ann. Surg. 83:79, 1926.

Beekman, E., and Sullivan, J. E.: Analysis of immediate postoperative complications in 2000 cases of inguinal hernia. Surg. Gynecol. Obstet. 68:1052, 1939.

Davis, L.: Complications and sequelae of the operation for inguinal hernia. J.A.M.A. 67:480, 1916.

Glenn, F.: The surgical treatment of 1,545 hernias. Ann. Surg. 25:72, 1947.

Goldstein, I. R., and Potts, W. J.: Inguinal hernia in female infants and children. Ann. Surg. 148:819, 1958.

Iason, A. H.: Hernia. Philadelphia, The Blakiston Co., 1941.

Kahnan, D. R.: Accidents of hernia operations. N.Y. State J. Med. 13:200, 1913.

Levy, A. H., Wren, R. S., and Friedman, M. N.: Complications and recurrences following inguinal hernia repair. Ann. Surg. 133:533, 1951.

Longmire, William P., Jr.: Cited in Nyhus, L. M., and Condon, R. E.: Hernia (2nd ed.). Philadelphia, J. B. Lippincott Co., 1978.

MacLaughlin, W. S., Jr., Kron, I. L., and Sager, G. F.: Experiences with 100 patients hospitalized for incarcerated hernia. J. Maine Med. Assoc. 67:319, 1976.

Moosman, D. A., and Oelrich, T. M.: Prevention of accidental trauma to the ilioinguinal nerve during herniorrhaphy. Am. J. Surg. 133:146, 1977.

Nissen, H. M.: Constriction of the femoral vein following inguinal hernia repair. Acta Chir. Scand. 141:279, 1975.

Nyhus, I. M., and Condon, P. E.: Hernia (2nd ed.). Philadelphia, J. B. Lippincott Co., 1978, pp. 264–275.

Richardson, W. R.: Inguinal hernia of the internal genitalia in female infants and children. Am. Surg. 29:446, 1963.

Stevenson, J. K., and Johnson, L. P.: Groin hernias in infants and children. In Nyhus, L. M., and Harkins, L. H.: Hernia. Philadelphia, J. B. Lippincott, 1964, pp. 73–91.

Swanson, J. A., and Chapler, F. K.: Infertility as a consequence of bilateral herniorrhaphies. Fertil. Steril. 28:1118, 1977.

Watson, L. F.: Hernia (3rd ed.). St. Louis, C. V. Mosby Co., 1948, pp. 520, 572.

Zimmerman, L. M., and Anson, B. J.: Anatomy and Surgery of Hernia. Baltimore, Williams & Wilkins Co., 1967, pp. 194–196.

## Additional Readings

Arnhein, E. E., and Linder, J. M.: Inguinal hernia in the pelvic viscera in female infants. Am. J. Surg. 92:486, 1956.

Condon, R. E., and Nyhus, L. M.: Complications of groin hernia and hernia repair. Surg. Clin. North Am. 51(6):1325, 1971.

Donovan, E. J., and Stanley-Brown, E. G.: Inguinal hernia in female infants and children. Surg. Gynecol. Obstet. 107:663, 1958.

Farah, Riah: Personal communication.

Gessner, N. B.: Some experimental work on circulation of the testicle. Am. J. Urol. 11:104, 1915.

Jones, T. I.: A comparative study of inguinal herniorrhaphy. Am. Surg. 41:20, 1975.

Koontz, A. R.: Atrophy of the testicle as a surgical risk. Surg. Gynecol. Obstet. 120:511, 1965.

Pick, J. W., Anson, B. J., and Ashley, F. L.: The origin of the obturator artery. Am. J. Anat. 70:317, 1942.

Ramos, R. L., and Burton, C. C.: The results of treatment of bilocular and direct inguinal hernias. Surg. Gynecol. Obstet. 70:953, 1940.

Rydell, W. B.: Inguinal and femoral hernia. Arch. Surg. 87:151, 1963.

# 28

# Early and Late Postoperative Complications and Their Management

The purpose of this chapter is to direct attention to both the possibility of fatality and the numerous complications that may follow hernia repair (Table 28–1). It is conceded that fatalities are rare in healthy patients undergoing repair of uncomplicated hernias; however, the death rate becomes significant when elderly patients must undergo surgical correction of strangulation-obstruction due to incarcerated hernias. As can be seen in Table 28–1, I found the reported death rate to range from 0.34 to 3 percent in various series. Those who operate upon infants and healthy adults will claim zero mortality, and surgeons who perform herniorrhaphies under local anesthesia will likewise have impressively low death rates.

On the other hand, those surgeons who must attempt to salvage elderly patients suffering from advanced cardiovascular disease plus strangulated hernias containing gangrenous bowel will report significant rates of mortality (MacLaughlin et al., 1976).

## POSTOPERATIVE FATALITIES

Although deaths occurring in healthy patients during herniorrhaphy are extreme-ly rare, the possibility exists, nevertheless. Deaths in the postoperative period are usually due to deterioration in health that occurs with aging or to such complications as strangulation. Patients and their families will, from time to time, challenge the surgeon with the unrealistic question, "There is no danger in this operation — is there?" Or, they may further betray their lack of knowledge with the statment, "This is a minor operation — isn't it?" Both questions demand a clear, honest, and realistic answer. The increased incidence of aged patients alters the fatality rate, since they often have advanced arteriosclerotic heart and severe lung disease. Even under local anesthesia, there is a minimal danger to those patients with less than optimal health. The greatest danger of sudden unexpected death, in my surgical experience, has been with the patient suffering from arteriosclerotic heart disease and angina. Furthermore, those patients with incarceration, strangulation, and gangrene of the bowel are at an even greater risk. A massive pulmonary embolus occurring in the postoperative period can be disastrous in an elderly patient. The patient and his family must be cognizant of the fact that a hernia repair cannot be considered a minor procedure, since the procedure involves abdominal section and entry into the peritoneal cavity in nearly every case. Furthermore, hernias often contain abdominal viscera that must be properly managed. Although it is possible to successfully operate on many patients over a period of months or even years, now and then, a death does occur in the postoperative period.

I examined the fatality rate for each type of hernia studied and observed the following: the death rate following repair of congenital indirect inguinal hernias (Chapter 10) was zero percent; for femoral hernias, 0.6 percent (Chapter 15); for incisional hernias, 0.63 percent (Chapter 21); and for umbilical hernias (Chapter 22), 0.58 percent.

Davis in 1916 reported 8 fatalities among 1,500 patients, for a mortality of 0.53

**Table 28–1.  INCIDENCE OF POSTOPERATIVE COMPLICATIONS REPORTED IN LITERATURE**

| | DAVIS (1916) | BEEKMAN AND SULLIVAN (1939) | GLENN (1947) | LEVY ET AL.[*] (1951) | LJUNGDAHL (1973) | MACLAUGHLIN ET AL. 1976[**] |
|---|---|---|---|---|---|---|
| **Wound** | | | | | | |
| Ecchymosis | Not listed | Not listed | Not listed | | | |
| Hematoma | 7.5% | 0.8% | 0.17 | 2.1 | 0 | 1 |
| Infection | 4.0% | 4.9% | 1.1% | 1.7% | | 4 |
| Seroma | | | | | 0.24 | |
| **Scrotal–Testicular** | | | | | | |
| Hematoma | 7.5% | 0.7% | | | | |
| Swelling | | | 0.32 | [*] | 0.47 | 5.0 |
| Atrophy | | | | | 0.47 | |
| Sterility | | (Incidence not reported) | | | | |
| Bilateral atrophy | | (Incidence not reported) | | | | |
| Orchidectomy | 0.33% | | | | | |
| Hydrocele | | | | | 2.59 | |
| **Genitourinary** | | | | | | |
| Retention | | | 0.71 | 0.3 | 1.42 | 2 |
| Infection | | 0.1% | 0.13 | | | 6 |
| Obstruction | | | | | 0.47 | |
| Infection | | | | | | |
| **Pulmonary** | | | | | | |
| Atelectasis | 9.2% | 8.5% | 0.76 | 2.4 | | |
| Pneumonitis | 0.5% | | 0.39 | | 0.24 | |
| Tracheobronchitis | 6.6% | | | | | |
| Pulmonary embolus | 0.13 | | 0.26 | 0.2 | 0.24 | |
| **Extremities** | | | | | | |
| Phlebothrombosis | 0.13 | 0.3% | 0.32 | 0.2 | 0.47 | |
| **Gastrointestinal** | | | | | | |
| Ileus | | 0.3% | | 0.5 | 0.24 | 1.0 |
| Acute gastric dilatation | | 0.05% | | | | |
| **Cardiac Complications** | | | | | | 2 |
| Neuropathy | | | | | 0.47 | |
| Headache | | 0.2% | | | | |
| **Dermatitis** | | 0.1% | | | | |
| **Postoperative Psychosis** | | 0.05% | | | | |
| **Recurrences** | 4.0% | | | | 4.0 | |
| **Deaths** | 0.53% | | 0.34 | | | 3[°] |

[*] Levy et al.: "Swelling of the scrotum and spermatic cord was the most frequent postoperative complication."
[**] MacLaughlin, et al., operated upon elderly patients with complications.

percent. Glenn in 1947 reported 6 deaths among 1,385 patients operated on — 3 patients died of peritonitis; 2, of pulmonary embolism, and 1 of coronary occlusion. Beekman and Sullivan (1939) reported 5 deaths among 2,000 cases operated on; pneumonia accounted for 2 of these deaths and pulmonary emboli for 3 others. Levy (1951) reported no deaths in 1,001 operations for hernia. MacLaughlin and coworkers (1976) reported 3 deaths among 100 patients operated on; however, more critical inspection of the findings revealed that 37 of those patients had incarcerated hernias. Thus, for those selected patients, the rate was actually 6.6 percent. The causes of death in the cases studied by MacLaughlin are of interest. One patient, aged 77 years, had a cardiac arrest; another, aged 66 years, aspirated gastric contents; the third, aged 70 years, had a strangulation obstruction with death of the bowel, septicemia, and a fatal gram-negative septicemia.

As a result of my studies, it is clear that a simple answer to the question of the fatality rate following hernia repair cannot be accurately assessed. Obviously, the rate will vary with the age of the patient, his general health at the time of surgery, and the presence of incarceration and strangulation.

There are lessons to be gained from a brief review of records of patients who died as a result of complications following hernia repairs.

## Postoperative Death — Arteriosclerotic Heart Disease and Pneumonitis (Case in Point)

This particular patient's record was drawn from our microfilm files. Although the quality of the tapes left much to be desired, it was possible — through great patience and determination — to obtain some useful information.

The patient was a 74-year-old male who came to Henry Ford Hospital for repair of a huge, scrotal, sliding, indirect inguinal hernia, which had become increasingly troublesome. Repair was advised and accomplished in 1947.

Preoperative evaluation revealed that

the patient had arteriosclerotic heart disease.

Repair of the large, scrotal, sliding, indirect inguinal hernia was accomplished under local anesthesia. Postoperatively, the patient developed severe swelling along the cord and in the testicle. Also, distention due to an ileus was an early complication. He developed tachycardia, cardiac arrhythmia, and increasing respiratory difficulty and was digitalized without improvement. Diffuse, moist rales were present in both lung fields. His condition continued to deteriorate, and he died on the eighth postoperative day. Death was attributed to arteriosclerotic heart disease, but pneumonitis was also present.

### Comment

This patient's record is presented in order to illustrate the type of patient who might present problems in the postoperative period.

First of all, he was an aged patient with evidence of arteriosclerotic heart disease. Second, he had a large, scrotal, sliding, indirect hernia. Third, dissection of the sliding component led to a hematoma along the cord. Fourth, manipulation of the bowel contributed to his ileus and distention which, no doubt, probably interfered with venous blood return to the heart. In the presence of initial marginal cardiac function, the patient experienced more difficulty with his heart. He subsequently developed pulmonary edema and pneumonitis and expired eight days following repair of the hernia.

Elderly patients must be carefully selected and prepared for any operative procedure. Extreme care in management of sliding hernias is necessary. Finally, when operations are being performed on patients who represent increased surgical risks, some fatalities will occur.

One other lesson might be learned from this case — i.e., an earlier operation might have been successful. Delay in accepting surgical repair eventually becomes counterproductive (although, no doubt, a younger patient could have tolerated the repair).

Occasionally, overwhelming sepsis develops that could claim the life of a patient, and the surgeon finds himself in a complicated situation in which decisions must be made promptly. The next case illustrates the seriousness of infection in complicated hernias.

### Postoperative Death — Sepsis (Case in Point)

The patient was an obese, 72-year-old male who presented with an incarcerated hernia and a tender distended abdomen. He reported that a physician attempted to aspirate "pus" from the groin. At operation, the patient had an incarcerated mass of preperitoneal fat and an inguinal hernia. Gangrenous, foul-smelling material was obtained from the mass. The abdomen was explored through a separate incision in order to establish viability of the intestine. The prevesical space was examined and later drained. The hernia was repaired with wire and catgut sutures. The wounds were thoroughly drained. The patient had a septic course postoperatively in spite of vigorous antibiotic therapy. He became comatose and developed convulsive seizures. Cardiac arrest occurred on the third day, and the patient could not be resuscitated.

Autopsy findings demonstrated retroperitoneal cellulitis, peritonitis, and septicemia. Bacteroides was recovered from the blood culture, and coliforms were found at the site of aspiration. The patient had advanced arteriosclerosis, but the cause of death was felt to be overwhelming sepsis.

### Comment

The dangerous practice of aspiration of groin masses still emerges from time to time. What structures were injured by the aspiration is not entirely clear, but the resultant infection with bacteroides and coliform organisms indicates that bowel was injured. Yet, at exploration the bowel was found to be intact. Extensive dissection at operation disseminated the organisms widely and septicemia followed. If viability of the bowel could have been determined without extensive surgical exploration, local drainage might have been a more desirable approach.

This case illustrates that aged patients tolerate complications poorly. Hernias

should be repaired before they become life-threatening to the patient.

In reviewing the surgical literature, it becomes apparent that it is the elderly patient with complications developing secondary to herniation whose life is in jeopardy. Strangulation-obstruction is more than some elderly patients can endure, regardless of appropriateness of treatment.

### Postoperative Death — Strangulation–Obstruction (Case in Point)

The patient was a 59-year-old female who had been acutely ill for three days before admission to the hospital. She had chronic lung disease and was in pulmonary edema secondary to arteriosclerotic heart disease. A right hydrothorax was present. The abdomen was greatly distended, and a large incisional hernia was present in the right lower quadrant — the site of an appendectomy 32 years before. The diagnosis was incarcerated and strangulated incisional hernia in a patient with congestive heart failure. She received emergency supportive treatment, including right thoracentesis.

At operation the large hernia contained ileum, cecum, and ascending colon. Resection was necessary, but only an exteriorization resection was elected by the surgeon. The patient had a stormy postoperative course and died of peritonitis and septicemia.

### Comment

Incisional hernias cause much discomfort and can, through complications, cause death. This patient delayed seeking help too long. In three days, she developed gangrene of the bowel and infection had established itself. She was, at best, a poor surgical risk; her cardiac disease and pulmonary edema further contributed to her demise. In this case, the hernia was present for 32 years before illness overcame the patient.

Aged patients with hypertension or cardiovascular and renal disease should be offered surgical treatment only after a thorough exploration of every option has been made. Occasionally, even after thorough preoperative evaluation, the patient will tragically fall into an inter-related web of complications that results in death. The following case report shows such a chain of events.

## Postoperative Death—Hypertensive–Cardiovascular Disease (Case in Point)

This patient, a 68-year-old female, was obese and had a large umbilical hernia and a small incisional hernia. The contents of the sac were omentum and small intestine, and incarceration was present. She had hypertension and both mitral insufficiency and aortic stenosis. The indications for surgical intervention included intermittent obstructive symptoms. After thorough clinical and laboratory investigations were complete the large umbilical defect and smaller incisional hernia were repaired. The hernia contained incarcerated small

bowel and omentum. Numerous adhesions were present.

Her postoperative course was stormy as indicated in the clinicopathologic correlation, and she developed cardiac, pulmonary, and renal complications. She received vigorous supportive and antibiotic therapy, but she succumbed on the twenty-fourth postoperative day.

A clinicopathologic correlation in this case might appear as that shown in Figure 28–1.

The cause of death was related to multiple factors including renal failure due to acute tubular necrosis, cerebral infarction, and acute myocardial infarction. Patients with advanced arteriosclerosis are at significant risk, even when modest operative procedures are performed. It is recommended that the matter of operative risk be discussed with responsible family members prior to surgical intervention.

In the four cases presented, there is an eloquent argument for early elective repair of hernias. Deferring operative treatment

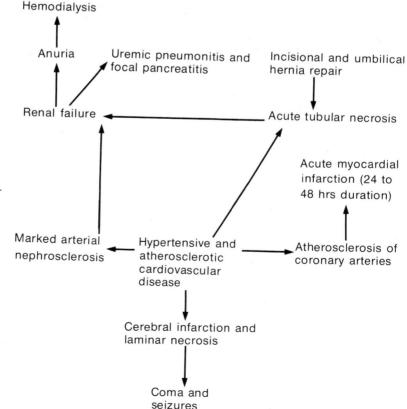

**Figure 28–1.** Clinicopathologic correlation.

too often leads to life-threatening complications. Aged patients with degenerative cardiovascular and pulmonary disease are poor candidates for major emergency surgical procedures.

## EARLY WOUND COMPLICATIONS

### Introduction

In looking over the chapter on intraoperative complications (Chapter 27) it can be seen that many postoperative complications are the direct consequence of some surgical-technical misadventure. Many of the complications can be eliminated and others reduced in number through improvement in technical skill and implementation of knowledge available to all surgeons. With thorough evaluation and appropriate treatment of cardiac, pulmonary, genitourinary tract, and metabolic diseases, further reduction in complications can be achieved. Obesity is too often overlooked as a hazard to patients requiring herniorrhaphy.

A postoperative complication rate of 10 percent is accepted by many surgeons as a reasonable incidence of undesirable sequelae to herniorrhaphy. This figure is probably lower than the actual rate because of incomplete recording and omission of many minor complications. More complete and uniform reporting of all complications is highly desirable.

The potential for complications will vary with the age of the patient, his general health, and the complexity of his hernia.

In the current era of "informed consent," it is useful to recognize the enormous numbers of postoperative complications that might develop following hernia repair. Table 28–2 presents an impressive list of complications, which I have divided into "early" and "late" complications. The early complications are seen in the immediate postoperative period or before the patient is discharged from the hospital. With the current practice of early discharge of patients from the hospital, it might be useful to consider those complications occurring within 10 to 14 days as "early." Those complications appearing after patients are well on the road to recovery can be considered "late" complications. Late complications may occur a few weeks or

even years following herniorrhaphy. Such complications as recurring infection, sinus formation, testicular atrophy, and recurrence of the hernia are considered late complications. In my surgical experience, I have seen nearly every complication listed in Table 28–2. Although the table includes most of the complications, it does not include all of the possibilities. The incidence of postoperative complications will vary directly with the accuracy of reporting and inversely with the knowledge, experience, and skill of the surgeon.

In examining Table 28–2, it is evident that while those complications arising from the operative effort may be disabling, the serious complications arise as a result of involvement and malfunction of remote organ systems. The need for careful postoperative evaluation of every patient about to undergo herniorrhaphy is clear.

### Ecchymosis

Of all the wound complications, ecchymosis is the most common, especially when local anesthesia is used. In most instances, the suffusion of blood into the subcutaneous tissues and epidermis is minimal and presents no danger, and complete recovery within two to three weeks can be expected. The bluish-black discoloration occasionally seen looks ominous to the patient and, hence, must be explained. In most cases, only reassurance is needed. Prevention of ecchymosis is sometimes a difficult task, but careful hemostasis is the best preventative measure.

Warm tub baths are comforting to the patient later in the recovery period. Interference with wound healing by fruitless exploration of the incision is ill-advised, since ecchymosis in most cases is a minor wound complication.

### Hematoma

Extravascular blood in the operative site is a more serious problem than is ecchymosis. Hematomas have been reported as occurring in from 0.17 percent to 7.5 percent of surgical wounds. The patient will be concerned with the conspicuous swelling in the incision and wonder if the hernia has recurred. Hematomas delay healing of the wound and predispose to infection. Larger hematomas can delay recovery for several days and, occasionally, for a few weeks.

Hematomas are the result of imperfect hemostasis. This does not imply that the operation was carelessly performed, for the blood vessel can commence bleeding after

## Table 28–2.  POSTOPERATIVE COMPLICATIONS

|  | *Early* | *Late* |
|---|---|---|
|  | Fatalities | Fatalities (see individual chapters) |
| *Wound* | Ecchymosis<br>Hematoma<br>Stitch abscess<br>Infection (cellulitis, suppuration)<br>Peritonitis (sepsis – death)<br>Minor wound separation<br>Wound disruption | Induration<br>Seroma<br>Wound pain – neuroma<br>Chronic sinus tracts<br>Recurring abscesses<br>Extrusion of mesh<br>Numbness<br>Keloid formation<br>Recurrent herniation* |
| *Scrotal and Testicular* | Swelling<br>Hematoma | Induration of testes<br>Hydrocele<br>Low-riding testicles<br>High-riding testicles<br>Post-vasectomy pain<br>Atrophy<br>Impotence<br>Sterility – male and female |
| *Genitourinary* | Retention<br>Obstruction<br>Infection | Obstruction<br>Recurring infection<br>Urinary tract fistula |
| *Pulmonary* | Atelectasis<br>Acute upper respiratory tract infection<br>Pneumonia<br>Embolus | Fatal pulmonary embolus |
| *Extremities* | Phlebothrombosis<br>Thrombophlebitis | Fatal pulmonary embolus<br>Chronic edema and stasis ulcer |
| *Nervous System* | Disorientation<br>Backache<br>Stroke<br>Paresis, femoral nerve<br>Pain in legs | Chronic backache (debility)<br><br>Partial paralysis or fatality |
| *Cardiac* | Hypotension<br>Cardiac arrhythmia<br>Cardiac failure | Myocardial infarction and death |
| *Gastrointestinal* | Distention – gaseousness<br>Constipation<br>Nausea – vomiting<br>Ileus<br>Acute gastric dilatation<br>Fecal fistula (Glenn) | Intestinal obstruction |
| *Allergies and Drug Reactions* | Sensitivity to drugs<br>Tape reaction<br>Reaction to antiseptic<br>Hypotension | Recurring allergic reactions |

*Recurrent hernias are considered a complication, but because of their importance they are considered separately in individual chapters.

the wound has been completely closed. At other times, a small and apparently insignificant blood vessel may continue bleeding for some time. The largest hematomas occur when larger vessels, such as the superficial circumflex iliac or deep inferior epigastric arteries, continue to bleed. Most hematomas present no major threat to wound healing and are best served by observation only.

Larger hematomas have an adverse effect upon the healing wound. If there is evidence of continued bleeding, the wound is probably best explored under aseptic conditions in the operating room. The skin should be carefully prepared, the sutures removed, and the abundant clot evacuated. At this point, it may be necessary to inject a local anesthetic solution about the periphery of the wound. The wound is then irrigated with saline, and all bleeding points clamped and ligated with fine absorbable suture material. If the bleeding vessel is not identified at the subcutaneous level, dissection is carried out through the external oblique aponeurosis and the search for the bleeding point continued.

The wound is not closed until hemostasis is complete. A drain is unnecessary if the bleeding has been controlled. Broad-spectrum antibiotics are administered in selected cases.

In my personal experience, those wounds from which hematomas have been evacuated heal better than wounds treated expectantly. It should be recalled that blood outside the vascular system is "dead tissue," which must either undergo organization or become liquefied and subsequently absorbed. To reiterate, small hematomas are best observed.

### Infection (Stitch Abscesses, Cellulitis, and Suppuration)

Wound infections may be considered major and minor. They have been noted to occur in from 1.1 to 4.9 percent of hernia repairs (Table 28–1).

Minor wound infections are those involving the skin and superficial portions of the subcutaneous tissues. When suture-approximation of the wound—utilizing silk sutures—was popular, small foci of infection due to staphylococci appeared as "stitch abscesses". These decreased in number when monofilament nonabsorbable sutures became available. Minor wound infections rarely require more than warm sterile saline compresses or warm tub baths following removal of skin sutures. Now, with tape closure of the epidermis, such minor infections need not occur.

Major wound infections are largely of two varieties—those due to staphylococci and those due to the mixed flora of the intestine. Such infections are uncommon in modern practice; but at one time, as recently as 25 years ago, the rate of infection ranged from 2 to 5 percent. Currently, the accepted rate of infection following herniorrhaphy is under one percent. Proper use of germicidal soaps on the evening prior to operation and again on the day of repair will help attain this goal. Povidone-iodine (Betadine) preparation is also an excellent agent for skin antisepsis. Major wound infections are serious problems; and in addition to the pain and suffering, it has been estimated that financial loss with each postoperative infection varies from $1000 to $7000. The second sum may seem exorbitant—but not when one considers loss of employment in addition to a hospital bill. I am citing such figures to emphasize the need for careful performance of every detail in the preparation and performance of herniorrhaphy.

In an occasional wound, there is considerable redness and diffuse swelling; this is located on the skin and subcutaneous fat. With application of warm sterile saline compresses, improvement usually occurs within 72 hours. Continued observation is necessary; for in some of these patients, suppuration does develop and treatment must be modified accordingly.

Deep-seated infections are manifested by pain, chills, fever, swelling and, in some cases, redness. If the infection is deep to the external oblique aponeurosis, redness may not appear until later; but swelling and edema may be apparent. Deep wound infections should be suspected when the patient fails to thrive after the fourth or fifth day. Fever and leukocytosis are demonstrable, and the patient will have pain, increasing rather than decreasing, which will be quite severe. Malaise and anorexia are not uncommon.

The source of staphylococci in major wounds may be from the patient's skin or the surgeon's hands. There are other possible sources, but those just cited are the most important.

Major wound infection, sepsis, and death occur from time to time when strangulation-obstruction results in gangrene and extension of infection into surrounding tissues. In these cases, cultures will reveal a mixed intestinal flora including some combination of these organisms: bacteroides, clostridium, enterococcus, coliform, bacillus, *Pseudomonas aeruginosa*, and *Proteus*.

The patient with a wound infection secondary to gangrenous intestine is likely to be elderly and suffering from arteriosclerotic cardiovascular disease. Not infrequently, the patient might be diabetic as well.

Besides the signs and symptoms already described, the patient with infection due to mixed intestinal flora is likely to have ileus and, hence, distention. When the infection has established itself deeply and into the peritoneal cavity, gram-negative sepsis and death are possible events. It is these potentially fatal complications that remind us that a hernia operation cannot be considered a minor procedure.

Deep-seated mixed infections require wide opening of the wound, well into the depths of the incision. Drains are indicated, especially if a foul-smelling purulent exudate is present. Culture of the wound is mandatory for identification of the organisms and selection of appropriate broad-spectrum antibiotics. A nasogastric tube is indicated in the presence of ileus and distention, and intravenous fluids must be given. Bed rest, warm tub baths, and local sterile warm compresses are other useful adjunctive measures.

## Minor Wound Separation

The complication of minor wound separation is of a trivial nature and does not cause a great deal of concern. However, the occasional patient who sees less than perfect healing will worry about the possibility of infection. If the surgeon proceeds with careful attention to detail and with accurate approximation of the epidermis, perfect healing can occur. Therefore, care must be taken that the epidermis is not inverted and that wound edges are precisely approximated.

Minor wound separations will heal nicely with minimal care. The area may be cleansed with alcohol or surgical soap and protected with a small dressing. *Betadine* ointment may be applied for further protection.

## Peritonitis—Sepsis—Death

This chain reaction is rare, but it does occur occasionally with catastrophic results. It may be seen in complicated hernias in which incarceration, strangulation, and gangrene of the intestine have occurred. These events are too often seen in elderly patients with some combination of cardiovascular, renal, or pulmonary disease. Femoral, incisional, and umbilical hernias are not rarely the underlying defects that entrap the bowel. The impact of sepsis on the wound has been reviewed in Chapter 20 (see Fig. 20–2, p. 334).

When the surgeon is faced with the strong likelihood of sepsis, the wound should be closed loosely and drained amply. I resort to monofilament wire when repairing hernias that are likely to be followed by wound infection. Broad-spectrum antibiotics are started promptly. If postoperative ileus is considered to be a possible complication, nasogastric suction is applied and intravenous fluids are administered.

Once deep-seated wound infection is recognized, skin sutures must be removed and the wound widely opened, including the aponeurotic layers (if a substantial collection of infection lies beneath them).

## Wound Disruption

This subject is of such fundamental importance that Chapter 20 deals with the problem and measures for prevention of this complication in depth. It will be obvious that abdominal incisions occasionally burst under excessive increase in intra-abdominal pressure.

## Induration

In a small number of patients the area of the incision remains hard and indurated for three or four weeks. The patient, concerned about the state of healing, will wish to know if his tissues will regain their normal texture. Such induration may be due to an occult hematoma, or it may reflect a surgical technique that is less than gentle. Vigorous traumatic retraction, blunt lacerating type of dissection, use of large clamps (such as Kelly's) for grasping small vessels, clamping of unnecessarily large bits of tissue, use of heavy ligatures, and prolonged exposure of the wound to the air are all factors that tend to produce such induration. Induration is also prominent in many wounds following operation for recurrent hernias.

Conversely, sharp scalpel dissection, use of small-pointed hemostats, use of fine suture material for precise ligation of vessels, and minimal exposure of the wound to air are factors favoring uneventful wound healing.

Treatment of induration begins with an explanation to the patient that some induration is a part of the healing process and that, with the passage of time, tissues will regain their normal consistency. Warm tub baths are also comforting to the patient.

## Complications of Nervous System Origin

Disorientation is occasionally seen in aged patients, especially those older than 80 years. Premedication must be given in minimal doses. Older patients tolerate pain very well and require very little medication. Barbiturates are not recommended. Use of restraints causes these individuals to become more disturbed. It is preferable to have members of the family stay with such patients for reassurance. Adequate fluids should be given, but overloading the vascular system with salt and water should be avoided.

Headache is an occasional problem following spinal anesthesia. Spinal anesthesia should be administered through a small bore needle, and postoperatively the patient must be well hydrated. If the headache is severe, the patient must be kept in the supine position. The simple measures of providing adequate hydration and placing the patient at bed rest will result in recovery. Analgesics are helpful. This is an annoying complication of spinal anesthesia

and can be avoided by use of local anesthesia.

### Stroke

Many patients with large hernias are aged, and in addition they are commonly found to have advanced arteriosclerotic cardiovascular disease. If for any reason these patients sustain a significant fall in blood pressure, myocardial infarction or stroke might be the result.

### Paresis of Femoral Nerve

It is interesting that in an attempt to achieve the desirable goal of a long-acting local anesthesia, a possible result may be undesirable side effects. If excessive quantities of long-acting local anesthetics are injected into the region of the femoral nerve, its function might be impaired. When short-acting agents are used, the anesthetic effect is dissipated before the patient becomes ambulatory. With long-acting agents, the anesthetic effect may persist for 8 to 12 hours, depending somewhat upon the use of epinephrine. The flexors of the thigh — including the rectus femoris, satorius, and quadriceps — are supplied by the femoral nerve. When this nerve is partially anesthetized inadvertently, the patient will be unable to flex his thigh effectively, and walking will be accomplished with difficulty — if at all.

Although I have seen this complication on two occasions (each time with recovery in a matter of 14 hours postoperatively), to the best of my knowledge, there have been no such cases reported in the literature. This complication is preventable. Local solution should not be injected laterally to the femoral artery except in minimal amounts. Furthermore, it is unnecessary to inject the solution deep to the inguinal ligament and under the iliac fascia.

### Injury to Femoral Nerve

The anatomic location of the femoral nerve should be clear to the surgeon who must repair complicated groin hernias. The femoral nerve lies outside of, and lateral to, the femoral sheath. Ordinarily, it is well protected by the dense iliac fascia. In complicated recurrent hernias, normal landmarks are often destroyed. Excisional therapy for malignancies in the area may expose the femoral nerve. Complications following vascular operations sometimes predispose to the formation of unusual recurrent hernias, which protrude into the prevascular space or lateral to it. I am aware of injuries to the femoral in two patients with complicated hernias.

## Gastrointestinal Complications

Gastrointestinal symptoms occur infrequently following repair of uncomplicated inguinal hernias, especially with local anesthesia. Hernias in which incarceration or strangulation of intestine is present result in ileus in a number of patients (Fig. 28–2). The incidence of postoperative ileus has been variously reported as between 1.24 and 1.0 percent. In such patients, distention is present and bowel sounds are minimal or absent. Nasogastric suction is indicated, and intravenous fluids are administered. Oral fluids and food are temporarily interdicted. Constipation and gaseousness are minor complaints and generally are easily relieved with a small saline-type enema.

Fecal fistulas are rare and result from injury to the bowel due to repair of complicated hernias. In such hernias, the bowel might have been incarcerated or strangulated in an incisional or femoral hernia. Fecal fistulas require individual-ized treatment; but antibiotics, intravenous fluids, and nasogastric suction are basic requirements. The Miller-Abbott tube may be indicated in some patients. Intravenous hyperalimentation is another important adjunctive measure.

## Allergies and Skin Reactions

An occasional patient will develop hypotension following injection of local anesthetic solution; this problem is discussed at length in Chapter 8. Sensitivity to antibiotics is occasionally a problem. Urticaria is seen from time to time and, generally, will respond to antihistaminic drugs such as Benadryl. Three types of skin reactions may be seen. These occur more often in blond, pale-skinned individuals than in people with brown or black skin.

First, a few patients will develop severe reactions to the antiseptic (such as iodine), which appear within a few hours of application (Fig. 28–3). The area of distribution of such an inflammatory response is characteristic in that it appears only in those areas exposed to the offending antiseptic agent. Unfortunately, the patient may not be aware of such sensitivity prior to exposure at the time of the operative procedure. Prevention through a careful clinical history, as well as subsequent avoidance of irritating germicides, is the ideal course to follow. Whenever the possibility of such untoward reactivity of the skin is even suspected, bland agents (such

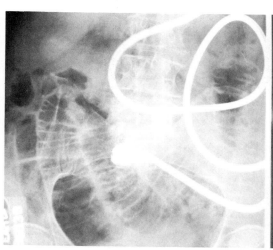
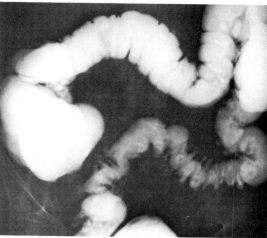

**Figure 28–2.** Following repair of a left indirect sliding inguinal hernia, this patient developed severe ileus as shown in flat film. Later barium enema examination revealed significant diverticular disease.

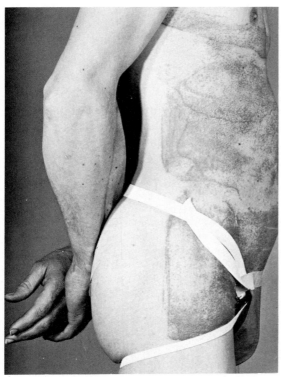

**Figure 28–3.** Some patients are highly sensitive to iodine. The skin reaction occurred in the area painted with tincture of iodine. We currently use povidone-iodine as a scrub or solution.

as chlorhexidine gluconate (Hibiclens) should be used in skin preparation. If an unusual erythema appears during application, the offending agent should be re-moved promptly with 70 percent alcohol. Treatment should consist of systemic therapy and local measures. I find that antihistaminic drugs such as Benadryl are helpful and may be administered in doses of 50 mg two to four times daily. Locally, methyl prednisolone acetate (Medrol) may be lightly rubbed into involved areas two or three times daily with good effect.

The second type of skin sensitivity occurs with the application of either the older type of adhesive tape or some of the new elastic types of tape. Again, the fair-haired, light-skinned individual is more vulnerable to the adverse effects of adhesive tape. Several hours after application of the dressing, the patient will complain of itching or burning beneath the dressing. Inspection will show that the reaction occurs in that portion of skin in contact with the adhesive (Fig. 28–4). Too often, the patient is unaware of such sensitivity prior to his operative procedure. Fortunately, newer adhesive tapes with a low potential for allergic responses are available. Currently, these are used in almost every patient.

Treatment consists of removal of the tape, cleansing of the skin, and local application of a steroid cream. Systemic antihistaminic drugs such as Benadryl are useful.

A third type of skin lesion is seen in relation to post-herniorrhaphy dressing. If the elastic tape is drawn too tightly, ex-

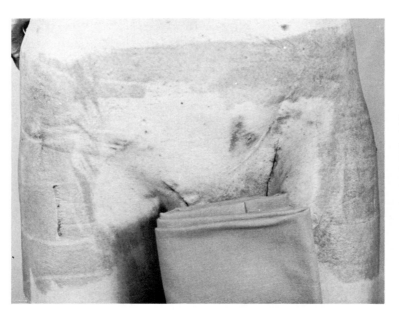

**Figure 28–4.** The older varieties of adhesive tape often caused severe skin reaction. Note distribution of reaction to areas where tape was applied. Excellent paper tape of low allergenicity is currently available.

coriation of the skin will result and produce, in effect, a "tape burn"; this lesion has the characteristics of a second degree thermal burn. Prevention is a simple matter: the elastic adhesive tape must not be drawn too tightly during application. Once the excoriation and burnlike lesion occur, the area may be treated much as a second degree burn. I then apply a nonadherent dressing, such as rayon, which is not removed until healing has occurred.

## Pulmonary Complications

Among the important pulmonary complications are atelectasis, pneumonitis, tracheobronchitis, and pulmonary embolism. The number of pulmonary complications reported prior to 1939 was quite high, ranging from 8.5 to 9.2 percent (see Table 28–1, p. 588). Currently, the incidence of pulmonary complications ranges from 0.2 percent to 0.76 percent.

Patients about to undergo herniorrhaphy should give up smoking for several days prior to repair. In patients with known pulmonary pathology, local anesthesia is preferred.

The operative repair is followed by immediate active pulmonary exercises and physical therapy.

In patients who develop fever, malaise, and a productive cough, sputum cultures are obtained and antibiotic therapy instituted. Pulmonary embolism is rarely seen in patients undergoing hernia repair under local anesthesia.

### Phlebothrombosis and Pulmonary Embolism

The threat of death to elderly patients from pulmonary embolism is ever-present. According to Trowbridge (1968), 40,000 deaths occur each year as a result of this complication. It has long been recognized that the great majority of thrombi form in the veins of the lower extremities.

It is true that the recorded incidence of phlebothrombosis is quite low following herniorrhaphy. The incidence in available reports varies from 0.3 to 0.47 percent. Pulmonary embolism occurred in 0.13 to

0.26 percent of the patients who had hernia repairs (see Table 28–1, p. 588). Landrum and Shaalan (1959) cited the incidence of thromboembolic phenomena to be 0.5 to 1.0 percent of all surgical operations.

Following phlebothrombosis, the rare patient develops chronic leg edema and stasis ulceration. The results can be chronically disabling in some patients.

Fatalities due to pulmonary embolism still occur, even though they are infrequently reported. Early ambulation following repair under local anesthesia is an important preventive measure in both phlebothrombosis and pulmonary embolism. Nissen (1975) pointed out that it is possible to constrict the femoral vein during hernia repair. This can occur during McVay repair of a femoral hernia. Brown and colleagues (1980) identified ipsilateral deep vein thrombophlebitis in five patients, four of whom developed pulmonary embolism.

## Cardiovascular Complications

Aged patients frequently have advanced cardiovascular disease along with complicated hernias, and cardiac arrhythmias are not at all rare. In a few patients, the cardiac rate becomes quite slow and treatment becomes necessary. Sapala and coworkers (1975) found that among 416 patients with documented heart disease, 24 developed complications—including myocardial infarction, myocardial ischemia, and postoperative arrhythmia.

Sapala and colleagues studied the operative and nonoperative risks in cardiac patients. Patients with anginal attacks following infarction were intermediate risks, in terms of complications and mortality. Those patients with previous infarction and accompanied with arrhythmia, A-V block, bundle-branch block, or congestive heart failure represented the highest risk. They found that the presence of severe A-V block was an indication for pacemaker insertion prior to attempts at diagnostic or therapeutic procedures. It was recommended that three months elapse before any elective procedures be undertaken following recent myocardial infarction. Sapala and coworkers observed that the well-compensated patient with normal rhythm and normal conduction tolerated surgical procedures well.

## LATE WOUND COMPLICATIONS

### Seroma

Occasionally following repair of a hernia, a soft, fluctuant, painless swelling appears in the operative area. The wound otherwise appears to be healing normally. The patient is concerned about the possibility of recurrence. Small collections of a serous or serosanguineous fluid require no active treatment, for they will become absorbed. Larger seromas may be aspirated under aseptic conditions. Pain is minimal if the 18-gauge needle is inserted through the incision, since sensory nerve supply has not yet regenerated at the site. Rarely, two or three aspirations at weekly intervals will be necessary. Pressure dressings do not seem to eliminate this complication.

### Pain — Neuroma — Neuralgia — Nerve Entrapment

The most important factor in avoiding complications of the ilioinguinal and iliohypogastric nerves is an accurate knowledge of the anatomy of these structures. Andrews (1926) and Moosman and Oerlich

(1977) pointed out important anatomic details.

Fortunately, the appearance of a postoperative neuroma following repair of an inguinal hernia is rare (Fig. 28–5). I see annually only one or two patients with such a complication. The patient with postoperative pain is usually a somewhat fragile type of individual with a low pain threshold, and one who is unhappy with his lot in life.

Pain is the symptom that the patient complains about, sometimes bitterly, localizing the pain to a limited area in the incision and toward the inguinoscrotal region. Examination usually reveals satisfactory healing without recurrence of the hernia. The patient has previously tried a variety of scrotal supports and analgesics for relief of pain. Tub baths at best offer only temporary relief. Physical activity usually aggravates the pain, and employers and plant physicians are annoyed at the result.

Not all postoperative pain is to be explained by nerve entrapment. A rather thin patient presented with postoperative incisional pain. Wire sutures could be palpated through the skin. Removal of the sutures was recommended (Fig. 28–6). An excessively large number of heavy wire sutures accounted for the patient's pain, and removal resulted in a cure.

In order to assess the possible benefit of

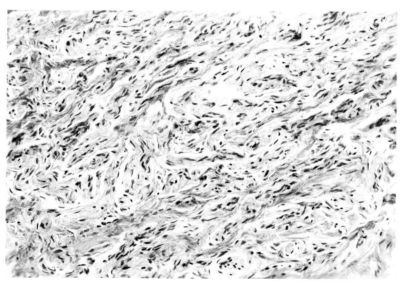

**Figure 28–5.**    This photomicrograph of an excised nerve shows dense scar tissue and disorganized nerve fibers. The ilioinguinal nerve was excised with relief of pain. (×320)

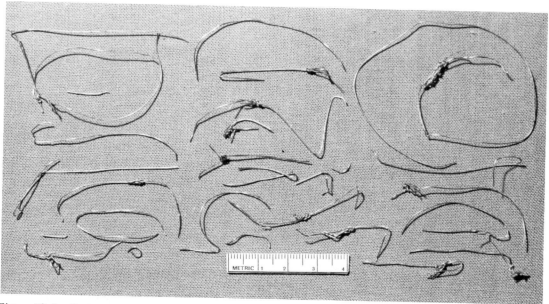

**Figure 28–6.** Postoperative pain can be caused by use of heavy wire in a patient with a thin abdominal wall. These sutures were removed from a midline epigastric incision. The number of heavy wire sutures for a short incision seems excessive.

neurectomy, I perform a nerve block of the ilioinguinal nerve and observe the patient for several hours postinjection. Also, nerve block can assist in the determination of possible involvement of the affected nerve in a cicatrix. If relief of pain is obtained by injection of local anesthetic agents, it is reasonable to expect benefit by excision of the ilioinguinal or iliohypogastric nerve and any associated neuroma. The patient and his wife must understand that anesthesia in the area will be the result of neurectomy and that no guarantee of complete freedom from discomfort can be made. Before embarking upon neurectomy, it is most important to understand how the patient feels about his job and work environment.

In a rare patient, nerve entrapment and scarring will result in pain and paresthesia along the path of the involved nerve. Whenever a patient complains of severe postoperative pain long after healing is complete, a careful history and thorough examination are both necessary. Other causes for the pain—orthopedic, urologic, or gastrointestinal in nature—must be considered. Also, a few of these patients will exaggerate their symptoms when they face an unpleasant work situation or an unhappy marital life. The surgeon should examine the patient on several occasions in order to fully appreciate the degree of the patient's discomfort and also to determine his reliability as a historian. Great pains should be taken to arrive at a precise diagnosis. As previously stated, if nerve block affords relief of pain, neurectomy should prove beneficial. However, in the occasional patient, complaints of pain will continue after neurectomy. The rapport that the surgeon establishes with such patients becomes important in postoperative management. Whenever neurectomy is contemplated, it is suggested that the matter be discussed with the patient and his wife. They should be told that anesthesia may occasionally be annoying following neurectomy and that there is no guarantee that all pain will be relieved by such a procedure.

Neuropathy involving the genitofemoral nerve following inguinal herniorrhaphy has been described by Laha and colleagues (1977). The patient was treated successfully, surgically, by extraperitoneal exposure and resection of the nerve.

The ilioinguinal nerve has also been involved in scar tissue with resulting postoperative pain. Such cases have been described by Kopell and colleagues (1962), Mumenthaler and colleagues (1965), and Westman (1970). Rao and coworkers (1977) described an unusual case of neuralgia paresthetica secondary to inguinal herniorrhaphy. The lateral femoral cutaneous nerve exits from the pelvis medial to the anterior superior iliac spine and passes beneath the inguinal ligament into the thigh. Injury to this nerve must be exceedingly rare during herniorrhaphy. I have now had experience with four such cases. I consider the results to be excellent in two, indifferent in the others. Therefore, I suggest that the diagnosis of nerve entrapment be approached with caution and that surgical treatment only be offered after all conservative measures have been exhausted.

## Granuloma — Chronic Sinus Tracts — Recurrent Abscesses — Extrusion of Mesh

A variety of late wound complications can develop following wound infection. Serious problems develop when infection supervenes in wounds closed with heavy braided sutures such as number 2–0 silk. Organisms find a favorable domicile in the braids of nonabsorbable sutures. Antibiotics have the ability to discourage bacterial growth. Too frequently, however, once the antibiotic is discontinued, the bacteria reassert themselves; and pain, redness, and chronic drainage from a sinus tract are the results. The braided suture material may eventually be extruded, but this takes many months. This phenomenon has been vividly described as "the spitting of silk"; however, other braided, nonabsorbable materials may act in a similar manner.

The problem of recurrent drainage can be eliminated more readily by surgical exploration of the wound and removal of all offending sutures. The wound may then be packed or closed loosely. Appropriate antibiotics are administered prior to and during operative treatment and for a minimum of 10 days postoperatively.

Chronic sinus tracts persist because of infection and because of the presence of braided, nonabsorbable sutures or mesh (or both). Again, pain, redness, recurrent swelling, and repeated purulent discharge are presenting complaints. In many cases, these symptoms and signs have recurred several times over a period of years. It then becomes necessary to remove the braided suture material and any infected prosthetic material surgically, if complete healing is to be expected. The surgical approach is similar to that described earlier. To reiterate, once a synthetic or metallic mesh has eroded the skin, removal is necessary if complete healing is to be expected. I have never seen skin grow over partially extruded mesh that became infected. The presence of heavy braided, nonabsorbable suture material adds to the persistence of this complicated situation; hence, it must be removed.

### Chronic Draining Sinus (Case in Point)

The patient, a 12-year-old boy, had a left orchidopexy performed elsewhere at the age of 3 years. He apparently required a second operation for the same problem at the age of 10 years. One year later, he had a right inguinal hernia repaired and an orchidopexy performed at another hospital.

Since that time, he had repeated episodes of swelling, pain, and drainage from the right groin. When seen at Henry Ford Hospital, the patient presented with multiple draining sinuses. The mother stated that with antibiotic therapy, the drainage decreased — only to return with cessation of therapy. She stated that a few silk sutures had been extruded.

Cultures were taken and revealed the presence of *Staphylococcus aureus* strains, which were resistant to penicillin and ampicillin but sensitive to erythromycin, tetracycline, and methacillin. With therapy (which included erythromycin, rest, and compresses), the infection was controlled.

Surgical excision was recommended and accepted by the parents. The specimen included dense scar tissue, which showed acute and chronic inflammation on microscopic examination. The heavy silk sutures were also removed (Fig. 28–7).

The heavy scar formation and intense cellular response seen in such cases is shown in a microscopic section of a chronic suture granuloma (Fig. 28–8). Repeated exacerbations of localized infection are common in such cases.

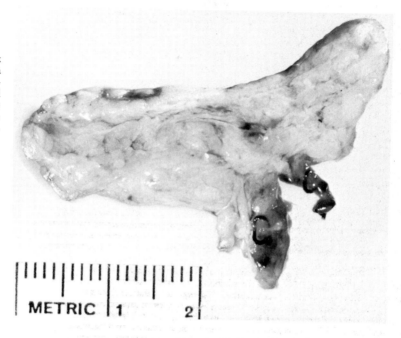

**Figure 28–7.** Heavy cicatrix excised from a groin incision in a young boy. Repeated exacerbations of pain, redness, and swelling with later drainage were due to infected heavy silk sutures. Excision resulted in relief of symptoms.

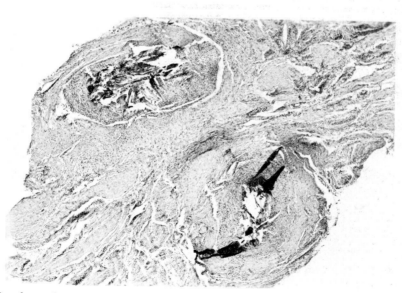

**Figure 28–8.** Note heavy layer of connective tissue about the sutures. There was a heavy cellular infiltrate in this patient with a chronically draining groin wound.

*Comment*

One of the undesirable aspects of silk sutures is that, in the presence of infection, the organisms are difficult to eliminate. They find refuge within the braids, and antibiotics have not been found effective in eliminating the bacteria; hence, surgical excision is desirable. The 12-year-old boy described here had prompt healing following surgical excision.

Conservative therapy of tub baths, compresses, rest, and antibiotics will control the acute phase of an infection, but, once these are discontinued, there is an exacerbation. Furthermore, it requires many months, even years, for the drainage to cease; and this will occur only when all the involved silk sutures have been extruded.

### Anesthesia–Paresthesia

A few patients will complain of annoying anesthesia for some weeks following hernia repair. After some explanation and reassurance, complete recovery follows. Injury to the ilioinguinal or iliohypogastric nerves, or both, is the cause. Occasionally, the period of anesthesia lasts for some months. The patient, who must be given a reasonable explanation, is told that during surgical procedures small sensory nerves are occasionally severed; he is also advised that these nerves will either regenerate or that other nerves in the area will assume sensory function in the area of operation. Fortunately, anesthesia in the area of incision is seldom much of a problem, and explanation and reassurance are helpful in alleviating the patient's concerns.

Paresthesia is less common as a postoperative complaint than is anesthesia. Careful examination of the patient presenting with such a complaint will reveal no significant abnormality. Again, reassurance does much to alleviate the patient's concern.

### Keloid Formation

Potentially, keloids might develop in any incision; as a rule, they require no particular treatment. Itching and burning at the incisional site tend to subside with the passage of time. Local application of a steroid cream gives symptomatic relief in some patients.

Dr. Donald M. Ditmars (of the staff of Plastic Surgery at Henry Ford Hospital) has had extensive experience with keloids. His observations and helpful suggestions on management of keloids are included in the following paragraphs.

Keloids occur mainly in blacks; however, they are prevalent in Oriental races and in the very oily skinned peoples of the world (such as those originating from the Mediterranean area). Keloids can occur after minor injuries or operative procedures.

After a keloid has developed along with the usual symptoms of enlargement, pruritus, irritation, and pain, our first method is to inject the lesion, using a Dermajet (spray injector) or a fine needle. The solution we have found most successful to date is triamcinolone acetonide (Kenalog), 10 mg per ml. Higher concentrations cause subcutaneous atrophy. The patient's symptoms are tremendously improved using this; however, the size of the lesion may diminish only slightly. These injections are carried out at monthly intervals for up to 8 months. Usually by this time, the balance between the benefit of symptomatic relief and the detrimental effects of tissue atrophy has been achieved.

The keloid after steroid injection is usually soft and asymptomatic. If the cosmetic deformity is unsatisfactory, then excision can be done at this time. Usually at the time of excision, the wound edges are infiltrated with Kenalog in the same concentration.

An alternative method is to excise the keloid and irradiate the wound edges. Although the radiation is relatively safe, I personally prefer the longer course using steroids due to the future potential for malignant change, especially in younger patients.

### Recurrence

Recurrence of a hernia must be accepted as a late wound complication. The reappearance of a hernia following repair varies with age of the patient, type of hernia, type of repair, number of previous repairs, and numerous other factors. In Table 28–3, I have summarized the recurrence rates

## Table 28–3. RECURRENCE RATES FOLLOWING REPAIR OF VARIOUS TYPES OF HERNIAS

| Type of Hernia | Recurrence Rates (Percent) |
|---|---|
| Indirect | |
|   Congenital | 0.67 |
|   Adults | 0.91 |
|   Sliding | 2.0 |
|   Recurrent indirect | 1.98 |
| Direct | 1.8 |
|   Recurrent direct | 6.0 |
|   Recurrent inguinal and femoral | |
|     repaired with mesh | 2.9 |
| Femoral | 3.0 to 8.4 |
| Umbilical | 1.54 |
| Incisional | 9.0 |
|   Incisional with mesh | 4.9 |

following repair of various types of hernias discussed in this volume.

The numerous factors that contribute to recurrence have been considered in some detail in Chapters 12, 14, 16, and 17, and need not be repeated here.

## Experimental Study of the Circulation of the Testes

The effects on the testes produced by ligature of spermatic vessels in dogs was studied experimentally by Griffiths (1895). His observations are consistent with the variations seen in man. Ligation of all the spermatic veins in dogs caused great swelling and engorgement of the veins. Extravasation of blood and necrosis of seminal tubules followed, resulting in an atrophic gland.

Ligation of both spermatic artery and veins led to great swelling followed by atrophy. The ligation of both vessels in full-grown dogs led to testicular sloughing, atrophy, and temporary fatty degeneration in some animals. In the last group, complete recovery is possible.

Clinically, there is variation in the response of the testicle to compromise of blood supply. Certain testes show great swelling, with scrotal swelling as well. Here, interference with venous return is suspected. In other patients, the testicle is moderately swollen, indurated, and painful. Interference with arterial circulation in such cases is most likely the cause.

In view of the importance of scrotal and testicular swelling, a brief review of the arterial and venous circulation as it concerns the testes is in order.

### Arterial Supply

The testicle derives its main arterial supply from the aorta via the internal spermatic or testicular artery. Both testicular arteries arise from the aorta in the lumbo-iliac region, and descend on the posterior abdominal wall to join the cord at the internal abdominal ring.

Additional arterial supply to the area is

**Figure 28–9.** The blood supply to the testicle as shown in a schematic representation by Neuhof and Mencher. The cremasteric artery is shown as a key vessel between the testiculocremasteric-deferential-arterial system on the one hand and the scrotal-arterial system on the other. (Reproduced by permission of *Surgery* from Neuhof, H., and Mencher, W. H.: The viability of the testis following complete severance of the spermatic cord. Surgery 8:675, 1940.)

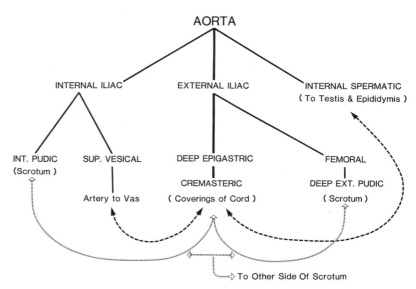

derived from the external spermatic artery. During hernia repair, its origin can be seen from the deep inferior epigastric artery, which in turn arises from the external iliac artery. The external spermatic arteries largely supply the cremasteric muscle but also have a function in the development of collateral circulation (Fig. 28–9).

The third source of arterial blood supply to the area is via the artery of the vas deferens, which originates from the superior vesical artery. This artery closely accompanies the ductus deferens and anastomoses extensively with the internal spermatic or testicular artery. For this reason, severance of the testicular artery will not jeopardize the viability of the testicle, provided that the artery to the vas deferens is preserved.

Additional collateral blood supply to the testicle should not be overlooked. Distally,

beyond the external ring, the vesical and prostatic arteries may anastomose with the internal spermatic and differential arteries. These anastomoses occur distally near the testicle.

Even further down at the lower pole of the testicle, the scrotal arterial branches anastomose with the internal spermatic and deferential arteries.

Under some circumstances, arterial blood could reach the testicle from the femoral artery via the external pudendal artery.

Koontz (1945) and Neuhof and Mencher (1940) pointed out the wisdom in preserving the testicle in its normal location unless there is some reason for its inspection or treatment. The collateral circulation is thereby preserved. Koontz (1965) explained that the anastomosis between the deferential, spermatic, and scrotal arteries

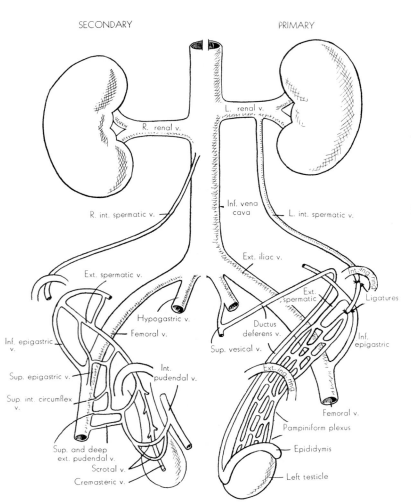

**Figure 28–10.** Venous drainage of the testis and epididymis. (Reproduced by permission of *Surgery, Gynecology and Obstetics* from Javert, C. T., and Clark, R. L.: A combined operation for varicocele and inguinal hernia; a preliminary report. Surg. Gynecol. Obstet. 79:645, 1944.)

is sufficient to maintain viability after ligation of the spermatic artery and veins in treatment of varicocele.

In summary, it is clear that the testicle has a rich blood supply and that an extensive collateral system is available. The internal spermatic artery provides the chief blood supply to the testicle together with the artery of the vas deferens. The vesical, prostatic, scrotal, and external spermatic and pudendal arteries are collateral sources of blood to the testes (Fig. 28–9).

## Venous Drainage from the Testicle

Like the arterial blood supply to the testicle, the venous blood has alternate routes it may follow to the inferior vena cava.

Javert and Clark (1944) have studied the venous drainage of the testicle in detail. The veins leaving the testicle form a rich, multi-channeled pampiniform plexus. These veins coalesce; and at the inguinal ring, an internal spermatic vein is usually formed. On the left, this vein ascends to empty into the left renal vein. On the right side, the internal spermatic vein empties into the inferior vena cava (Fig. 28–10).

Besides the major channels of drainage, the superficial and deep epigastric veins, the superficial internal circumflex veins, the scrotal and internal pudendal veins provide alternate channels for drainage of venous blood. Considering the arterial supply and venous drainage of blood to and from the testicle, it is little wonder that the viability of the testicle is infrequently compromised.

## Division of the Spermatic Cord in Herniorrhaphy

The sectioning of the spermatic cord during herniorrhaphy has been advocated for over four decades. Burdick and Higginbotham in 1935 completely divided the cord in repair of 200 inguinal hernias, including 59 recurrent hernias. They reported a staggering infection rate of 17.5 percent. In four patients, orchidectomy was necessary because of testicular necrosis. Six patients died in the postoperative period. The incidence of testicular atrophy

was difficult to assess; however, 11 of the patients had slight atrophy while 11 more demonstrated testes one-half their normal size.

Under similar circumstances, the incidence of testicular atrophy was much higher in the experience of Neuhof and Mencher (1940). They found testicular atrophy in 6 of 19 patients.

Bodhe in 1959 ligated the cord at the internal ring in 27 patients. He avoided mobilization of the testicle and administered antibiotics in the postoperative period. He concluded that, while testicular swelling suggested a certain amount of damage, it was insufficient to cause complete atrophy.

Morton (1967) described a case in which the patient developed gas gangrene of the testicle secondary to an infection that followed division of the spermatic cord. Orchidectomy, débridement, and therapy with antibiotics and antisera resulted in recovery of the patient.

Neuhof and Mencher (1940) took a critical look at the matter of severance of the cord during herniorrhaphy. They reviewed the circulation to the testicle in detail (Fig. 28–8) and recommended a careful technique in which the cord structures were individually ligated after being divided between the internal and external abdominal rings. Neuhof and Mencher cautioned against manipulation beyond the external ring, fearing disruption of collateral vascular channels to the testicle. Even with such care, they reported that obvious testicular atrophy occurred in six patients, or 32 percent of individuals in whom the cord was ligated.

Heifetz (1971) reported his experience of 20 years with resection of the spermatic cord in selected inguinal hernias. He reported atrophy of testes in 39 of 112 patients in whom the spermatic cord was resected. In 23 individuals, the testes were found to be in an abnormally high position, while firmness of the testicle was reported in 33 patients. Four patients developed hydroceles. Heifetz acknowledged that resection of the cord was not a method of repairing inguinal hernias. I would point out that section of the cord expedites closure of the internal abdominal ring and, therefore, is most applicable in repair of indirect inguinal hernias. It is generally accepted that indirect inguinal hernias are comparatively easily repaired. It would be advisable to inform the patient in whom the spermatic cord is to be divided that the risk to the testicle is substantial. Many patients would be reluctant to accept a testicular atrophy rate of 35 percent, as noted by Heifetz (1971), or 32 percent, as reported by Neuhof and Menscher (1940).

Koontz, in an editorial in 1957, stated that in certain oft-recurrent hernias, the cord may be extremely difficult to identify. In such unusual situations, he preferred to divide the cord and ligate remnants at the internal and external abdominal rings. Grace and Johnson (1937) noted that in such situations, necrosis of the testicle followed mobilization of the testicle out of its normal position. It is at least theoretically possible that branches of the vesical and prostatic arteries may provide blood to the testicle in such situations. The major blood supply to the testicle is depicted in Figure 2–12, page 30.

### Early Scrotal and Testicular Swelling — Hematoma

*Swelling Due to Arterial Occlusion*

Operative treatment of inguinal hernia always places the arterial supply to the testes in some jeopardy. In infants the structures comprising the spermatic cord are small; and injury can occur to the blood vessels, especially during dissection of large complicated hernias. In adults with large, sliding or scrotal hernias, the structures are densely adherent. If incarceration and gangrene are present, identification of cord structures may be exceedingly difficult.

Recurrent hernias are associated with heavy scar tissue formation, compounding the surgeon's problem. In spite of these risks to the testes, repair of hernias is advisable. A complicated hernia may endanger the patient's very life, while an unavoidable injury to the arterial supply of the testicle may cause the organ to atrophy.

In a very few cases, the patient will endure unusual pain in the inguinal and scrotal areas postoperatively. Some temperature elevation is likely as well. Examination will show that the testicle is slightly to moderately swollen and unusually tender. The testicle is firm to hard on palpation. The operative wound shows no abnormality, such as hematoma or ecchymosis. In this type of situation, it is likely that the arterial supply has been compromised to the testicle. Useful measures include a scrotal suspensory and application of an ice bag to the scrotum. Narcotic analgesics are necessary and ambulation is uncomfortable. Bed rest is permitted and bathroom privileges are allowed.

The patient is followed with patience and understanding. The discomfort slowly subsides, and in several weeks or months atrophy of the testicle is recognizable. Management at this point must be individualized, but the patient can be assured that one functional testicle is adequate for both sexual and reproductive functions.

*Swelling Due to Venous Obstruction*

I have reviewed the circumstances under which the arterial supply to the testicle might be injured. The same events could lead to venous obstruction. Although such a complication is rare, occasionally the scrotum is swollen and a large bulbous testicle is palpable. A hematoma of the wound is not identified and ecchymosis is also absent. In this type of case, the swelling is largely confined to the lower cord, scrotum, and testicle. Again, pain is a prominent symptom and fever is present as well.

The average patient with scrotal swelling and testicular pain and swelling will actually have some combination of both arterial and venous occlusion. As I have indicated, treatment is individualized and conservative therapy is favored. Most testicles showing some degree of swelling will recede and return to normal. Just as there is no operative procedure with a zero mortality rate, so the surgeon cannot promise survival of every testicle.

Some swelling of the scrotum and testicle is present in a large number of post-herniorrhaphy patients. Levy and coworkers (1951) felt that swelling of the scrotum and spermatic cord was the most frequent complication following herniorrhaphy. This is particularly true if, during repair, the cord was vigorously manipulated. In some patients a large inguinoscrotal hernia makes it difficult to dissect the peritoneal sac without some postoperative scrotal edema. Such scrotal swelling is usually self-limited and subsides within two weeks.

Prevention of scrotal swelling begins with a knowledge of its causes. Hence, gentle handling of the spermatic cord is of great importance. This is especially true for patients with recurrent hernias or for patients with a single functioning testicle. Unnecessary stripping of the cremaster muscle and blunt avulsion of the peritoneal sac from the cord will contribute to the severity of scrotal swelling. The distal sac need not always be freed all the way to the testicle. Sharp dissection of the sac from the cord is recommended practice. Needless to say, great care should be used in clamping bleeding points. Only the use of fine-pointed hemostats and fine suture material for ligatures should be tolerated.

If a normal testicle is palpable through the scrotal swelling, reassurance will do much to relieve the patient's concern about his condition. A scrotal support and tub baths are both helpful.

## Hematoma

Occasionally a patient will bleed excessively, even without an easily demonstrable coagulopathy. Great care must be exercised in hemostasis. Every tiny vessel must be clamped and ligated. On occasion—as, for instance, during repair of a recurrent hernia—difficult dissection must be carried out through heavy cicatrix. In such patients, oozing or bleeding from small vessels continues until a large accumulation of blood finds its way into the scrotum. This is especially likely to happen if the testicle has been dislocated from the scrotum and subsequently replaced. In other patients the surgeon might have operated for hydrocele or performed a testicular biopsy. The groin, lower abdomen, and scrotum are ecchymotic and swollen. The scrotum varies somewhat in size but may assume frightening proportions. Strangely, although the scrotum is markedly swollen when a scrotal hematoma is present, pain is not especially severe. On the other hand, when testicular blood supply is compromised, pain is unusually severe.

In dissection of certain large hernial sacs

completely out of the scrotum, it is possible to damage venules of the pampiniform plexus. Because of the laxity of tissues in the area, a large amount of blood can accumulate in the scrotal sac. The smaller scrotal hematomas can be treated conservatively with scrotal support and warm tub baths.

Rarely, the collection of blood is so large that conservatism will result in a greatly prolonged recovery period. In such situations, consideration should be given to evacuation of the extravascular blood under aseptic conditions in the operating room. Hemostasis must be complete. Recovery is hastened considerably by this decisive approach to an annoying problem.

## Late Scrotal and Testicular Complications

Some attempt should be made to differentiate the various types of scrotal swelling and testicular abnormalities seen following herniorrhaphy. I am personally satisfied that as I have become more conservative in disposing of the cremaster muscle, the incidence of scrotal swelling, as well as testicular abnormalities, has decreased.

In Table 28–2 (p. 593), I have listed both early and late complications as they involve the scrotum and testicles.

Induration of the testes without significant compromise of testicular blood supply results in little or no functional abnormalities.

## Hydrocele

Obney (1956) reviewed his experiences with hydroceles as influenced by herniorrhaphy. Nine patients, or 1.2 percent, of 730 operations for repair of hernia and hydrocelectomy developed testicular atrophy. Also, the hydroceles recurred in 44, or 6 percent, of 730 patients having hydrocelectomies. More recently, the recurrence rate of hydroceles was reduced to 2.4 percent with an altered operative procedure.

An embarrassing cause for postoperative swelling following herniorrhaphy is an occasional overlooked hydrocele. The hydrocele results in a swelling, which can ordinarily be identified as separate from the hernia. Digital examination will reveal that the protrusion originates at the internal ring, if the hernia is indirect, and through the floor of Hesselbach's triangle, if it is direct. Furthermore, the hydrocele, if it is sufficiently large, can easily be transilluminated. A careful preoperative examination will clarify the diagnosis, and it is a simple matter to include hydrocelectomy along with herniorrhaphy. It is recommended that the surgeon who is to perform the herniorrhaphy examine the patient preoperatively. In the occcasional case, it is advisable to deliver the testicle for direct inspection. If a small hydrocele is overlooked at the time of hernia repair, it may be observed if asymptomatic. Hydrocelectomy is indicated in the larger symptomatic hydroceles.

Finally, an occasional hydrocele will develop several months following hernia repair. The exact etiology of such hydroceles is difficult to establish. It is possible that, in some cases, leaving the distal peritoneal sac intact may result in an endothelial membrane, which becomes filled with fluid. Permanent success with aspiration of hydroceles has not been great in my experience. If the hydrocele is large and troublesome, I advise surgical excision of at least a portion of the sac.

### Low-Riding Testicle

Now and then, a patient will be seen complaining that his testicles are so low in the scrotal sac as to be embarrassing; this observation may be made during warm weather when the cremaster muscles are relaxed. On the other hand, the habit of complete stripping of the cremaster muscle with severance of nerves will result in testes occupying a dependent position in the scrotal sac.

Reassuring the patient that the testicle is normal and advising him to wear a suspensory will usually take care of the complaint.

### High-Riding Testicle

A more annoying problem than the low-riding testicle is the testicle that is located high in the scrotum or even over the pubic bone. This unhappy event may follow an attempt at correction of cryptorchidism, treatment of a hydrocele, or herniorrhaphy. The testicle in the high position interferes with physical activity, such as participation in sports, and it is subject to trauma during intercourse. This complication is rare but is most annoying to a few individuals.

Prevention, of course, is the desirable objective. Every precaution should be taken to place the testicle low in the scrotum during orchidopexy. Following hernia repair and hydrocelectomy, the position of the testicle in the scrotum should be noted. The testicle must be replaced in its normal habitat if the complication of high-riding testicle is to be avoided.

Early treatment consists of careful examination and a frank discussion of the problem. A lengthy period of follow-up is indicated, during which the degree of disability is evaluated. In the meantime, tub baths are encouraged. Finally, in selected cases an attempt at surgical correction of the abnormality is warranted. The incision and dissection is similar to that used in herniorrhaphy. Dissection of the cord toward the scrotum and fixation of the testicle in the lower scrotum may be necessary.

Another term has been applied to the postoperative state just described. Kaplan (1976) labeled it "iatrogenic cryptorchidism" and identified nine boys in whom normally located testes became iatrogenically undescended following herniorrhaphy. In seven of the boys, reoperation was performed in order to correct the testicular malposition. Kaplan advised that prevention is the best treatment. Care should be taken to place the testicle in its proper scrotal position during repair; and, at the completion of the procedure, the final location should be confirmed by testicular palpation.

### Postvasectomy Pain

An increasing number of patients are seen in today's practice requesting a vasectomy to control fertility; nevertheless, this procedure should not be undertaken lightly. Although it is technically simple, it may be accompanied by complications in a few patients. Also its effectiveness must be substantiated by postoperative sperm counts to establish sterility. Annoying pain is described by some of these patients before and after intercourse; reassurance and analgesics are helpful as a rule.

Therefore, the consequences of a vasectomy procedure should be made clear to the patient and, if he is married, to his wife as well. I make it a point to review and discuss the procedure with both partners.

## Postvasectomy Pain (Case in Point)

The patient had bilateral direct inguinal hernias repaired and bilateral vasectomy. Postoperatively, he complained of a burning sensation in the inguinal region; this sensation radiated to the base of the penis. It occurred only with ejaculation; and if the patient had intercourse two or three nights in succession, the pain would be almost incapacitating. On examination, the hernia repair was intact and no other urologic abnormalities were found. Nerve block was performed with effective anesthesia. The patient was advised to take tub baths and given a non-narcotic analgesic. He was seen three years following operation without significant complaints.

## Testicular Atrophy

A most annoying postoperative complication is that of testicular atrophy. Patients are increasingly aware of the size, shape, and consistency of their gonads. Although atrophy of a single testicle is an unhappy event, the fact that procreation and all that it implies can be achieved with a unilateral testicle causes far less concern among patients than does bilateral atrophy.

The presence of bilaterally atrophic testicles following hernia repair leads to litigation almost without exception. When embarking upon bilateral hernia repair, it is advisable to at least discuss the possibility of impaired testicular function. When litigation occurs, one question arises, "Was the patient informed?" Each surgeon should reflect on the potential for complications in the individual case and present a reasonable list of possible postoperative problems.

The risk of postoperative atrophy of the testicle is greater in patients requiring operative repair of recurrent hernia. Furthermore, I have confirmed the fact that risk to the testicle increases with repeated attempts at repair. This fact is well documented in Chapter 11 on recurrent inguinofemoral hernia. In patients requiring re-operation, scar tissue may be quite dense, resulting in difficult dissection. The cord structures may be more or less randomly distributed in the cicatrix. Bleeding from the pampiniform plexus may be troublesome. In difficult cases, it may be necessary to identify the cord as it enters the upper scrotum.

Great caution is necessary in approaching a contralateral hernia repair when an atrophic testicle has been demonstrated on the opposite side. In young patients with recurrent inguinal hernias, it would be prudent to repair one side and observe the patient for healing. Then, after three months, the second side could be repaired in the absence of testicular atrophy. On the other hand, in a male during the reproductive phase of his life, it might be desirable to defer repairing a second recurrent hernia if an atrophic testicle is already proven to be present on the opposite side.

## Atrophy, Sterility, Impotence

Late testicular abnormalities are found more frequently than most surgeons would care to admit. In some stoic individuals who do not indulge in self-examination, an atrophic testicle may be discovered during physical examination long after a hernia has been repaired. In a few, the atrophic testicle might have been the result of a congenital abnormality. Bilaterally atrophic testicles, if present, should be recognized and the fact recorded preoperatively. Also, if atrophy has occurred following mumps orchitis, this information should also be recorded.

The surgeon interested in the repair of hernias should be increasingly aware of the danger of litigation that might evolve following the complication of testicular atrophy. It behooves the surgeon to be aware of the statistics of Baumrucker (1946) on the incidence of testicular pathology. He reported findings on 10,000 army inductees between the ages of 18 to 37 years.

Any testicle measuring one-half the size of a normal mate was considered atrophic. Some testes were almost completely atrophied (being pea-sized).

Baumrucker found either bilateral or unilateral testicular atrophy in 152, or 1.7 percent, of 10,000 men examined. In his patient population, 12 individuals had bilateral atrophy. Five of the twelve men with atrophic testicles secondary to mumps were married; and, while claiming normal sexual relations, these individuals were unable to have children. Baumrucker noted that undescended testicles, even when bilaterally atrophic, did not cause impotence. He suggested that, for this reason, it might be preferable to avoid orchiectomy when possible. Sterility, of course, would remain when bilateral atrophic testes are present, but potency would be preserved.

While mumps orchitis is the most common cause of testicular atrophy, other causes include trauma, herniorrhaphy, gonorrheal epididymo-orchitis, congenital abnormality, scarlet fever, and trauma associated with wearing a truss.

The need for a careful history and physical examination to establish the functional state of the testes is clear. Furthermore, consideration should be given to the consequences of repair of a second hernia, virginal or recurrent, when an atrophic testicle is present on the opposite side.

The surgeon must be aware of any coexistent testicular abnormality. Hydroceles of the testes are common and are easily corrected during hernia repair. Recognition of the hydrocele may spare the patient a subsequent operative procedure. Tumors of the testes are rare in my experience, but the possibility should be considered.

The two most common *nonoperative* causes for testicular atrophy are, in my experience, congenital atrophy and atrophy secondary to mumps orchitis.

Seen more often than congenital or postinfectious atrophy is testicular atrophy secondary to operative procedures. The anatomic details of testicular circulation and various types of postoperative complications are shown, respectively, in Figure 28–9 and Table 28–2 (pp. 605 and 593). The clinical course of testicular atrophy resulting from inadvertent or deliberate compromise of the blood supply to the testicle may vary somewhat in degree among different individuals but follows a recognizable pattern. Some surgeons deliberately ligate and divide the cord in repair of selected hernias. I do not resort to this technique.

The patient, while in the hospital, develops pain and marked swelling of the scrotum and testicle. Although a low-grade fever follows almost every hernia repair, in this group of patients there is significant temperature elevation. Loss of appetite, malaise, and a reluctance to move about are other complaints.

Examination will reveal the painful swelling; rarely, the testicle may merely exhibit moderate swelling. Not all testicular swelling is followed by atrophy; hence, conservative management is indicated.

Bed rest and icepacks are employed as early measures. Narcotic analgesics are required to control pain. A large hydrocele scrotal suspensory is helpful. Later, tub baths are helpful, and the medication is changed to non-narcotic analgesics. In time, the testicle will decrease in size and pain will cease to be a problem.

The patient deserves an explanation of the course of events. He should understand that the complication should not impair his sexual or reproductive functions, provided that he has a remaining viable and functioning testicle on the opposite side.

Care must be taken initially to inform the patient that, in every projected herniorrhaphy, there is some risk to the viability of the testicle, especially in complicated hernias. This danger to the survival of the testicle is much greater when dealing with an oft-recurrent hernia. (In Chapter 19 on complicated inguinofemoral hernias, I noted that an absent or atrophic testicle was found in 7 out of 9 patients with such hernias.)

Testicular atrophy following herniorrhaphy is an unavoidable complication in a small number of patients and does not imply lack of knowledge or carelessness.

### Testicular Atrophy (Case in Point)

The need for careful preoperative examination of the patient who is undergoing hernia repair has assumed great importance in current practice. It is advisable that the history include a note about any previous history of testicular abnormalities. In a rare patient, the testes will be congenitally atrophic. Mumps orchitis is followed by an atrophic testicle with surprising frequency.

The patient was a 25-year-old male who was first seen three years earlier for an attack of acute tonsillitis. During this hospitalization, it was found that both testicles were atrophic (the right being smaller than the left). Fortunately, these observations were recorded.

The patient was hospitalized for repair of a right indirect and femoral hernia. A combination Moschcowitz-Bassini repair was performed under spinal anesthesia. Subsequently, the patient developed a seroma that required aspiration. No specific reference was made to the condition of the testes at two separate examinations. The patient was reluctant to return to work, and a variety of complaints—including headaches and backaches—followed. He was encouraged to return to work after an absence of five months. The patient, who continued to complain of scrotal swelling and pain, went to a doctor in his neighborhood and was treated with penicillin shots, without relief.

A consultation with a urologist confirmed the presence of bilateral testicular atrophy, which had been present prior to hernia repair. An explanation of his condition to the patient together with symptomatic treatment resulted in cessation of complaints. He was advised to wear a scrotal support and to use sitz baths as necessary. Simple non-narcotic analgesics were prescribed.

*Comment*

This case of bilateral testicular atrophy prior to any surgical procedure could have been a serious problem to the surgeon, for the atrophy could have been ascribed to the operative procedure. It bears repeating that careful description of the testes is advised prior to any operative procedure for groin hernia. It is recommended that such important findings be discussed with the patient prior to the operative procedure. This approach is helpful in postoperative management of such unfortunate individuals.

### Postoperative Hypogonadism

The occasional occurrence of bilateral testicular atrophy in post-herniorrhaphy patients is deceptively important. Even though the problem is uncommon, when it does occur, the pathophysiologic consequence becomes most disturbing to the patient and physician and of great interest to the legal profession.

Informed consent should be assured before repair is embarked upon, for testicular atrophy occasionally follows a benign surgical procedure. Such permission becomes more important when an atrophic testicle already exists on the contralateral side. Once bilateral testicular atrophy has been identified, the consequences should be appreciated.

A discussion by Dr. Raymond Mellinger (Head of the Department of Endocrinology at Henry Ford Hospital) on the matter of testicular atrophy and infertility is included here. Testicular atrophy is a major complication of inguinal herniorrhaphy. Bilateral involvement may cause testosterone deficiency and sterility although severe oligospermia may result without serious hormone deficit. Impaired Leydig cell function can be satisfactorily treated by testosterone administration, but seminiferous tubular failure is irreversible. The affected testis is usually painful and swollen in the early postoperative period, presumably as a result of impaired venous blood flow. With subsidence of the swelling, the gland will shrink to less than normal size as the seminiferous tubules atrophy. If this ischemic phase is severe, Leydig cell function is also lost. The occurrence and the extent of atrophy is unpredictable in the early postoperative days, but significant reduction of testicular volume indicates the loss of seminiferous tubules. Viable Leydig cells occupy a small mass, and atrophic testes measuring less than two centimeters in size may secrete quite normal amounts of testosterone.

Any involvement of either testis should be followed by diagnostic evaluation after convalescence. Even if the swollen testis apparently returns to normal size and function, the patient should be offered diagnostic studies. The testis that involutes to less than its preoperative size must be evaluated. Every patient who experiences impaired sexual potency or reduced fertility merits study and treatment. Untreated male hypogonadism often leads to serious complications. Not only does the hypogonadal man suffer in the sphere of sexual potency, but also he often encounters other emotional problems such as loss of well-being, reduced initiative, and mental depression. Physical effects of hypogonadism include anemia, reduced strength, a tendency to adiposity, hair loss, reduced skin turgor and sebaceous activity, and disabling osteoporosis with pathologic bone fractures. Despite the potential seriousness of this complication, some surgeons may dismiss testicular involvement after the herniorrhaphy with statements of misguided reassurance to the patient and to themselves.

### Infertility in Females as a Result of Bilateral Hernia Repairs

In the chapters on congenital indirect inguinal hernias (Chapter 10) and sliding hernias (Chapter 18), I dealt with sliding hernias in female infants. Tubal obstruction has long been identified as a cause of sterility, but herniorrhaphy during infancy has not been generally recognized as a cause of such obstruction.

Swanson and Chapler (1977) noted that 20 to 30 percent of infantile female hernias are of the sliding type; furthermore, 15 to 25 percent are bilateral. The delicate tubes can be easily injured during herniorrhaphy. The surgeon must handle the fimbriae delicately and replace the intact tubes into the peritoneal cavity (see Fig. 27–11, p. 585), if sterility is to be avoided as a late complication.

### Impotence

I am surprised at how often post-herniorrhaphy patients — my own as well as others I have seen following referral — include impotence among their complaints. To begin with, the surgeon must be aware of what the patient expects of his operative procedure. A careful history will help identify a few patients who are losing their sexual prowess. If the symptoms are swelling or protrusion with discomfort in the area and if a hernia is present, the repair will be helpful. If, on the other hand, the patient has a variety of exaggerated complaints — including penile, scrotal, and perineal pain — then other explanations must be sought for his disability. Some such patients will complain of low back and rectal pain as well.

In the management of such patients, careful attention to the patient's complaints, plus repeated examinations, is essential. Special examinations, such as urologic consultation, are indicated. Laboratory work, including urinalysis, must be repeated later, since a few of these patients will be found to be diabetic.

Treatment of urologic diseases or of any systemic disease (such as diabetes) will prove helpful. When the hormone levels are found to be depressed, replacement therapy has proven useful.

### EVALUATION

The degree of possible testicular impairment is assessed by semen analysis along with the determination of serum testosterone and the pituitary gonadotropins. Testicular biopsy may be useful in some cases.

Without preoperative semen analysis, the postoperative evaluation may not be conclusive. However, if a previously fertile man is found to have severe oligospermia or azoospermia postoperatively, the reproductive failure is probably the result of the surgery. Unilateral testicular involvement, of course, could not produce oligospermia or androgen deficiency unless there had been prior abnormality of the contralateral gonad. Decreased number and viability of sperm with normal semen volume usually indicate that involvement of the seminiferous tubules has occurred without impaired Leydig cell function. In patients with testosterone deficiency, the volume of the ejaculate usually diminishes in proportion to the degree of hypoandrogenism. Sperm motility is usually impaired along with the reduction in sperm numbers.

Serum testosterone less than 350 mg/dl in a mature male of any age indicates probable testosterone deficiency. If the blood level is persistently below normal, replacement therapy is indicated on a regular and indefinite basis.

Gonadotropin assay provides inferential information about testicular function and is, therefore, less essential to the diagnostic study. Impaired seminiferous tubular function in either testis may be associated with increased secretion of the follicle-stimulating hormone (normal FSH equals 3 to 12 mIu/ml). Thus, a patient with one functionally normal testis could have elevated secretion of FSH. LH, on the other hand, correlates with androgen secretion and does not rise in level unless there is testosterone deficiency (normal LH equals 4 to 16 mIu/ml). Accordingly, elevated levels of LH indicate impaired hormonal secretion by both gonads.

Testicular biopsy might be indicated when a patient is demonstrated to have azoospermia with apparently normal-sized testes. Under these circumstances, obstructed vas deferens may be suspected and the diagnosis confirmed if the testicular biopsy is normal. When oligospermia results from seminiferous tubular damage, however, these tubules are found to be atrophic; and no germinal functions will be present. In very severe testicular atrophy, the Leydig cells are absent, having been replaced by fibroblasts.

The only treatment possible in such cases is testosterone replacement; this is best accomplished by the administration of long-acting intramuscular preparations in a dosage of 300 to 400 mg each month. The injections are given at intervals of two to four weeks. Oral androgen preparations are equally effective but carry the risk of possible induced impairment of hepatic function. Either methyltestosterone (10 to 25 mg.) or fluoxymesterone (5 to 10 mg.), daily, may be prescribed. There is no available treatment for reproductive failure.

Replacement therapy with testosterone is usually completely effective in restoring health. In some patients, the return of sexual functions is not entirely satisfactory. Deficiency of libido or orgasmic ability may result from the psychologic impact of infertility and, in some ways, may be considered as "a castration complex." If hypogonadism has been neglected to the point of disabling osteoporosis, restoration of bone integrity is not considered possible, although progression of the disorder can be halted. Testosterone deficiency should be treated in a normal man of any age.

### Genitourinary Complications—Early and Late

The use of local anesthesia and immediate ambulation, particularly in elderly patients, will greatly minimize post-herniorrhaphy urinary retention. It is not the healthy male who develops retention but the aging individual who has some degree of obstruction to his urinary tract due to prostatic hypertrophy. Insertion of a catheter into the urethra of such an individual might result in infection or obstruction or, too frequently, both of these.

Most patients will void spontaneously if given adequate amounts of fluids. A small number will require indwelling catheters because of inability to void, and an occasional patient in this group will eventually require prostatic resection.

Haskell and colleagues (1974) found that 5, or 12 percent, of 41 men over 50 years of age required catheterization following hernia repair. Surprisingly, urinary tract infections did not develop in these patients. Haskell and coworkers found no disadvantage in leaving the catheter in situ for 24 hours in a group of cases requiring catheterization. However, they reported that three patients developed bacteriuria, which responded to appropriate antibiotic therapy.

It can be seen in Table 28–1 (p. 588) that the incidence of urinary retention ranged from 0.3 to 2.0 percent as reported by various authors. Infection occurred less frequently, varying between 0.1 to 0.13 percent as reported by two authors. Ljungdahl (1973) reported the incidence of obstruction to be 0.47 percent. MacLaughlin and coworkers (1976), in a more critically ill group of patients, reported the incidence of urinary tract infection to be 6 percent.

Antibiotic therapy is indicated when prolonged catheter drainage is necessary or when urinary tract infection is identified. Late complications involving the genitourinary tract include repeated infections and prostatic obstruction. If obstructive symptoms persist, then prostatic resection becomes necessary.

In an occasional patient, urinary tract symptoms may be due to a post-herniorrhaphy suture granuloma. These inflammatory masses may simulate bladder neoplasms. Such cases were reported by Brandt (1956), Helms and Clark (1977), and Daniel and colleagues (1973). They may appear as late as 11 years following hernia repair.

Kathan (1913) reported an extraordinary experience in which a patient developed chills, fever, and evidence of cystitis following herniorrhaphy. Three weeks later, this patient voided a large double-knot catgut suture.

## Management of Prostatism in the Hernia Patient

Dr. Riad Farah of the Department of Urology at Henry Ford Hospital makes these useful observations and helpful recommendations as to management of patients with prostatism:

Most common among elderly men is prostatism. In this group of patients with hernias, the increased abdominal pressure created during micturition aggravates their hernia problem. Based on this theory, a urologic evaluation is always recommended for patients with hernia prior to repair. An intravenous pyelogram as a preliminary study and, depending on the results, cystometry and cystoscopy followed by a prostatectomy may have to precede or be combined with the hernia repair. The latter concept has been recently advocated by some investigators. In our experience, we still advocate the two-stage management of the patient with hernia and prostatic hypertrophy.

In the case of urinary retention developing postoperatively, our management has been to insert a Foley catheter for 24 to 48 hours. Then, a trial of voiding is given. Depending on the results, the following steps will be taken:

1. If patient fails to urinate, the catheter will be inserted; and the patient will undergo a complete urologic evaluation, which includes IVP, cystometrogram, and cystoscopy. If the endoscopic evaluation reveals a partially open prostatic urethra, the patient should undergo a trial on bethanechol chloride, 28 mg every 6 hours, while the catheter is still in place for the first 24 hours, then, continue on with the medication after the catheter has been removed. This method has proven successful in most cases.
2. If the patient fails to void and the endoscopic evaluation reveals an obstructing prostate, a prostatectomy is recommended (preferably, a transurethral resection to avoid the site of hernia repair).

The prostatic surgery can be performed on the same admission.

3. If open prostatectomy is found to be the only possible surgery, then one should wait for 2 to 3 weeks while the patient is kept on catheter drainage and antibiotics.

In conclusion, a complete urologic history and, definitely, a digital rectal exam of the prostate prior to hernia repair will minimize the chances of postoperative complications of the lower urinary tract through discovery of possible obstructing lesions.

## Late Complications—Backache

One of the reasons that I have largely abandoned spinal anesthesia was due to the postoperative problem of backache. Spinal anesthesia is an excellent technique for anesthetizing the patient for hernia repair, but the occasional patient complains bitterly of the late consequences. Such individuals will date their disabling backache to the time "the needle was put in my back." From then on, all ordinary measures are of no avail.

Not every patient with a postoperative backache exaggerates his complaints. Arthritis, prostatism, and rectal and pelvic tumors have been discovered in such patients. Therefore, the history and physical examination must be repeated with thoroughness. Special studies and consultations are in order. Those with specific causes for the backache usually respond to appropriate treatment. Orthopedic evaluation is always obtained in individuals with the problem of refractory back pain.

Prevention of the problem begins with avoidance of spinal anesthesia in apprehensive individuals. Local anesthesia permits prompt and continued ambulation. If not vigorously ambulated, even occasional patients with local anesthesia will complain of back discomfort.

## Backache After Spinal Anesthesia (Case in Point)

It matters little whether or not there is an organic basis for the patient's complaint of backache after spinal anesthesia insofar as employment for the patient is concerned.

There are few more annoying complications than postspinal backache.

The patient was a 24-year-old male assembly-line worker in an automobile plant. He underwent successful repair of a femoral hernia under spinal anesthesia. He insisted that for two years since his operation, he had experienced pain in the lumbosacral area, which was aggravated by activity, coughing, and sneezing. There were no symptoms referable to the genitourinary tract.

Physical examination revealed inconsistent straight leg raising signs — bilaterally positive at 45 degrees; at other times, varying to almost 90 degrees with different tests. He held his back rigidly during the examination and showed increased motion of the back in getting off the table compared to that elicited when he was lying on his back. He could heel and toe walk very well. The neurologic examination was negative. The examining physician felt that the patient's symptoms were obviously exaggerated. X-ray examination of the spine and basic laboratory studies were negative.

The orthopaedic surgeon who saw the patient concluded that if the patient had any organic pathology, it was impossible to evaluate because of added functional complaints. The patient was placed on strict bed rest, sedatives, and tranquilizers. He allegedly never fully recovered, although he was ambulatory.

In 1961, five years after his operation, a letter was received from the Department of Health, Education and Welfare inquiring about the nature of his backache. At 29 years of age, he had applied to the government for determination of disability under the Social Security Act.

Such experiences led me to the frequent use of local anesthesia in the repair of hernias. If the patient is emotionally unable to accept local anesthesia, then a general anesthetic would be recommended.

## SUMMARY

The best assurance of an acceptable postoperative result following herniorrhaphy comes from thorough clinical and appropriate laboratory evaluation of the patient and precise technical performance of a well-chosen method of repair based on a sound knowledge of normal and pathologic anatomy of the region.

Systemic diseases should be treated to a point of maximum improvement, whenever possible. Obese patients should be urged to lose weight.

Local anesthesia provides safe and effective analgesia for most patients requiring herniorrhaphy. Pulmonary, genitourinary, and musculoskeletal symptoms (such as backache) are seen infrequently in patients who can be mobilized promptly.

The incidence of major and minor complications is higher than most surgeons realize. Great care in the performance of every detail of the operative procedure is of paramount importance in decreasing the rate of wound complications.

Wound infections can be reduced to well below one percent by thorough preparation of the skin. A 10-minute tub bath with generous use of a surgical soap on the evening prior to repair is recommended. Shaving is done just prior to the operative procedure. Meticulous surgical technique must be utilized in every repair, with emphasis on gentleness, sharp scalpel dissection, and use of fine-pointed instruments for grasping bleeding vessels. Only number 4–0 suture material, or finer, should be used as ligatures. The wound must not be exposed any longer than absolutely necessary. Repair must be effective and prompt.

Recurrences can be reduced if accurate diagnosis is followed by use of an effective method of repair. Monofilament nonabsorbable suture material is preferred because of its long-term strength.

Fortunately, most complications following herniorrhaphy are relatively minor, but they are annoying to the patient. Hence, each complication must be treated with patience and understanding to a point of maximum improvement.

## REFERENCES

Andrews, E.: The iliohypogastric nerve in relation to herniotomy. Ann. Surg. 83:79, 1926.

Baumrucker, George O.: Incidence of testicular pathology. Bull. U.S. Army Med. Dept. 5(3):312, 1946.

Beekman, F., and Sullivan, John E.: Analysis of immediate postoperative complications in 2,000 cases of inguinal hernia. Surg. Gynecol. Obstet. 68:1052, 1939.

Bodhe, Y. G.: Condition of testicle after division of

cord in treatment of hernia. Br. Med. J. *1*:1507, 1959.

Brandt, W. E.: Unusual complications of hernia repairs: Large symptomatic granulomas. Am. J. Surg. *92*:640, 1956.

Brown, R. E., Kinateder, R. J., and Rosenberg, N.: Ipsilateral thrombophlebitis and pulmonary embolism after Cooper's ligament herniorrhaphy. Surgery *87*(2):230, 1980.

Burdick, C. G., and Higginbotham, N. L.: Division of the spermatic cord as an aid in operating on selected types of inguinal hernias. Ann. Surg. *102*:863, 1935.

Daniel, W. J., Aarons, B. J., Hamilton, N. T., and Duggy, D. B.: Paravesical granuloma presenting as a late complication of herniorrhaphy. Aust. N.Z. J. Surg. *43*:38, 1973.

Davis, L.: Complications and sequelae of the operations for inguinal hernia. J.A.M.A. *67*:480, 1916.

Ditmars, Donald M., Jr.: Personal communication.

Farah, Riad: Personal communication.

Glenn, F.: The surgical treatment of 1,545 hernias. Ann. Surg. *125*:72, 1947.

Grace, R. V., and Johnson, V. S.: Results of herniotomy in patients more than fifty years of age. Ann. Surg. *106*:347, 1937.

Griffiths, M. A.: The effects upon the testes of ligature of the spermatic artery, spermatic veins and of both artery and veins. J. Anat. Physiol. *30*:81, 1895.

Haskell, D. L., Sunshine, B., and Heifetz, C. J.: A study of bladder catheterization with inguinal hernia operations. Arch. Surg. *109*(3):378, 1974.

Heifetz, C. J.: Resection of the spermatic cord in selected inguinal hernias. Arch. Surg. *102*:36, 1971.

Helms, C. A., and Clark, R. E.: Post-herniorrhaphy suture granuloma simulating a bladder neoplasm. Radiology *124*(1), 56, 1977.

Javert, C. T., and Clark, Randolph, L.: A combined operation for varicocele and inguinal hernia: A preliminary report. Surg. Gynecol. Obstet. *79*:644, 1944.

Kaplan, G. W.: Iatrogenic cryptorchidism resulting from hernia. Surg. Gynecol. Obstet. *142*:671, 1976.

Kathan, D. R.: Accidents of hernia operation. N.Y. J. Med. *13*:200, 1913.

Koontz, A. R.: Atrophy of the testicle as a surgical risk. Surg. Gynecol. Obstet. *120*:511, 1965.

Koontz, A. R.: Resection of the cord in inguinal hernia repair. Am. Surg. *23*:1072, 1957.

Kopell, H. B., Thompson, W. A. L., and Postel, A. H.: Entrapment neuropathies of the ilioinguinal nerve. N. Eng. J. Med. *266*:16, 1962.

Laha, R. K., Rao, S. P., Pidgeon, C. N., and Dujovny,

M.: Genito-femoral neuralgia. Surg. Neurol. *8*(4): 280, 1977.

Landrum, S., and Shaalan, A. K.: Phlebothrombosis, pulmonary embolism, thrombophlebitis: Etiological factors, clinical manifestations, medical and surgical management — House Staff Lectures, Henry Ford Hospital. Gen. Surg. Rev. 72:1, 1959.

Levy, A. H., Wren, R. S., and Friedman, M. N.: Complications and recurrences following inguinal hernia repair. Ann. Surg. *133*(4):533, 1951.

Ljungdahl, I.: Inguinal and femoral hernias. Personal experience with 502 operations. Acta Chir. Scand. Suppl. 1–81, 1973.

MacLaughlin, W. S., Jr., Kron, I. L., and Sager, G. F.: Experience with 100 patients hospitalized for incarcerated groin hernia. J. Maine Med. Assoc. *67*(11):319, 1976.

Mellinger, R.: Personal communication.

Moosman, D. A., and Oelrich, T. M.: Prevention of accidental trauma to the ilioinguinal nerve during inguinal herniorrhaphy. Am. J. Surg. *133*(2):145, 1977.

Morton, Anthony: Testicular gas gangrene after hernia repair with cord division. Med. J. Aust. *2*:605, 1967.

Mumenthaler, V. A., Mumenthaler, M., Luciana, G., and Kramer, J.: Das ilioinguinalis syndrome. Dtsch. Med. Wochenschr. *90*:1073, 1965.

Neuhof, Harold, and Mencher, William, H.: The viability of the testis following complete severance of the spermatic cord. Surgery *8*:672, 1940.

Nissen, H. M.: Constriction of the femoral vein following inguinal hernia repair. Acta Chir. Scand. *141*:279, 1975.

Obney, N.: Hydroceles of the testicle complicating inguinal hernias. Can. M. A. J. *75*:733, 1956.

Rao, T., Kim, H., Mathrubhutham, M., and Lee, K. N.: Peralgia paresthetica: Unusual complication of inguinal herniorrhaphy. J.A.M.A. *237*(23):2525, 1977.

Riccitelli, M. L.: Pulmonary embolism: Modern concepts and diagnostic techniques. J. Am. Geriatr. Soc. *18*(9):714, 1970.

Sapala, J. A., Ponka, J. L., and Duvernoy, W. F.: Operative and non-operative risks in the cardiac patient. J. Am. Geriatr. Soc. *23*(12):529–534. 1975.

Swanson, J. A., and Chapler, F. K.: Infertility as a consequence of bilateral herniorrhaphies. Fertil. Steril. *28*(10):1118, 1977.

Trowbridge, P.: Thromboembolic disease. (The Hartford Hospital Inter-Departmental Conference.) Conn. Med. *32*:881, 1968.

Westman, Mats: Ilioinguinalis — och Genitofemoralis–Neuralgi. Lakartidningen *67*(47):5525, 1970.

# 29

# Concluding Remarks

*It is interesting to speculate on what changes the future may hold for herniorrhaphy. Has the last important chapter on the subject been written? Living constantly in the present we are most likely to believe that it has and that the ultimate has been reached in our modern anatomical repairs. Yet, with a glance backward at the many peaks already passed, we cannot but feel that there must be some quite large ones still ahead.*

Taylor, 1933

Great progress in the repair of hernias has been made over the last 50 years, and further progress is still possible. But before that progress can be achieved, two extremely difficult obstacles must be overcome—apathy and complacency. Taylor speculated on what changes the future might hold for herniorrhaphy when he made the statement quoted at the beginning of this chapter. It is the element of inquisitiveness that is required to stimulate further progress. Despite the progress that has already been made, improvements toward reduced complications and decreased mortality can still be made.

Taylor's statement proved to be prophetic in that truly large steps have been made in improved treatment of hernias since 1933 in the fields of anatomy, pathology, anesthesiology, bacteriology, and technology. And it is expected that the future will see more effective application of the known knowledge in these disciplines as they apply to hernia repair. Such an approach would, in my opinion, produce a significant improvement in results.

## ANATOMY

Surgeons who devote a significant amount of time to the hernia problem know that important anatomic details have been identified for over 175 years. Cooper in 1804 and 1807 described the internal abdominal ring, inguinal canal, spermatic cord, transversalis fascia, femoral sheath, and of course, Cooper's ligament. Also, he recognized that certain hernias developed at the internal abdominal ring. Hesselbach (1814) described the inguinal ligament, the transversus abdominis muscle, and transversalis fascia.

I will not refer here to significant and numerous contributions of many surgeons and anatomists already detailed in Chapters 1 and 2. From an anatomic point of view, however, two of the most significant contributions have been the identification of the transversus abdominis layer together with its components, and the appreciation of the inter-relationships of the lamina of the abdominal wall.

Two instructive and informative articles

have appeared in the current decade. Condon (1971) described the surgical anatomy of the transversus abdominis and transversalis fascia as it applies to direct, indirect, and femoral hernias. The second important publication is historically oriented and more detailed. McVay (1974) presented his views on the anatomic basis for inguinal and femoral hernioplasty, along with an excellent historical review.

Modern contributions to the advancement of anatomical knowledge as it applies to hernia repair are those of McVay (1941); McVay and Anson (1942); Lytle (1945); Fruchaud (1956); Nyhus (1964); Nyhus, Stevenson, Listerud, and Harkins (1959); Anson, Morgan, and McVay (1949 and 1960); Condon (1971); and McVay (1974).

The importance of transversalis fascia and the transversus abdominis layer has been repeatedly emphasized and the knowledge implemented in repair of hernias. Perhaps history will prove this fact to be the most important anatomic contribution of the last half century insofar as resolution of the hernia problem is concerned.

Hesselbach (1814) and Thomson recognized the iliopubic tract as a significant anatomic structure; however, as noted, full importance of this structure is of recent origin. Harrison (1920) identified the transversalis fascia as being of great importance in protecting the integrity of the abdominal wall. The anatomy of the transversalis fascia is reviewed in some detail in Chapter 2.

The anatomic observation that the posterior abdominal wall attaches to Cooper's ligament (not the inguinal ligament) not only was of practical importance to surgeons who repair hernias (McVay, 1941) but also led to an accurate description of the femoral ring as well — the medial margin of the femoral ring being formed by the attachment of the posterior abdominal wall along Cooper's ligament (McVay and Anson, 1942).

Surgeons who repair hernias should be expert anatomists. Chapter 2 deals briefly with those essential anatomic details applicable to surgical repair of hernias.

## PATHOLOGY

Protrusions of the abdominal wall have been of interest to mankind since early recorded history. As indicated in Chapter 1, Celsus described umbilical hernias in the first century B.C.; and slowly over a period of 2000 years, various types of hernias were identified. Not until the seventeenth century was it recognized that actual rupture of the peritoneum did not occur in hernia.

Differentiation among direct, indirect, and femoral hernias was made long before suitable methods of repair were developed. Stromayr in 1559 (according to Zimmerman and Veith, 1967) clearly depicted such hernias. This information was to lie fallow for 300 years, to be revived after the discovery of anesthesia and the development of the science of bacteriology.

Recognition that certain hernias were actually congenital anomalies was attributed to Percival Pott in 1756. According to Watson, William and John Hunter recognized such hernias independently in 1762. Important differences between direct and indirect inguinal hernias were clearly recognized and illustrated by Andrews and Bissel in 1934.

A logical division of hernias into congenital and acquired protrusions followed, but currently this concept is being questioned and re-evaluated. The concept that increased intra-abdominal pressure from work or disease on a weakened portion of the abdominal wall resulted in herniation seemed to explain hernias occurring in adults and aging individuals. Interest in the nature of biochemical changes that occur in support tissue is of recent origin and will be dealt with later in this chapter.

## ANESTHESIOLOGY

The science of anesthesiology is a comparatively recent development. While general anesthesia was clearly established in 1846, it was not until 1884 that Köller introduced cocaine as a local anesthetic agent.

Once pain was eliminated as a limiting factor, surgeons could evaluate hernias and repair them with deliberation. Great successes in surgical repair of hernia were reported following introduction of anesthesia.

An effective method of achieving local anesthesia was introduced by Cushing in 1900. Local anesthesia has proven safe and effective in elderly and poor risk patients. Ponka and Brush (1974) reported operative experiences with 200 patients, 70 years of age or older, with only one death occurring due to a cerebrovascular accident.

Among the effective and safe local anesthetic solutions, chlorprocaine (Nesacaine) 0.5% is excellent; but its action is of short duration. In selected cases, it is practical to prolong the anesthetic effect with the addition of epinephrine, 0.5 cc of a 1:1000 cc solution, per 100 cc of local anesthetic solution. I do not add the vasoconstrictor to patients with hypertension or with cardiac arrhythmias. Lidocaine (xylocaine) in a 0.5% solution will usually provide anesthesia up to two hours; mepivacaine (Carbocaine) 0.5% solution will induce local anesthesia for up to three hours. Tetracaine (Pontocaine) provides longer duration of analgesia, well over three hours. A 0.25% solution of bupivacaine (Marcaine) is an excellent local anesthetic agent because of its safety. The duration of anesthesia following its use is four to six hours. With epinephrine added to bupivacaine, Ponka and Sapala (1976) found that the anesthetic effects last for up to 12 hours.

Immediately following repair under local anesthesia, the patient is able to walk about, void, and continue oral intake of liquids. Early ambulation was advocated by Leithauser and Bergo in 1941, Shouldice in 1945, Lichtenstein in 1964, and Gaster in 1970. The importance of prompt mobilization of the patient following hernia repair cannot be overemphasized. Besides minimizing such complications as urinary retention and pulmonary complications, I have found through utilization of this approach that pulmonary embolism is greatly decreased in incidence. It is interesting to note here that in 1930 Gibson and Felter reported· 8 deaths among 1618 patients operated upon — 4 of which resulted from pulmonary embolism — and that these procedures were performed before early ambulation was considered to be a desirable practice.

With a regimen of prompt mobilization, postoperative complications are minimal. Almost all uncomplicated inguinal hernias in adults could be repaired on an out-patient basis once postoperative pain and apprehension are effectively controlled without such side effects as weakness, vertigo, nausea, vomiting and hypotension.

In my practice, the patient is not permitted to return to his home until the patient's vital signs are stable and he is fully ambulatory. The patient must void prior to leaving the ambulatory surgical center. Needless to say, the patient must have a stable home environment, and a responsible family member must be in attendance for at least 48 hours.

The science of anesthesiology will have a significant bearing on the management of patients with hernias in the future. Newer agents will, no doubt, offer freedom or dissociation from pain with minimal untoward effects. Also, better analgesic drugs will become a reality and will result in greater comfort for the patient and a shorter hospital stay (which will, in turn, result in obvious economic advantages).

## BACTERIOLOGY

With application of the facts provided by progress through the science of bacteriology, there has been a significant decrease in wound infection following hernia repair. Development of effective antibiotic therapy has reduced the mortality. In 1931, Frankau reported a mortality of 53 percent following treatment of patients with strangulated hernia with gangrenous bowel. In 1978, Stewardson and colleagues reported a zero mortality following management of similar cases.

There can be no doubt that prompt surgical treatment of incarcerated hernias will forestall development of gangrene. Once necrosis of bowel wall supervenes, the danger of wound infection and peritonitis is substantial. At this point, effective antibiotic therapy is life-saving.

In modern surgical practice, the rate of wound infection should be reduced well below one percent.

## TECHNOLOGY

There is no need to review the numerous techniques that have been developed for repair of various types of hernias, since these have been described in detail elsewhere in this text — i.e., congenital indirect inguinal hernia (Chapter 10), indirect sliding inguinal hernias (Chapter 18), indirect inguinal hernia in adults (Chapter 11), and femoral hernias (Chapter 15). Rather than utilizing a single procedure for repair of all hernias, I recommend careful evaluation of the defect at hand, then selection of a procedure that will correct the particular deficiency. The fundamentals to follow include: high ligation of the sac, closure of the defect in the transversalis fascia, and multilayered reconstruction of the abdominal wall. Bassini (1888 and 1890) and Halsted (1893) initiated the modern era of surgical treatment of hernia independently. In addition, I have described various methods available for repair of incisional hernias in Chapter 21.

One important contribution insufficiently recognized is that made by Lucas Championnière in 1892 when he opened the aponeurosis of the external oblique. This maneuver permitted accurate visualization of the cord and the internal ring. It became possible to intercept and repair the hernia at its origin at the internal ring or in the floor of the inguinal canal. Few authors stress the great significance of this particular detail.

It is worthwhile to recall that a hernia repair consists of a number of orderly steps designed to repair a specific defect. High ligation of the peritoneal sac is curative in the infant with a patent processus vaginalis and a normal abdominal wall. In opening the peritoneal sac, the surgeon gains access to the peritoneal cavity, permitting exploration for other defects such as femoral or direct hernias.

The importance of identifying and closing the transversus abdominis layer accurately cannot be overemphasized.

In trying to bridge certain defects, such as those seen in indirect inguinal hernias, it is necessary to shift tissues under some tension. To avoid any excessive tension, the relaxing incision (as described in detail in Chapter 25) is recommended. Furthermore, it assumes greater importance in the repair of bilateral direct inguinal hernias.

If defects cannot be closed effectively even with relaxing incisions without resulting in abnormal tension at the suture line, then a prosthetic implant should be used. Results in surgical management of difficult and recurrent inguinal hernias would improve if prosthetic meshes were used more liberally.

Recognition of the great importance of suture material in repair of hernias is comparatively recent in its development. I have described the characteristics of various suture materials in Chapter 20. Included in the list of desirable qualities is that of enduring strength (among other attributes). The synthetic absorbable sutures (polyglactin or Vicryl and polyglycolic acid or Dexon) and catgut are of temporary value. Silk, contrary to popular opinion, is not a "nonabsorbable suture"; it does undergo phagocytosis and eventually disappears from the incision. Adamson and Enquist (1963) found that in experimental animals, wounds were always stronger with sutures in place than when sutures had been removed. As a result of such evidence and clinical observation, certain hernias should be repaired with wire or synthetic nonabsorbable sutures.

In repair of congenital indirect inguinal hernias, the choice of suture material is not as important as it is in repair of direct inguinal hernias. In the former, the abdominal wall is of adequate strength; in the latter, continuous approximation of tissues is desirable to maintain the repair.

Surgeons are constantly in search of "the method" or "a technique" that will offer promise of success in every surgical endeavor. In this effort, it is possible that insufficient attention is being given to the numerous and well-known principles of surgical technique promulgated by Lister (1867), Halsted (1891), Reid (1938), Dunphy (1960), and Wheeler (1974). I consider these technical details to be of such great importance that they bear repetition here: rigid adherence to rules of asepsis; sharp scalpel dissection; careful hemostasis; gentleness in wound management; use of fine-pointed hemostats; use of fine suture material for ligature of vessels; and the avoidance of mass ligature of tissues, as well as the avoidance of prolonged wound exposure. All maneuvers should be done with dexterity and without procrastination. Excellent exposure of the area to permit identification of all structures, avoidance of excessive tension at the suture line, and avoidance of suture strangulation of tissues are also important factors. Use of synthetic nonabsorbable sutures (polyester and polypropylene) or wire is recommended for enduring strength. Catgut and synthetic absorbable sutures do not meet this objective.

Approximation of tissues should accomplish the objective at hand—for instance, closure of the transversalis fascial lamina is the first line of defense in repair of the internal ring.

Use of prosthetic materials has proven effective in repair of many direct, recurrent inguinal, femoral, and incisional hernias. Conversely, there is no indication for use of implants in small indirect inguinal hernias.

If these details are painstakingly implemented in the conduct of herniorrhaphies, excellent healing will follow. The surgeon must be equipped to carry out a method of repair that has proven to be effective. A number of suitable techniques for repair are described and illustrated in this book.

## ON THE TEACHING OF SURGERY OF HERNIA

Even though many outstanding herniologists have pointed out the error of delegating hernia repair to the most inexperienced member of the surgical team, this important matter has not received a great deal of consideration.

The house officer or resident who is interested in hernias should know the details on anatomy and pathology of all types of hernias. It is of paramount importance that the house officer learns to appreciate the endless variabilities of hernias and that he understands the anatomic relations as three-dimensional rather than as flat surfaces. Anatomic details of the groin are not easily understood and must be pointed out to the resident by a surgeon who is an experienced anatomist. Even in this enlightened era, there are surgeons who would dispute the existence of the iliopubic tract.

The inexperienced house officer should not be expected to conduct a herniorrhaphy without the assistance of a well-trained surgeon. Only after junior house officers have had repeated exposure to the procedure and opportunities to assist an experienced surgeon should they attempt a hernia repair. At this stage in the house officer's career, he should be knowledgeable about surgical bacteriology, physiology, and wound healing. He would also be expected to be well informed about the

usefulness and limitations of various suture materials.

A word must be said about manual dexterity. This quality is not bestowed upon the medical student automatically on graduation from medical school; it must be acquired through long hours of practice. This means repetition of a skill such as knot tying until it becomes a reflex action.

Each of the details described in the preceding review of techniques must be pointed out to the house officer many times. It is difficult to justify an operative time of two to three hours for repair of an ordinary indirect inguinal hernia! A well-planned operative procedure can, and should, be carefully executed in a reasonable amount of time (including that allowed for teaching).

Finally, I am firmly convinced that care in execution of every detail of the procedure—from skin preparation to wound closure—has a great deal to do with minimizing operative and postoperative complications. In this regard, Schilling (1976) estimates that about one-half of all postoperative complications are wound complications, and approximately one-half of these can be directly attributed to abuse of basic principles of operative technique. He also called attention to the importance of a "tissue conscience" in the surgeon, to which I would like to amend "and suture conscience." The dictum should be *Approximation not strangulation.*

Madsen in 1953 carried out an experimental and clinical evaluation of suture materials. He studied the effect of minimal trauma, such as insertion of a needle, and found that even the prick of a needle produced an inflammatory response for approximately 5 days. Healing and scarring continued for 10 to 15 days, and the scar was visible 20 days postinjury. He found that more severe trauma, such as tying a ligature, caused compression of tissue with an increased area of tissue reaction. The period of exudation was prolonged and resulted in a wider cicatrix. These observations can be supported clinically and emphasize the need for gentleness in handling tissue on the part of the surgeon. The skill needed to insure accurate approximation requires judgment and dexterity, which are not acquired without the expenditure of effort. Should the findings at operation prove to be unusual, or should a complication develop, the experienced surgeon can take corrective steps. Properly managed operative complications usually cause little or no increase in morbidity.

## BIOCHEMISTRY OF HERNIA

Progress in the science of medicine has taken a recognizable course in many fields. Gross pathology became important beginning with the contributions of Morgagni (1769). Cellular pathology became established with the contributions of Virchow (1860). At present, there is no question that medical scientists are looking at disease at subcellular or biochemical levels. In the past, morphology commanded attention by investigators; currently, the biochemical aberrations that cause morphologic changes in the abdominal wall are being studied.

### Historical Background

Early interest in biochemical changes that could contribute to the better understanding of hernia stems from unusual sources. Lathyrism due to ingestion of seeds of *Lathyrus odoratus* has been known to produce connective tissue lesions in most mammals. In 1933 Geiger and coworkers (*Journal of Nutrition*)reported that, while hernias in stock colony rats were very unusual, the incidence in these animals was 25 percent when they were on a lathyrogenic diet. In 1952 Ponseti and Baird noted that scoliosis and dissecting aneurysms were seen in rats fed *Lathyrus odoratus* seeds. They suggested that the mesodermal structures were involved. Medial necrosis was seen in the wall of the thoracic aorta, and in some cases a saccular aneurym of the aorta was seen.

Bachhuber and Lalich (1955) studied the effect of sweet pea meal on rat aorta. They identified edema, swelling, and fragmentation of elastic fibers. With weakening of the wall, dilatation and dissection of the aorta followed. According to the authors, the toxic factor was isolated by Dupuy and Lee later synthesized by Schilling and Strong. It was proven to be B(N-y-L-glutamyl) aminoproprionitrile.

Wirtschafter and Bentley (1964) noted that hernias did not occur in stock colony Long-Evans rats. They related the occurrence of such hernias to a defect in collagen metabolism.

In 1966 Peacock and Madden studied the effect of B-aminoproprionitrile on collagen in wounds. They found that the administration of B-aminoproprionitrile between the fourteenth and nineteenth days of sutured wound healing in rats stopped the increase in wound strength. Increase in extractable collagen occurred without alteration of the amount of insoluble collagen. Madden and Peacock (1968) continued their basic studies on the rate of collagen synthesis and deposition in cutaneous wounds of rats. They noted that the rate of collagen deposition could be related to gain in wound strength during the initial ten weeks of healing.

Read in 1970 identified attenuation of the rectus sheath in patients with inguinal hernia. He identified presenile aponeurotic atrophy of unknown etiology as a cause of both onset and recurrences of inguinal hernias in adults. In 1971 Wagh and Read further investigated the collagen in rectus sheath of patients with hernias. They found decreased amounts of collagen in the rectus sheath of patients with hernia. In another significant study in 1971, Madden and Peacock studied the biology of collagen in the healing skin wound. They found that during the first three weeks, there is a correlation between burst strength and collagen accumulation; after this time, there is no such correlation. They made a remarkable observation; after three weeks, the skin wound had gained less than 20 percent of its eventual strength; hence, 80 percent of the wound strength developed when total collagen content failed to increase. They concluded that quantitative changes in collagen are not the only factors responsible for wound strength.

Conner and Peacock (1973) produced inguinal hernias in rats through both inducing lathyrism and by injury to the internal ring. Enlargement of the external ring in rats fails to produce hernias in these animals. Even creating a peritoneal lining in a scrotal sac failed to produce an inguinal hernia in rats. The combination of lathyrism, achieved by injecting B-aminoproprionitrile, and enlargement of the internal ring proved effective in producing hernias.

Thus, in this study, the combination of an anatomic area of weakness and induction of a metabolic defect in cross linkage of collagen resulted in both direct and indirect inguinal hernia in rats.

More recently, Wagh and colleagues (1974) indicated that direct inguinal hernias in men represent a disease of collagen. They identified ultrastructural abnormalities and a deficiency in hydroxyproline content. In 1971, these authors demonstrated a quantitative deficiency of collagen in rectus sheaths of men with direct inguinal hernias. They indicated that a biochemical explanation for this phenomenon could be the presence of a defect in hydroxylation of the collagen molecule in these individuals. Wagh and coworkers found the hydroxyproline:proline ratio to be altered. This, they said, could be due to a failure of certain prolyl groups in the collagen molecule to undergo hydroxylation.

## COMMENT

The references just cited on the biology of hernia open up new vistas for the surgeon interested in the basic sciences as they relate to hernia. The suggestion that congenital hernias might be induced by chemical agents is most interesting, and the idea would be supported by the appearance of hernias in young rats on a meal of *Lathyrus* seeds.

Is the human infant in utero exposed to substances that result in congenital hernias? Are hernias seen in adults the result of the same chemical abnormalities responsible for hernias in infants? If so, why must 50 or more years elapse before direct inguinal hernias appear in adults? Will it become possible for the physician or surgeon to alter the disturbed collagen metabolism, so that the defect in the abdominal wall is corrected? While seeking answers to the hernia problem through biochemical analyses, the authors cited have raised many relevant questions as to the precise chemical aberrations seen in man and animals with hernia.

Until further progress in this area provides surgeons with curative measures, they must depend upon principles that have been established through centuries of trial and error. Gross anatomic defects must be recognized and repaired by any of a number of effective methods. Regardless of eponymic designations, the following details in performance of herniorrhaphy continue to be important:

1. Identification of the peritoneal sac.
2. Opening of the peritoneal sac at the internal ring, with digital exploration for other locules.
3. Closure of the peritoneum, with high ligation being an important detail.
4. Performance of a Hoguet maneuver in direct or femoral hernias.
5. Removal of lipomas of the cord or excessively hypertrophied cremaster muscle.
6. Accurate identification of the transversalis fascia at the internal ring, permitting its snug closure.
7. In direct inguinal hernias, the attenuated transversalis will not suffice as barrier to herniation. The transversus arch should be utilized in the repair. Here aponeurosis, and not attenuated fascia, should be depended on for strength.
8. The principle of multilayered closure of Bassini-Halsted continues to be useful.
9. In certain hernias, Cooper's ligament is a preferred anchoring site.
10. Nonabsorbable sutures should be depended on for long-term strength. Catgut, synthetic absorbable sutures, and silk do not meet this requirement.
11. The relaxing incision is a simple and effective method of avoiding tension at the suture line.
12. There should be less reluctance to use prosthetic implants in direct, recurrent hernias, certain femoral and incisional hernias.

With intelligent application by the surgeon of the knowledge gained through the efforts of many contributors and through painstaking attention to numerous technical details, herniorrhaphy should be a safe and effective procedure.

## REFERENCES

Adamson, R. J., and Enquist, I. F.: The relative importance of sutures to the strength of healing wounds under normal and abnormal conditions. Surg. Gynecol. Obstet. *117*:396, 1963.

Andrews, E. A., and Bissel, A. D.: Direct hernia. A record of surgical failures. Surg. Gynecol. Obstet. 58:753, 1934.

Anson, B. J., Morgan, E. H., and McVay, C. B.: The anatomy of the hernial regions. 1. Inguinal hernia. Surg. Gynecol. Obstet. 89:417, 1949.

Anson, B. J., Morgan, E. H., and McVay, C. B.: Surgical anatomy of the inguinal region based on a study of 500 body-halves. Surg. Gynecol. Obstet. 111:707, 1960.

Bachhuber, T. E., and Lalich, J. J.: Effect of sweet pea meal on the rat aorta. Arch. Path. 59:247, 1954.

Bassini, E.: Uber de Behandlung des Leistenbruches. Arch. Klin. Chir. 40:429, 1890.

Bassini, E.: Sopra 100 casi cura radicale dell 'hernia inguinale operata col metodo dell'autore. Arch. Atti. Soc. Ital. Chir. 5:315, 1888.

Cushing, H.: The employment of local anesthetics and the radical cure of certain cases of hernia with a note on the nervous anatomy of the inguinal region. Ann. Surg. 31:1, 1900.

Condon, R. E.: Surgical anatomy of transversus abdominis and transversalis fascia. Ann. Surg. 173:1, 1971.

Conner, W. T., and Peacock, E. E., Jr.: Some studies on the etiology of inguinal hernia. Am. J. Surg. 126(6):732, 1973.

Cooper, A. P.: The Anatomy and Surgical Treatment of Abdominal Hernias. (2 vols). London, Longman & Co, 1804.

Fruchaud, H.: Anatomie Chirurgicale des Hernies de l'Aine. Paris, G. Doin & Cie, 1956.

Dunphy, J. E.: On the nature and care of wounds. Ann. Roy. Coll. Surg. Engl. 26:69, 1960.

Gaster, J.: Hernia. Darien, Conn., Hafner Publishing Co., 1970.

Geiger, B. J., Steenbock, H., and Parsons, H. T.: Lathyrism in the rat. J. Nutr. 6:427, 1933.

Gibson, C. L., and Felter, R. K.: End results of inguinal hernia operations. Ann. Surg. 92:744, 1930.

Halsted, W.: The treatment of wounds. Johns Hopk. Hosp. Rep. 2:255, 1891.

Halsted, W. S.: The radical cure of inguinal hernia in the male. Bull. Johns Hopk. Hosp. 4:17, 1893.

Harrison, P. W.: Inguinal hernia: A study of the principles involved in surgical treatment. Arch. Surg. 4:680, 1922.

Hesselbach, F. C.: Neuste anatomisch pathologische untersuchungen uber den ursprung und das Fortschreiten der Leistenund. Schenkelbuche. Wurzburg, Joseph Stabel, 1814.

Hoguet, P.: Direct inguinal hernia. Ann. Surg. 72:671, 1920.

Keith, A.: On the origin and nature of hernia. Br. J. Surg. 11:455, 1923.

Köller, Karl: Uber die locale anwendung des cocains am auge. Klin. MBL. Heilk. 22:443, 1884.

Leithauser, D. J., and Bergo, H. L.: Early rising and ambulatory activity after operation: A means of preventing complications. Arch. Surg. 42:1086, 1941.

Lichtenstein, I. L.: Local anesthesia for hernioplasty. Immediate ambulation and early return to work: A preliminary report. Cal. Med. 100:106, 1964.

Lister, J.: On the antiseptic principle in the practice of surgery. Lancet 2:353, 1867.

Sucas-Championnière, J.: Cure Radicale des Hernies;

Avec une Étude statistique de deux cents soixante-quinze operations et cinquante figures intercalées dans le Text. Paris, Reuff et Cie., 1892.

Lytle, W. J.: The internal ring. Br. J. Surg. 32:441, 1945.

Madden, J. W., and Peacock, E. E., Jr.: Studies on the biology of collagen during wound healing. Surgery 64(1):288, 1968.

Madden, J. W., and Peacock, E. E., Jr.: Studies on the biology of collagen during wound healing. III. Dynamic metabolism of scar collagen and remodeling of dermal wounds. Ann. Surg. 174:511, 1971.

MacGregor, W. W.: The demonstration of a true internal inguinal sphincter and its etiologic role in hernia. Surg. Gynecol. Obstet. 49:510, 1929.

Madsen, E. T.: An experimental and clinical evaluation of suture materials. Surg. Gynecol. Obstet. 97:73, 1953.

McVay, C. B.: An anatomic error in current methods of inguinal herniorrhaphy. Ann. Surg. 113:1111, 1941.

McVay, C. B., and Anson, B. J.: A fundamental error in current methods of inguinal herniorrhaphy. Surg. Gynecol. Obstet. 74:746, 1942.

McVay, C. B.: The anatomic basis for inguinal and femoral hernioplasty. Surg. Gynecol. Obstet. 139:931, 1974.

Merritt, W., Peacock, E. E., Jr., and Chvapil, M.: Comparative biology of fascial autografts and allografts. Surg. Forum 25:524, 1974.

Morgagni, G. B.: DeSedibus et Causis Morborum per Anatomen Indagitis, 1761. Translated by B. Alexander. London, A. Miller, 1769. (Reprinted: New York, Hafner Publishing Co., 1960.)

Nyhus, L. M.: An anatomic reappraisal of the posterior inguinal wall: Special considerations of the iliopubic tract and its relation to groin hernias. Surg. Clin. North Am. 44:1305, 1964.

Nyhus, L. M., Stevenson, J. K., Listerud, M. B., and Harkins, H. N.: Preperitoneal herniorrhaphy: A preliminary report in fifty patients. West. J. Surg. 67:48, 1959.

Ponka, J. L., and Brush, B. E.: Experiences with repair of groin hernia in 200 patients aged 70 years or older. J. Am. Geriatr. Soc. 22:18, 1974.

Ponka, J. L., and Sapala, J. A.: Bupivacaine as a local anesthetic for hernia repair. H.F.H. Med. Jour. 24:31, 1976.

Peacock, E. E., and Madden, J. W.: Some studies on the effect of B-aminopropionitrile on collagen in healing wounds. Surgery 60:7, 1966.

Peacock, E. E., Madden, J. W., and Trier, W. C.: Some studies on the treatment of burned hands. Ann. Surg. 171:903, 1970.

Ponseti, I., and Baird, W. A.: Scoliosis and dissecting aneurysm of the aorta in rats fed with Lathyrus odoratus seeds. Am. J. Path. 28:1059, 1952.

Pott, P. A.: A Treatise on Ruptures. London, Hitch and Hawes, 1756.

Read, R. C.: Preperitoneal exposure of inguinal herniation. Am. J. Surg. 116:653, 1968.

Read, R. C.: Attenuation of the rectus sheath in inguinal herniation. Am. J. Surg. 120:610, 1970.

Reid, M. R., and Stevenson, J.: The treatment of fresh wounds. Surg. Gynecol. Obstet. 66:313, 1938.

Schilling, J. A.: Wound healing. Surg. Clin. North Am. 56(4):859, 1976.

Shouldice, E. E.: Surgical treatment in hernia. Ontario Med. Rev. *4*:43, 1945.

Stewardson, R. H., Bombeck, C. T., and Nyhus, L. M.: Critical operative management of small bowel obstruction. Ann. Surg. *187*:189, 1978.

Thomson, A.: Cause anatomique de la hérniae inguinale externe. J. Conn. Med. Prat. *4*:137, 1836.

Taylor, F. W.: The evolution of hernirrhaphy. Am. J. Surg. *21*:131, 1933.

Virchow, R.: *Cellular Pathology as Based Upon Physiological and Pathological Histology* (translated by F. Chance). New York, R. M. Dewitt, 1860.

Wagh, P. V., and Read, R. C.: Collagen deficiency in rectus sheath of patients with inguinal herniation (35582). Proceed. Soc. Exp. Biol. Med. *137*:382, 1971.

Wagh, P. V., Leverich, A. P., Sun, C. N., White, H. J., and Read, R. C.: Direct inguinal herniation in men: A disease of collagen. J. Surg. Res. *17*:425, 1974.

Watson, L. F.: *Hernia* (3rd ed.). St. Louis, C. V. Mosby Co., 1948.

Wheeler, E. S.: The development of antibiotic surgery. Am. J. Surg. *127*:573, 1974.

Wirtschafter, Z. T., and Bentley, J. P.: Hernias as a collagen maturation defect. Ann. Surg. *160*:852, 1964.

Wirtschafter, Z. T., and Bentley, J. P.: The influence of age and growth rate on the extractable collagen of skin of normal rats. Lab. Invest. *11*:316, 1962.

Zimmerman, L. M., and Veith, I.: *Great Ideas in the History of Surgery* (2nd rev. ed.). New York, Dover Publications, 1967.

# index

Note: Page numbers in *italics* refer to
illustrations. Page numbers followed by (t) refer to
tables.

## A

Abdomen, burst. See *Wound disruption*.
  flat films, 65–68, *65–67*
  preoperative examination of, 58
Abdominal approach, inguinal incision in, 12
  to femoral hernia repair, 249
Abdominal ring
  external, anatomy of, *20*, 21
    ligation of hernial sac at, 10
  internal, closure of, 12
    defect of, and hernia, 5
    in indirect inguinal hernia repair, 185
Abdominal wall
  anatomy of, description of, 6
  anterolateral, muscles of, anatomy of,
    20–26, *20*
  blood vessels of, 19
  defects of, embryology of, 418–421, 418(t),
    *419, 420*, 509(t)
  direct infiltration of, for local anesthesia,
    94, *97*
  hernias of. See *Hernia(s)*.
  maldevelopment of, and hernia, 42
  reconstruction of, in lumbar hernia repair,
    472
  sinuses of, incisional hernia repair and,
    392(t), 393
  tumors of, vs. epigastric hernia, 445
Abscess(es)
  recurrent, 602
  stitch, 594
  vs. hernia, 52
  vs. lumbar hernia, 471
ACTH, and wound healing, 343
Adhesive strips. See *Tape*.
Adrenocorticotropic hormone, and wound
  healing, 343
Adults
  clinical appraisal of, 54
  history of, 55
  indirect inguinal hernia in. See *Indirect
    inguinal hernia*.
  umbilical hernia in. See *Umbilical hernia,
    in adults*.

Age. See also *Infants; Children;* and *Adults*.
  and appendectomy and herniorrhaphy, 518,
    518(t)
  and congenital indirect inguinal hernia,
    146, 147(t)
  and direct inguinal hernia, 210, *210*
  and direct-indirect-femoral hernia, 279(t),
    280
  and epigastric hernia, 442, *442*
  and femoral hernia, 240, *240*, 253
  and hernia, 42
  and incisional hernia, 373, *373*
  and incisional hernia requiring implants,
    547, *548*
  and indirect inguinal hernia, 168, 169(t)
  and management of cryptorchidism, 142
  and recurrent direct inguinal hernia, 232,
    232(t)
  and recurrent direct-indirect-femoral
    hernia, 285, 285(t)
  and recurrent femoral hernia, 269, 269(t)
  and recurrent indirect inguinal hernia, 187,
    187(t)
  and recurrent inguinal and femoral hernia
    repair with prostheses, 563, 565(t)
  and sliding inguinal hernia, 312
  and Spigelian hernia, 483, 485(t)
  and umbilical hernia, in adults, 408, 409(t)
    in infants and children, 402, 403(t)
  and wound disruption, 332, 358, *359*
Aged, clinical appraisal of, 55
  history of, 55
  surgery in, 53
Allergy
  and postoperative complications, 597
  prosthetics, 536
  to local anesthesia, 104
    management of, 104–105
Allografts, 538(t), 541
Amniocele. See *Omphalocele*.
Amniotic hernia. See *Omphalocele*.
Anatomy, 18–39
  abdominal wall, description of, 6
  and hernia in female, 82–83
  for local anesthesia, 93–97, *93–97*

Anatomy (*Continued*)
 of direct inguinal hernia, 197–198
 of epigastric hernia, 438–439
  pathologic, 439–441, *440*
 of femoral hernia, 238–240, *239*
 of hernia, progress in, 619–620
  understanding of, 4–7
 of Littre's hernia, 502–503
 of lumbar hernia, 466–469, *466*
 of relaxing incision, 530–532, *531*
 of Spigelian hernia, 479–480, *480–482*
 of supravesical hernia, 488–489, *488*
Anemia, and wound healing, *333, 338,* 341
Anesthesia
 considerations before, 76–78
 development of, 7
 in congenital indirect inguinal hernia in
  repair, 148
 in direct inguinal hernia repair, 210 210(t)
 in direct-indirect-femoral hernia repair, 281
 in epigastric hernia repair, 447
 in femoral hernia repair, 256
 in incisional hernia repair, 390
  with prostheses, 553, 555(t)
 in indirect inguinal hernia repair, 169,
  169(t)
 in recurrent direct inguinal hernia repair,
  232
 in recurrent femoral hernia repair, 269
 in recurrent indirect inguinal hernia repair,
  188 188(t)
 in sliding inguinal hernia repair, 313
 in umbilical hernia repair, in infants and
  children, 405
 in wound disruption, 363, 363(t)
 local, 91–107
  advantages and disadvantages of,
   105–106, 106(t)
  anatomy for, 93–97, *93–97*
  armamentarium for, 97–100, *100, 101*
  drugs for, 100, 102(t), 103(t)
  historical background of, 91–93
  in inguinal and femoral hernia repair,
   108–117
  pharmacologic considerations in, 100–104
  reactions to, 104
   management of, 104–105
 postoperative, 604
 preparation for, 76–81
  emergency vs. routine, 78
 spinal, and backache, case history of, 616
  and headache, in femoral hernia repair,
   261
Anesthesiology, progress in, 620–621
Anorchia, bilateral, 122
Antimetabolites, and wound healing, 343
Antisepsis, 8
Aorta, as homograft, 541
Aponeurosis, external oblique, in direct
 inguinal hernia repair, 208, *209*
 vs. fascia, 7
Appendectomy, and herniorrhaphy, 514–521
 clinical study of, 518–520, 518(t)
 complications of, 520
 in femoral hernia, 257
 in indirect inguinal hernia, 174
Appendicitis, acute, and incarcerated indirect
 inguinal hernia, 519

Appendix
 in hernia, 514
  clinical features of, 516–517, *517*
  historical background of, 515–516, *515*
  operative findings in, 519
  operative treatment of, 518
 in indirect inguinal hernia, 174
 incarcerated, in direct inguinal hernia, 519
 inflammation of, acute, and incarcerated
  indirect inguinal hernia, 519
 removal of. See *Appendectomy.*
Arteriosclerosis, and postoperative death,
 case history of, 589
 in preoperative evaluation of elderly, 56
Artery
 accessory obturator, injury to,
  intraoperative, 578–579, *578*
 deep inferior epigastric, bleeding from,
  intraoperative, 575, *576*
 deferential, injury to, intraoperative, 579,
  *579*
 femoral, injury to, intraoperative, 576, *576*
 occlusion of, and scrotal and testicular
  swelling, 608
 spermatic, external, injury to,
  intraoperative, 579, *579*
  internal, injury to, intraoperative, 579,
   *579*
 supplying testes, 605, *605*
Ascorbic acid, deficiency of, and wound
 healing, 342
Asepsis, 8
 and wound healing, 350
Atrophy, testicular, 611
 case history of, 612
 division of spermatic cord and, 607
Autografts, 538–541, 538(t)


                              **B**

Backache, postoperative, 616
 spinal anesthesia and, case history of, 616
Bacteriology, progress in, 621
Bandelette iliopubienne, 5
Barium enema examination of colon, 68–70,
 *68, 69*
 in inguinal hernia and carcinoma, 522, *524*
Bassini, Eduardo, 13, *13,* 156
Bassini repair
 of direct-indirect-femoral hernias, 281(t),
  282
 of femoral hernia, 247, *254, 259*
 of indirect inguinal hernia, 170, 170(t)
 vs. indirect inguinal hernia repair, 168
Bassini-Halsted repair, of direct inguinal
 hernia, 199(t), 200
Bassini-Kirschner repair, of femoral hernia,
 247, *247*
 of recurrent femoral hernia, 270(t), 271
Berger, relaxing incision of, 527, *527*
Biliary tract, disease of, vs. epigastric hernia,
 444
Bladder, urinary
 contrast studies of, 70–71, *72, 73*
 hernias about. See *Supravesical hernia.*

Bladder, urinary (*Continued*)
    in sliding hernia, 297, *298, 299*
        developmental and anatomic
            considerations in, 301
        historical considerations of, 291
        repair of, 310
        injury to, intraoperative, 580–581, *580*
Bleeding, from pampiniform plexus,
        intraoperative, 576
    from superficial blood vessels,
        intraoperative, 575, *575*
Blood supply
    of colon, in sliding hernia, 300, *300*
    of spermatic cord, 29
    testicular, experimental study of, 605, *605*
        injury to, intraoperative, 579–580, *579*
Blood vessels. See also *Artery;* and *Vein.*
    abdominal wall, 19
    disease of, and postoperative death, case
        history of, 591, *591*
        postoperative, 599
    femoral, injury to, intraoperative, 576, *576,
        577*
    injury to, intraoperative, 576–578, *576, 577*
    superficial, bleeding from, intraoperative,
        575, *575*
Bowel. See *Intestine.*
Brüche, darmwand. See *Richter's hernia.*
    lateral. See *Richter's hernia.*
    partial. See *Richter's hernia.*
Bupivacaine, in local anesthesia, 101, 102(t),
    103(t)

C

Canal
    inguinal, anatomy of, 27–30
        description of, 5
        in recurrent direct inguinal hernia, 223,
            *224*
    of Nuck, cysts of, 120
        in sliding hernia, developmental and
            anatomic considerations in, 301
Cancer. See *Carcinoma;* and *Tumors.*
Carcinoma
    and inguinal hernia, 522–524, *524*
        historical background of, 522–523
    and wound disruption, 332(t), *333,* 336
    colonic, and hernia, 42, 56
        vs. diverticulitis, 523, *524*
        vs. hernia, 51, *51*
    stomach, vs. epigastric hernia, 444
Cardiac disease. See *Heart, disease of.*
Cardiovascular disease, and postoperative
        death, case history of, 591, *591*
        postoperative, 599
Catheters, suction, in incisional hernia repair,
    388, 389
Cecum, in sliding hernia, developmental and
        anatomic considerations in, 300
        historical considerations in, 290
    wall of, Richter's hernia of, 462
Cellulitis, postoperative, 594
Celosomias, 420
    upper, 420

Chemical factors, and wound healing,
    340–343
Chest, preoperative examination of, 57, *57*
    preoperative x-ray of, 58, *60*
Children
    clinical appraisal of, 54
    congenital indirect inguinal hernias in, 118
    direct inguinal hernia in, 128
    femoral hernias in, 128–129
    hydrocele in, management of, 135
    preoperative medication for, 80, 81(t)
    surgery in, 53
    umbilical hernia in. See *Umbilical hernia,
        in infants and children.*
Chloroprocaine, in local anesthesia, 101,
    102(t), 103(t)
Cirrhosis, and wound disruption, 337
    Laennec's, and wound disruption, *333,* 337
    with umbilical hernia, 412, *413*
Cloth, definition of, 535
Colon
    ascending, in sliding hernia,
        developmental and anatomic
            considerations in, 300
    barium enema examination of, 68–70, *68,
        69*
        in inguinal hernia and carcinoma, 522,
            *524*
    carcinoma of, and hernia, 42
        vs. diverticulitis, 523, *524*
        vs. hernia, 51, *51*
    in sliding hernia, 300
        blood supply to, 300, *300*
        historical considerations in, 291
        injury to, intraoperative, *581,* 582
    sigmoid, in sliding hernia, developmental
            and anatomic considerations in, 300
        historical considerations in, 290
        repair of, 307–312, *308–310*
Colostomy, and peri-stomal hernias, 389
    performance of, 390
Congenital factors, and hernia, 41
    direct inguinal, 42
Congenital hernia. See also *Infants;* and
        *Indirect inguinal hernia, congenital.*
    description of, 3
    lumbar, 469, 469(t)
Conjoined tendon, 6
Connective tissue phase, of wound healing,
    339, 339(t), 340
Constipation, and hernia, 42
Cooper, Astley, 4, *5*
Cooper's ligament
    anatomy of, *34,* 35
    description of, 5
    in direct inguinal hernia repair, 200
    in femoral hernia repair, 12
    in recurrent groin hernia repair with mesh,
        565, *566*
    injection of, in local anesthesia, 111, *115*
Cooper's ligament repair. See
    *Lotheissen-McVay repair.*
Cord, spermatic. See *Spermatic cord.*
    umbilical, hernia in, 418(t), 419, *420*
        vs. gastroschisis, *506*
Coughing, and wound disruption, 335, *335*
Cremaster muscle
    excision of, 14

Cremaster muscle (*Continued*)
  failure of, 184
    in indirect inguinal hernia repair, 183,
     *183*
  in indirect inguinal hernia repair, 161, *161*
Cryptorchidism, 121, *121*
  consequences of, 139
  failure of spermatogenesis in, 139
  iatrogenic, 610
  malignancy of testes in, 139
  management of, 140, 150
    principles of, 142–146
    technique for, 143, *144–145*
  psychologic abnormalities in, 140
  testicular torsion in, 140
  testicular trauma in, 140
  with congenital indirect inguinal hernia,
    139
Cutaneous. See *Skin.*
Cutis grafts, 539
  and cyst, 539, *539, 540,* 541(t)
Cyst(s)
  cutis graft and, 539, *539, 540,* 541(t)
  of canal of Nuck, 120
  skin graft and, 539, 541(t)
  vs. hernia, 52
Cystograms, 70–71, *72, 73*


D


Dacron mesh, for prosthesis, 546
  placement of, technique for, 553, *553*
Darmwand brüche. See *Richter's hernia.*
Dead space, avoidance of, 352
Deaths. See *Mortality.*
Deferential artery, injury to, intraoperative,
  579, *579*
Dehiscence, wound. See *Wound disruption.*
Dermatologic lesions, preoperative treatment
  of, 62
Devitalized tissues, removal of, 351
Diabetes mellitus, and wound disruption, 337
Diaphragmatic hernia, description of, 4
Diastasis recti, vs. epigastric hernia, 445, *446*
Differentiation phase, of wound healing, *339,*
  339(t), 340
Digestive tract. See *Gastrointestinal tract.*
Direct inguinal hernia, 196–215, *197*
  anatomic considerations in, 197–198
  clinical pathologic correlation and
    considerations of, 196–197
  clinical study of, 209–213
  congenital factors and, 42
  description of, 3
  historical background of, 196
  in females, incidence of, *85,* 86–87
  in infants and children, 128
  incarcerated appendix in, 519
  physical examination in, 44, *46*
  recurrent, 216–237
    causes of, 225–226, 225(t)
    classification of, 222, *222–224*
    clinical study of, 232–235
    factors in, 220
    historical background of, 216–218, *217,*
     *218*
    incidence of, 218–221, 219(t)

Direct inguinal hernia (*Continued*)
  recurrent, large, 223, *224*
    repair of, 230, *230, 231*
    medial, *222,* 223
     repair of, 228, *229*
    recurrence of, 234
    repair of, 228–232, *229–231*
     clinical study of, 232
     complications of, 233, 234(t)
     technical errors in, case history of, 226
     type of, 233 233(t)
    small, 223, *223*
     repair of, 229
    time of, 219
    types of, 222–225
  repair of
    additional procedures with, 212 212(t)
    multilayered closure in, 199(t), 200
    preperitoneal approach to, 199(t), 203,
     *250–251,* 252
    and recurrence, 219
    results of, 213
    single-layered closure in, 199, 199(t)
    technical details of, 204–209, *204–209,*
     233, 233(t)
    techniques for, 198–204, 199(t), 210,
     211(t)
     details of, 211, 211(t)
  site of, 198
Direct-indirect-femoral hernia. See
  *Multilocular inguinal hernia.*
Dissection, sharp, 351
Diverticular disease, and hernia, 42
Diverticulitis, vs. colonic carcinoma, 523, *524*
Drains, 353
Drugs. See also names of specific drugs.
  for local anesthesia, 100, 102(t), 103(t)
  preoperative, 76–81
    for ambulatory surgery, 79
    for children, 80, 81(t)
    standard dose of, 80
    timing of, 79
Duodenum, ulcer of, vs. epigastric hernia,
  444


E


Ears, preoperative examination of, 57
Ecchymosis, postoperative, 592
Ectopia, *120,* 121
EKG, preoperative, 60
Elderly, clinical appraisal of, 55
  history of, 55
  surgery in, 53
Electrocardiograms, preoperative, 60
Embolism, pulmonary, femoral hernia repair
  and, 261
Embryology, 122–128
  of abdominal wall defects, 418–421, 418(t),
    *419, 420,* 509(t)
  of gastroschisis, 507–509, 509(t)
Embryonic folds, maldevelopment of, 420
Emergency, and preparation for surgery and
  anesthesia, 78
En masse reduction. See *Reduction en*
  *masse.*
Endometriosis, vs. hernia, 52
Enterocele, partial. See *Richter's hernia.*

Epigastric artery, deep inferior, bleeding
    from, intraoperative, 575, 576
Epigastric hernia, 435–454
    anatomic considerations in, 438–439
    clinical characteristics of, 441–447
    clinical history in, 442
    definition of, 372, 435
    differential diagnosis of, 444
    historical background of, 435–438
    incidence of, 89
    location of, 444, 444(t)
    operative findings in, 452, 452(t)
    pathologic anatomy and clinical picture in,
        439–441, 440
    recurrence of, 453
    repair of, 447–453
        complications of, 453
        technique for, 447(t), 448
Epinephrine, reactions to, 104
Etiology, of hernia, 41–43, 41(t)
Examination, physical. See Physical
    examination.
Exomphalos. See Omphalocele.
Extra-aponeurotic hernia, 494, 495
Extraperitoneal sliding hernia, 295(t), 297,
    297–299
Extremities, preoperative examination of, 58
Exudative phase, of wound healing, 339, 339,
    339(t)
Eyes, preoperative examination of, 57


                            F

Fabric, definition of, 534
Fallis, relaxing incision of, 528, 529
Fallopian tube, in sliding hernia, historical
    considerations in, 293
    injury to, intraoperative, 584–585, 585
Falx inguinalis, 6
Fascia
    as heterograft, 541
    enteroabdominal. See Transversalis fascia.
    external oblique, in indirect inguinal
        hernia repair, 160, 161
        incision of, 11
        injection of, in local anesthesia, 111, 113
    lumbodorsal, closure of, in lumbar hernia
        repair, 472
    transversalis. See Transversalis fascia.
    vs. aponeurosis, 7
Fascia lata
    as autograft, 538
    as homograft, 541
    sheets of, in lumbar hernia repair, 472
    strips of, in lumbar hernia repair, 472
Female. See also Sex.
    direct inguinal hernias in, incidence of, 85,
        86–87
    hernia in, 82–90
        incidence of, 83, 84(t)
            statistical analysis of, 84–86, 85
        indirect inguinal hernia in, 86
        infertility in, bilateral hernia repair and,
            614
        processus vaginalis in, embryology of, 127
        sliding hernias in, 86
            historical considerations in, 293

Female (Continued)
    sliding hernias in, repair of, 310, 311
        intraoperative complications of, 584,
            585
Femoral approach, to femoral hernia repair,
    12
Femoral artery, injury to, intraoperative, 576,
    576
Femoral hernia, 238–263
    after inguinal hernia repair, 264–265, 265(t)
    anatomy of, 238–240, 239
    and intestinal strangulation, 256, 257, 258
    bilateral, 255
    clinical features of, 255, 255(t)
    clinical study of, 252–262
    combined with inguinal hernia. See
        Multilocular inguinal hernia.
    definition of, 238
    errors in diagnosis of, 253, 253(t)
    etiologic factors in, 240–241
    historical considerations in, 241–243, 241
    in infants and children, 128–129
    incidence of, 85, 87
    inguinal incision of upper approach in, 12
    location of, 255
    overlooked, 266–267
    physical examination in, 44, 46, 47
    recurrent, 264–274
        clinical study of, 269–273
        etiology of, 265–268, 266(t)
        multiple factors and, case history of, 267
        number of previous repairs of, 269, 269(t)
        repair of, 269
            and recurrence, 272
            complications of, 272
            inadequate, case history of, 268
            prosthesis in. See Prosthesis, in
                recurrent femoral hernia repair.
            technique for, 269, 270(t)
        technical factors and, 266(t), 267
    repair of, 256
        abdominal or posterior approach to, 249
        and recurrence, 258, 258(t), 265, 265(t)
        complications of, 259, 260(t)
        femoral or lower approach to, 12
        local anesthesia for, 108–117
        preperitoneal approach to, 13, 249
            technique for, 249, 250–251, 259
        techniques for, 243
        types of, 258, 258(t)
    with incarceration and strangulation, 256,
        257, 258
Femoral nerve, injury to, 596
    lateral cutaneous, injury to, intraoperative,
        582, 583
    paresis of, postoperative, 596
Femoral ring, in femoral hernia, 238
Femoral sheath, anatomy of, 32, 33, 34
    description of, 5
Femoral vein, injury to, intraoperative, 576,
    576, 577, 578
Ferguson repair, in congenital indirect
    inguinal hernia, 149, 149(t)
    in indirect inguinal hernia, 170, 170(t)
Fibroblastic phase, of wound healing, 339,
    339(t), 340
Fibroma, vs. lumbar hernia, 471
Filigree, definition of, 534
    silver, 544
Folds, embryonic, maldevelopment of, 420
    peritoneal, 37

Fossa supravesicalis, hernia into. See *Supravesical hernia.*
Fossae, pelvic peritoneal, anatomy of, 37–38, *38*
Fovea supravesicalis. See *Supravesical hernia.*

# G

Gastrointestinal tract. See also *Intestine;* and *Stomach.*
  and postoperative complications, 597
  disease of, and wound disruption, 332(t), 336
    functional, vs. epigastric hernia, 445
    in preoperative evaluation of elderly, 56
  preoperative studies of, 61, *62*
  upper, x-ray of, 70
Gastroschisis, 421, 504–514
  and hernia, 42
  anomalies associated with, 509–510
  clinical features of, 509
  definition of, 505, *506*
  embryology of, 507–509, 509(t)
  historical background of, 505–507
  repair of, 510–512, *511*
  treatment of, 510
    immediate nonoperative, 510
  vs. omphalocele, 417, *506*
Genitourinary tract
  disease of, and hernia, 43
    in preoperative evaluation of elderly, 56
  complications of, femoral hernia repair and, 260, 260(t)
    postoperative, early and late, 615
  preoperative examination of, 60, *61*
Geriatric. See *Elderly.*
Gibson incision, 370, *371*
Gimbernat, lacunar ligament of, anatomy of, *21, 22, 22*
  description of, 5
Gloves, rubber, use of, 9
Gonadotropins, pituitary, 614
Graft(s)
  auto-, 538–541, 538(t)
  cutis, 539
    and cyst, 539, *539, 540,* 541(t)
  hetero-, 538(t), 541–542
  homo-, 538(t), 541
  musculofascial flap, in lumbar hernia repair, 473, *474*
  skin, and cyst, 539, 541(t)
  whole skin, 539
Granuloma, postoperative, 602
Gubernaculum testis, 123, *123*

# H

Halsted, William Stewart, 14, *15*
  relaxing incision of, 527, *528*
Halsted repair
  of congenital indirect inguinal hernia, 149, 149(t)

Halsted repair (*Continued*)
  of direct inguinal hernia, 204–209, *205–209*
  of direct-indirect-femoral hernias, 281, 281(t)
  of indirect inguinal hernia, 170, 170(t)
  of recurrent direct inguinal hernia, 231
Halsted-Bassini repair, of direct inguinal hernia, 199(t), 200
Hampton, Caroline, 9, *10*
Headaches, spinal, femoral hernia repair and, 261
Heart
  disease of, and hernia, 42
    and postoperative death, case history of, 591, *591*
    and wound disruption, 338, *338*
    arteriosclerotic, and postoperative death, case history of, 589
    in preoperative evaluation of elderly, 56
    postoperative, 599
  preoperative examination of, 58, *59*
Hematoma
  and scrotal and testicular swelling, 609
  incisional hernia repair and, 392, 392(t)
  postoperative, 592
  vs. lumbar hernia, 471
Hemorrhage, intraoperative, 574(t), 575
Hemostasis, 351
Henry-Cheatle-Nyhus repair, of indirect inguinal hernia, 170(t), 171
  of recurrent femoral hernia, 270(t), 272
Hernia(s)
  amniotic. See *Omphalocele.*
  anterior retroperitoneal. See *Supravesical hernia.*
  biochemistry of, 624–625
    historical background of, 624
  classification of, 41(t)
  combined direct-indirect-femoral. See *Multilocular inguinal hernia.*
  congenital. See also *Infants;* and *Indirect inguinal hernia, congenital.*
    description of, 3
  contributions to understanding and treatment of, 1–17, *2*
  diagnosis of, 40–52
    differential, 49–52
  diaphragmatic, description of, 4
  differentiation of direct, indirect, and femoral, 3
  early treatment of, 1
  epigastric. See *Epigastric hernia.*
  extra-aponeurotic, 494, *495*
  femoral. See *Femoral hernia.*
  hiatal, incidence of, 89
    vs. epigastric hernia, 445
  hypogastric. See *Supravesical hernia.*
  iatrogenic, 179
  incisional. See *Incisional hernia.*
  inguinal. See *Inguinal hernia.*
    direct. See *Direct inguinal hernia.*
    indirect. See *Indirect inguinal hernia.*
  interparietal. See *Interparietal hernia.*
  interstitial, *493, 494, 494*
  into fovea or fossa supravesicalis. See *Supravesical hernia.*
  intravesical. See *Supravesical hernia.*
  Littre's. See *Littre's hernia.*

Hernia(s) (*Continued*)
  masked. See *Richter's hernia;* and
    *Spigelian hernia.*
  multilocular inguinal. See *Multilocular*
    *inguinal hernia.*
  muscle, vs. lumbar hernia, 471
  nipped. See *Richter's hernia.*
  obturator, description of, 4
  of Meckel's diverticulum. See *Littre's*
    *hernia.*
  overlooked, 178, 266–267
    case report of, 182
  paravesical. See *Supravesical hernia.*
  pathology of, progress in, 620
    understanding of, 2–4
  perineal, description of, 3
  peri-stomal, 389
  pinched. See *Richter's hernia.*
  preoperative evaluation of, 53–63
  prevesical. See *Supravesical hernia.*
  properitoneal supravesical. See
    *Supravesical hernia.*
  recurrence of, 604, 605(t)
    classification of, 178, 178(t)
    definition of, 177
    incidence of, 179
  sliding. See *Sliding hernia.*
  Spigelian. See *Spigelian hernia.*
  spontaneous lateral ventral. See *Spigelian*
    *hernia.*
  suprapubic. See *Supravesical hernia.*
  unusual, 455–524, 455(t), *456*
    incidence of, 278, *278*
  vesicopubic. See *Supravesical hernia.*
Hernia justavesicalis. See *Supravesical*
  *hernia.*
Hernial sac
  description of, 3
  ligation of, at external abdominal ring, 10
  pathology of, in indirect inguinal hernia,
    171, *171,* 172(t)
Hernie partiale. See *Richter's hernia.*
Herniography, 71–75
Herniorrhaphy. See also *Surgery;* and names
  of specific types of hernias.
  adjuncts to, 7–10
  and appendectomy. See *Appendectomy,*
    *and herniorrhaphy.*
  and fatalities, 587–592
  anesthesia for. See *Anesthesia.*
  combination of techniques in, 12
  complications of, early and late
    postoperative, 587–618, 588(t), 593(t)
    intraoperative, 573–586, 574(t)
  evaluation of hernia prior to, 53–63
  experience and, 221–222
  teaching of, 623–624
  technical contributions to, 10–16
  technology for, progress in, 621–623
Herzfeld, Gertrude, 130, *130*
Hesselbach's triangle, 197, *197*
  anatomy of, 27, *28*
  description of, 5
  in direct inguinal hernia, 196, *204,* 216
  in indirect inguinal hernia repair, 186
  in recurrent direct inguinal hernia, 223,
    *223*
Heterografts, 538(t), 541–542
Hiatal hernia, incidence of, 89
  vs. epigastric hernia, 445

History, clinical, 55–56
  in epigastric hernia, 442
  in diagnosis of hernia, 43–44
  in incisional hernia, 374
  in incisional hernia requiring implants,
    548
  in preoperative evaluation, 55–56
  preoperative evaluation of, 77
Hoguet maneuver, 14
  in direct inguinal hernia repair, 203, *205*
  in direct-indirect-femoral hernia repair,
    282, *283,* 283(t)
  in femoral hernia repair, 257
  in sliding hernia repair, 305, *306*
Homografts, 538(t), 541
Hormone, adrenocorticotropic, and wound
  healing, 343
  in treatment of cryptorchidism, 141
Hunter's gubernaculum, 123, *123*
Hydrocele, 119, 609
  in infants and children, management of,
    135
  indirect inguinal hernia with, 173
  vs. congenital indirect inguinal hernia, 148
  vs. hernia, 47, 50, *50*
    in infants, 48
Hydrocelectomy, 150
Hypertension, and postoperative death, case
  history of, 591, *591*
Hypogastric hernia, definition of, 435
  retroperitoneal. See *Supravesical hernia.*
Hypogonadism, postoperative, 613
Hypoproteinemia, and wound healing, *333,*
  341
Hypotension, local anesthetics and, 105
Hypothyroidism, and wound disruption, 338


# I

Ileostomy, and peri-stomal hernias, 389
  performance of, 390
Ileum, in sliding hernia, historical
  considerations of, 291
Ileus, femoral hernia repair and, 260
  postoperative, 597, *597*
  Richter's hernia and, 463
Iliohypogastric nerve, in local anesthesia, *93,*
  *94, 94,* 98, *110,* 111
  injury to, intraoperative, 582, 583, 600
Ilioinguinal nerve, in local anesthesia, *93, 94,*
  *94, 99,* *110,* 111
  injury to, intraoperative, 582, 583, 600, *600*
Iliopubic tract, 5. See also *Transversalis*
  *fascia.*
  in direct inguinal hernia, 198
Implant(s)
  definition of, 534
  in incisional hernia repair, 554, 556(t)
    clinical study of, 547–553
    operative findings in, 556, 556(t)
  in lumbar hernia repair, 473
  prosthetic. See *Prosthesis.*
Impotence, 611
  postoperative, 614
Incarceration
  and postoperative death, case history of,
    590

Incarceration (*Continued*)
  femoral hernia with, 256, 257, *258*
  indirect inguinal hernia with, 173
    and acute appendicitis, 519
  of appendix, in direct inguinal hernia, 519
Incision
  and incisional hernias, 375, *376*, 382, *382*
  and wound disruption, 352–355, *354*
  Gibson, 370, *371*
  groin or scrotal, 10
  in indirect inguinal hernia repair, 160, *160*
  in sliding hernia repair, 301
    historical considerations in, 292
  inguinal, *19*, 20
    of upper (abdominal) approach, 12
  long oblique, and wound disruption, 355
  McBurney's, and wound disruption, *354*,
    355
  multiple, and wound disruption, 355
  of external oblique fascia, 11
  pararectus, and wound disruption, 355
  postoperative disruption of. See *Wound
    disruption.*
  previous, and wound disruption, 355
  rectus, and wound disruption, 354, *354*
  relaxing. See *Relaxing incision.*
  subcostal, and wound disruption, 354, *354*
    excessively long, and wound disruption,
      355
  transverse, and wound disruption, 352, 354,
    *354*
    in epigastric hernia repair, 448, *449*
  vertical midline, and wound disruption,
    353, 354, *354*
    in epigastric hernia repair, 448, *450, 451*
Incisional hernia, 330, 369–396
  clinical history in, 374
  clinical study of, 372–394
  definition of, 372, 372(t)
  etiologic factors in, 380, 381(t)
  incidence of, 85, 88, 371–372
  historical summary of, 369–371
  number of previous laparotomies and, 380
  onset of, 378, 378(t)
  physical examination in, 374
  recurrences of, 393
    after repair with implants, 557
    prevention of, 394–395
  repair of, 383–389, 383(t), *384–388*
    complications of, 391, 392(t)
    one-layer closure of, 383, *387*
    prosthesis in. See *Prosthesis, in
      incisional hernia repair.*
    side-to-side closure of, 388, *389*
    transverse closure of, 383, *386*
    two-layer closure of, 383, *384–385*
  requiring prosthesis
    of lower abdomen, 559, *562–564*
    previous repair of, 550, 550(t)
    site of, 550, 551(t)
    supraumbilical, 558, *559–561*
    time of appearance of, 550, 550(t)
  site of, 378, 379(t)
  size of, 380
  strangulated-incarcerated, and
    postoperative death, case history of, 590
Incremental phase, of wound healing, *339*,
  339(t), 340

Indirect inguinal hernia, 118, 155–175
  clinical study of, 168–175
  congenital
    and related abnormalities, 118–154
    clinical picture of, 147
    clinical study of, 146–152
    complications of, 151
    contralateral exploration for, 138
    cryptorchidism with, 139
    incidence of, 119
    management of, principles of, 132–135
    recurrence of, 151
    repair of
      contralateral, 135–138
      experience in, 148, 148(t)
      historical notes on, 129–132
      procedures in, 149, 149(t)
      technique for, 132, *133*
  history of, 155–158
  in female infants, 86
  incarcerated, 173
    and acute appendicitis, 519
  incidence of, 85, *85*, 168
  physical examination in, 44, *45*
  recurrent, 175, 176–195
    bilateral indirect inguinal hernia repair
      and, 192
    clinical study of, 187–189
    enigma of, 179–187, *180*
    etiology of, 191, 191(t)
    interval between original repair and, 192,
      192(t)
    number of previous repairs in, 192, 192(t)
    repair of
      and recurrence, 193
      complications of, 193, 193(t)
      principles of, 189–193
      technique for, 188(t), 189, 189(t)
    site of, 180
    statistics and, 176–179
  repair of, 158–159, 169
    bilateral, and recurrence, 192
    complications of, 174, 174(t)
    findings in, 172, 172(t)
    preperitoneal approach to, *250–251*, 252
    technique for, 159–165, *160–165*, 169,
      170(t)
      current, 159
      obsolescent, 159
      obsolete, 159
    vs. Bassini repair, 168
Induration, postoperative, 595
Infants
  clinical appraisal of, 54
  congenital indirect inguinal hernia in. See
    *Indirect inguinal hernia, congenital.*
  direct inguinal hernia in, 128
  female, indirect inguinal hernias in, 86
    sliding hernias in, 86
      historical considerations in, 293
      repair of, 310, *311*
        intraoperative complications of, 584,
          585
  femoral hernias in, 128–129
  hernias in, 47–48
  history of, 55
  hydrocele in, management of, 135
  lumbar hernias in, 469, 469(t)

Infants (*Continued*)
  surgery in, 53
  umbilical hernia in. See *Umbilical hernia,
    in infants and children.*
Infection, wound. See *Wound, infection of.*
Infertility, 611
  in females, bilateral hernia repair and, 614
Inflammatory phase, of wound healing, 339,
  *339*, 339(t)
Inguinal canal, anatomy of, 27–30
  description of, 5
  in recurrent direct inguinal hernia, 223,
    *224*
Inguinal hernia
  and carcinoma, 522–524, *524*
    historical background of, 522–523
  combined with femoral hernia. See
    *Multilocular inguinal hernia.*
  direct. See *Direct inguinal hernia.*
  direct-indirect, 277
    incidence of, 276
    recurrent, repair of, technique for,
      278–279
  indirect. See *Indirect inguinal hernia.*
  internal. See *Supravesical hernia.*
  recurrent, repair of, prosthesis in. See
    *Prosthesis, in recurrent inguinal and
    femoral hernia repair.*
  repair of, and femoral hernia, 264–265,
    265(t)
    local anesthesia for, 108–117
    preperitoneal approach to, 13
  sliding. See *Sliding hernia.*
  vs. epigastric hernia, 445
Inguinal ligament
  anatomy of, *21, 22*
  and transversalis fascia, 6
  description of, 6
  in direct inguinal hernia repair, 200
Inguinal region, anatomy of, *24, 35, 36, 37*
Inguinal ring. See *Abdominal ring.*
Inguinal shutter, 157
Inguinal triangle. See *Hesselbach's triangle.*
Inguinofemoral hernia, recurrent, 272,
    319–329, *319, 322*
  case histories of, 326–328
  clinical features of, 321–322
  description of, 285, 285(t), 319–320
  historical background of, 320–321
  initial operative procedures and, 321
  repair of, principles of, 322–326
    results of, 328–329
    technique for, 323, *324, 325*
  subsequent operative procedures in, 321
Inguinofemoral region, anatomy of, 30–35, *31*
Injections, of local anesthetic, for inguinal
  and femoral hernia repair, 108, *109–116*
Interparietal hernia, 491–496, *493*
  clinical features of, 494–495
  definition of, 492
  historical background of, 492
  treatment of, 495
  types of, 492
Interstitial hernia, *493, 494, 494*
Intestine. See also *Colon;* and
    *Gastrointestinal tract.*
  incarceration and strangulation of, femoral
    hernia with, 256, *257, 258*

Intestine (*Continued*)
  injury to, intraoperative, 574(t), 581–583,
    *581*
  obstruction of. See *Ileus.*
  prolapse of, 331
  small, x-ray of, 70
Intra-abdominal pressure, and femoral hernia,
  241
  rise in, and hernia, 43
    and wound disruption, 335, *335*
Intravesical hernia. See *Supravesical hernia.*
Iodine, skin reaction to, 597, *598*
Ivalon, for prosthesis, 547


K

Keloid, formation of, 604
Kirschner-Bassini repair, of femoral hernia,
  247, *247*
  of recurrent femoral hernia, 270(t), 271


L

La Roque approach, in sliding inguinal
  hernia repair, historical considerations in,
  292
Laboratory examinations, preoperative, 58
Lacunar ligament, anatomy of, *21, 22, 22*
  description of, 5
Laennec's cirrhosis, and wound disruption,
  *333,* 337
Lag phase, of wound healing, 339, *339,* 339(t)
Langer's lines, 18, *18*
Laparocéles spontanées. See *Spigelian
  hernia.*
Laparotomy. See also *Incision.*
  number of previous, and incisional hernia,
    380
Lathyrism, 624
Lidocaine, in local anesthesia, 101, 102(t),
  103(t)
Ligament
  Cooper's. See *Cooper's ligament.*
  Gimbernat's, anatomy of, *21, 22, 22*
    description of, 5
  inguinal. See *Inguinal ligament.*
  lacunar, anatomy of, *21, 22, 22*
    description of, 5
  Poupart's. See *Inguinal ligament.*
  round, in indirect inguinal hernia, 173
  Thomson's, 5
    in direct inguinal hernia, 198
Line(s), Langer's, 18, *18*
Linea alba, 438, *438*
  hernias of. See *Epigastric hernia.*
Linea semilunaris, hernia of. See *Spigelian
  hernia.*
Lipomas
  indirect inguinal hernia with, 172
  vs. epigastric hernia, 445, *445*
  vs. hernia, 49, *49*
  vs. lumbar hernia, 470

Lister, Joseph, 8, *8*
Littre's hernia, 4, 459, 500–504, *501*
    anatomic and pathological features of,
        502–503
    definition of, 500
    historical background of, 500–501, *502*
    incidence of, 501–502, 502(t)
    treatment of, 503
Lotheissen, Georg, 320
Lotheissen-McVay repair
    of direct inguinal hernia, 202
    of femoral hernia, 244–245, *244*
    of recurrent femoral hernia, 269, 270(t)
    of recurrent inguinofemoral hernia, 321
Lucas-Championnière, Just, 11, *11*
Lumbar hernia, 465–478
    acquired, 469, 469(t), 476
    anatomic considerations in, 466–469, *466*
    anatomic relationships of, 468, *468*
    classification of, 469–470, 469(t)
    clinical cases of, 475–477, 476(t)
    congenital, 469, 469(t)
    definition of, 465
    description of, 4
    differential diagnosis of, 470
    diffuse, 468
    historical background of, 465–466
    repair of, 471
        technique for, 472, *474*, *475*, 476, 476(t)
    spontaneous, 469, 469(t)
    symptoms and signs of, 470
    traumatic, 469, 469(t)
        postoperative, 469(t), 470
    treatment of, 471–475
Lumbar triangle, 6
    inferior, 467, *467*
    superior, 467, *467*
Lumbodorsal fascia, closure of, in lumbar
    hernia repair, 472
Lung. See *Pulmonary disease.*
Lymph nodes, inflammation of, vs. hernia, 49,
    *50*
    inguinal, *31*, 32
Lymphadenitis, vs. hernia, 49, *50*

# M

Male. See also *Sex.*
    incidence of hernia in, 83, 84(t)
        statistical analysis of, 84–86, *85*
    processus vaginalis in, embryology of, 125,
        *126*, *127*
Malignancy. See *Carcinoma;* and *Tumors.*
Malnutrition, and wound disruption, 333, *333*
    and wound healing, 340–343
Marcaine, in local anesthesia, 101, 102(t),
    103(t)
Marlex mesh, 544. See also *Prosthesis.*
    in recurrent direct-indirect-femoral hernia
        repair, 287, 287(t)
    in recurrent femoral hernia repair, 267
    placement of, technique for, 552, *552*
Masked hernia. See *Richter's hernia;* and
    *Spigelian hernia.*
Master stitch, in direct inguinal hernia repair,
    208, *208*
    in recurrent direct inguinal hernia repair,
        229, *229*

McBurney's incision, and wound disruption,
    *354*, *355*
McVay, Chester, 6, *7*
McVay repair, of direct-indirect-femoral
        hernias, 278, 281, 281(t)
    of femoral hernia, 243, 258
    of indirect inguinal hernia, 170(t), 171
Meckel's diverticulum, hernia of. See *Littre's
    hernia.*
Medication. See *Drugs;* and names of
    specific drugs.
Mersilene mesh, 546. See also *Prosthesis.*
    placement of, technique for, 553, *553*
Mesh, synthetic. See also *Prosthesis.*
    definition of, 535
    extrusion of, 602
    in femoral hernia repair, 565, 565(t)
    in incisional hernia repair. See
        *Prosthesis, in incisional hernia repair.*
    in lumbar hernia repair, 473, *475*
    in multistaged omphalocele repair, 428,
        *430–432*
    in recurrent inguinal and femoral hernia
        repair. See *Prosthesis, in recurrent
        inguinal and femoral hernia repair.*
    in recurrent inguinofemoral hernia
        repair, 323, *325*
        case history of, *322*, 327
    Marlex. See *Marlex mesh.*
    Mersilene (Dacron), 546
        placement of, 553, 552–555
Metallic prostheses, 538(t), 542–544
Mortality
    congenital indirect inguinal hernia repair
        and, 151
    direct inguinal hernia repair and, 213,
        213(t)
    femoral hernia and, 257
    femoral hernia repair and, 261
    gastroschisis repair and, 512
    herniorrhaphy and, 587–592
        case histories of, 589–591
        peritonitis and sepsis and, 595
    incisional hernia repair and, 394
    incisional hernia repair with implants and,
        556
    indirect inguinal hernia repair and, 174,
        175(t)
    intraoperative, 575
    omphaloceles and, 429
    recurrent indirect inguinal hernia repair
        and, 193
    reduction en masse and, 499
    Richter's hernia repair and, 464
    sliding inguinal hernia repair and, 317
    umbilical hernia repair in adults and, 416
    wound disruption and, 364, 364(t)
Moschcowitz repair, of direct-indirect-femoral
        hernias, 281(t), 282
    of femoral hernia, 245–247, *246*, 259
    of recurrent femoral hernia, 270, 270(t)
Mouth, preoperative examination of, 57
Multilocular inguinal hernia, 275–288
    clinical study of, 279–284, *280*
    incidence of, 84(t), 87, 276–278, *278*
    number of previous repairs of, 285, 285(t)
    recurrent, 275–288. See also
        *Inguinofemoral hernia, recurrent.*
    factors leading to, 286, 286(t)
    repair of, 286, 287(t)

Multilocular inguinal hernia (*Continued*)
  recurrent, repair of, complications of, 287, 288t
    technical details of, 287, 287(t)
      types of, 285, 285(t)
  repair of, complications of, 283, 284(t)
    technical details of, 282, 283(t)
      types of, 281, 281(t)
  types of, 280, 281(t)
Muscle(s)
  abdominal, attachment and arrangement of, and hernia, 42
  cremaster. See *Cremaster muscle.*
  external oblique, anatomy of, 20, *20,* 35
  internal oblique, anatomy of, *20,* 23, 35, *36*
  of anterolateral abdominal wall, anatomy of, 20–26, *20*
  pyrimidalis, in relaxing incision, 530, *531*
  rectus abdominis, anatomy of, 25, *25*
    in relaxing incision, 530, *531*
  transversus abdominis, anatomy of, 23, *23, 24,* 36, *37*
    in direct inguinal hernia repair, 204, *207, 208*
Muscle hernias, vs. lumbar hernia, 471
Musculofascial pedicle, in lumbar hernia repair, 473, *474*


**N**

Neonates. See also *Infants.*
  clinical appraisal of, 54
  history of, 55
  surgery in, 53
Neoplasms. See *Tumors.*
Nerve(s)
  abdominal, anatomy of, 23, 26, *26*
  entrapment of, 600
  femoral, injury to, 596
    lateral cutaneous, injury to, intraoperative, *582, 583*
    paresis of, postoperative, 596
  iliohypogastric, in local anesthesia, 93, 94, *94, 98, 110,* 111
    injury to, intraoperative, *582, 583,* 600
  ilioinguinal, in local anesthesia, 93, 94, *94, 99, 110,* 111
    injury to, intraoperative, *582, 583*
  in local anesthesia, 93, *93–99*
  intercostal, in local anesthesia, 93, *93,* 95, *96*
  of spermatic cord, 30
Nervous system, and postoperative complications, 596
Nesacaine, in local anesthesia, 101, 102(t), 103(t)
Netting, definition of, 534
Neuralgia, postoperative, 600
Neuroma, postoperative, 600, *600*
Nipped hernia. See *Richter's hernia.*
Nose, preoperative examination of, 57
Nuck, canal of, cysts of, 120
  in sliding hernia, developmental and anatomic considerations in, 301
Nutrition, and wound disruption, 333, *333*
  and wound healing, 340–343
Nylon, for prosthesis, 546


**O**

Obesity
  and hernia, 42, 82
  and incisional hernias, 374, *375*
  and wound disruption, 337
  preoperative treatment of, 62
Obturator artery, accessory, injury to, intraoperative, 578–579, *578*
Obturator hernia, description of, 4
Omphaloceles, 417–434
  anomalies associated with, 421
  delayed closure of, 424, *426–428*
  description of, 3
  historical background of, 417–418
  management of, 423–429
    conservative, 422
  multistaged repairs of, 426, *430–432*
  primary closure of, 424, *425*
  vs. gastroschisis, 417, *506*
  vs. umbilical hernia, 397, 417
Omphalomesenteric duct, patent, 418, 418(t), *419*
Operation. See *Herniorrhaphy;* and *Surgery.*
Orchidectomy, 150
Orchiectomy, 150
Orchidopexy, 140, 150
  principles of, 142–146
  technique for, 143, *144–145*
Orchiopexy. See *Orchidopexy.*
Orthopedic examination, preoperative, 61, *63*
Ovary
  descent of, 124
  in sliding hernia, historical considerations in, 293
  injury to, intraoperative, 584–585, *585*
  origins and development of, 122
Oxygen, and wound healing, 342


**P**

Pain
  history of, 43
  postoperative, 600, 616
  postvasectomy, 610
    case history of, 611
  spinal anesthesia and, 261, 616
Pampiniform plexus, bleeding from, intraoperative, 576
  varicosity of, vs. hernia, 51
Pantaloon hernia, 277
Pararectus incision, and wound disruption, 355
Paravesical hernia. See *Supravesical hernia.*
Paresis, femoral nerve, postoperative, 596
Paresthesia, postoperative, 604
Pasteur, Louis, 8, *8*
Patient
  clinical appraisal of, 54–55
  physical status of, 77
  position of, for lumbar hernia repair, 471
Pediatric. See *Infants;* and *Children.*
Pelvic peritoneal fossae, anatomy of, 37–38, *38*
Pericardium, as heterograft, 541

Perineal hernia, description of, 3
Peri-stomal hernia, 389
Peritoneal sac
  closure of, in indirect inguinal hernia
      repair, 182, *182*
  conversion of direct into indirect. See
      *Hoguet maneuver.*
  high ligation of, 11
    in congenital indirect inguinal hernia
        repair, 129
    in indirect inguinal hernia repair, 163,
        *163*, 181
    in sliding hernia repair, 305, *306*
  in congenital indirect inguinal hernia
      repair, *133*, 134
  in indirect inguinal hernia repair, 162, *162*
  simple ligation of, 11
Peritoneum, injection of, in local anesthesia,
    111, *116*
  rupture of, in hernia, 3
  vaginal process of. See *Processus vaginalis.*
Peritoneography, 71–75
Peritonitis, postoperative, 595
Petit, 3
Physical examination
  in congenital indirect inguinal hernia, 147
  in diagnosis of hernia, 44–47, *45–47*
  in direct inguinal hernia, 44, *46*
  in epigastric hernia, 442
  in femoral hernia, 44, *46, 47*
  in incisional hernia, 374
  in incisional hernia requiring implants, 548
  in indirect inguinal hernia, 44, *45*
  in preoperative evaluation, 56–58
Pincement herniaire de l'intestine. See
    *Richter's hernia.*
Pincement lateral. See *Richter's hernia.*
Pinched hernia. See *Richter's hernia.*
Pituitary gonadotropins, 614
Plastic materials, for prosthesis, 538(t),
    544–547
Plateau phase, of wound healing, *339,* 339(t),
    340
Pneumonitis, and postoperative death, case
    history of, 589
Polyethylene, high-density. See *Marlex mesh.*
Posterior approach, to femoral hernia repair,
    249
  technique for, 249–252, *250–251*
Potts procedure, in congenital indirect
    inguinal hernia, 149, 149(t)
Poupart's ligament. See *Inguinal ligament.*
Pregnancy, and hernia, 43, 82
  and umbilical hernia, 402, *402,* 409
Preperitoneal approach
  in direct inguinal hernia repair, 199(t), 203,
      *250–251,* 252
    and recurrence, 219
  femoral hernia repair, 13, 249
    technique for, 249, *250–251,* 259
  in indirect inguinal hernia repair, *250–251,*
      252
  in inguinal hernia repair, 13
Preperitoneal hernia, 492–493, *493, 494*
Pressure, intra-abdominal, and femoral
    hernia, 241
  rise in, and hernia, 43
    and wound disruption, 335, *335*
Prevesical hernia. See *Supravesical hernia.*
Processus vaginalis
  embryology of, in female, 127
    in male, 125, *126, 127*

Processus vaginalis (*Continued*)
  patent, and congenital indirect inguinal
      hernias, 118
    herniography of, 74
    incidence of, 118
Proctosigmoidoscopy, preoperative, 58
Proliferative phase, of wound healing, *339,*
    339(t), 340
Properitoneal hernia, 492–493, *493, 494*
  supravesical. See *Supravesical hernia.*
Prostatism, and hernia, 42
  management of, 616
Prosthesis
  classification of, 537–538, 538(t)
  definition of, 534
  desirable qualities in, 535, 535(t)
  durability of, 535
  ease of handling of, 536
  ease of sterilization of, 536
  economy of, 537
  flexibility and pliability of, 536
  implantation of, alterations following, 537
    principles of, 568–569
  in direct inguinal hernia repair, 199(t), 212
  in femoral hernia repair, 565, 565(t)
  in hernia repair, 534–572
    indications for, 550, 551(t)
    placement of, 553, 555, 555(t)
      technique for, 551, *552–555*
  in incisional hernia repair, 553–563, 556(t)
    and recurrence, 557
    clinical study of, 547–553
    complications of, 556, 557(t)
    location of, 391
    operative findings in, 556, 556(t)
  in lumbar hernia repair, 473, *475*
  in recurrent direct inguinal hernia repair,
      231
    case history of, 227
  in recurrent inguinal and femoral hernia
      repair, 272, 565, 565(t), 566–567
    and recurrences, 566
    clinical experience with, 563–566
    clinical features of, 564
    complications of, 566
    indications for, 567–568, 568(t)
    methods of, 565, *566, 567*
  in recurrent inguinofemoral hernia repair,
      323, *325*
    case history of, *322, 327, 328*
  metallic, 538(t), 542–544
  nonfragmentation of, 536
  nonwandering of, 536
  plastic, 538(t), 544–547
  porosity of, 536, *537*
  strength of, 535
  tolerance of, 536
Protein, and wound healing, *333,* 341
Psychologic abnormalities, in cryptorchidism,
    140
Pubic tubercle, recurrent direct inguinal
    hernia near, *222, 223*
Pulmonary disease
  and hernia, 42
  and wound disruption, 335,336
  femoral hernia repair and, 260(t), 261
  in preoperative evaluation of elderly, 56
  postoperative, 599
Pulmonary embolism, femoral hernia repair
    and, 261
Pulse, and wound disruption, 360
Pyelograms, intravenous, *61,* 70, *71*

Pyramidalis muscle, in relaxing incision, 530, *531*

**R**

Race, and umbilical hernia in infants and children, 402
Radiography. See *X-ray studies.*
Rectal examination, preoperative, 58
Rectus abdominis muscle, anatomy of, 25, *25*
  in relaxing incision, 530, *531*
Rectus incision, and wound disruption, 354, *354*
Rectus sheath, anatomy of, *23, 25, 25*
  in relaxing incision, 530, *531*
Reduction en masse, 496–500
  clinical features of, 497
  definition of, 496
  historical background of, 496–497
  in Richter's hernia, 463
  incidence of, 497
  pathology of, 497, *498, 499*
  treatment of, 499
Relaxing incision, 14, 525–533
  advantages of, 532
  anatomy of, 530–532, *531*
  historical background of, 525–530, *526–529*
  in direct inguinal hernia repair, 204, 207, *208*
  in femoral hernia repair, 257
  technique for, 532
Rejection, of prosthesis, 536
Remodeling phase, of wound healing, *339*, 339(t), *340*
Resorptive phase, of wound healing, *339*, 339(t), *340*
Respiratory tract. See also *Pulmonary disease.*
  disease of, and wound disruption, *335, 335*
Retention sutures, 356, *356, 357*
Richter's hernia, 456–465, *457*
  anatomic sites of, 457–459, *458*, 459(t)
  case reports of, 462–463
  clinical and pathologic correlation of, 461–462
  definition of, 459
  description of, 3
  diagnosis of, 47, *248, 253*
  historical background of, 459–460
  incidence of, 457
  operative treatment of, 463–464
  pathogenesis of, 460–461
  synonyms for, 459
  umbilical, in adults, 415, *416*
  x-ray of, *65, 67*
Ring, abdominal. See *Abdominal ring.*
  femoral, in femoral hernia, 238
  inguinal. See *Abdominal ring.*
Risk, 77
Roentgenography. See *X-ray studies.*
Ronsil, 4

**S**

Saddlebag hernia, 276
Scopolamine, preanesthetic, 79
Scrotum, postoperative complications of, 609
  swelling of, femoral hernia repair and, 260, 260(t)

Scrotum (*Continued*)
  swelling of, postoperative, 608
Sedation, preanesthetic
  for ambulatory surgery, 79
  for children, 80, 81(t)
  standard dose of, 80
  timing of, 79
Semen, analysis of, 614
Seminiferous tubules, in cryptorchidism, 140
Sepsis, and postoperative death, case history of, 590
  postoperative, 595
  prevention of, 8
Seroma, incisional hernia repair and, 391, 392(t)
  postoperative, 600
Sex. See also *Female;* and *Male.*
  and appendectomy and herniorrhaphy, 518
  and congenital indirect inguinal hernia, 147
  and direct inguinal hernia, 209
  and direct-indirect-femoral hernia, 279
  and epigastric hernia, 442
  and femoral hernia, 255
  and hernia, 41, 82, 82(t)
    incidence of, 83–84, 84(t)
  and incisional hernia, 373
  and incisional hernia requiring implants, 547
  and indirect inguinal hernia, 169, 169(t)
  and recurrent direct inguinal hernia, 232
  and recurrent direct-indirect-femoral hernias, 284
  and recurrent femoral hernia, 269
  and recurrent femoral hernia repair with prostheses, 563
  and recurrent indirect inguinal hernia, 188
  and recurrent inguinal hernia repair with prostheses, 563
  and sliding inguinal hernias, 312
  and umbilical hernia, in infants and children, 402, 403(t)
  and wound disruption, 332, 358
Shouldice repair, of direct inguinal hernia, 202
Shutter, inguinal, 157
Sigmoid, in sliding hernia, developmental and anatomic considerations in, 300
  intestinal, 574(t), 581–583, *581*
  testicular, in cryptorchidism, 140
  to Fallopian tubes and ovaries, intraoperative, 584–585, *585*
  to nerves, intraoperative, 582, *583*
  to vas deferens, intraoperative, 583, *584*
  vascular, intraoperative, 576–580, *576–579*
Triangle
  Hesselbach's. See *Hesselbach's triangle.*
  inguinal. See *Hesselbach's triangle.*
  lumbar, 6
    inferior, 467, *467*
    superior, 467, *467*
Tube, fallopian, in sliding hernia, historical considerations in, 293
  injury to, intraoperative, 584–585, *585*
Tubules, seminiferous, in cryptorchidism, 140
Tumors. See also *Carcinoma;* and *Lipomas.*
  abdominal wall, vs. epigastric hernia, 445
  malignant, testicular, in cryptorchidism, 139
  vs. hernia, 51, *51*
  vs. lumbar hernia, 471

Sigmoid, in sliding hernia (*Continued*)
 historical considerations in, 290
 repair of, 307–312, *308–310*
Silver wire, for prosthesis, 544
Sinuses, abdominal wall, incisional hernia
 repair and, 392(t), 393
 chronic draining, 602
 case history of, 602, *603*
Skin
 closure of, in indirect inguinal hernia
 repair, 165–167
 problems with, 167
 grafts of, 539
 and cyst, 539, 541(t)
 incision of. See *Incision.*
 lesions of, preoperative treatment of, 62
 preparation of, for lumbar hernia repair,
 471
 for surgery, 350
 reactions of, 597, *598*
Sliding hernia
 bladder in. See *Bladder, urinary, in sliding
 hernia.*
 cecal, developmental and anatomic
 considerations in, 300
 historical considerations in, 290
 classification of, 294–297, 295(t)
 diagnosis of, 48–49
 extraperitoneal, 295(t), 297, *297–299*
 in female infants, 86
 historical considerations in, 293
 repair of, 310, *311*
 intraoperative complications of, 584,
 *585*
 indirect inguinal, and postoperative death,
 case history of, 589
 inguinal, 312–317
 clinical features of, 312
 description of, 3
 duration of, 312, 313(t)
 preoperative diagnosis of, 313, 313(t)
 recurrence of, 316
 repair of, 314, 315(t)
 complications of, 315
 findings in, 314, 314(t)
 inguinal and femoral, 289–318
 definition of, 289
 developmental and anatomic
 considerations in, 297–301
 historical considerations in, 289–294
 repair of, historical considerations in, 292
 inguinal approach for, 301–307,
 *302–307*
 sigmoid, historical considerations in, 290
 repair of, 307–312, *308–310*
 simple, 295, *295, 299*
 vesicomesenteric, 295(t), 296, *297, 298*
 vesicoparietal, 295(t), 296, *296*
Smead-Jones suture technique, 356, *356*
Spermatic artery, external, injury to,
 intraoperative, 579, *579*
 internal, injury to, intraoperative, 579, *579*
Spermatic cord
 anatomy of, 27–30, *29, 30*
 and hernias, 184
 division of, 607
 in indirect inguinal hernia repair, 161, *161*
 in sliding hernia repair, 302, *302*

Spermatic cord (*Continued*)
 injection of, in local anesthesia, 111, *114*
 lipomas of, indirect inguinal hernia with,
 172
 transplantation of, 14
Spermatoceles, indirect inguinal hernia with,
 173
Spermatogenesis, failure of, in
 cryptorchidism, 139
Spigelian hernia, 478–486
 anatomic considerations in, 479–480,
 *480–482*
 clinical experience with, 483–485
 clinical features of, 481–482
 definition of, 478
 differential diagnosis of, 482–483
 etiologic factors in, 481
 historical background of, 479
 incidence of, 479
 synonyms for, 478
 treatment of, 483, *484*
Spinal anesthesia, and backache, case history
 of, 616
 and headache, in femoral hernia repair, 261
Sponge, definition of, 535
Steel, stainless, for prosthesis, 542
Sterility, 611
 in females, bilateral hernia repair and, 614
Steroids, and wound healing, 343
Stitch, master, in direct inguinal hernia
 repair, 208, *208*
 in recurrent direct inguinal hernia repair,
 229, *229*
Stitch abscess, 594
Stoma, and hernia, 389
Stomach. See also *Gastrointestinal tract.*
 carcinoma of, vs. epigastric hernia, 444
 in epigastric hernias, 436
 ulcer of, vs. epigastric hernia, 444
 x-ray of, 70
Strangulation
 and postoperative death, case history of,
 590
 femoral hernia with, *256, 257, 258*
 indirect inguinal hernia with, 173
 release of, 10
Stroke, postoperative, 596
Subcostal incision, and wound disruption,
 354, *354*
 excessively long, and wound disruption,
 355
Subcutaneous tissue, closure of, in indirect
 inguinal hernia repair, 165–167
Substrate phase, of wound healing, 339, *339,*
 339(t)
Suction catheters, in incisional hernia repair,
 388, *389*
Suppuration, postoperative, 594
Suprapubic hernia. See *Supravesical hernia.*
Supravesical hernia, 486–491
 anatomy of, 488–489, *488*
 clinical features of, 489–490
 definition of, 487
 external, 487
 historical background of, 487–488
 internal, 487
 pathology of, 489, *489, 490*
 treatment of, 490

Surgery. See also *Herniorrhaphy*; and names of specific surgical procedures.
  ambulatory, 79–81
  and wound disruption, 361, 361(t)
  considerations before, 76–78
  gentleness in, 351
  in aged, 53
  in infant or neonate, 53
  medication prior to, 76–81
  orders prior to, 76–81, 80
  preparation for, emergency vs. routine, 78
  prior, and hernia, 82
    and incisional hernia, 374, 375(t), *376*
    and incisional hernia requiring prosthesis, 548, 549(t)
    and recurrent inguinofemoral hernia, 321
    complications of, 377, 377(t)
      and incisional hernia requiring prosthesis, 549, 549(t)
  technique for, principles of, and wound disruption, 349–352
Suture(s)
  absorbability of, 348
  and wound disruption, *339*, 343–349, *344*
  as refuge for organisms, classification of, 343, 344(t), 345(t)
  ease of handling of, 345
  excessive tension on, and recurrent direct inguinal hernia, 220, 225(t)
    case history of, 225
  and recurrent femoral hernia, 266(t), 267
  in congenital indirect inguinal hernia repair, 149
  in direct inguinal hernia repair, 210
  in epigastric hernia repair, 451
  in femoral hernia repair, 256
  in incisional hernia repair, 391
  in incisional hernia repair with prostheses, 554
  in indirect inguinal hernia repair, 164, *165, 166,* 169
  in sliding inguinal hernia repair, 314
  knot slippage in, 345
  retention, 356, *356, 357*
  Smead-Jones, 356, *356*
  strength of, 347, *347*
    enduring, 348
  tissue reaction to, 347
  wire, and postoperative pain, 600, *601*
Synthetic implant. See *Prosthesis.*
Synthetic mesh. See *Mesh, synthetic;* and *Prosthesis.*

T

Tanner, relaxing incision of, 529, *529,* 533
Tantalum gauze, for prosthesis, 543, *544*
Tape
  in skin closure, in indirect inguinal hernia repair, 166, *167*
    problems with, 167
  in wound disruption, 364
  skin reaction to, 598 *598*
Teflon, for prosthesis, 547
Temperature, and wound disruption, 360
Tendon, as autograft, 538
  as heterograft, 541
  conjoined, 6

Testis(es)
  absence of, bilateral, 122
  atrophy of, 611
    case history of, 612
    division of spermatic cord and, 607
  blood supply to, experimental study of, 605, *605*
  injury to, intraoperative, 579–580, *579*
  descent of, 124, *125*
    and hernia, 42
    failure of. See *Cryptorchidism.*
  ectopic, *120, 121*
  excision of, 150
  high-riding, 610
  low-riding, 610
  malignancy of, in cryptorchidism, 139
  mislocated, 120
  origins and development of, 122, *123*
  postoperative complications of, 609
  retractile (or bashful), 120
  swelling of, postoperative, 608
  torsion of, in cryptorchidism, 140
  trauma to, in cryptorchidism, 140
  undescended. See *Cryptorchidism.*
Testosterone, 614
Textiles, definition of, 535
Thomson's ligament, 5
  in direct inguinal hernia, 198
Thorax, preoperative examination of, 57, *57*
Throat, preoperative examination of, 57
Thrombophlebitis, femoral hernia repair and, 261
Tissue
  acceptance of prosthesis, 535
  devitalized, removal of, 351
  reaction to sutures, 347
  subcutaneous, closure of, in indirect inguinal hernia repair, 165–167
Transversalis fascia
  anatomy of, 24, *24*
  and inguinal ligament, 6
  closure of, 12
    failure of, 12, 186
    in indirect inguinal hernia repair, 185
  importance of, 5
  in indirect inguinal hernia repair, 163, *164,* 185
  triangulation of, at internal ring, in indirect inguinal hernia repair, 163, *164*
    in recurrent indirect inguinal hernia repair, 190
  in direct inguinal hernia repair, 206, *207*
  in sliding hernia repair, 305, *307*
Transverse closure, in incisional hernia repair, 383, *386*
Transverse incision, and wound disruption, 352, 354, *354*
  in epigastric hernia repair, 448, *449*
Transversus abdominis arch, in direct inguinal hernia repair, 204, *207, 208*
Transversus abdominis muscle, anatomy of, 23, *23, 24, 36, 37*
  in direct inguinal hernia repair, 204, *207, 208*
Trauma
  and hernia, 43
  and lumbar hernias, 469, 469(t)
    postoperative, 469(t), 470
  bladder, intraoperative, 580–581, *580*

# U

Ulcer, duodenal and gastric, vs. epigastric hernia, 444
Umbilical cord, hernia in, 418(t), 419, *420*
 vs. gastroschisis, *506*
Umbilical eventration. See *Omphalocele.*
Umbilical hernia
 definition of, 372
 history of, 398–399
 in adults, 408–417
  diseases with, 410, 411(t)
  duration of, 409
  operative findings in, 415, *416*
  physical findings in, 410, *410, 411*
  recurrences of, 415
  repair of, 412, *414*, 415(t)
   complications of, 415
   indications for, 411, *411–413*
  symptoms of, 409
 in infants and children, 397–417
  clinical features of, 403
  clinical study of, 402–408
  operative findings in, 407
  physical findings in, 404
  recurrences of, 408
  repair of, complications of, 408
   indications for, 404
   technique for, 406, *406*, 407(t)
 incidence of, *85*, 88
 natural history of, 399–402, *401, 402*
 repair of, transverse overlapping technique for, 14
 vs. epigastric hernia, 445
 vs. omphalocele, 397, 417
Umbilicus, defects of, embryology of, 418–421, 418(t), *419, 420*
Urachus, patent, 418, 418(t), *419*
Urinary bladder. See *Bladder, urinary.*
Urine, retention of, 615
Urogenital tract. See *Genitourinary tract.*
Urologic examination, preoperative, 60, *61*
Uterus, in sliding hernia, historical considerations in, 293


# V

Vaginal examination, preoperative, 58
Varicoceles, vs. hernia, 51
Varix, saphenous, vs. hernia, 50
Vas deferens, injuries to, intraoperative, 583, *584*
Vascular. See *Blood vessels.*
Vasectomy, and pain, 610
 case history of, 611
Vein
 draining testes, *606*, 607
 femoral, injury to, intraoperative, 576, *576, 577, 578*
 obstruction of, and scrotal and testicular swelling, 608
 varicose, vs. hernia, 50
Ventral hernia, definition of, 372
Vertical midline incision, and wound disruption, 353, *354, 354*
 in epigastric hernia repair, 448, *450, 451*
Vesicoinguinal hernia. See *Supravesical hernia.*
Vesicomesenteric sliding hernia, 295(t), 296, *297, 298*
Vesicoparietal sliding hernia, 295(t), 296, *296*
Vesicopubic hernia. See *Supravesical hernia.*
Vital functions, preoperative evaluation of, 56
Vitamin C, deficiency of, and wound healing, 342


# W

Wall, abdominal. See *Abdominal wall.*
Weight, preoperative, 57
Wire, silver, for prosthesis, 544
Wölfler, relaxing incision of, 525, 527
Woman. See *Female.*
Wound
 closure of, and wound disruption, 355–358, *356, 357*
  secondary, 352
 complications of, early, 592–600
  femoral hernia repair and, 260, 260(t)
  late, 600–614
 contamination of, 350
 healing of, and wound disruption, 338–340
  nutritional and chemical factors in, 340–343
  phases of, 339, *339*, 339(t)
 induration of, incisional hernia repair and, 392(t), 393
 infection of, 594
  and wound disruption, 332(t), 333, *333, 334*, 361
  incisional hernia repair and, 392, 392(t)
  understanding of, 8
 minor separation of, 595
Wound disruption, 330–368, 595
 abdominal incisions and, 352–355, *354*
 and principles of operative technique, 349–352
 and wound healing, 338–340
 clinical conditions with, 332–338, 332(t)
 clinical picture of, 359
 clinical study of, 358–365
 closure of abdominal wounds and, 355–358, *356, 357*
 complete, 331
 correction of, 363
 definition and description of, 330–331
 incidence of, 331–332, 331(t)
 management of, 362
 organ systems operated on and, 361, *361*
 partial, 330
 prevention of, 364, 365(t)
 signs and symptoms of, 359, 360(t)
 site of, 362, 362(t)


# X

Xenograft, 538(t), 541–542
X-ray studies, 64–75, 64(t)
 abdominal, 65–68, 65–67
 chest, preoperative, 58, *60*
 in en masse reduction, 498
 of bladder, 70–71, *72, 73*
 of upper gastrointestinal tract and small bowel, 70
Xylocaine, in local anesthesia, 101, 102(t), 103(t)